IMPORTANT:

HERE IS YOUR REGISTRATION CODE TO ACCESS
YOUR PREMIUM McGRAW-HILL ONLINE RESOURCES.

MCGRAW-HILL
ONLINE RESOURCES

For key premium online resources you need THIS CODE to gain access. Once the code is entered, you will be able to use the Web resources for the length of your course.

If your course is using **WebCT** or **Blackboard**, you'll be able to use this code to access the McGraw-Hill content within your instructor's online course.

Access is provided if you have purchased a new book. If the registration code is missing from this book, the registration screen on our Website, and within your WebCT or Blackboard course, will tell you how to obtain your new code.

Registering for McGraw-Hill Online Resources

TO gain access to your McGraw-Hill web resources simply follow the steps below:

1. USE YOUR WEB BROWSER TO GO TO: http://www.mhhe.com/anspaugh5e/
2. CLICK ON **FIRST TIME USER**.
3. ENTER THE REGISTRATION CODE* PRINTED ON THE TEAR-OFF BOOKMARK ON THE RIGHT.
4. AFTER YOU HAVE ENTERED YOUR REGISTRATION CODE, CLICK **REGISTER**.
5. FOLLOW THE INSTRUCTIONS TO SET-UP YOUR PERSONAL UserID AND PASSWORD.
6. WRITE YOUR UserID AND PASSWORD DOWN FOR FUTURE REFERENCE.
   KEEP IT IN A SAFE PLACE.

TO GAIN ACCESS to the McGraw-Hill content in your instructor's **WebCT** or **Blackboard** course simply log in to the course with the UserID and Password provided by your instructor. Enter the registration code exactly as it appears in the box to the right when prompted by the system. You will only need to use the code the first time you click on McGraw-Hill content.

Thank you, and welcome to your McGraw-Hill online Resources!

aficionado-58282165

REGISTRATION CODE

* YOUR REGISTRATION CODE CAN BE USED ONLY ONCE TO ESTABLISH ACCESS. IT IS NOT TRANSFERABLE.

0-07-281911-1 ANSPAUGH: WELLNESS; CONCEPTS AND APPLICATIONS 5/E

Wellness

Concepts and Applications

Wellness

Concepts and Applications

Fifth Edition

David J. Anspaugh, PED, EdD, CHES

TRI-STATE UNIVERSITY

Michael H. Hamrick, EdD, CHES, FAAHE

THE UNIVERSITY OF MEMPHIS

Frank D. Rosato, EdD

THE UNIVERSITY OF MEMPHIS

Boston   Burr Ridge, IL   Dubuque, IA   Madison, WI   New York   San Francisco   St. Louis
Bangkok   Bogotá   Caracas   Kuala Lumpur   Lisbon   London   Madrid   Mexico City
Milan   Montreal   New Delhi   Santiago   Seoul   Singapore   Sydney   Taipei   Toronto

McGraw-Hill Higher Education

A Division of The McGraw-Hill Companies

WELLNESS: CONCEPTS AND APPLICATIONS
FIFTH EDITION

Published by McGraw-Hill, a business unit of The McGraw-Hill Companies, Inc., 1221 Avenue of the Americas, New York, NY 10020. Copyright © 2003, 2000, 1997, 1994, 1991 by The McGraw-Hill Companies, Inc. All rights reserved. No part of this publication may be reproduced or distributed in any form or by any means, or stored in a database or retrieval system, without the prior written consent of The McGraw-Hill Companies, Inc., including, but not limited to, in any network or other electronic storage or transmission, or broadcast for distance learning.

Some ancillaries, including electronic and print components, may not be available to customers outside the United States.

This book is printed on acid-free paper.

3 4 5 6 7 8 9 0 QPD/QPD 0 9 8 7 6 5 4 3

ISBN 0–07–246166–7

Vice president and editor-in-chief: *Thalia Dorwick*
Publisher: *Jane E. Karpacz*
Executive editor: *Vicki Malinee*
Developmental editor: *Lynda Huenefeld*
Senior marketing manager: *Pamela S. Cooper*
Project manager: *Christine Walker*
Production supervisor: *Enboge Chong*
Designer: *Matthew Baldwin*
Cover image: *GettyImages/Jim Cummins*
Senior photo research coordinator: *John C. Leland*
Photo research: *Mary Reeg*
Senior supplement producer: *David A. Welsh*
Media technology producer: *Lance Gerhart*
Compositor: *Shepherd Inc.*
Typeface: *10/12 Sabon*
Printer: *Quebecor World Dubuque, Inc.*

The credits section for this book begins on page 491 and is considered an extension of the copyright page.

Library of Congress Cataloging-in-Publication Data

Anspaugh, David J.
   Wellness : concepts and applications / David J. Anspaugh, Michael H. Hamrick,
Frank D. Rosato. — 5th ed.
   p.   cm.
   Includes bibliographical references and index.
   ISBN 0–07–246166–7
   1. Health. 2. Self-care, Health. 3. Medicine, Preventive. I. Hamrick, Michael H.
II. Rosato, Frank D. III. Title.

RA776 .A57 2003
613—dc21
                                    2001052194
                                    CIP

The Internet addresses listed in the text were accurate at the time of publication. The inclusion of a website does not indicate an endorsement by the authors or McGraw-Hill, and McGraw-Hill does not guarantee the accuracy of the information presented at these sites.

www.mhhe.com

To my wife Susan, the light of my life. To my children, Jay, Aimee and Zeb, and to my grandson, Conner, who will always be special.

David J. Anspaugh

To Harrison Scott Bingham, June 21, 1998, Kate Elizabeth Bingham, June 7, 2001, and Virginia Rhea Hensley, Circa March, 2002, who give "mops" and "pops" a reason to smile each day.

Michael H. Hamrick

To my wife, Pat, for her continued patience and support during this and all of my professional endeavors.

Frank D. Rosato

What's in This for You?

Looking for wellness and fitness information online? Working hard to get in shape? Trying to improve your grade? The great features in *Wellness: Concepts and Applications* will help you do all this and more! Let's take a look . . .

Online Learning Center Resources

Want to get a better grade? This box reminds you about the study aids and other resources available at McGraw-Hill's free Online Learning Center and describes some of the useful study tools you'll find there.

Goals for Behavior Change

The opening page of each chapter contains a list of behavior change goals specific to that chapter to help you as you strive to achieve a better state of wellness.

Chapter Key Terms

The opening page of each chapter lists the main terms for that chapter, helping you to know which terms to pay close attention to as you study the chapter.

Chapter Objectives

The opening page of each chapter also lists the objectives for that chapter to help you understand what concepts you should know by the conclusion of the chapter. This will help you in test preparation.

Real-World Wellness

These question-and-answer boxes show you how to put wellness concepts into practice. Helpful tips give practical advice for initiating behavior change and staying motivated to follow a wellness lifestyle.

ood health is one of our most cherished possessions, one that is often taken for granted until it is lost. Some people convincingly argue that everything else in life is secondary to good health. For many, it is not difficult to recall instances when life's goals, whether academic, career, or family; small or large; immediate or long-range, seemed unimportant because of sudden illness or a long-term debilitating health crisis.

Fortunately, the prospects of good health for Americans have never been better. The extent to which good health is realized is contingent on many factors. Chief among these factors are our actions and the choices we make. We can make choices that will promote health and well-being, prevent or delay the premature onset of many chronic illnesses, and improve our quality of life (see Real-World Wellness: Benefits of Living a Wellness Lifestyle). Staying healthy is not just a matter of common sense. Rather, it is a lifelong process that requires self-awareness, introspection, reflection, inquiry, accurate information, and action. This process relies on the concept of wellness and implies that each of us has the opportunity and the obligation to assume responsibility for factors that are under our control and to shape our health destiny. The wellness approach represents a formidable challenge because the processes leading to today's serious health threats are insidious, often originate in childhood or adolescence, flourish throughout adulthood, and finally culminate in full-blown disease in middle age or later. Lifestyle interventions initiated late in life produce limited success, but begun early in life they have maximum effect.

Components of Wellness

Wellness is defined as a lifelong process that at any given time produces a positive state of personal well-being; of feeling good about yourself; of optimal physical, psychological, and social functioning; and the control and minimization of both internal and external risk factors for both diseases and negative health conditions.[1] Wellness is a process rather than a goal. It implies a choice, a way of life. It means integrating the body, mind, and spirit. It symbolizes acceptance of yourself. It suggests that what you believe, feel, and do has an influence on your health. However, it does not imply that we make the best choice in every situation.

Consider the brief profiles of David, Susan, Carlos, and Maria. How would you rate each of them in terms of health and wellness?

David is physically active, places a high priority on his social life, barely makes passing grades in school, and engages in binge drinking almost every weekend. Susan is a perfectionist and her grades reflect it. To her, a B means

Real-World Wellness
Benefits of Living a Wellness Lifestyle

I am a full-time student, work twenty plus hours a week, and help with family responsibilities. At the same time, I'm trying to maintain my academic scholarship. There just isn't enough time in the day to be concerned about health and wellness. What am I to gain from a wellness lifestyle?

A wellness lifestyle offers the following benefits:

- Increases energy level and productivity at work and school
- Decreases absenteeism from school and work
- Decreases recovery time after illness or injury
- Supplies the body with proper nutrients
- Improves awareness of personal needs and the ways to meet them
- Expands and develops intellectual abilities
- Increases the ability to communicate emotions to others and to act assertively rather than aggressively or passively
- Promotes the attitude that life's difficulties are challenges and opportunities rather than overwhelming threats
- Acts from an internal locus of control
- Increases ability to cope with stress and resist depression
- Improves the cardiorespiratory system
- Increases muscle tone, strength, flexibility, and endurance
- Improves physical appearance
- Helps prevent or delay the premature onset of some forms of chronic disease
- Regulates and improves overall body function
- Promotes self-confidence
- Delays the aging process
- Promotes social awareness and the ability to reach out to, understand, and care about others

failure. She spends an inordinate amount of time studying, regularly skips meals, has no physical activity outlet, and rarely socializes. Her family tells her to "get a life." She needs the entire weekend to recover from the stress of academics. Carlos runs 3 miles every day, works out with weights 3 times a week, eats a balanced diet almost every day, has a close circle of friends, refuses to use his seat belt when driving, and smokes an average of two packs of cigarettes daily. Maria is a worrier. She makes good grades but is rarely satisfied. Her eating practices

---

Nurturing Your Spirituality

These boxes cover such topics as living well with cancer, making decisions about sex, and enjoying healthy pleasure, showing how wellness goes beyond just the physical dimension.

Nurturing Your Spirituality
Can Spirituality Improve Your Physical Health?

It's all in your mind. Or is it in your body? Or both? The interconnections between mind and body are the bases for many types of alternative health practices. Spirituality is believing in a source of value that transcends the boundaries of the self but also nurtures the self. Mind-body medicine builds upon spirituality, encouraging methods for improving the body by altering the mind. The National Institutes of Health (NIH) suggests the following spiritual practices:

- *Psychotherapy* focuses on the mental and emotional health of the patient and has been proven to reduce the amount of time required to recover from an illness.
- *Support groups* give patients the consolation that others have endured similar health challenges and survived, instilling hope.
- *Meditation*, formerly associated solely with religious practice, is a self-governed exercise for relaxation. Regular practice of meditation is recommended for reducing blood pressure and anxiety and increasing the quality of life and longevity.
- *Imagery* includes use of all the senses to encourage attitude change, behavior, or physiological responses. Uses of imagery include pain control in cancer patients and increasing immunity in elderly patients.
- *Hypnosis* is an ancient practice molded to fit modern needs. Today physicians, dentists, psychologists, and other mental health professionals use hypnosis to help people overcome addictions, control pain, and deal with phobias.
- *Biofeedback* provides patients with a picture of what is occurring physiologically in their bodies and an understanding of how trial-and-error adjustments of mental processes can affect these physiological behaviors. This technique is used in treatment for a wide variety of disorders, such as epilepsy, respiratory diseases, migraines, vascular disorders, and hypertension.
- *Yoga* is a disciplined practice of altering mental and physiological processes previously thought to be outside an individual's control. These alterations, performed on a regular basis, can reduce anxiety, lower blood pressure, treat arthritis, and increase the efficiency of the heart.

Enjoyable physical activity improves wellness inside and out.

- *Dance therapy* uses body movement for therapeutic purposes. It is proven effective for achieving such goals as improving self-concept and self-esteem, minimizing fears, reducing bodily tension, improving circulatory and respiratory functions, promoting healing, and reducing depression.
- *Music therapy* puts to good use the power of music on the psyche. Do you ever listen to music to make you feel better? So do stroke, Parkinson's, brain-injury, cancer, anxiety, cerebral palsy, and burn patients.
- *Art therapy* uses self-expression through art to enhance healing. Art therapy is used with patients being treated for burns, emotional problems, chemical addictions, and sexual abuse.
- *Prayer and mental healing* involves communication with some form of higher power. A wide variety of healing techniques fall within this category. Examples are being physically touched by a religious healer or experiencing healing through personal prayer or attendance at church. Studies link regular church attendance with reduced chance of dying from stroke or heart disease, lower blood pressure, lower suicide rates, and reduced depression.

healthy body fat level, and avoid abusing alcohol and other drugs or using tobacco products. In general, physical health is an investment in positive lifestyle habits. Separate chapters in this text are devoted to many of these physical dimensions of wellness.

Emotional

Emotional wellness is the ability to control stress and to express emotions appropriately and comfortably. It is the ability to recognize and accept feelings and not be defeated by setbacks and failures. Achieving emotional

Just the Facts

Special material in these boxes will encourage you to delve into a particular topic or more closely examine an important health issue.

Just the Facts

Eliminating Health Disparities: Three Examples

Despite notable progress in the overall health of the nation, American Indians, Alaskan Natives, Latinos, African Americans, and Pacific Islanders continue to shoulder more of the burden of illness and death compared with the U.S. population as a whole. These disparities are even greater if comparisons are made between each racial and ethnic group and the Caucasian population. Three examples follow.

- Heart disease is the leading cause of death for all racial and ethnic groups. Disparities exist among population groups, with a disproportionate burden of death and disability in minority and low-income populations. The age-adjusted death rate for heart disease for the total population declined by 20 percent from 1987 to 1995; for African Americans, the overall decrease was only 13 percent. Racial and ethnic minorities have higher rates of hypertension, tend to develop hypertension at an earlier age, and are less likely to undergo treatment to control their high blood pressure. Also, the rates for regular screening for cholesterol show disparities for certain racial and ethnic minorities—only 50 percent of American Indians and Alaska Natives, 44 percent of Asian Americans, and 38 percent of Mexican Americans have had their cholesterol checked within the past two years.

- Infant mortality is an important measure of a nation's health and worldwide indicator of health status. Although infant mortality in the United States has declined steadily over the past several decades and is at a record low of 7.2

per 1000 live births, the United States still ranks 24th in infant mortality compared with other industrialized nations. Infant mortality rates vary substantially among and within racial and ethnic groups. Infant death rates among American Indians and Alaska Natives, Hispanics, and African Americans in 1995 or 1996 were above the national average. The greatest disparity exists for African Americans, whose infant death rate is 14.2 per 1000 live births. The overall infant death rate for American Indians (9.0) and Hispanics (7.6) does not reflect the diversity among this group.

- Cancer disparities exist in mortality and incidence rates. Native Hawaiian men have elevated rates of lung cancer compared with white men. Alaska Native men and women suffer disproportionately higher rates of cancers of the colon and rectum than do whites. Vietnamese women in the United States have a cervical cancer incidence rate more than five times greater than white women. Hispanic women also suffer elevated rates of cervical cancer. African Americans have an overall cancer death rate 35 percent higher than that for whites. Death rate for lung cancer is about 27 percent higher for African Americans than for whites. The prostate cancer mortality rate for African American men is more than twice that of white men.

source: National Institute of Health. (2001). What are health disparities? (http://healthdisparities.nih.gov/whatare.html)

---

usually treatable, and often disappear in a short time. Appendicitis, pneumonia, and influenza are examples of acute illnesses.

Diseases are not the only causes of death. Accidents, homicide, and suicide are the leading killers of Americans between the ages of 15 and 24. Most (75 percent) accidental deaths among this age group involve motor vehicle accidents, many of which are alcohol related. For young adults 25 to 44 years old, accidents, cancer, heart disease, suicide, human immunodeficiency virus (HIV) infection, and homicide are the leading causes of death.

For too many Americans these conditions reflect the dangers of negative lifestyle choices. Despite this, much of Americans' health-related anxiety involves exotic diseases. The current fear that some sort of strangely mutated disease will soon pose the greatest threat to life on Earth ironically coincides with a reduction in attention to chronic diseases that do kill in large numbers. The fear of bizarre pathogens leading to runaway deaths in the United States has been fueled primarily by

newspaper headlines, fictional books, and movies. Five recent headlines serve as examples:

- "Is mad-cow disease a threat in the U.S.?"
- "Animal disease shuts Irish tourist sites"
- "Foot and mouth disease causes crisis in England"
- "'Bird flu' causes Hong Kong to slaughter every chicken"
- "Kenya disease killing humans, animals"

Although the appearance of an unstoppable, overwhelming disease is possible and the spread of new viruses in a global community is a genuine concern, the real threats to Americans are mundane and are less likely to be featured as the lead stories in the evening news. As scary as some exotic diseases sound, the chances of getting them are infinitesimally remote, especially when comparing them to the chance of getting illnesses that people can take practical steps to avoid.[17]

Healthy lifestyles that involve diet, physical activity, and personal health habits offer the most potential for

---

Wellness Across the Generations

These boxes address wellness concepts throughout the life span by looking at issues such as childhood origins of heart disease, alcohol and drug use among young women, and strength training for older adults.

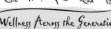

Wellness Across the Generations

Tips for Staying Physically Active

Sedentary lifestyles are the most formidable wellness challenge for Americans of all ages. More people are at risk for premature death and/or morbidity due to physical inactivity than to any of the other risk factors. For years, medical experts have advised regular exercise to improve fitness and health, to prevent disease and disability, even to lengthen life. Unfortunately, most people starting an exercise program drop out, usually within the first six months. About one-fourth of Americans succeed in making exercise a regular part of their lives. How do they do it? What are they doing right? What are the basic principles of their success stories? Here are some tips from leading exercise experts who practice what they preach.

1. Team up. People who exercise regularly often team up with at least one other person. It might be a roommate, spouse, neighbor, or friend. It might be a workout at the fitness club with a half-dozen friends; it might be a midday break to shoot baskets; it might be an early-morning walk with a member of the family.

2. Use exercise as a pick-me-up. Tired from the demands of work, many people resist expending energy on exercise. However, many experts do the opposite by turning to exercise as a source of energy. For them, exercise is a tranquilizer; it makes them more productive at work and home, it refreshes and relaxes them, and it helps them sleep.

3. Get a jump on the day. Many people are more consistent in their exercise routines when they exercise early. Quoting one expert: "You can't plan how your day is going to end, but you can plan how it will start."

4. Break up your workout. Exercise recommendations call for thirty minutes of moderate exercise most days of the week. But it doesn't have to be in one shot. Short bursts scattered throughout the day count, too. Look for opportunities to add exercise to your daily regimen. For example, use the stairs instead of the elevator; park farther away and walk briskly to class; or when shopping, grab the first parking space (which is usually farther away); if you're waiting for someone, walk while you wait.

5. Seek variety. Engage in a variety of activities. If you work inside all day, you might exercise outside. Try seasonal activities. Catch the evening news while working out on a treadmill. Remember, if you enjoy your workout, you are more likely to continue working out.

6. Revel in your success. The more you make exercise feel like an accomplishment rather than a chore, the more you'll look forward to each session. One lifelong jogger logs his mileage because it boosts his lifetime record. A walker wears a pedometer so he can monitor his progress as he attempts to walk at least 10,000 steps each day.

source: Consumer Union. (1999). Success stories: How the experts stay active. Consumer Reports on Health 11(4);8–9.

---

emphasis from intensive aerobic exercise to a broader range of health-enhancing physical activity regardless of age (see Wellness Across the Generations: Tips for Staying Physically Active). For those who are inactive, even small increases in physical activity are associated with measurable health benefits (see Just the Facts: Physical Activity and Health—Selected Highlights). The benefit of physical activity is the underlying theme of this text and, ideally, will serve as an impetus for you to establish an active lifestyle.

Achieving Lifestyle Change: A Self-Help Approach

A fundamental assumption underlying lifestyle-change programs is that behavior is a learned response. For example, we are not born with a taste for some foods and a dislike for others. And using seat belts is not a function of heredity. Like most other behaviors, health be-

haviors are learned responses to both obvious and subtle influences. This learning begins at birth and continues throughout life. This is as true for behaviors that promote wellness as for behaviors that diminish it.

Examples of obvious influences that help shape behavior include parents and family, role models, advertising, and social norms. In many instances these influences are combined to form a single powerful influence on behavior, such as exemplified by an advertisement for cigarettes using "ideal" masculine or feminine models, depending on the brand of cigarettes and the target population. Advertisers are successful not only at marketing products but also at influencing people to think they need those products.

Subtle forces also shape behavior. A good example is *subliminal advertising*, a technique in which messages, words, and symbols are embedded or hidden in the pictures, sounds, or words used in advertisements. Theoretically these messages, though not directly observable,

Wellness on the Web

These behavior change activities take you to quizzes, questions, and self-assessments on the text's Online Learning Center. Completing these activities will help you assess your current practices and design a more wellness-oriented lifestyle.

Health and Human Performance Website

www.mhhe.com/hhp McGraw-Hill's Health and Human Performance Website provides a wide variety of information—including articles about current issues, articles that celebrate our diversity, study tips, online study guides, scholarship information, and exam preparation materials. It also includes professional organization and career information.

Preface

ellness: Concepts and Applications assumes that health is not a destination but a journey. Wellness is not a static condition, but a continual balancing of the different dimensions of human needs—spiritual, social, emotional, intellectual, physical, occupational, and environmental. Because each of us is responsible for our growth in these areas, this edition continues to strive to emphasize the importance of self-responsibility. And because we know that knowledge alone stimulates change for very few people, the reader will be challenged to be actively involved in the learning process by constantly assessing how the information presented affects lifestyle from a personal perspective.

Wellness: Concepts and Applications is neither a fitness book nor a personal health text. Instead, this text is designed to help students gain knowledge and understanding in a variety of areas, with the goal of taking that information and using it to make behavioral changes that will have a positive impact on their lives. In many cases these changes are necessary if people are to develop the skills, attitudes, beliefs, and habits that will ultimately result in the highest possible level of health and wellness.

Audience

When the fitness and wellness concept appears in university courses and programs, it is usually a scaled-down model of the traditional personal health course or an upscale version of physical fitness courses. In some cases, it is a hybrid of personal health and fitness courses, with emphasis on self-participation in the medical marketplace. Wellness: Concepts and Applications is a hybrid because the physical components of wellness are blended with its many other components. The primary objectives of this text are to present cogni-

tive health and wellness information appropriate for today's college students and to offer suggestions for their application. These suggestions relate to lifestyle behaviors over which people can exert some control. The emphasis is on self-responsibility, and this theme is implemented through a strong self-analysis and assessment component.

Approach

Important features unique to Wellness: Concepts and Applications distinguish it from other texts.

Balanced approach: Unlike other approaches that emphasize only physical fitness as a route to wellness, Wellness: Concepts and Applications provides a balanced presentation of the health benefits of exercise, diet, and cardiovascular wellness, along with the management of lifestyle change and consumer responsibility to achieve lifetime wellness.

Complete lifestyle decision-making information: Along with Goals for Behavior Change, Real-World Wellness boxes, Wellness on the Web Behavior Change Activities, and Assessment Activities that help apply the content, coverage of substance use, sexually transmitted diseases, cancer, and chronic health conditions is provided to enable and encourage responsible student decision making.

Consumer-oriented: Chapter 15, "Becoming a Responsible Health Care Consumer," offers information to help students become wise consumers.

Interdisciplinary author team: Two health educators and a fitness educator currently teaching wellness courses have combined their expertise to provide the most balanced presentation possible.

Full-color: A full-color format is used in the photographs, line drawings, and design of the text to increase visual appeal and to enhance the teaching-learning process.

Highlights of This Edition

Every chapter of *Wellness: Concepts and Applications* has been carefully updated. New tables, figures, and issues found in this edition are highlighted here.

New Photographs

The fresh, updated look of the many new photographs in this new edition offer a detailed look at the many exercises and assessments described in the text. The new photographs also reflect the diversity of college students of all ages.

Online Learning Center

In every chapter, the chapter-opening page contains an Online Learning Center box directing the reader to additional online information and study resources for that chapter.

Wellness on the Web: Behavior Change Activities

The text includes activities in every chapter that take students to online quizzes, questions, and self-assessment activities. This feature has been completely revised from the previous edition, with the reader being directed to the Online Learning Center at **www.mhhe.com/anspaugh5e** to complete the activities. This ensures that the links will be active when the reader tries to access them.

HealthQuest Activities

The HealthQuest CD-ROM that accompanies each new copy of *Wellness: Concepts and Applications* contains many useful health and wellness self-assessments. HealthQuest Activities have been incorporated throughout the text.

Just the Facts

Special material in newly-written Just the Facts boxes encourages students to delve into a particular topic or closely examine an important health issue.

Wellness Across the Generations

New content appears in the Wellness Across the Generations feature throughout the textbook.

New or Expanded Topics

We are committed to making this textbook the most up-to-date wellness text available. Following is a sampling of topics that are either completely new to this edition or are covered in greater depth than in the previous edition:

Chapter 1: Wellness and Fitness for Life
- New and updated figures and tables.
- New information on a seventeen-year study and how it relates to the social aspect of wellness.
- New information on a study performed and how it relates to the emotional aspect of wellness.
- New information on Leading Health Indicators (LHIs) as identified in the landmark document *Healthy People 2010*.
- New Just the Facts box on eliminating health disparities.
- New Wellness Across the Generations box on tips for staying physically active.

Chapter 2: Preventing Cardiovascular Disease
- New and updated figures and tables.
- Updated information from *Healthy People 2010*.
- New Just the Facts box on detecting and lowering high cholesterol.
- New section on high sensitivity C-reactive protein (hs-CRP).

Chapter 3: Increasing Cardiorespiratory Endurance
- New and updated figures and tables.
- New definition on physical fitness, physical activity, and exercise as defined by the American College of Sports Medicine (ACSM).
- Updated formula for calculating the target zone for exercise.
- Information on the "Talk Test."
- Explanation of the FIT principle as a means to remember the first three principles of exercise.

Chapter 4: Building Muscular Strength and Endurance
- New and updated figures and tables.
- Revised Just the Facts box on muscle fiber types.
- New content on the preferred order of exercise associated with resistance training.
- Additional information on creatine.

Chapter 5: Improving Flexibility
- New and updated figures and tables.
- New Wellness on the Web Behavior Change Activities box.

Chapter 6: Forming a Plan for Good Nutrition
- New and updated figures and tables.
- New Just the Facts box on unscrambling nutrition acronyms.
- Information on macronutrients versus micronutrients.
- New information on the trace mineral selenium.
- New Just the Facts box called "Bottled Water Comes with Many Names."

- New Just the Facts box on functional foods.
- Updated information on insoluble fiber as a protectant against colon cancer.
- New Just the Facts box on whole-grain foods.
- Inclusion of the *2000 Dietary Guidelines for Americans.*
- New sections on aiming for a healthy weight and being physically active every day.
- New Just the Facts box on using variety when choosing foods.
- New section on keeping food safe to eat.
- New Just the Facts box on foodborne illness.
- New section on sugar intake, glycemic index, and diabetes mellitus.
- New Just the Facts box called "Glycemic Index (GI)."
- Inclusion of the ten FDA approved health claims that link foods to diseases.

Chapter 7: *Understanding Body Composition*

- New and updated figures and tables.
- New guidelines from the ACSM on taking skinfold measurements.
- New information on air-displacement plethysmography.

Chapter 8: *Achieving a Healthy Weight*

- New and updated figures and tables.
- New Just the Facts box on waist size.
- New Just the Facts box called "Can You Be Fat and Fit?"
- New Just the Facts box on adult obesity.
- Rewritten section on heredity.
- New Just the Facts box on viral infections and obesity.
- New Just the Facts box on body shape.
- New information based on the Surgeon General's report on physical activity and health.
- New information from the National Heart, Lung, and Blood Institute on the treatment of obesity.
- New Just the Facts box on yo-yo dieting and toxicity.
- Inclusion of the Mayo Clinic Healthy Weight Pyramid.
- New Just the Facts box on restaurant dining.
- New Just the Facts box on solid calories versus liquid calories.
- New sections on low-carbohydrate diets and novelty diets.
- New section on diet supplements and herbal remedies.
- New section on eating disorders and disordered eating.
- New section on the female athlete triad.
- Revised basic principles of weight maintenance and loss.
- New Just the Facts box on calories.

Chapter 9: *Coping with and Managing Stress*

- New and updated figures and tables.
- New section called Attitude and Stress.
- New section called Gender and Stress.
- New section on time management.

Chapter 10: *Taking Charge of Your Personal Safety*

- New and updated figures and tables.
- New Real-World Wellness box on apartment and dormitory insurance.
- New Just the Facts box on air pollution.
- New Just the Facts box on exercise safety.

Chapter 11: *Taking Responsibility for Drug Use*

- New and updated figures and tables.
- Revised section on binge drinking among college students.
- Guidelines for reducing the risk associated with heavy or binge drinking.
- New sections on Rohypnol, GHB, and ketamine.

Chapter 12: *Preventing Sexually Transmitted Diseases*

- New and updated figures and tables.
- Revised Wellness Across the Generations box on HIV and AIDS.
- New data on AIDs-related deaths in 2000.

Chapter 13: *Reducing Your Risk of Cancer*

- New and updated figures and tables.
- New data on cancer-related deaths in 2000.
- Revised Just the Facts box on cancer prevention.
- New information on cancer treatment.
- New Just the Facts box on the power of synergy.

Chapter 14: *Managing Common Conditions*

- New and updated figures and tables.
- New Just the Facts box on diabetes in youth.
- Included information in the headache section on experiencing an "aura."

Chapter 15: *Becoming a Responsible Health Care Consumer*

- New and updated figures and tables.
- Updated section on understanding health information.
- New Just the Facts box called "The Making of a Medical Flip-Flop."
- New information on iatrogenic conditions.
- New Just the Facts box on when to visit a doctor.
- New Just the Facts box on polypharmacy problems.
- New information on a study regarding patient-doctor communication.
- New Just the Facts box on fecal occult-blood tests.

Successful Pedagogical Features

Wellness: Concepts and Applications continues to use a variety of learning aids to enhance student comprehension.

Key Terms: The most important terms for student retention have been set in boldface type in the text for easy identification.

Chapter Objectives: These are introduced at the beginning of each chapter. They help the student identify the chapter's key topics. Accomplishing the objectives indicates fulfillment of the chapter's intent.

Goals for Behavior Change: These are listed at the beginning of each chapter, giving students objectives that help them apply what they learn in the text. They reinforce the concept of self-responsibility on which the text is based.

Nurturing Your Spirituality: These boxes cover such topics as living well with cancer, making decisions about sex, and enjoying healthy pleasure, showing students that wellness goes beyond the physical dimension.

Wellness on the Web: These are activities that take students to quizzes, questions, and self-assessments on the text's online learning center. Completing these activities will help the students assess their current practices and design a more wellness-oriented lifestyle.

Wellness Across the Generations: These boxes address wellness concepts throughout the life span by looking at issues such as childhood origins of heart disease, alcohol and drug use among young women, and strength training for older adults.

Real-World Wellness: These question-and-answer boxes show students how to put wellness concepts into practice. Helpful tips give students practical advice for initiating behavior change and staying motivated to follow a wellness lifestyle.

Just the Facts: Special material in these boxes encourages students to delve into a particular topic or closely examine an important health issue.

Chapter Summaries: These identify the main parts of the chapter and reinforce the chapter objectives.

Review Questions: Questions are provided to help students review and analyze material for overall understanding.

References: Accurate and current documentation is given at the end of the chapters.

Suggested Readings: Additional current resources are provided for students to obtain further information.

Assessment Activities: Each chapter concludes with at least two Assessment Activities to help students apply the content learned in the chapter to their decision making. The text is perforated for easy removal of the Assessment Activities.

Appendix: Food Composition Table—More than 1200 common foods and fast foods are analyzed. This comprehensive table will help students complete Assessment Activities in Chapter 6.

Glossary: A comprehensive glossary is provided at the end of the text that includes all key terms, as well as additional terms, used in the text.

Technology: The Key to Teaching and Learning

Just a quick glance through the pages of *Wellness: Concepts and Applications* will show you that technology is woven through every chapter. Similarly, the ancillary package that accompanies the text emphasizes technology while acknowledging the merit of the printed ancillaries. Together, the text and its ancillaries offer the ideal approach to teaching and learning—one that integrates the best tools that technology has to offer, challenging both instructors and students to reach higher.

Ancillaries

An extensive ancillary package is available to qualified adopters to enhance the teaching-learning process. We have made a concerted effort to produce supplements of extraordinary utility and quality. This package has been carefully planned and developed to help instructors derive the greatest benefit from the text. We encourage instructors to examine them carefully. Many of the products can be packaged with the text at a discounted price. Beyond the following brief descriptions, additional information about these ancillaries is available from your McGraw-Hill sales representative.

Course Integrator Guide
ISBN 0-07-246168-3

This manual includes all the features of a useful instructor's manual, including learning objectives, suggested lecture outlines, suggested activities, media resources, and weblinks. It also integrates the text with all the wellness resources McGraw-Hill offers, such as the HealthQuest CD-ROM, the Online Learning Center (OLC), the AIDS booklet, the video clips CD-ROM, and the Health and Human Performance Discipline Page. The guide also includes references to relevant print and broadcast media.

Test Bank
ISBN 0-07-253325-0

This printed manual includes more than 2000 questions, including multiple choice, true/false, and short essay. The questions have been entered into the computerized test bank.

Computerized Test Bank
ISBN 0-07-246171-3

Available on Hybrid CD-ROM for Windows and Macintosh, the latest version of our computerized testing software is available. This allows instructors to custom design tests, use the expanded test bank, and add testing questions.

Overhead Transparency Acetates
ISBN 0-07-246167-5

Sixty of the text's most important illustrations, diagrams, tables, and charts are available as full-color transparency acetates. These useful tools facilitate learning and classroom discussion and were chosen specifically to help explain difficult concepts. This package is also available to qualified adopters of the text.

Online Learning Center (OLC)

www.mhhe.com/anspaugh5e

This website offers resources to students and instructors. It includes downloadable ancillaries, weblinks, student quizzing, additional information on topics of interest, and much more.

Resources for the instructor include:

- Downloadable PowerPoint presentation with annotated lecture notes
- Lecture outlines
- Interactive links
- Links to professional resources

Resources for the student include:

- Flashcards of chapter key terms
- Downloadable PowerPoint presentation
- Interactive activities
- Self-grading quizzes

HealthQuest® 4.0 by Bob Gold and Nancy Atkinson
ISBN 0-07-253052-9

HealthQuest 4.0 comes free with new texts and helps students explore the behavioral aspects of wellness through a state-of-the-art interactive CD-ROM. Students will be able to assess their current health and wellness status, determine their health risks, and explore options to improve the behaviors that will impact their health.

Image Presentation CD-ROM
ISBN 0-07-246172-1

The Image Presentation CD-ROM is a bank of images for use in the classroom and in the accompanying PowerPoint presentation. A slide editor tool allows the user to create customized slide shows.

Health and Human Performance Website www.mhhe.com/hhp

McGraw-Hill's Health and Human Performance Discipline Page provides a wide variety of information for instructors and students—including articles about current issues, articles that celebrate our diversity, text ancillaries, a "how-to" guide on technology, study tips, and exam preparation materials. It includes professional organization, convention, and career information, and explains how to become a McGraw-Hill author. Additional features of the Discipline Page include:

- This Just In—Offers information on the latest hot topics, the best web resources, and more.
- Faculty Support—Presents online course supplements such as lecture outlines and PowerPoint presentations, and allows instructors to create a course website with PageOut.
- Student Success Center—Offers students online study guides and other resources to improve their academic performance. Students can also explore scholarship opportunities and learn how to launch their career.
- Author Arena—Interested in writing a textbook or supplement for the college market? Read the McGraw-Hill proposal guidelines and links to the editorial and marketing teams, and meet and converse with our current authors.

PageOut®: The Course Website Development Center www.pageout.net

PageOut enables instructors to develop a website for their course. The site includes:

- A course home page
- An instructor home page
- A syllabus (interactive and customizable, including quizzing, instructor notes, and links to the Online Learning Center)
- Weblinks
- Discussions (multiple discussion areas per class)
- An online grade book
- Student webpages
- Design templates

This program is now available to registered adopters of McGraw-Hill textbooks. Contact your sales representative for assistance.

Primis Online

www.mhhe.com/primis/online

Primis Online is a database-driven publishing system that allows instructors to create content-rich textbooks, lab manuals, or readers for their courses directly from our website. The customized text can be delivered in printed or electronic (eBook) form. A Primis eBook is a digital version of the customized text (sold directly to students as a downloadable file to their computer or accessed online by a password).

Video Library

Choose from the McGraw-Hill videotape library, which contains many quality videotapes, including selected Films for Humanities and all videos from the award-winning series *Health Living: Road to Wellness*. Digitized video clips are also available.

Foodwise College Edition
ISBN 0-07-240786-7

Based on the widely tested professional version of Food-Works, this dietary analysis software has been developed for use in college courses. It offers a variety of functions based on the latest release of the USDA database. It is easy to use and allows the user to add foods to the database. Available for Windows and for networks.

Fitsolve II Software
ISBN 0-697-33950-5

This software package enhances learning of wellness concepts by personalizing information and explaining the meaning of results rather than just "grading" students as other programs do. It begins with a coronary heart disease risk questionnaire, followed by input of fitness test scores. Features include score summary, heart attack risk categorization, and health-related fitness status.

The AIDS Booklet by Frank Cox
ISBN 0-697-29428-5

This booklet provides current facts about AIDS and HIV: what it is, how the virus is transmitted, its prevalence among various population groups, symptoms of HIV infection, and strategies for prevention. It also covers the legal, social, medical, and ethical issues related to HIV and AIDS. Ongoing updates are posted to the website at **www.mhhe.com/catalogs/sem/hhp/ student/updates/aids.mhtml**. This booklet is available for $1.00 when combined with any McGraw-Hill product to create a package.

Testwell by the National Wellness Institute
ISBN 0-697-21131-2

This is a self-scoring, pencil-and-paper wellness assessment developed by the National Wellness Institute in Stevens Point, Wisconsin, and distributed exclusively by McGraw-Hill Publishers. It adds flexibility to any wellness course by allowing adopters to offer preassessments and postassessments at the beginning, end, or at any time during the course.

Diet and Fitness Log by McGraw-Hill
ISBN 0-8151-2524-0

This logbook helps students track their diet and exercise programs. It serves as a diary to help students log their behaviors. Each log offers a brief introduction, followed by an evaluation section in which they can assess their improvements and setbacks. It may be packaged with your textbook for an additional $1.00.

Acknowledgments

We wish to thank the following people for modeling for the photos for this edition:

Scott T. Belzer

Shonteh Henderson

Holly Ruth Henry

Chad Kirksick

Stacy Lancaster

Christopher Rasmussen

We wish to thank the reviewers, whose contributions have added significantly to the text. To the following, a grateful acknowledgement of their expertise and assistance:

For the Fifth Edition

John Bratcher
Lee University (Tennessee)

John Burgess
Suffolk County Community College (New York)

Kenneth L. Cameron
United States Military Academy, West Point (New York)

Lisa Hicks
University of Indianapolis (Indiana)

Mary LaRue
University of Wisconsin, Eau Claire (Wisconsin)

Sandra Mull
Northwest Missouri State University (Missouri)

Michael Nordvall
Marymount University (Virginia)

Sharon Woodard
Wake Forest University (North Carolina)

David J. Anspaugh

Michael H. Hamrick

Frank D. Rosato

Brief Contents

1 Wellness and Fitness for Life   1

2 Preventing Cardiovascular Disease   33

3 Increasing Cardiorespiratory Endurance   65

4 Building Muscular Strength and Endurance   97

5 Improving Flexibility   133

6 Forming a Plan for Good Nutrition   155

7 Understanding Body Composition   215

8 Achieving a Healthy Weight   235

9 Coping with and Managing Stress   275

10 Taking Charge of Your Personal Safety   309

11 Taking Responsibility for Drug Use   337

12 Preventing Sexually Transmitted Diseases   363

13 Reducing Your Risk of Cancer   381

14 Managing Common Conditions   407

15 Becoming a Responsible Health Care Consumer   423

A Appendix A: Food Composition Table   455

B Appendix B: Nutritional Content of Popular Items from Fast-Food Restaurants   465

C Appendix C: A Self-Care Guide for Common Medical Problems   470

D Appendix D: Resources for Self-Care   478

Glossary   482

Credits   491

Index   493

Contents

Preface   x

1 Wellness and Fitness for Life   1

Components of Wellness   2

The Wellness Challenge   7

Achieving Lifestyle Change:
A Self-Help Approach   11

Assessment Activities

1-1   Lifestyle Assessment Inventory   23

1-2   Health Locus of Control   29

1-3   Assessing Your Health Behavior   31

2 Preventing Cardiovascular Disease   33

Circulation   34

Cardiovascular Disease: A Twentieth-Century
Phenomenon   36

Risk Factors for Heart Disease   38

Preventing and Reversing Heart Disease   53

Other Possible Risk Factors   54

Medical Contributions   55

Assessment Activities

2-1   What's Your Heart Attack Risk?   61

2-2   Case Study of Bill M.   63

3 Increasing Cardiorespiratory Endurance   65

The Components of Physical Fitness   66

Cardiorespiratory Endurance   67

Cardiorespiratory Endurance and Wellness   70

Principles of Conditioning   71

Other Exercise Considerations   76

Environmental Conditions   78

Assessment Activities

3-1   The Rockport Fitness Walking Test   85

3-2   The 1.5-Mile Run/Walk Test   89

3-3   The 3-Minute Bench Step Test   91

3-4   Calculating Target Heart Rate   93

3-5   Design an Exercise Program   95

4 Building Muscular Strength and Endurance   97

The Health Benefits of Resistance Training   98

Anaerobic Exercise   99

Muscular Strength   99

Muscle Contraction and Resistance Training   100

Muscular Endurance   112

Principles of Resistance Training   112

Ergogenic Aids   114

Keeping a Daily Training Log   116

Assessment Activities

4-1   Calculation of Strength (Selected
Muscle Groups)   121

4-2   Muscular Endurance   123

4-3   Abdominal Muscular Endurance—the Canadian
Trunk Strength Test   125

4-4   Assessing Muscular Strength and Endurance
with Selected Calisthenic Exercises   127

4-5   Resistance Training Log   131

5 Improving Flexibility   133

Flexibility and Wellness   134

Developing a Flexibility Program   134

When to Stretch   134

Types of Stretching   135

Flexibility Assessment 140

Preventing Back and Neck Pain 140

Assessment Activities

5-1 Sit-and-Reach Test 147

5-2 Shoulder Flexion Test 149

5-3 Sling Test 151

5-4 Trunk Extension 153

6 Forming a Plan for Good Nutrition 155

Nutrition and Health 156

Essential Nutrients 157

Other Nutrients with Unique Health Benefits 173

Putting Nutrition to Work 178

Other Nutrition Issues of Concern 190

Food Labels 193

Changes in American Eating Patterns 195

Planning a Nutrition Strategy for Wellness 196

Assessment Activities

6-1 Assessing Your Carbohydrate
and Protein RDA 201

6-2 Assessing Your Maximum Fat and Saturated
Fat Intakes 203

6-3 Nutrient Intake Assessment 205

6-4 How Does Your Diet Compare
with the Recommended Diet? 209

6-5 Do You Have Fatty Habits? 211

6-6 Eating Behaviors to Consider 213

7 Understanding Body Composition 215

Obesity 216

Overweight 218

Regional Fat Distribution 218

Methods for Measuring Body-Weight Status 220

Measurement of Body Fat 221

Selected Methods for Measuring Body
Composition 223

Assessment Activities

7-1 Using BMI to Estimate Body-Weight Status
and Calculate Desirable Body Weight 231

7-2 Calculating Desirable Body Weight from Percent
Body Fat 233

8 Achieving a Healthy Weight 235

Americans' Obsession with Body Weight 236

Defining the Problem 237

Health Aspects of Obesity 238

Weight Loss: A New Attitude Emerges 239

Development of Obesity 239

Causes of Obesity 241

Dieting and Exercise: Strategies for Weight
Maintenance or Weight Loss 245

Regular Exercise Is the Key to Weight Management:
Make It Fun 256

Eating Disorders and Disordered Eating 257

Principles of Weight Management:
Putting It All Together 260

Assessment Activities

8-1 Assessing Your Body Image 267

8-2 Calculating Caloric Expenditure
Through Exercise 269

8-3 Estimating Your Basal Metabolic Rate 271

8-4 Assessing Calorie Costs of Activities 273

9 Coping with and Managing Stress 275

What Is Stress? 276

Sources of Stress and Warning Signs 278

Factors Generating a Stress Response 279

Physiological Responses to Stress 279

Self-Esteem and Stress 282

Attitude and Stress 282

Gender and Stress 284

Personality and Stress 284

Dealing with Stress 285

Relaxation Techniques 286

Selecting a Stress-Reducing Technique 291

Assessment Activities

9-1 Life Stressors 295

9-2 How Stressed Are You? 297

9-3 Stress Style: Mind, Body, Mixed? 299

9-4 Identification of Coping Styles 301

9-5 How Hardy Are You? 303

9-6 Goals and Priorities 305

9-7 Analyzing Your Use of Time 307

10 Taking Charge of Your Personal Safety 309

Home Safety 310

Recreational and Outdoor Safety 312

Vehicle Safety 315

Violence and Intentional Injury 319

Assessment Activities

10-1 How Safe Is Your Home? 329

10-2 Recreational Safety—How Safe Are You? 331

10-3 Road Rage and You 333

10-4 Encounters of the Dangerous Kind 335

11 Taking Responsibility for Drug Use 337

Reasons for Drug Use 338

Drug Classification 339

Commonly Abused Substances 341

Illegal Drugs 351

Other Drugs of Concern 353

A Final Thought 354

Assessment Activities

11-1 Do You Have a Drinking Problem? 359

11-2 What Are Your Reasons for Drug Use? 361

12 Preventing Sexually Transmitted Diseases 363

Safer Sex 364

Sexually Transmitted Diseases (STDs) 366

Viral Diseases 367

Bacterial Diseases 373

Other Common STDs 374

Assessment Activities

12-1 Are You at Risk for a Sexually Transmitted Disease? 377

12-2 Making a Decision 379

13 Reducing Your Risk of Cancer 381

Causes and Prevention 384

Cancer Site 387

Exercise and Cancer Prevention 388

Cancers of Concern to Everyone 388

Treatment 398

Assessment Activities

13-1 Cancer Early Detection Inventory 403

13-2 Are You Practicing Cancer Prevention? 405

14 Managing Common Conditions 407

Diabetes Mellitus 408

Arthritis 411

Osteoporosis 412

Asthma 413

The Common Cold 415

Influenza 415

Headaches 415

Inflammatory Bowel Disease 417

Assessment Activities

14-1 Are You at Risk for Diabetes? 419

14-2 Managing Your Asthma 421

15 Becoming a Responsible Health Care Consumer 423

Understanding Health Information 424

Guidelines for Evaluating Health Information 424

Managing Health Care 430

Alternative Medicine 439

Assessing Your Health 440

Paying for Health Care 444

Assessment Activities

15-1 Are You Communicating with Your Physician? 449

15-2 Assessing the Results of Diagnostic Tests 451

15-3 Self-Care Inventory 453

A Appendix A: Food Composition Table 455

B Appendix B: Nutritional Content of Popular Items from Fast-Food Restaurants 465

C Appendix C: A Self-Care Guide for Common Medical Problems 470

D Appendix D: Resources for Self-Care 478

Glossary 482

Credits 491

Index 493

1

Wellness and Fitness for Life

Online Learning Center

Log on to our Online Learning Center (OLC) for access to these additional resources:

- Chapter key term flashcards
- Learning objectives
- Additional goals for behavior change
- Concentration game
- Self-scoring chapter quizzes

- Additional lab activities

The OLC also offers weblinks for study and exploration of wellness topics. Access these links through **www.mhhe.com/anspaugh5e**, click on "Student Center," click on "Chapter 1," and then click on "Web Activities."

Goals for Behavior Change

- Implement four new health-promoting behaviors.
- Increase physical activity to improve overall wellness.
- Choose and implement three countering strategies.
- Formulate a self-help plan for lifestyle change.

Key Terms

contracting
countering
health-behavior gap
health disparities
Leading Health Indicators
  (LHI)
lifestyle diseases
locus of control

psychosomatic diseases
risk factors
self-efficacy
self-help
shaping up
transtheoretical model of
  behavior change
wellness

Objectives

After completing this chapter, you will be able to do the following:

- Discuss the wellness approach to healthy living.
- Identify benefits of living a wellness lifestyle.
- Describe the dimensions of wellness.
- Cite evidence of the relationship between physical health problems and social, emotional, and spiritual stressors.
- Identify health disparities that exist in the United States.
- Compare and contrast the major influences on the health of Americans today with those of Americans of the past.

- Identify and discuss the main wellness challenges for Americans.
- Identify obvious and subtle factors that help shape behavior.
- Discuss some of the underlying assumptions of lifestyle change.
- Identify and describe the six stages of change.
- Describe strategies that can be useful in designing and implementing an action plan for change.

ood health is one of our most cherished possessions, one that is often taken for granted until it is lost. Some people convincingly argue that everything else in life is secondary to good health. For many, it is not difficult to recall instances when life's goals, whether academic, career, or family; small or large; immediate or long-range, seemed unimportant because of sudden illness or a long-term debilitating health crisis.

Fortunately, the prospects of good health for Americans have never been better. The extent to which good health is realized is contingent on many factors. Chief among these factors are our actions and the choices we make. We can make choices that will promote health and well-being, prevent or delay the premature onset of many chronic illnesses, and improve our quality of life (see Real-World Wellness: Benefits of Living a Wellness Lifestyle). Staying healthy is not just a matter of common sense. Rather, it is a lifelong process that requires self-awareness, introspection, reflection, inquiry, accurate information, and action. This process relies on the concept of wellness and implies that each of us has the opportunity and the obligation to assume responsibility for factors that are under our control and to shape our health destiny. The wellness approach represents a formidable challenge because the processes leading to today's serious health threats are insidious, often originate in childhood or adolescence, flourish throughout adulthood, and finally culminate in full-blown disease in middle age or later. Lifestyle interventions initiated late in life produce limited success, but begun early in life they have maximum effect.

Components of Wellness

Wellness is defined as a lifelong process that at any given time produces a positive state of personal well-being; of feeling good about yourself; of optimal physical, psychological, and social functioning; and the control and minimization of both internal and external risk factors for both diseases and negative health conditions.[1] Wellness is a process rather than a goal. It implies a choice, a way of life. It means integrating the body, mind, and spirit. It symbolizes acceptance of yourself. It suggests that what you believe, feel, and do has an influence on your health. However, it does not imply that we make the best choice in every situation.

Consider the brief profiles of David, Susan, Carlos, and Maria. How would you rate each of them in terms of health and wellness?

David is physically active, places a high priority on his social life, barely makes passing grades in school, and engages in binge drinking almost every weekend. Susan is a perfectionist and her grades reflect it. To her, a B means

Real-World Wellness

Benefits of Living a Wellness Lifestyle

I am a full-time student, work twenty plus hours a week, and help with family responsibilities. At the same time, I'm trying to maintain my academic scholarship. There just isn't enough time in the day to be concerned about health and wellness. What am I to gain from a wellness lifestyle?

A wellness lifestyle offers the following benefits:

- Increases energy level and productivity at work and school
- Decreases absenteeism from school and work
- Decreases recovery time after illness or injury
- Supplies the body with proper nutrients
- Improves awareness of personal needs and the ways to meet them
- Expands and develops intellectual abilities
- Increases the ability to communicate emotions to others and to act assertively rather than aggressively or passively
- Promotes the attitude that life's difficulties are challenges and opportunities rather than overwhelming threats
- Acts from an internal locus of control
- Increases ability to cope with stress and resist depression
- Improves the cardiorespiratory system
- Increases muscle tone, strength, flexibility, and endurance
- Improves physical appearance
- Helps prevent or delay the premature onset of some forms of chronic disease
- Regulates and improves overall body function
- Promotes self-confidence
- Delays the aging process
- Promotes social awareness and the ability to reach out to, understand, and care about others

failure. She spends an inordinate amount of time studying, regularly skips meals, has no physical activity outlet, and rarely socializes. Her family tells her to "get a life." She needs the entire weekend to recover from the stress of academics. Carlos runs 3 miles every day, works out with weights 3 times a week, eats a balanced diet almost every day, has a close circle of friends, refuses to use his seat belt when driving, and smokes an average of two packs of cigarettes daily. Maria is a worrier. She makes good grades but is rarely satisfied. Her eating practices

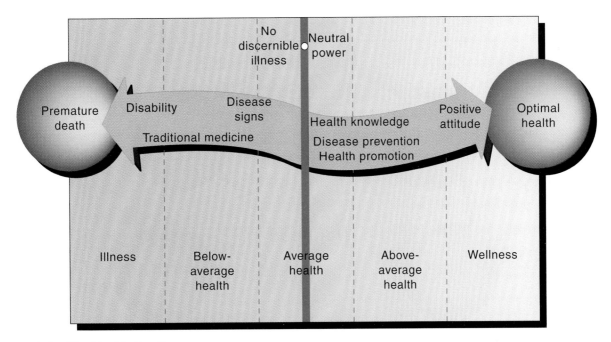

Figure 1-1 The Health Continuum

are exemplary, but she is constantly counting fat grams and calories and rarely looks forward to mealtime. She is self-conscious about her weight and occasionally engages in bulimic practices.

Figure 1-1 depicts how health moves along a continuum from optimal health to premature death. Your position on this continuum is always subject to change and is affected by many factors, including physical health, activity level, nutritional patterns, personal demands, career goals, time of year, and effectiveness in managing stress. The direction you move on the continuum and your place on the continuum at any time are largely determined by the activities you pursue and your attitudes toward these activities. These activities and attitudes can prevent illness and promote health or can destroy peace of mind and physical well-being. Because your behaviors are intrinsic to your health, you must learn to assume responsibility for your health by developing the skills and acquiring the knowledge to improve it.

In the past, medicine approached wellness from a different perspective. It emphasized the treatment of diseases rather than their prevention. It demanded no more than passive participation by the patient in the decision-making process. Now people are encouraged to become active participants in their health care, to exercise control over wellness **risk factors** (factors or conditions that threaten wellness and increase the chances of developing or contracting disease), to shape their lifestyles to promote health, and to serve as partners with health care providers in making medical decisions. This approach places the responsibility for wellness on the individual.

HealthQuest Activities

- Use the Wellboard to report your life score (number of years out of 114) and the score percentages for each of the eight health areas.

- Fill out the Wellboard using data from a fictional college student. On the first assessment screen, change the demographics to show how gender, ethnicity, age, marital status, and community affect average life expectancy.

Achieving a high level of wellness requires constant balance and maintenance of certain components (figure 1-2): spiritual, social, physical, emotional, intellectual, occupational, and environmental.

Spiritual

Spirituality is a belief in a source of value that transcends the boundaries of the self but also nurtures the self. Everyone has a personal perception of spirituality. The spiritual component provides meaning and direction in life and enables you to grow, learn, and meet new challenges. Spiritual wellness includes developing a strong sense of values, ethics, and morals. It overlaps with the emotional component of wellness (described later). While spirituality may relate to religious precepts, it does not necessarily adhere to any particular

Figure 1-2 The Seven Components of Wellness

religious structure (see Nurturing Your Spirituality: Can Spirituality Improve Your Physical Health?).

Social

Being social means having the ability to interact successfully with people and one's personal environment. Social health is the ability to develop and maintain intimacy with others and to have respect and tolerance for those with different opinions and beliefs. Numerous studies report on the advantage patients surrounded by a network of family and friends have over patients without a social support system in recovering from surgery or coping with chronic conditions.

In one study for example, researchers monitored the health of nearly 7000 participants for more than seventeen years. They found that those lacking social connections were two to three times more likely to experience premature death than their socially connected peers.[2] The same study found that older people who stay socially connected to others by volunteering live longer than those who don't volunteer. Social activities, such as visiting friends; attending church, a movie, a play, a sporting event, a club, or other group event; or playing games, forestall infections and protect against disease. Researchers concluded that adults, young and old, should stay connected either to other people, a pet, or a favorite hobby.[3]

Social contacts are even being studied in terms of communicable diseases. Researchers from Carnegie Mellon University gave 276 healthy volunteers nasal sprays containing one of two cold viruses. Volunteers with large relationship networks developed fewer cold symptoms and infections than did people with smaller networks. Researchers pointed out that what mattered was not the number of friends, but the number of types of relationships. People with six or more relationship types (parents, siblings, schoolmates, coworkers, roommates, and community acquaintances) had 4.2 times fewer colds than did those who had one to three types. The study defined a relationship as speaking with a person at least every two weeks.[4] The investigation revealed that a lack of diverse social contacts is a stronger risk factor for colds than is smoking, low vitamin C intake, or elevated stress hormones.[5]

Physical

The physical component of wellness involves the ability to carry out daily tasks, develop cardiorespiratory and muscular fitness, maintain adequate nutrition and a

Nurturing Your Spirituality

Can Spirituality Improve Your Physical Health?

It's all in your mind. Or is it in your body? Or both? The interconnections between mind and body are the bases for many types of alternative health practices. Spirituality is believing in a source of value that transcends the boundaries of the self but also nurtures the self. Mind-body medicine builds upon spirituality, encouraging methods for improving the body by altering the mind. The National Institutes of Health (NIH) suggests the following spiritual practices:

- *Psychotherapy* focuses on the mental and emotional health of the patient and has been proven to reduce the amount of time required to recover from an illness.

- *Support groups* give patients the consolation that others have endured similar health challenges and survived, instilling hope.

- *Meditation,* formerly associated solely with religious practice, is a self-governed exercise for relaxation. Regular practice of meditation is recommended for reducing blood pressure and anxiety and increasing the quality of life and longevity.

- *Imagery* includes use of all the senses to encourage attitude change, behavior, or physiological responses. Uses of imagery include pain control in cancer patients and increasing immunity in elderly patients.

- *Hypnosis* is an ancient practice molded to fit modern needs. Today physicians, dentists, psychologists, and other mental health professionals use hypnosis to help people overcome addictions, control pain, and deal with phobias.

- *Biofeedback* provides patients with a picture of what is occurring physiologically in their bodies and an understanding of how trial-and-error adjustments of mental processes can affect these physiological behaviors. This technique is used in treatment for a wide variety of disorders, such as epilepsy, respiratory diseases, migraines, vascular disorders, and hypertension.

- *Yoga* is a disciplined practice of altering mental and physiological processes previously thought to be outside an individual's control. These alterations, performed on a regular basis, can reduce anxiety, lower blood pressure, treat arthritis, and increase the efficiency of the heart.

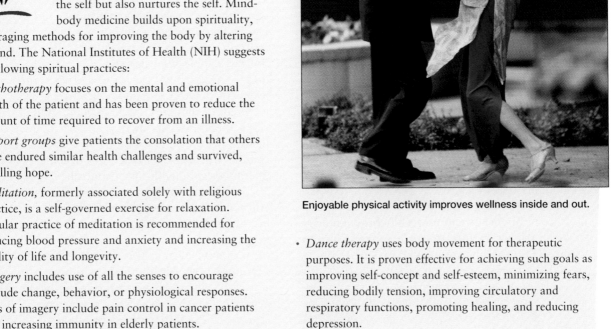

Enjoyable physical activity improves wellness inside and out.

- *Dance therapy* uses body movement for therapeutic purposes. It is proven effective for achieving such goals as improving self-concept and self-esteem, minimizing fears, reducing bodily tension, improving circulatory and respiratory functions, promoting healing, and reducing depression.

- *Music therapy* puts to good use the power of music on the psyche. Do you ever listen to music to make you feel better? So do stroke, Parkinson's, brain-injury, cancer, anxiety, cerebral palsy, and burn patients.

- *Art therapy* uses self-expression through art to enhance healing. Art therapy is used with patients being treated for burns, emotional problems, chemical addictions, and sexual abuse.

- *Prayer and mental healing* involves communication with some form of higher power. A wide variety of healing techniques fall within this category. Examples are being physically touched by a religious healer or experiencing healing through personal prayer or attendance at church. Studies link regular church attendance with reduced chance of dying from stroke or heart disease, lower blood pressure, lower suicide rates, and reduced depression.

healthy body fat level, and avoid abusing alcohol and other drugs or using tobacco products. In general, physical health is an investment in positive lifestyle habits. Separate chapters in this text are devoted to many of these physical dimensions of wellness.

Emotional

Emotional wellness is the ability to control stress and to express emotions appropriately and comfortably. It is the ability to recognize and accept feelings and not be defeated by setbacks and failures. Achieving emotional wellness allows you to experience life's ups and downs with enthusiasm and grace and maintain satisfying relationships with others.[6]

Many studies report on the connection between wellness and emotional health. Anger, for example, is a powerful emotion that has consistently been found to increase the risk of heart attacks. In a recent study involving men who had both coronary heart disease and high scores for anger and hostility, participants who participated in an eight-week anger management course were less angry and their blood pressure dropped significantly. The benefits were still apparent two months later. Participants in the control group whose anger score remained the same experienced an increase in blood pressure.[7] Other large-scale studies involving thousands of men and women now acknowledge that anger-prone people have a nearly threefold higher risk than others of suffering a heart attack or dying from heart disease.[8]

Many other health problems are rooted in emotional stressors. Health conditions ranging from hives to cancer may have as their origin a breakdown in the body's immune system caused by the body's response to emotional stressors. These stressors, by disrupting the body's delicate balance of powerful hormones, may serve as the triggering mechanism for myriad health problems. The growing acceptance of stress-coping techniques, like those presented in Chapter 9 of this text, is evidence of the trend toward nonphysical strategies for preventing and treating many health problems.

Intellectual

The intellectual component of wellness involves the ability to learn and use information effectively for personal, family, and career development. Intellectual wellness means striving for continued growth and learning to deal with new challenges effectively. It means acting on accepted principles of wellness and assuming responsibility for eliminating the discrepancy between knowledge and behavior, often referred to as the **health-behavior gap.** For example, people know that they should wear their seat belts and that they should not smoke, yet many people do not buckle up and continue to use tobacco products. For wellness to occur, people must internalize information and act on it.

An intellectually well person understands and applies the concepts of locus of control and self-efficacy. **Locus of control** refers to a person's view or attitude about his or her role in wellness and illness. A person's locus of control may be either internal or external. When people view problems concerning their health or other parts of their lives as generally out of their control (when they view themselves as being at the mercy of other people, places, and events), they have an external locus of control. On the other hand, people who

have an internal locus of control view their own behaviors as having significant effects, feel that they are at least partially the masters of their fate, and recognize that they can change the course of their health. People with an internal locus of control are more likely to succeed in wellness activities, because they assume the necessary responsibility for their actions.

Locus of control serves as a simple but powerful yardstick of the relationship between health perceptions and mortality. Numerous studies have established a strong link between how people perceive their health and how likely they are to die sooner rather than later. People whose self-assessments are bleak have a higher mortality rate than those whose self-assessments are upbeat. People who perceive their health as excellent and believe they can have a direct influence on longevity have a mortality rate that is 2 to 3 times lower than that of comparable individuals who perceive themselves as having little influence on their health.[9] Assessment Activity 1-2 at the end of this chapter will help you determine whether you have an internal or external locus of control.

Another influence on intellectual wellness is self-efficacy. **Self-efficacy** refers to a person's belief in his or her ability to accomplish a specific task or behavior. Perhaps the most important influence on the achievement of a wellness goal is the perception that it can be accomplished. Although the support of others is a source of encouragement, success is likely to require generating a personal sense of competence. Self-efficacy is not earned, inherited, or acquired; it is something you bestow on yourself.

For high-level wellness to be achieved, people must see themselves as successful and believe that they can accomplish a task. Although locus of control establishes an attitude toward one's role in achieving wellness, self-efficacy establishes behavior. Self-efficacy links knowing what to do and accomplishing the task. Together, an internal locus of control and a strong sense of self-efficacy are powerful tools in promoting wellness and coping with illness.

Occupational

Occupational wellness is the ability to achieve a balance between work and leisure time. Attitudes about work, school, career, and career goals greatly affect work or school performance and interactions with others. Striving for occupational wellness adds focus to your life and allows you to find personal satisfaction in your life through work.

Environmental

Environmental wellness is the ability to promote health measures that improve the standard of living and quality of life in the community, including laws and agencies that safeguard the physical environment.

To illustrate the impact of environment on wellness, consider the differences in mortality (incidence of deaths) and morbidity (incidence of sickness) between earlier times and today. At the beginning of the twentieth century, the average life span of Americans was 47 years. Today, it is 76.7 years,[10] an all-time high. In 1900, communicable or infectious diseases (diseases that can be transmitted from one person to another) were the major causes of death. Influenza, pneumonia, tuberculosis, smallpox, polio, diphtheria, and dysentery were often fatal and were greatly feared. Only 50 percent of children were expected to reach their fifth birthday. Environmental conditions were appalling; water was dirty and food was often unsafe for consumption. People generally had little control over their health, and prospects for a long life were greatly influenced by fate and circumstance. By comparison, children born today have a 99 percent rate of survival to their fifth birthday. Governmental agencies at the federal, state, and local levels now assume responsibility for protecting health and preventing infectious diseases. Vaccinations have eradicated many dreaded diseases. The world food supply has more than doubled.[11] Adult literacy has increased. Mind-boggling advancements in medical technology have given rise to diagnostic and surgical procedures far beyond the wildest imaginations of early–twentieth–century physicians. Still, even with all of the discoveries of modern medicine, the greatest improvement in the health of Americans is due to a much more basic element of the environment: safe water. No other factor, not even vaccinations or antibiotics, has had as significant an impact on mortality reduction and population growth as safe water.[12]

Today, environmental influences include more than safe water, food, and air. Recent changes in countries such as Russia, where the death rate in 1995 outstripped the birth rate by 1.6 times and the mortality rate was as much as 77 percent higher than it was in 1990,[13] are grim reminders of the effect of the political environment on health and wellness. Here in the United States, subtle influences such as the socioeconomic factors of income, housing, and education play a critical role in the health status of various population groups.

Health disparities refers to differences in the incidence, prevalence, mortality, and burden of diseases and other adverse health conditions that exist among specific population groups in the United States.[14] The National Institutes of Health has identified six focus areas in which racial and ethnic minorities experience serious disparities in health access and outcomes:

1. Infant mortality
2. Cancer screening and management
3. Cardiovascular disease
4. Diabetes
5. HIV Infection/AIDS
6. Immunizations

These areas were selected for emphasis because they reflect areas of disparity known to affect multiple racial and ethnic minority groups at all life states (see Just the Facts: Eliminating Health Disparities: Three Examples). Research on health disparities related to socioeconomic status will be addressed later in this text.

An important assumption of the wellness approach to living is that good health is best achieved by balancing each of the seven components. The body, mind, and spirit are inseparably linked. When they work together in a fully unified, integrated biological system, the body can ward off or overcome many diseases. When any of these components breaks down, wellness is threatened. Although the association between disease and physical causes (such as pathogens) is obvious, some people are reluctant to accept the association between illness and its mental, social, and spiritual aspects.

Nonphysical causes of illness are intangible and difficult to assess. Many people experience poor health because of guilt, anger, hostility, poor interpersonal skills, loneliness, anxiety, and depression. Any of these factors can interfere with the body's immune system and lay the foundation for the disease process. Medical records are replete with examples of **psychosomatic diseases,** in which physical (soma) symptoms are caused by mental and emotional (psycho) stressors. Such symptoms are just as real as if caused by disease-producing germs. Every disease involves interplay among the components of wellness. Fortunately, after a long-standing obsession with medical technology, many health care providers are beginning to focus on treating the whole person, and more people are demanding more than test-tube medical care.

Assessment Activity 1-1 at the end of this chapter provides an evaluation of various aspects of wellness.

The Wellness Challenge

The most serious health problems of today are largely caused by the way people live and are referred to as **lifestyle diseases.** Almost half of all premature deaths in the United States and other developed countries are caused by lifestyle-related problems.[15] The leading causes of death in the United States among all age groups are heart disease, cancer, and stroke; they account for 61 percent of all deaths (table 1-1).[16] These are chronic diseases that are often caused by behaviors established early in life. *Chronic diseases* are health conditions that often begin gradually, have multiple causes, and usually persist for an indefinite time. Heart disease, diabetes, arthritis, and hypertension are examples of chronic illnesses. By contrast, *acute illnesses* come on suddenly, often have identifiable causes, are

Just the Facts

Eliminating Health Disparities: Three Examples

Despite notable progress in the overall health of the nation, American Indians, Alaskan Natives, Latinos, African Americans, and Pacific Islanders continue to shoulder more of the burden of illness and death compared with the U.S. population as a whole. These disparities are even greater if comparisons are made between each racial and ethnic group and the Caucasian population. Three examples follow.

• Heart disease is the leading cause of death for all racial and ethnic groups. Disparities exist among population groups, with a disproportionate burden of death and disability in minority and low-income populations. The age-adjusted death rate for heart disease for the total population declined by 20 percent from 1987 to 1995; for African Americans, the overall decrease was only 13 percent. Racial and ethnic minorities have higher rates of hypertension, tend to develop hypertension at an earlier age, and are less likely to undergo treatment to control their high blood pressure. Also, the rates for regular screening for cholesterol show disparities for certain racial and ethnic minorities—only 50 percent of American Indians and Alaska Natives, 44 percent of Asian Americans, and 38 percent of Mexican Americans have had their cholesterol checked within the past two years.

• Infant mortality is an important measure of a nation's health and worldwide indicator of health status. Although infant mortality in the United States has declined steadily over the past several decades and is at a record low of 7.2

per 1000 live births, the United States still ranks 24th in infant mortality compared with other industrialized nations. Infant mortality rates vary substantially among and within racial and ethnic groups. Infant death rates among American Indians and Alaska Natives, Hispanics, and African Americans in 1995 or 1996 were above the national average. The greatest disparity exists for African Americans, whose infant death rate is 14.2 per 1000 live births. The overall infant death rate for American Indians (9.0) and Hispanics (7.6) does not reflect the diversity among this group.

• Cancer disparities exist in mortality and incidence rates. Native Hawaiian men have elevated rates of lung cancer compared with white men. Alaska Native men and women suffer disproportionately higher rates of cancers of the colon and rectum than do whites. Vietnamese women in the United States have a cervical cancer incidence rate more than five times greater than white women. Hispanic women also suffer elevated rates of cervical cancer. African Americans have an overall cancer death rate 35 percent higher than that for whites. Death rate for lung cancer is about 27 percent higher for African Americans than for whites. The prostate cancer mortality rate for African American men is more than twice that of white men.

SOURCE: National Institute of Health. (2001). What are health disparities? **(http://healthdisparities.nih.gov/whatare.html)**

usually treatable, and often disappear in a short time. Appendicitis, pneumonia, and influenza are examples of acute illnesses.

Diseases are not the only causes of death. Accidents, homicide, and suicide are the leading killers of Americans between the ages of 15 and 24. Most (75 percent) accidental deaths among this age group involve motor vehicle accidents, many of which are alcohol related. For young adults 25 to 44 years old, accidents, cancer, heart disease, suicide, human immunodeficiency virus (HIV) infection, and homicide are the leading causes of death.

For too many Americans these conditions reflect the dangers of negative lifestyle choices. Despite this, much of Americans' health-related anxiety involves exotic diseases. The current fear that some sort of strangely mutated disease will soon pose the greatest threat to life on Earth ironically coincides with a reduction in attention to chronic diseases that do kill in large numbers. The fear of bizarre pathogens leading to runaway deaths in the United States has been fueled primarily by

newspaper headlines, fictional books, and movies. Five recent headlines serve as examples:

- "Is mad-cow disease a threat in the U.S.?"
- "Animal disease shuts Irish tourist sites"
- "Foot and mouth disease causes crisis in England"
- "'Bird flu' causes Hong Kong to slaughter every chicken"
- "Kenya disease killing humans, animals"

Although the appearance of an unstoppable, overwhelming disease is possible and the spread of new viruses in a global community is a genuine concern, the real threats to Americans are mundane and are less likely to be featured as the lead stories in the evening news. As scary as some exotic diseases sound, the chances of getting them are infinitesimally remote, especially when comparing them to the chance of getting illnesses that people can take practical steps to avoid.[17]

Healthy lifestyles that involve diet, physical activity, and personal health habits offer the most potential for

Table 1-1 Ten Leading Causes of Death in 1900 and Today for All Ages and for Ages 25–44

All Ages, 1900[*][1]			All Ages, Today[*][2]			Ages 25–44[*][2]		
Cause	Rank	%	Cause	Rank	%	Cause	Rank	%
Pneumonia and influenza	1	12	Heart disease	1	21	Accidents	1	21
			Cancer	2	23	Cancer	2	16
Tuberculosis	2	11	Stroke	3	7	Heart disease	3	13
Diarrhea and enteritis	3	8	Chronic obstructive lung disease	4	5	Suicide	4	9
Heart disease	4	8				HIV infection	5	7
Stroke	5	6	Accidents	5	4	Homicide and legal intervention	6	6
Nephritis	6	5	Pneumonia and influenza	6	4			
Accidents	7	4				Liver disease and cirrhosis	7	3
Cancer	8	4	Diabetes	7	3			
Diptheria	9	2	Suicide	8	1	Stroke	8	2.5
Meningitis	10	2	Nephritis	9	1	Diabetes	9	2
			Liver disease and cirrhosis	10	1	Pneumonia and influenza	10	1.5
All other causes		38	All other causes		20	All other causes		19
Total		100			100			100

[*]Percentage mortality: i.e., percentage of all deaths in that year
[1]Novartis Nutrition and McGraw-Hill. (2000). Obesity: a modern epidemic. *Innovations: Nutrition Updates and Applications.* McGraw-Hill.
[2]Murphy, S. L. (2000). Deaths: final data for 1998. *National Vital Statistics Reports,* 48(11):26.

preventing health problems or delaying them until much later in life. More specifically, the following ten health issues have been identified in the landmark document *Healthy People 2010*[18] as priority areas. These priority areas are referred to as **Leading Health Indicators (LHIs)**[19] and are discussed in detail in this text. The LHIs are:

1. Physical activity
   - Vigorous physical activity in adolescents
   - Moderate physical activity in adults
2. Overweight and obesity
   - Overweight and obesity in children and adolescents
   - Obesity in adults
3. Tobacco use
   - Cigarette smoking by adolescents
   - Cigarette smoking by adults
4. Substance abuse
   - Alcohol and illicit drug use by adolescents
   - Illicit drug use by adults
   - Binge drinking by adults
5. Responsible sexual behavior
   - Responsible adolescent sexual behavior
   - Condom use by adults
6. Mental health
   - Treatment for adults with recognized depression
7. Injury and violence
   - Deaths from motor vehicle crashes
   - Homicides
8. Environmental quality
   - Ozone pollution exposure
   - Exposure to environmental tobacco smoke
9. Immunization
   - Fully immunized children aged 19 to 35 months
   - Flu and pneumococcal vaccination in high-risk adults
10. Access to health care
   - Persons with health insurance
   - Source of ongoing care
   - Early prenatal care

The risk factor most strongly associated with premature death and chronic disease is cigarette smoking.[20] In studies that try to pinpoint the cause of death, tobacco use is responsible for 20 percent of deaths. Experts state that it is the single most preventable cause of death and disease in the United States. It is followed in descending order by poor diet and lack of exercise, alcohol, infectious agents, pollutants, firearms, risky sexual behavior, motor vehicles, and illicit drug use (see figure 1-3). The seriousness of tobacco use is reflected in the following quote in a testimony to the U.S. Senate:

Today, nearly 3,000 young people across our country will begin smoking regularly. Of these 3,000 young people, 1,000 will lose that gamble to the diseases caused by smoking. The net effect of this is that among children living in America today, 5 million will die an early preventable death because of a decision made as a child.[21]

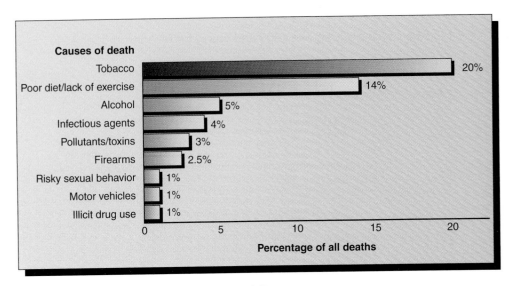

Figure 1-3 Underlying Causes of Death in the United States

For the smoker, his or her primary wellness challenge is to stop smoking; if that proves impossible, significant reduction in the frequency and duration of smoking will attenuate some of the risk factors that threaten health.

Second in importance to the smoker and first in importance to the nonsmoker as a wellness challenge are improvements in diet and an increase in physical activity. When physical inactivity is combined with poor diet, the impact on health is devastating, accounting for an estimated 300,000 deaths per year. Tobacco use is the only behavior that kills more people.[22]

The most formidable wellness challenge for Americans of all ages, however, is neither smoking cessation nor improvements in dietary habits. It is related to sedentary lifestyles. More people are at risk due to physical inactivity than to any of the other risk factors.[22] Less than 10 percent of the U.S. adult population reports regular, vigorous physical activity for twenty minutes or longer three or more days per week. Only about 25 percent of adults report physical activity on five or more days per week for thirty minutes or longer, and another 25 percent of adults do not participate in any regular physical activity.[23] Americans' propensity for sedentary lifestyles comes at a time when evidence of the benefits of an active lifestyle is compelling. Physically active people outlive those who are inactive, and physical activity enhances the quality of life for people of all ages. Physical inactivity is regarded by many respected researchers as a risk factor for heart disease comparable to cigarette smoking, high blood pressure, and high blood cholesterol.

The Surgeon General's hallmark report *Physical Activity and Health*[23] brought a historic new perspective to exercise, fitness, and physical activity by shifting the

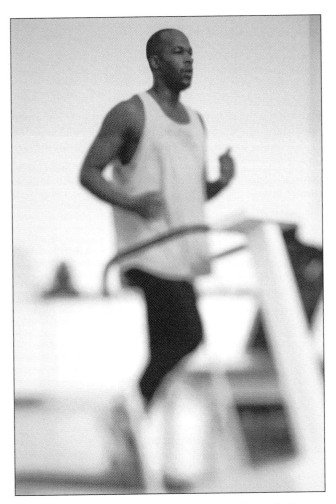

Running is a challenging activity that builds cardiorespiratory endurance.

Sedentary lifestyles are the most formidable wellness challenge for Americans of all ages. More people are at risk for premature death and/or morbidity due to physical inactivity than to any of the other risk factors. For years, medical experts have advised regular exercise to improve fitness and health, to prevent disease and disability, even to lengthen life. Unfortunately, most people starting an exercise program drop out, usually within the first six months. About one-fourth of Americans succeed in making exercise a regular part of their lives. How do they do it? What are they doing right? What are the basic principles of their success stories? Here are some tips from leading exercise experts who practice what they preach.

Wellness Across the Generations
Tips for Staying Physically Active

1. Team up. People who exercise regularly often team up with at least one other person. It might be a roommate, spouse, neighbor, or friend. It might be a workout at the fitness club with a half-dozen friends; it might be a midday break to shoot baskets; it might be an early-morning walk with a member of the family.

2. Use exercise as a pick-me-up. Tired from the demands of work, many people resist expending energy on exercise. However, many experts do the opposite by turning to exercise as a source of energy. For them, exercise is a tranquilizer; it makes them more productive at work and home, it refreshes and relaxes them, and it helps them sleep.

3. Get a jump on the day. Many people are more consistent in their exercise routines when they exercise early. Quoting one expert: "You can't plan how your day is going to end, but you can plan how it will start."

4. Break up your workout. Exercise recommendations call for thirty minutes of moderate exercise most days of the week. But it doesn't have to be in one shot. Short bursts scattered throughout the day count, too. Look for opportunities to add exercise to your daily regimen. For example, use the stairs instead of the elevator; park farther away and walk briskly to class; or when shopping, grab the first parking space (which is usually farther away); if you're waiting for someone, walk while you wait.

5. Seek variety. Engage in a variety of activities. If you work inside all day, you might exercise outside. Try seasonal activities. Catch the evening news while working out on a treadmill. Remember, if you enjoy your workout, you are more likely to continue working out.

6. Revel in your success. The more you make exercise feel like an accomplishment rather than a chore, the more you'll look forward to each session. One lifelong jogger logs his mileage because it boosts his lifetime record. A walker wears a pedometer so he can monitor his progress as he attempts to walk at least 10,000 steps each day.

SOURCE: Consumer Union. (1999). Success stories: How the experts stay active, *Consumer Reports on Health* 11(4):8–9.

emphasis from intensive aerobic exercise to a broader range of health-enhancing physical activity regardless of age (see Wellness Across the Generations: Tips for Staying Physically Active). For those who are inactive, even small increases in physical activity are associated with measurable health benefits (see Just the Facts: Physical Activity and Health—Selected Highlights). The benefit of physical activity is the underlying theme of this text and, ideally, will serve as an impetus for you to establish an active lifestyle.

Achieving Lifestyle Change: A Self-Help Approach

A fundamental assumption underlying lifestyle-change programs is that behavior is a learned response. For example, we are not born with a taste for some foods and a dislike for others. And using seat belts is not a function of heredity. Like most other behaviors, health be-

haviors are learned responses to both obvious and subtle influences. This learning begins at birth and continues throughout life. This is as true for behaviors that promote wellness as for behaviors that diminish it.

Examples of obvious influences that help shape behavior include parents and family, role models, advertising, and social norms. In many instances these influences are combined to form a single powerful influence on behavior, such as exemplified by an advertisement for cigarettes using "ideal" masculine or feminine models, depending on the brand of cigarettes and the target population. Advertisers are successful not only at marketing products but also at influencing people to think they need those products.

Subtle forces also shape behavior. A good example is *subliminal advertising,* a technique in which messages, words, and symbols are embedded or hidden in the pictures, sounds, or words used in advertisements. Theoretically these messages, though not directly observable,

Just the Facts

Physical Activity and Health—Selected Highlights

Here are selected highlights from the Surgeon General's Report:

- *Mortality:* Higher levels of physical activity are associated with lower mortality rates. Those who are moderately active on a regular basis have lower mortality rates than do those who are least active.

- *Cardiovascular disease:* Regular physical activity decreases the risk of cardiovascular disease. Regular physical activity is comparable to not smoking in decreasing risk of heart disease.

- *Cancer:* Regular physical activity is associated with a decreased risk of colon cancer.

- *Non–Insulin-Dependent Diabetes Mellitus:* Regular physical activity lowers the risk of developing non–insulin-dependent diabetes mellitus.

- *Osteoarthritis:* Weight-bearing physical activity is necessary for maintaining normal muscle strength, joint structure, and joint function.

- *Falling:* Promising evidence suggests that strength training and other forms of exercise in older adults preserve their ability to maintain independent living status and reduce the risk of falling.

- *Obesity:* Low levels of activity, resulting in fewer kilocalories used than consumed, contribute to the high prevalence of obesity in the United States. Physical activity may favorably affect body fat distribution.

- *Mental health:* Physical activity appears to relieve symptoms of depression and anxiety and improve mood. Regular physical activity may reduce the risk of developing depression, although further research is needed on this topic.

- *Health-related quality of life:* Physical activity appears to improve the health-related quality of life by enhancing psychological well-being and by improving physical functioning in people compromised by poor health.

- *Adverse effects:* Most musculoskeletal injuries related to physical activity are believed to be preventable by gradually working up to a desired level of activity and by avoiding excessive amounts of activity. Serious cardiovascular events can occur with physical exertion, but the net effect of regular physical activity is a lower risk of mortality from cardiovascular disease.

SOURCE: U.S. Department of Health and Human Services. 1996. *Physical Activity and Health: A Report of the Surgeon General.* Atlanta, Ga.: U.S. Department of Health and Human Services, Centers for Disease Control and Prevention, National Center for Chronic Disease Prevention and Health Promotion.

---

can be perceived by the subconscious mind in such a way as to influence behavior.

Much of our behavior is also motivated by psychological needs. An infant whose main source of attention and stimulation comes during feeding time may learn to associate food with the deeper psychological needs of love and affection. A parent who consistently uses food to appease an unhappy child may be inadvertently establishing a preoccupation with food that will endure far beyond childhood.

Sometimes, behavior is motivated in response to force or coercion. *Reactance motivation,* a theory of behavior that has been associated with drinking among college students, suggests that telling people to abstain completely from doing something often produces the opposite reaction. For many people it isn't difficult to recall instances in their lives in which they behaved a certain way primarily because they were told that they could not or should not behave that way. Coercion in particular leads to the arousal of reactance, which in turn tends to reduce compliance.

These examples help to explain the myriad complex forces that contribute to behavior and illustrate why successful lifestyle change is so difficult to achieve. The hope and promise of any lifestyle-change program is that, while easier said than done, bad habits can be unlearned and new habits can be learned.

A Self-Help Plan

A **self-help** approach assumes that individuals can manage their lifestyle changes and can learn to control those features in the environment that are detrimental to health. In other words, expensive, long-term, professional help is not a prerequisite for everyone trying to make a lifestyle change. The self-help approach puts you in control of your health, requires your involvement, and permits you to determine what to do and how and when to do it. However, to be successful, this approach requires considerable time and thought devoted to planning. Successful lifestyle change is almost impossible to achieve without a plan.

The self-help approach that follows is based on the **transtheoretical model of behavior change.**[24] This model of lifestyle change is presented in six stages (figure 1-4), as described next along with recommended

Stage	1. Precontemplation	2. Contemplation	3. Preparation	4. Action	5. Maintenance	6. Termination
Characteristic	Lack of awareness Denial	Awareness of the need to change Thinking about changing	Planning to change within a month Thinking about the future	Engaging in strategies Commitment to change	Greater difficulty than action stage Duration from six months to a lifetime	Problem behavior no longer an issue
Goal	Feedback on need to change Consciousness raising	More consciousness raising Emotional arousal	Public affirmation of change Development of a plan	Application of strategies Changes in environment Forming of or joining support groups Establishment of rewards Countering	Application of same strategies as in action stage	Exit from cycle of change
Stage	1. Precontemplation	2. Contemplation	3. Preparation	4. Action	5. Maintenance	6. Termination

Figure 1-4   Stages, Characteristics, and Goals of Lifestyle Change

strategies. In applying this model of change, it is helpful to remember several important assumptions:

1. Each of the six stages is well defined and entails a series of tasks that need to be completed before moving to the next stage.

2. A linear progression through the stages of change, although possible, is rare. Most people lapse at some point, and it is possible to get stuck at one stage or another. However, the important thing is to formulate a plan and act on it. Even if a relapse takes you back temporarily to an earlier stage, you are twice as likely to succeed during the next six months as a person who never tried at all.[25]

3. A key to successful change is knowing what stage you are in for the health issue or behavior at hand. Behavioral research reveals that people who try to accomplish changes they are not ready for set themselves up for failure. Similarly, too much time spent on a task already mastered—such as understanding your problem—may result in an indefinite delay in taking action.

4. Although nearly all change begins with precontemplation, only the most successful ends in termination. But you cannot skip stages. Most people who succeed follow the same road for every problem. However, you may be at different stages of change for different problems.

5. Successful behavior change does not typically happen all at once; it takes time.

Precontemplation stage

In this stage, individuals have no intention of changing in the near future. Precontemplators may be unaware of the health risks associated with their behaviors. Or they may feel a situation is hopeless; maybe they've tried to change before without success. They often use denial and defensiveness to keep from going forward. They feel safe in precontemplation because they can't fail there.

Strategies.   Consciousness raising is a key strategy. Sometimes it comes from a visit to the doctor, a health-threatening diagnosis, a headline news story, or feedback from others. One way to encourage consciousness raising is to take an inventory of personal health habits and practices. A good way to start is to make a list of your health-promoting behaviors, practices you engage in to maintain or improve your level of wellness (see

Wellness On the Web Behavior Change Activities

Your Wellness Profile

How much do you really know about your family's health history and the resulting risks to your own personal health? The knowledge of your family's health history should influence the lifestyle choices you make every day. Go to the Online Learning Center at **www.mhhe.com/anspaugh5e**, select Student Center, then Chapter 1, then Wellness on the Web, then Activity 1 and answer several questions about your own health history.

   Is there a history of heart disease or other cardiovascular problems in your family?

   Have either of your parents suffered a heart attack before the age of 60?

   Is there a history of cancer in your family?

   Is there a history of stroke in your family?

   Is there a history of diabetes in your family?

   Is there a history of high blood pressure in your family?

The Health-Behavior Gap

The discrepancy between knowing what behavior is good for your health and actually doing it is called the health-behavior gap. The key to striving for high-level wellness is motivation, since no single principle or incident can provide the stimulus necessary to institute change and maintain positive lifestyle habits.

   It is also important to recognize the links between your physical, spiritual, emotional, social, and intellectual health. What are some of the changes you can make in your own life to shrink the ever-widening health-behavior gap? Go to the Online Learning Center at **www.mhhe.com/anspaugh5e**, select Student Center, then Chapter 1, then Wellness on the Web, then Activity 2 and answer the questions found there regarding your own wellness.

   Do you think of yourself as a confident person?

   Do you have high self-esteem?

   Do you make time in your schedule for relaxation?

   Do you read for your own enjoyment?

   Do you engage in activities that keep your body and mind active?

   Do the people you surround yourself with serve as positive health role models?

   Do the people in your life support you in your quest for a healthier lifestyle?

Just the Facts

Examples of Health-Promoting Behaviors

Specific behaviors conducive to good health:

- I avoid the extremes of too much or too little exercise.
- I get an adequate amount of sleep.
- I avoid adding sugar and salt to my food.
- I include 15 to 20 g of fiber in my diet each day.
- I plan my diet to ensure consumption of an adequate amount of vitamins and minerals.
- I brush and floss my teeth after eating.
- I avoid driving under the influence of alcohol or drugs.
- I drive within the speed limit.
- I wear my seat belt whenever traveling in an automobile.
- I avoid the use of tobacco.
- I consume fewer than two alcoholic drinks per day.
- I know the instructions provided with any drug I take.
- I do my part to promote a clean and safe environment.
- I feel positive and enthusiastic about my life.
- I can express my feelings of anger.
- I can say "no" without feeling guilty.
- I engage in activities that promote a feeling of relaxation.
- I am able to develop close, intimate relationships.
- I am interested in the views of others.
- I am satisfied with my study habits.
- I am satisfied with my spiritual life.
- I am tolerant of the values and beliefs of others.

Just the Facts: Examples of Health-Promoting Behaviors). Make another list of health-inhibiting behaviors, practices that may be detrimental to your health (see Assessment Activity 1-3). If your lists are specific and identify behaviors that relate to wellness in its broadest sense (that is, the physical, social, emotional, and psychological aspects of health), comparing the two should give you insight into and information about your lifestyle.

   Detailed, comprehensive lifestyle questionnaires, such as in Assessment Activity 1-1, can provide even more information about specific health practices and behavioral tendencies that can be targeted for change. Many of these questionnaires are similar to those you might complete for your physician. Regardless of the tool you use, remember that the goal is to learn more about yourself.

Contemplation stage

Contemplators have a sense of awareness of a problem behavior and begin thinking seriously about changing it. However, it is easy to get stuck in the contemplation stage for years. Perhaps making a change requires more effort than someone is willing to expend or the rewards or pleasures of the current behavior seem to outweigh the benefits of change. Traps[25] include the search for absolute certainty (nothing in life is guaranteed); waiting for the magic moment (you need to make the moment); and wishful thinking (hoping for different results without changing your behavior).

Strategies. Contemplators need more consciousness raising. Reading, studying, and enrolling in courses are good ways to promote an awareness of the potential problems associated with certain behaviors. (One goal of this text, for example, is to increase your consciousness of habits and practices that promote wellness and of risk factors that may threaten your health.) Getting involved in activities that expose you to information about various aspects of health and wellness allows you to focus on the negatives of your current health practices and to imagine the consequences down the line if your behavior doesn't change.

Cognitive dissonance, the internal conflict that occurs when people feel that their behavior is inconsistent with their intentions or values (such as exhibited by a smoking parent who doesn't want his or her child to smoke), helps in this stage. Also, *emotional arousal,* sometimes accomplished by watching a movie or news story on the subject in question (such as about the sudden death of a child caused by drunken driving), spurs someone to action. Social strategies also help. For example, a problem drinker might attend an Alcoholics Anonymous meeting as a way of experiencing social support for behaving differently.

Preparation stage

Most people in this stage are planning to take action within a month. They think more about the future than about the past, more about the pros of a new behavior than about the cons of the old one. Many people motivate themselves by making their intended change public rather than keeping it to themselves. This stage involves developing a plan customized to a person's unique circumstances and personality.

Most people make two serious mistakes when starting a lifestyle change. First, they expect miracles and set unrealistic goals. Setting goals that are too ambitious often guarantees failure. For many people the fear of failure easily discourages future efforts at a lifestyle change.

Second, people often view lifestyle change as a temporary goal rather than as a lifetime change. Perhaps

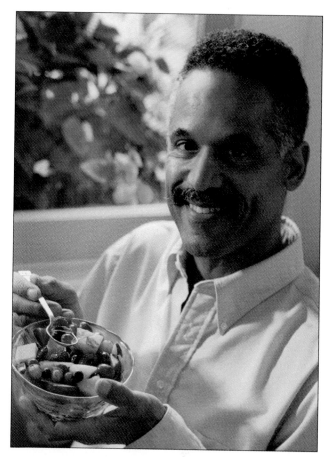

Behavior change, such as following a healthier diet, should be viewed as a lifetime goal, not a temporary fix.

more than anything else, this attitude accounts for the high *recidivism* (the tendency to revert to the original behavior) rate of many programs. One of the best examples is weight-loss programs. In weight-loss programs, for example, people typically set a goal, diet until they reach their goal, revert to their original eating habits, and invariably regain the lost weight. The proper way is to change eating habits so that they will endure for a lifetime. When people try to change some aspect of behavior, they have to deny themselves something that feels comfortable or that provides some source of enjoyment or pleasure. Denial often triggers a preoccupation that worsens the health behavior being changed. This is the reason dieters often become more interested in food during a diet (see Real-World Wellness: Are You Ready for a Lifestyle Change?).

No single strategy for lifestyle change is right for everyone. The key is to get involved in planning your personal program and to use your imagination to create the most suitable plan.

Strategies. In this stage a firm, detailed plan is developed that involves (1) assessing behavior and (2) setting specific, realistic goals.

Real-World Wellness

Are You Ready for a Lifestyle Change?

I've started an exercise program four times during the past two years. Each effort resulted in failure. I don't want to start again until I know I'm ready. How will I know that I'm ready to begin a lifestyle-change program?

If you can answer "yes" to the following questions, you are ready to begin a lifestyle-change program:

- Do you view lifestyle change as a lifetime goal rather than as a temporary, short-term goal?
- Are you willing to get personally involved in planning a lifestyle-change program?
- Are you prepared for some disappointments?
- Are you willing to experiment with different ideas?
- Do you have the patience to accept success in small increments stretched over a long period?
- Are you willing to set modest, realistic goals?
- Are you willing to establish some time benchmarks for success?
- Are you willing to make some changes in the way you live?
- Are you willing to tell others about your goals?
- Can you accept a relapse as a temporary setback rather than as a full-blown failure?
- Are you willing to formulate a plan that makes provisions for countering, avoidance, contracting, shaping up, reminders, and support?

Assess behavior. Behavior assessment, the collection of data on target behaviors, is the lifeline of any lifestyle-change plan. It involves the process of counting, recording, measuring, observing, and describing. Any behavior that can be qualified is assessed.

Assessment tools provide objective data regarding behavioral patterns, health changes, and/or results. They may be daily logs, journals, and diaries or medical diagnostic tools (e.g., blood pressure machine). Data should be collected long enough to note trends, usually for a minimum of one to two weeks. Often, people are surprised at what they learn about themselves. In a study of 235 nonexercising adults, participants were asked to record how much time they spend sitting or lying down. They were shocked when they found they were sleeping eight hours a day and spending fifteen of the remaining sixteen hours sitting down.[26]

Sometimes a behavior assessment will prompt a change in behavior without any other action. In most lifestyle-change programs a plan of action is not started until it is clear that assessment alone will not be enough to alter the behavior completely. For example, some people attach an electronic pedometer to their waistband to count the number of steps taken each day. The average sedentary person usually takes about 3000 steps a day (2000 steps equals a mile).[27] For some people the first step is the only step required. Counting serves as a sufficient intervention to behavior improvement. Several studies have shown that people who engage in self-assessment activities do better than people who don't, even if they don't write down everything. It's not so much that you write it down, but the act of recording that seems to make a difference, perhaps because it forces you to face your actions.[28]

The assessment phase also provides clues to a person's commitment to making a change in lifestyle. A thorough, detailed log is a good sign that a person has the motivation to carry out the plan.

When the assessment phase is finished, there should be sufficient information to form a behavioral profile, state specific goals, and customize an intervention program that matches goals and strategies to a person's unique circumstances and personality.

Set specific, realistic goals. Setting specific goals means setting goals that focus on concrete, observable, measurable behaviors. A behavioral goal to overcome shyness is different from a goal that requires someone to initiate a conversation with a different person each day for the next week. If goals are specific, you know precisely what you are trying to accomplish and where, when, and how often. By using specific goals, you get instant feedback on your progress. Another way to increase specificity is to establish a timetable for achieving goals. A timetable adds structure to the plan and provides a way to evaluate progress.

Realistic behavioral goals are reasonable and relate to personal circumstances. Setting realistic goals also means forming them in the context of correct information. For example, an informed dieter knows that setting a goal to lose 10 pounds in a week is not reasonable. A more achievable goal is 1 to 2 pounds.

When setting goals, starting off small is best. Setting a modest goal initially facilitates some degree of success, which increases confidence. For complex lifestyle changes, behavioral psychologists recommend breaking down an ambitious, long-range goal into a set of intermediate goals, beginning with the easier ones and then moving gradually to more difficult ones. Goals should be structured in moderation. Extreme goals promote the erroneous attitude that lifestyle change is temporary. They create a strong sense of denial, encourage preoccupation with target behaviors, and invariably lead to failure. Exceptions include cigarette smoking, alcoholism, and drug dependence, for which abstinence is still the primary treatment.

Action stage

In this stage a person overtly makes changes in behavior, experiences, or environment. This is the busiest stage of change. It's also the stage most visible to others. New behaviors, such as exercising, not smoking, or actively changing a dietary pattern, can be observed.

Strategies. People in the action stage implement their plan for change. In doing so, they apply their sense of commitment to the change. Rewards and incentives are important elements of this stage. **Countering,** or behavior substitution, in which a new behavior is substituted for the undesirable one, is the most common and one of the most powerful strategies available to people trying to make a change. When this technique is applied, the goal is to think of a behavior incompatible with the one being altered. Examples include chewing gum to suppress the urge to smoke, substituting diet colas for sweetened colas, and going for a walk instead of watching television. Some effective countering techniques are summarized in Just the Facts: Countering Strategies.

Making changes in the environment is another key element of the action stage. Avoidance, or the elimination of the circumstances associated with an undesirable behavior, is a fundamental technique of the control process. A smoker cannot smoke if there are no cigarettes, an ice cream binge is not possible if there is no ice cream parlor, and loud music cannot interfere with studying if the radio is put away.

Avoidance is not limited to objects. It may also include jobs, school, and even people. If taking eighteen hours of coursework while working twenty hours per week is compromising your academics, you may feel justified in dropping several courses or withdrawing from school if a reduction in your workload isn't possible. By the same token it may be necessary to associate less often with people who contribute to a problem behavior.

The use of reminders is also a key element of an action plan. These may be in the form of a daily planner, calendar, clocks, sticky notes, signs on a door, or a to-do list. During times when behavior change is not an issue, the list might read, "call home, library, 2:00–4:00 PM, racquetball, 4:30–5:30, dinner date, 6:00–8:30, study time, 9:00–11:00." If you are working on an action plan for lifestyle change, adding action goals is a natural extension. If, for example, you

Just the Facts

Countering Strategies

Here are some countering strategies you can use to replace problem behaviors:

- Exercising
- Cooking
- Playing a musical instrument
- Relaxing (see Chapter 9)
- Cleaning
- Doing crossword puzzles
- Walking
- Reading a book
- Calling a friend
- Going to a movie
- Keeping busy
- Learning to be more assertive
- Learning a new skill
- Joining a fitness club
- Organizing
- Playing a game
- Surfing the Internet
- Learning to use new software
- Watching a favorite television show
- Practicing thought stopping (counterthinking) by substituting positive thoughts for negative ones

are working on social skills, you might add, "initiate a conversation with a classmate" or "eat lunch with someone different." A positive benefit of reminders, in addition to their reinforcement of positive behaviors, is the satisfaction that results from checking something off a list.

Contracting is another common action strategy. Written contracts tend to be more powerful than spoken ones. They usually include a statement of long-range and intermediate health goals; target dates for completion of each goal; intervention strategies; and rewards and incentives, such as "I will deposit five dollars in my new car savings account for every day that I attend all of my classes between now and the end of the semester." These contracts are not legal documents, so simplicity and creativity are in order.

Shaping up is an another essential part of lifestyle change. It requires a person to allow him- or herself opportunities to practice desired behaviors, usually in small increments. The saying "Behavior begets behavior" is the essence of shaping up. This is also true for harmful behaviors. For example, cigarette smokers rarely enjoy their first cigarette; they learn to enjoy smoking by smoking. The same is true for most beer drinkers. Typically, shaping up occurs gradually until it becomes fully integrated into one's behavioral repertoire.

The acquisition of positive health behaviors occurs the same way. A step-by-step approach, with reinforcement following each successive movement, promotes success. In overcoming a fear of flying, a person might first visit the airport; the next step might be to tour an airplane; next the person may take a seat, fasten up, and visualize flying. Each step brings the person closer to flying, each step is reinforced, and any feelings of anxiety are countered with relaxation. People forget that problem behaviors are formed cumulatively and reflect many years of conditioning. It is only reasonable to expect that acquiring a preference for a new behavior will also require considerable time, thought, and reinforcement.

Another good strategy in an action plan is the formation of a support group, which may include a roommate, family, friends, classmates, or someone who can identify with the lifestyle goal. Dieting may be easier and more tolerable when done with a friend. Two people may accomplish their goals more effectively than either can alone. For example, two roommates may be more successful at maintaining their exercise regimen together than separately. Involving someone else in the process of change makes it easier to stick to your action plan, provides a source of encouragement, and holds you accountable for your goals.

Maintenance stage

The goal in this stage is to retain the gains made during the action and other stages and to try hard to prevent a relapse. Change never ends with action. Although people tend to view maintenance as a static stage, it is actually a continuation of the action stage and can last six months to a lifetime. Programs that promise easy change usually fail to acknowledge that maintenance is a long, ongoing process. This is why trendy, extreme programs, such as many diet programs, have a high recidivism rate. People may achieve their weight-loss goal, but they cannot maintain their strategy for losing weight for life. When this happens, a person may erroneously view the action plan as a temporary strategy. This is the opposite of maintenance and lifestyle change.

Most people experience a relapse and return to the precontemplation or contemplation stage of change,

maybe several times, before eventually succeeding in maintaining the change. People move through the change process at different paces, and relapse is a part of behavior change. Learn from any relapse instead of reacting to it by giving up. It is important to remember that the real test of a program's success is not how many people reach their goals but how many people successfully maintain that goal for at least two years.

Strategies.   Strategies used in the action plan should be continued in maintenance. Provisions for avoidance, reminders, contracting, countering, shaping up, and support groups apply during maintenance just as they do during the action stage.

Termination stage

The termination stage is the ultimate goal for people trying to make a lifestyle change. In this stage the problem behavior is no longer tempting. A person becomes confident that his or her problem behavior will never return; it becomes a nonissue. The cycle of change is exited.

Strategies.   Some experts believe that termination is impossible, that the most anyone can hope for is a lifetime of maintenance. The key strategy is to be aware of early warning signs of relapse, such as overconfidence, that can recycle the problem behavior.

Regardless of the results, maintaining the proper perspective about success and failure is important. Many people have the attitude that they either completely succeed or completely fail. This way of thinking can be devastating to a person's motivation. When goals are not fully realized, the proper attitude is to view the shortcoming as justification for making adjustments in the program. The goals may have been too general or unrealistic. The intervention strategies may have lacked relevance. Reshaping goals, setting a more realistic schedule, changing the rewards and penalties, or formulating different intervention strategies may be necessary.

Above all, you should maintain a healthy perspective about yourself and not burden yourself with guilt if you fall short of your goals. What seems important now becomes insignificant when viewed within a broader context. You may consider how significant this event is likely to be to you two years from now. Doing this helps establish the right perspective on your progress. More important than total success are the answers to the following questions: What did you learn from this experience? What did you learn about yourself? What can you do differently? Lifestyle change is a lifelong project that requires insight, skillful planning, and plenty of practice.

Summary

- Wellness is a lifelong process that requires self-awareness, introspection, reflection, inquiry, accurate information, and action. It means assuming attitudes and engaging in behaviors that promote health and well-being.
- Health is a constantly changing state of being that moves along a continuum from optimal health to premature death and is affected by an individual's attitudes and activities.
- Lifestyle diseases represent the major threat to the health and quality of life of Americans.
- Wellness requires the consistent balancing of spiritual, social, physical, emotional, intellectual, occupational, and environmental dimensions.
- An internal locus of control is the attitude that a person is in control of his or her life. An internal locus of control is consistent with the principles of wellness. An external locus of control is the belief that factors affecting health are outside one's control.
- *Self-efficacy* refers to the beliefs people have in their ability to accomplish specific tasks or behaviors. A strong sense of self-efficacy is consistent with the principles of wellness.
- The mind, body, and spirit are inseparably linked. A breakdown in any one of these can threaten health and wellness.
- Psychosomatic diseases occur when physical symptoms are caused by psychological, social, spiritual, or emotional stressors.
- *Healthy People 2010* has as one of its goals the elimination of health disparities that exist among population groups.

- Lifestyle diseases are those caused by the way people live. The major lifestyle diseases are heart disease, cancer, and stroke. Together these account for almost two-thirds of deaths among Americans.
- Chronic diseases are those that persist for an indefinite time.
- Accidents are the leading cause of death among Americans between 15 and 44 years of age.
- The risk factor most strongly associated with premature death and chronic disease in the United States is cigarette smoking.
- The risk factor most prevalent among Americans is physical inactivity.
- Physical inactivity as a risk factor for heart disease is comparable with cigarette smoking, high blood pressure, and high blood cholesterol.
- Lifestyle change is one of the most pervasive human endeavors.
- A fundamental belief in lifestyle-change programs is that health behavior is a learned response and therefore can be changed.
- Health behavior is influenced by many complex forces, including family, role models, social pressure, advertising, and psychological needs.
- The six stages of change are precontemplation, contemplation, preparation, action, maintenance, and termination.
- Action strategies include countering, avoidance, reminders, contracting, shaping up, and support groups.

Review Questions

1. How are the health problems of today different from those of fifty years ago? One hundred years ago?
2. This book suggests that wellness is a process rather than a goal. What does this mean? What are the implications of this statement?
3. What are the components of wellness? How are they similar? Dissimilar?
4. Define *psychosomatic diseases*. Cite four examples of psychosomatic conditions.
5. Cite some data that confirm the relationship between physical health problems and the spiritual, social, and emotional dimensions of wellness.
6. What are the differences between an internal locus of control and an external locus of control? Which of the two is more consistent with the principles of wellness?
7. Define the concept of self-efficacy. What is the relationship between the concepts of locus of control and self-efficacy?
8. How does the impact of environmental improvements compare with advancements in medical technology in increasing health and longevity among Americans?
9. To what does the concept *health disparities* refer? Give three examples.

10. How do the leading causes of mortality today compare with those of 100 years ago? How do the leading causes of mortality among all Americans compare with those of young adults between the ages of 25–44?
11. To what does the phrase Leading Health Indicator refer? Identify ten Leading Health Indicators.
12. What do medical experts consider the risk factor most strongly associated with premature death and chronic disease?
13. This book suggests that the most formidable wellness challenge for Americans of all ages is overcoming a sedentary lifestyle. What is the rationale for identifying physical activity as more important than diet or cigarette smoking?
14. Identify six benefits of physical activity as cited in the Surgeon General's Report *Physical Activity and Health*.
15. Identify and briefly describe the six stages of change as presented in the transtheoretical model of behavior change.
16. What are some common mistakes people make in trying to change or modify some aspect of their health behavior?
17. What is a major reason for the high recidivism rate in many lifestyle-change programs?

18. If a college student wants to use countering strategies as a way to cope with compulsive eating, what can he or she do or use?
19. Your roommate wants to improve his or her study habits. Identify for your roommate four strategies that

apply the techniques recommended in the action stage of lifestyle change.
20. Give an example of a specific and realistic lifestyle goal.
21. Identify three strategies experts recommend for staying physically active.

References

1. Wellness Program SUNY at Stony Brook. 2001. Wellness is . . . (http://naples.cc.sunysb.edu/pres/wellness.nst/pages/definition).
2. Mayo Clinic. 1999. Staying connected: close ties promote health. *Mayo Clinic Health Letter* 17(11):7.
3. New England Journal of Medicine. 2000. Exercising away depression. *HealthNews* 7(5):7.
4. New England Journal of Medicine. 1997. Can social contacts prevent colds? *HealthNews* 3(9):7.
5. Harvard Medical School. 1998. Emotions and health: can stress make you sick? *Harvard Health Letter* 23(6):1–3.
6. National Wellness Institute Inc. 1997. *Testwell: Making Wellness Work for You.* Madison, Wis.: WCB Brown and Benchmark.
7. New England Journal of Medicine. 1999. Anger and blood pressure. *HealthNews* 10(1):8.
8. Tufts University. 2001. The mind and the heart: they really are connected. *Tufts University Health & Nutrition Letter* 18(6):1, 4.
9. Consumer Union. 2000. Health perceptions predict mortality. *Consumer Reports on Health* 12(4):10.
10. Murphy, S. L. Deaths: final data for 1998. *National Vital Statistics Reports* 48(11). Hyattsville, Md.: National Center for Health Statistics.
11. Plotkin, S. L., and S. A. Plotkin. 1998. A short history of vaccination. In *Vac-

cines*, eds. S. A. Plotkin and E. A. Mortimer. Philadelphia: W.B. Saunders.
12. Knox, R. 1998. Longevity reshaping the glove. *The Commercial Appeal.* 159(132):2.
13. Associated Press. 1997. Racked with ill health, Russia shrinks. *The Commercial Appeal* 158(159):2.
14. American Alliance for Health, Physical Education, Recreation, and Dance. 1995. Cooper delivers stirring convention address. *Update* May/June: 1–4.
15. O'Donnell, M. P. 2001. Our history and philosophy. *American Journal of Health Promotion.* (www.healthpromotionjournal.com/).
16. Murphy, S. L. *op cit.*
17. Tufts University. 2001. Is mad-cow disease a threat in the U.S.? *Tufts University Health & Nutrition Letter* 18(12):1, 6.
18. U.S. Department of Health and Human Services. 2000. *Healthy People 2010* (2nd ed.). With *Understanding and Improving Health and Objectives for Improving Health.* 2 vols. Washington, D.C.: U.S. Government Printing Office.
19. U.S. Department of Health and Human Services. 2000. *Tracking Healthy People 2010.* Washington, D.C.: U.S. Government Printing Office.
20. U.S. Department of Health and Human Services. 2000. *Chronic Disease and Health Promotion: Adapted from the MMWR, Tobacco Topics

1990–1999.* Atlanta: Centers for Disease Control.
21. U.S. Department of Health and Human Services. 1998. *Targeting Tobacco Use: The Nation's Leading Cause Of Death, At A Glance—1998.* Atlanta: Centers for Disease Control.
22. U.S. Department of Health and Human Services. 2000. *Promoting Better Health for Young People Through Physical Activity and Sports.* Washington, D.C.: U.S. Government Printing Office.
23. U.S. Department of Health and Human Services. 1996. *Physical Activity and Health: A Report of the Surgeon General.* Atlanta: Centers for Disease Control and Prevention, National Center for Chronic Disease Prevention and Health Promotion.
24. Prochaska, J. 1994. *Changing for Good.* New York: William Morrow and Company.
25. Prochaska, J. 1996. "Just do it" isn't enough: Change comes in stages. *Tufts University Diet & Nutrition Letter* 14(7)4–6.
26. Consumer Union. 1999. Workouts that work. *Consumer Reports* 64(2):31–34.
27. Consumer Union. 2000. Try a movement motivator. *Consumer Report on Health* 12(10):3.
28. Environmental Nutrition. 1999. Combat holiday overeating: Nag Yourself. *Environmental Nutrition* 22(11):3.

Suggested Readings

Benson H., and M. Stark, 1997. *Timeless Healing—the Power and Biology of Belief.* New York: Fireside.
Drawing on twenty-five years as a physician and researcher, Dr. Benson reveals how affirming beliefs, particularly belief in a higher power, makes an important contribution to physical health. This book explains how anyone can, with the aid of a caring physician or

healer, use their beliefs and other self-care methods to heal over 60 percent of medical problems.
Brickey, M. P. 2000. *Defy Aging: Develop the Mental and Emotional Vitality to Live Longer, Healthier, and Happier Than You Ever Imagined.* Columbus, Ohio: New Resources Press.
Distilling thousands of scientific articles and hundreds of books in the field of health

and longevity, Dr. Brickey presents a refreshing new way of looking at life. Most books about longevity are about pills and diets and say little about the mental and emotional aspects that drive 70 percent of longevity. By attending to the mental aspects of aging, people can learn to live well while living long.
Wilcox, B. J., C. Wilcox, and M. Suzuki. 2001. *The Okinawa Program: How

the World's Longest-Lived People Achieve Everlasting Health, and How You Can Too, Crown Publishers. Many experts claim that the people of Okinawa are the world's healthiest people. Their rates of obesity; heart disease; osteoporosis; memory loss; menopause; and breast, colon, and prostate cancer rank far below the rates for these illnesses in America and other industrialized countries. Based on twenty-five years of study, the authors present a four-week plan, patterned according to the lifestyle of Okinawans to beat aging. The plan includes dietary recommendations, meditation, developing one's spirituality, doing volunteer work, and building a solid network of friends and family.

Name _____ Date _____ Section _____

Assessment Activity 1-1

Lifestyle Assessment Inventory

Directions: Wellness involves a variety of components that work together to build the total concept. Following are some questions concerning the different aspects of wellness. Using the scale, respond to each question by circling the number that best represents you at this time. At the end of each section, add up your response numbers and transfer the total to the appropriate section in the Wellness Assessment Summary. Save your results. Your instructor may ask you to complete this assessment again toward the end of the semester.

10 Yes/almost always (at least 90% of the time)
7   Very often (more than 50% but less than 90% of the time)
5   Sometimes (about 50% of the time)
3   Occasionally (less than 50% of the time but more than 10% of the time)
1   No/almost never (less than 10% of the time)

Physical Assessment

	Yes/Almost Always	Very Often	Sometimes	Occasionally	No/ Almost Never
1. I get at least thirty minutes of moderately intense physical activity most days of the week.	10	7	5	3	1
2. When participating in physical activities, I include stretching and flexibility exercises.	10	7	5	3	1
3. When driving or riding (in a vehicle), I wear a seat belt.	10	7	5	3	1
4. I engage in resistance-type exercises at least two times per week.	10	7	5	3	1
5. My physical fitness level is excellent for my age.	10	7	5	3	1
6. My body composition is appropriate for my gender (men, 10%–18% body fat; women 17%–25%).	10	7	5	3	1
7. I have appropriate medical checkups regularly and am able to talk to my doctor and ask questions that concern me.	10	7	5	3	1
8. I keep my immunizations up-to-date.	10	7	5	3	1
9. When operating a vehicle, I avoid talking on a cell phone.	10	7	5	3	1
10. I get eight hours of sleep each night.	10	7	5	3	1

Physical assessment score _____

Alcohol and Drugs Assessment

	Yes/Almost Always	Very Often	Sometimes	Occasionally	No/ Almost Never
1. I avoid smoking.	10	7	5	3	1
2. I avoid using smokeless tobacco products.	10	7	5	3	1
3. I avoid drinking alcohol or restrict my consumption to two drinks or fewer per day.	10	7	5	3	1
4. I avoid drinking alcohol to the point of intoxication.	10	7	5	3	1
5. I do not drive when drinking alcoholic beverages or taking medicines that make me sleepy.	10	7	5	3	1
6. I avoid using mood-altering substances.	10	7	5	3	1
7. I follow directions when taking medications.	10	7	5	3	1
8. I thoroughly read labels before taking a nonprescription drug.	10	7	5	3	1
9. I ask about warnings and side effects of prescription drugs before taking them.	10	7	5	3	1
10. I keep in my wallet or purse a record of drugs to which I am allergic.	10	7	5	3	1

Alcohol and drugs assessment score _____

Nutritional Assessment

	Yes/Almost Always	Very Often	Sometimes	Occasionally	No/ Almost Never
1. I eat at least three to five servings of vegetables and two to four servings of fruits each day.	10	7	5	3	1
2. My daily diet includes at least six to eleven servings from the bread, cereal, rice, and pasta food group.	10	7	5	3	1
3. I limit my daily intake of dairy products to two to three servings.	10	7	5	3	1
4. My daily intake of meats, eggs, and nuts is two to three servings.	10	7	5	3	1
5. I make a conscious effort to choose or prepare foods low in saturated fat.	10	7	5	3	1
6. When purchasing a food item, I read the labels to identify foods high in salt, hidden sugars, tropical oils, and saturated fat.	10	7	5	3	1
7. I avoid adding salt to my food without first tasting my food.	10	7	5	3	1
8. I avoid eating unless I'm hungry.	10	7	5	3	1
9. I stop eating before feeling completely full.	10	7	5	3	1
10. I avoid binge eating.	10	7	5	3	1

Nutritional assessment score _____

Social Wellness Assessment

	Yes/Almost Always	Very Often	Sometimes	Occasionally	No/ Almost Never
1. I have at least one person in whom I can confide.	10	7	5	3	1
2. I have a good relationship with my family.	10	7	5	3	1
3. I have friends at work or school from whom I gain support and with whom I talk regularly.	10	7	5	3	1
4. I am involved in school activities.	10	7	5	3	1
5. I am involved in my community.	10	7	5	3	1
6. I do something for fun and just for myself at least once a week.	10	7	5	3	1
7. I am able to develop close, intimate relationships.	10	7	5	3	1
8. I engage in activities that contribute to the environment.	10	7	5	3	1
9. I am interested in the views, opinions, activities, and accomplishments of others.	10	7	5	3	1
10. I provide social support to others.	10	7	5	3	1

Social wellness assessment score _____

Spiritual Wellness Assessment

	Yes/Almost Always	Very Often	Sometimes	Occasionally	No/ Almost Never
1. I know my values and beliefs.	10	7	5	3	1
2. I live by my convictions.	10	7	5	3	1
3. My life has meaning and direction.	10	7	5	3	1
4. I derive strength from my spiritual life daily.	10	7	5	3	1
5. I have life goals that I strive to achieve every day.	10	7	5	3	1
6. I view life as a learning experience and look forward to the future.	10	7	5	3	1
7. I have a sense of peace about my life.	10	7	5	3	1
8. I am tolerant of the values and beliefs of others.	10	7	5	3	1
9. I am satisfied with the degree to which my activities are consistent with my values.	10	7	5	3	1
10. Personal reflection is an important part of my life.	10	7	5	3	1

Spiritual wellness assessment score _____

Emotional Wellness Assessment

	Yes/Almost Always	Very Often	Sometimes	Occasionally	No/ Almost Never
1. I feel positive about myself and my life.	10	7	5	3	1
2. I am able to be the person I choose to be.	10	7	5	3	1
3. I am satisfied that I am performing to the best of my ability.	10	7	5	3	1

	Yes/Almost Always	Very Often	Sometimes	Occasionally	No/Almost Never
4. I can cope with life's ups and downs effectively and in a healthy manner.	10	7	5	3	1
5. I am nonjudgmental in my approach to others.	10	7	5	3	1
6. I feel there is an appropriate amount of excitement in my life.	10	7	5	3	1
7. When I make mistakes, I learn from them.	10	7	5	3	1
8. I can say "no" without feeling guilty.	10	7	5	3	1
9. I find it easy to laugh.	10	7	5	3	1
10. I avoid blaming others for my failures or problems.	10	7	5	3	1

Emotional wellness assessment score _____

Stress Control Assessment

	Yes/Almost Always	Very Often	Sometimes	Occasionally	No/Almost Never
1. I am easily distracted.	1	3	5	7	10
2. I tend to be nervous and impatient.	1	3	5	7	10
3. I prepare ahead of time for events or situations that cause stress.	10	7	5	3	1
4. I schedule enough time to accomplish what I need to do.	10	7	5	3	1
5. I set realistic goals for myself.	10	7	5	3	1
6. I can express my feelings of anger.	10	7	5	3	1
7. I avoid putting off important tasks to the last minute.	10	7	5	3	1
8. I participate in activities that provide relief from stress.	10	7	5	3	1
9. When working under pressure, I stay calm and patient.	10	7	5	3	1
10. I can make decisions with a minimum of stress and worry.	10	7	5	3	1

Stress control assessment score _____

Intellectual Wellness Assessment

	Yes/Almost Always	Very Often	Sometimes	Occasionally	No/Almost Never
1. I believe my education is preparing me for what I would like to accomplish in life.	10	7	5	3	1
2. I am interested in learning just for the sake of learning.	10	7	5	3	1
3. I like to be aware of current social and political issues.	10	7	5	3	1
4. I have interests other than those directly related to my vocation.	10	7	5	3	1
5. I am able to apply what I know to real-life situations.	10	7	5	3	1
6. I am interested in the viewpoint of others, even if it is very different from my own.	10	7	5	3	1
7. I seek advice when I am uncertain or uncomfortable with a recommended health or medical treatment.	10	7	5	3	1

	Yes/Almost Always	Very Often	Sometimes	Occasionally	No/Almost Never
8. I ask about the risks and benefits of a medical test before its use.	10	7	5	3	1
9. When seeking medical care, I plan ahead how to describe my problem and what questions I should ask.	10	7	5	3	1
10. I keep abreast of the latest trends and information regarding health matters.	10	7	5	3	1

Intellectual wellness assessment score _____

Occupational Wellness Assessment

	Yes/Almost Always	Very Often	Sometimes	Occasionally	No/Almost Never
1. I am aware of my skills, strengths, and weaknesses as they relate to possible occupational choices.	10	7	5	3	1
2. I have a good work ethic at school, home, and work.	10	7	5	3	1
3. I look for opportunities to learn about careers that may be of interest to me.	10	7	5	3	1
4. I am aware of the demands that future occupational choices may make on my personal life.	10	7	5	3	1
5. I am aware of the demands that future occupational choices may make on my family life.	10	7	5	3	1
6. I try hard to connect academics to the needs and demands of occupational choices.	10	7	5	3	1
7. I view occupational choices as a source of personal growth and fulfillment.	10	7	5	3	1
8. I consider money the only criterion for choosing a career.	10	7	5	3	1
9. I am aware of the need for continuing education in various careers of interest to me.	10	7	5	3	1
10. I am willing to spend extra personal time acquiring skills and knowledge required for occupational success.	10	7	5	3	1

Occupational wellness assessment score _____

Environmental Wellness Assessment

	Yes/Almost Always	Very Often	Sometimes	Occasionally	No/Almost Never
1. I try to conserve energy by turning off lights and electrical appliances when they are not being used.	10	7	5	3	1
2. I repair or report leaking faucets.	10	7	5	3	1
3. I avoid littering.	10	7	5	3	1
4. I avoid disposing of toxic chemicals or petroleum products illegally.	10	7	5	3	1
5. I look for recycled materials when purchasing products.	10	7	5	3	1

6. I store toxic chemicals in their original containers and out of the reach of small children.	10	7	5	3	1
7. I make sure that smoke detectors are in use and working properly.	10	7	5	3	1
8. I make sure that carbon monoxide detectors are in use and working properly.	10	7	5	3	1
9. I check for or inquire about radon concentrations when moving into a new house or apartment.	10	7	5	3	1
10. I wash my hands with soap for at least ten seconds after using the bathroom.	10	7	5	3	1

Wellness Assessment Summary

Transfer the total score for each section to the following spaces. Add the scores and divide by 10 to determine your average wellness score.

Physical assessment	_____
Alcohol and drugs assessment	_____
Nutritional assessment	_____
Social wellness assessment	_____
Spiritual wellness assessment	_____
Emotional wellness assessment	_____
Stress control assessment	_____
Intellectual wellness assessment	_____
Occupational wellness assessment	_____
Environmental wellness assessment	_____
Total	_____
Average wellness score (Divide total score by 10)	_____

90–100—Excellent. You are engaging in behaviors and attitudes that can significantly contribute to a healthy lifestyle and a higher quality of life. If you scored in this range, you are an example to many.

Environmental wellness assessment score _____

75–89—Good. You engage in many health-promoting attitudes and behaviors that should contribute to good health and a more satisfying quality of life. However, there are some areas that could use some upgrading to provide optimal benefits. If you are at this level, you are showing how much you care about yourself and your life.

65–74—Average. You are typical of the average American who tends to act without considering the consequences of behaviors. Now is the time to consider your lifestyle and the ramifications it is having on you now and will have in the future. Maybe there are some positive actions that you could consider taking to improve your quality of life.

45–64—Below average. Perhaps you lack current information about behaviors and attitudes that can enhance your health and quality of life. Now is the time to begin to learn about positive changes that can improve your life.

0–44—Needs improvement. It's good that you are concerned enough about your health to take this test, but indications are that your behaviors and attitudes may be having detrimental effects on your health. You can easily begin to take action now to improve your prospects for the future.

Follow-Up

Complete the following statements: In completing this wellness assessment,

1. I was surprised to learn that I _____

_____

2. I was disappointed that _____

_____

3. I have learned that the concept of wellness _____

_____

Name _____ Date _____ Section _____

Assessment Activity 1-2

Health Locus of Control

Locus of control is an important component of individual wellness. This activity will assist you in identifying your locus of control and its ability to affect your health. This rating scale is an adaptation of the Multidimensional Health Locus of Control Scales. The test is composed of three subscales:

1. The *Internal Health Locus of Control Scale (I)* measures whether you feel that you have control over your health.
2. The *Powerful Others Health Locus of Control Scale (P)* measures whether you feel that powerful individuals, such as physicians or other health professionals, control your health.
3. The *Chance Health Locus of Control Scale (C)* measures whether you feel your health is due to luck, fate, or chance.

Directions: For each answer, choose a number from 1 to 5 that best describes your feelings.

    5 = Strongly agree
    4 = Agree
    3 = Neither agree nor disagree
    2 = Disagree
    1 = Strongly disagree

Subscale 1: Internal Health Locus of Control (I)

_____ If I get sick, my behavior determines how soon I get well.
_____ I am in control of my health.
_____ When I get sick, I am to blame.
_____ If I take care of myself, I can avoid illness.
_____ If I take the right actions, I can stay healthy.
_____ Total

Subscale 2: Powerful Others Health Locus of Control (P)

_____ Having regular contact with my physician is the best way for me to avoid illness.
_____ Whenever I don't feel well, I should consult a medically trained professional.
_____ My family has a lot to do with my becoming sick or staying healthy.
_____ Health professionals control my health.
_____ When I recover from an illness, it's usually because other people, such as doctors, nurses, family, and friends, have been taking good care of me.
_____ Regarding my health, I can only do what my doctor tells me to do.
_____ Total

Subscale 3: Chance Health Locus of Control (C)

_____ No matter what I do, if I am going to get sick, I will get sick.
_____ Most things that affect my health happen to me accidentally.
_____ Luck plays a big part in determining how soon I will recover from an illness.
_____ My good health is largely a matter of good fortune.
_____ No matter what I do, I am likely to get sick.
_____ If it is meant to be, I will stay healthy.
_____ Total

To obtain your score for each subscale, add the numbers you chose.

1. A score of 23 to 30 on any subscale means you have a strong inclination toward that particular subscale. For example, a high C score indicates you hold strong beliefs that your health is a matter of chance.
2. A score of 15 to 22 means you are moderate on that particular subscale. For example, a moderate P score indicates you have moderate belief that your health is due to powerful others.
3. A score of 6 to 14 means you are low on that particular subscale. For example, a low I score means you generally do not believe that you control your health.

Name _____ Date _____ Section _____

Assessment Activity 1-3

Assessing Your Health Behavior

Before planning a lifestyle-change program, you should take an inventory of your health behaviors. This reveals important information about your lifestyle and should also help identify areas in need of improvement.

Directions: In this assessment, you are asked to make two lists. In the left column, list the things you do to maintain or improve your level of health. These are

your health-promoting behaviors. In the right column, list the things you do that may be detrimental to your health. These are your health-inhibiting behaviors. Try to be specific. Include the things that affect your mental, emotional, social, spiritual, and physical health. If you have a difficult time thinking of specific activities, you can refer to Assessment Activity 1-1.

Health-promoting behaviors	**Health-inhibiting behaviors**
1. _____	1. _____
2. _____	2. _____
3. _____	3. _____
4. _____	4. _____
5. _____	5. _____
6. _____	6. _____
7. _____	7. _____
8. _____	8. _____
9. _____	9. _____
10. _____	10. _____
11. _____	11. _____
12. _____	12. _____
13. _____	13. _____
14. _____	14. _____
15. _____	15. _____

Which health-inhibiting behavior would you be willing to change right now? _____

_____

2
Preventing Cardiovascular Disease

Online Learning Center

Log on to our Online Learning Center (OLC) for access to these additional resources:

- Chapter key term flashcards
- Learning objectives
- Additional goals for behavior change
- Concentration game
- Self-scoring chapter quizzes

- Additional lab activities

The OLC also offers weblinks for study and exploration of wellness topics. Access these links through **www.mhhe.com/anspaugh5e**, click on "Student Center," click on "Chapter 2," and then click on "Web Activities."

Goals for Behavior Change

- Choose three high-fat foods that you regularly eat and replace them with low-fat healthier foods.
- Find out your total cholesterol, LDL cholesterol, and HDL cholesterol. Select three or four lifestyle behaviors to change to improve your cholesterol profile.
- Find out your blood pressure. Select two or three behaviors to change (excluding taking medication) to lower it.
- If you use tobacco products, devise a plan for quitting the tobacco habit.
- If you are not currently active, make a list of physical activities to improve your health status and level of fitness. Determine how many calories you would attempt to expend per week.
- Plan and implement three strategies to help you deal with chronic stress.

Key Terms

aneurysm
atherosclerosis
cerebral hemorrhage
cholesterol
embolus
hypertension

ischemia
lipoprotein (a)
myocardial infarction
sedentary
thrombus

Objectives

After completing this chapter, you will be able to do the following:

- Describe the gross anatomy and function of the heart.
- Trace the development of cardiovascular disease during the twentieth century in the United States.
- Identify and differentiate among several types of cardiovascular disease.

- Identify the risk factors for coronary heart disease and discuss ways to reduce them.
- Explain the lifestyle behaviors that contribute to health and longevity.

ardiovascular disease encompasses a group of diseases that affect the heart and blood vessels. Cardiovascular disease—the leading cause of death in the United States—accounts for 41.4 percent of deaths.[1] About 25 percent of Americans (approximately 59 million people) have one or more forms of heart or blood vessel disease. Approximately 1.5 million heart attacks have occurred every year in the last few years, and about 500,000 of these end in death each year. At least 250,000 heart attack victims die within the first hour following the onset of symptoms. They fail to reach a hospital before death occurs. A significant number of these premature deaths could have been prevented with early recognition and treatment.

Of heart attack victims, 50 percent wait an average of two hours before seeking medical attention. Denying the possibility that a heart attack is occurring is the primary reason for the delay. The situation is complicated because the symptoms of a heart attack are similar to those of other physical ailments, and people are more prone to believe that it is one of the other problems than that it is a heart attack.

Although the figures are foreboding, substantial progress has occurred during the last forty-five years. The death rate for cardiovascular diseases has declined by more than 50 percent since 1950.[1] Although an impressive accomplishment, it is somewhat diminished by the fact that cardiovascular diseases remain by far the leading cause of death in the United States. Two types in particular, coronary heart disease and strokes, are the first and third leading causes of death. More than 50 percent of the premature deaths in our society are attributed to lifestyle habits.

Research has convincingly shown that following a heart-healthy lifestyle can significantly lower the risk for heart disease, and it has been a major contributor to the decline in heart disease mortality.[2] The medical profession, through the development and use of sophisticated diagnostic procedures and vastly improved after-the-fact treatments, have equally contributed to the downward trend in the death rate from cardiovascular disease.

Circulation

You can understand circulation better if you are familiar with the basic anatomy and function of the heart. The heart consists of cardiac muscle and weighs between 8 and 10 ounces. It is about the size of a fist and lies in the center of the chest. The heart is divided into two halves, or pumps, by a wall (the septum), and each half is subdivided into an upper chamber (the atrium) and a lower chamber (the ventricle). The right heart, or pulmonary pump, receives deoxygenated blood from

the tissues and pumps it to the lungs so that carbon dioxide can be exchanged for a fresh supply of oxygen. From the lungs, the oxygen-rich blood is sent to the left heart, or systemic pump, so that the oxygenated blood can be pumped to all the tissues of the body. Both pumps work simultaneously. The systemic pump carries the heavier workload of the two and thus has a more muscular ventricular wall. Figure 2-1 illustrates the circulatory system.

The arteries carry oxygenated blood away from the heart while the veins carry deoxygenated blood to the heart. There are two exceptions, one in the arterial system and one in the venous system. First, the pulmonary artery carries *deoxygenated* blood from the right heart to the lungs to exchange carbon dioxide for a fresh supply of oxygen. Second, the pulmonary vein carries *fully oxygenated* blood from the lungs to the left heart for distribution throughout the body.

The primary function of circulation is to provide a constant supply of blood and nutrients to the cells while removing their waste products. Under ordinary circumstances, the interruption of blood flow for as little as four to six minutes can result in irreversible brain damage due to oxygen deprivation.

The average heart beats seventy to eighty times per minute at rest. Endurance athletes often have resting

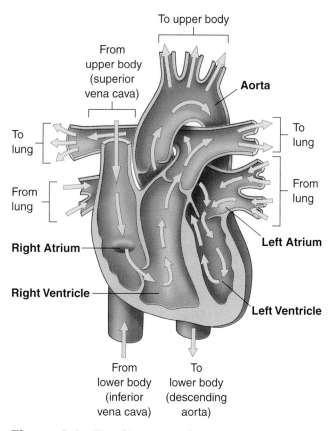

Figure 2-1   The Circulatory System

heart rates in the thirty and forty beat range, whereas some overweight and sedentary smokers have resting heart rates in the nineties. The low heart rates of endurance athletes reflect physiological adaptations to training that represent normal values for this group. The Framingham Heart Disease Study showed that a rapid resting heart rate increased the risk of death from heart attack. Mortality increased progressively with higher resting heart rates, especially among men.

The heart is self-regulating; it contains its own conduction system fully capable of establishing and maintaining the heart beat without outside neural stimulation. The heart's beating rate and rhythm are established by the sinoatrial node (SA node, or pacemaker), located in the right atrium, as shown in figure 2-2. The atria contract, forcing blood into the ventricles as the electrical impulse travels from the SA node to the atrioventricular node (AV node), located between the right atrium and right ventricle. The electrical impulse pauses for one-tenth of a second at the AV node to allow the ventricles to fill with blood and then resumes down the system and spreads throughout the ventricular walls. The ventricles contract during this time, ejecting blood from these chambers.

Blood that enters the chambers of the heart does not directly nourish the heart muscle because there are no direct circulatory routes from the heart's chambers into its muscular walls. Instead, blood must first be ejected from the heart to the aorta (the largest artery in the body) and then to the coronary arteries that supply the myocardium (heart muscle) with blood and oxygen.

The majority of blood is received by the myocardium during diastole (between beats) because the blood vessels dilate during this time, increasing their capacity to accept and deliver blood.

Coronary circulation is illustrated in figure 2-3. The left coronary artery supplies a major portion of the myocardium with blood, whereas the right coronary artery serves less of it. Both vessels divide and subdivide downstream and eventually culminate in a dense network of capillaries (the smallest blood vessels in the body). Blood supply to the myocardium is so important that every muscle fiber is supplied by at least one capillary. The coronary veins return deoxygenated blood to the right atrium so that it can enter pulmonary circulation. The veins bring deoxygenated blood from all tissues back to the right atrium.

Blood plasma is a clear, yellowish fluid that carries approximately 100 chemicals. Plasma represents 55 percent of the blood content. The remaining 45 percent consists of blood solids—the erythrocytes (red blood cells), the leukocytes (white blood cells), and the blood platelets. The red blood cells are the most abundant of the blood solids, composing about 99 percent of the total. These cells carry oxygen and carbon dioxide attached to hemoglobin, an iron-rich protein pigment and a main component of red blood cells. The white blood cells are an important part of the body's defense system against invading microorganisms and other foreign substances. The blood platelets are involved in the complex processes that lead to the formation of clots for repairing damaged blood vessels.

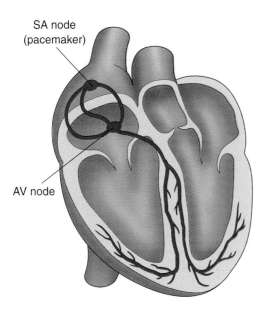

Figure 2-2 Electrical Conduction System of the Heart

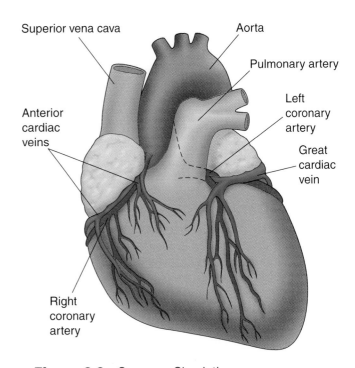

Figure 2-3 Coronary Circulation

Cardiovascular Disease: A Twentieth-Century Phenomenon

Cardiovascular disease, a relatively rare event 100 years ago, reached epidemic proportions during the middle of the twentieth century. The term *angina pectoris* (chest pain) was introduced into the medical literature by William Heberden, a British physician, in the latter part of the eighteenth century. He was unable to offer any treatment for this strange malady. It was not until 1910 that physicians made the connection between recurrent episodes of angina pectoris and heart disease. Chest pain and other manifestations of a heart attack were not identified with obstructions of the coronary arteries until the early 1900s. An American physician gave the first accurate description of the events associated with a heart attack in 1912. The illness he described, which afflicted a 55-year-old man with no previous evidence of disease, is now a common occurrence in American life. The man died three days after the onset of symptoms. A postmortem examination of the heart revealed that a clot had occluded, or blocked, one of the major coronary arteries. In 1912, this was a medical rarity.

Coronary heart disease is responsible for the majority of heart attack deaths, but other forms of heart disease contribute to disability and death. Congenital heart defects, which exist at birth, affect approximately 32,000 newborns annually. Approximately 4820 of these infants die from their defects.[1] Rheumatic heart disease, caused by a streptococcal infection of the throat or ear, is virtually 100 percent preventable. Antibiotic treatment during the infection stage arrests the processes that could lead to rheumatic heart disease. Congestive heart failure occurs when the heart muscle is so damaged that it can no longer contract with sufficient force to pump blood throughout the body. The leading causes of congestive heart failure are poorly controlled or uncontrolled long-standing hypertension or a history of previous heart attacks or both. Approximately 4.6 million Americans have congestive heart failure and about seventy-one thousand die annually of this condition.

Coronary Heart Disease

Coronary heart disease (also known as *coronary artery disease*) is a disease of the arteries that supply the heart with blood and nutrients. A diagnosis of coronary artery disease is made if any artery is narrowed by 60 percent. A heart attack, or **myocardial infarction** (death of heart muscle tissue), occurs when an obstruction or spasm disrupts or blocks blood flow to a portion of the heart muscle. The amount of heart muscle damage is determined by the location of the obstruction or spasm and the speed with which medical intervention is begun. Heart attacks of any magnitude produce irreversible in-

jury and myocardial tissue death. It usually takes five to six weeks to form a fibrous scar around dead cardiac tissue. This area of dead tissue can no longer contribute to the pumping of blood, resulting in a less efficient heart. Massive heart attacks that cause extensive muscle damage result in death.

Although most heart attacks occur after the age of 65, the dysfunctions leading to them often begin before adolescence. These processes occur most often without symptoms and often go undetected until, without warning, a heart attack occurs. The attack is sudden, but the circumstances leading to it develop over many years. There is considerable evidence that the silent phase of coronary heart disease begins as early as childhood.[3,4]

Risk factors are genetic predispositions, lifestyle behaviors, and environmental influences that increase one's susceptibility to disease. Elevated blood pressure and blood fats (cholesterol and triglycerides) that occur during adulthood can often be traced back to childhood. See Wellness Across the Generations: Childhood Origins of Heart Disease for more information about this connection.

The ongoing Framingham Study, which began in 1949, identified the risk factors connected with heart disease.[5] Cigarette smoking, high blood pressure, elevated cholesterol levels, diabetes, obesity, stress, physical inactivity, age, gender, and family history were found to be highly related to heart attack and stroke. As the risks were discovered, the realization evolved that heart disease was not the inevitable consequence of aging or bad luck but a preventable acquired disease. After a few years, researchers realized that preventive efforts should begin in childhood.

Autopsy studies of 18-year-olds who died in accidents have shown a positive relationship between blood cholesterol levels and the prevalence of fatty streaks on the walls of the coronary arteries and aorta. The evidence indicates that the average cholesterol level in children in overfed, underexercised societies such as the United States is too high.

Autopsy studies of American combat battle casualties, whose average age was 22 years, in the Korean and Vietnam wars showed obstructions in the coronary arteries. These obstructions are caused by **atherosclerosis,** a slow, progressive disease of the arteries that can originate in childhood.[4] It is characterized by the deposition of plaque beneath the lining of the artery (figure 2-4). Plaque consists of fatty substances, cholesterol, blood platelets, fibrin, calcium, and cellular debris. The atherosclerotic process is responsible for 80 percent of the coronary heart disease deaths in the United States. The lipid oxidation theory, the current theory of the development of atherosclerosis, is explained in the section dealing with cholesterol as a risk factor.

As many as one-third of heart attacks are silent; they have no obvious signs or symptoms.[5] These patients

Behavior patterns established during childhood that increase the likelihood of coronary heart disease may and often do persist into adulthood. A physically inactive child is likely to become a physically inactive adult.[6] Only 50 percent of young people in the United States (ages 12 to 21 years) regularly participate in vigorous physical activity, and one-fourth report no physical activity at all.[4] Physical inactivity is a primary contributor to the unprecedented explosion of overweight and obesity among children in the United States. The percentage of overweight youngsters today has doubled since 1980, and this trend shows no signs of abating or reversing in the near future.[7] Sixty-one percent of overweight 5- to 10-year-olds have one or more risk factors for cardiovascular disease and 27 percent have two or more.[8] One of the serious consequences of early obesity has been the emergence of Type 2 diabetes—a disease with life-threatening complications that in the recent past occurred almost exclusively to middle-aged adults—which is currently occurring among American adolescents. The two major reasons for this trend are: (1) overweight/obesity and (2) physical inactivity.[7] The American Diabetic Association and the American Academy of Pediatrics recommend that at-risk children should be screened with a blood test every two years starting at the age of 10.[9] An estimated 6 million teenagers and 100,000 youngsters under the age of 13 are regular smokers.[11] Smoking rates among high school students rose from 27.5 percent in 1991 to 34.8 percent in 1995.[12] These are major risks that begin in childhood and

Wellness Across the Generations
Childhood Origins of Heart Disease

continue into adulthood. More than 3000 children and teenagers take up the smoking habit.[4]

Leading health authorities presented a list of ten high priority public health concerns in *Healthy People 2010*. Topping the list was the need for Americans, young and old, to become more physically active. The second concern dealt with the unprecedented number of overweight and obese people in the United States.[10]

A recent study using sophisticated measuring techniques has found that children 9 to 11 years old whose cholesterol was higher than normal had blood vessels stiffer than expected for their young age. Arterial dilation was less than normal in these children while resistance to blood flow was greater than normal in response to the heart's contractions.[13]

Another recent study found that young males with elevated levels of blood cholesterol "have a much greater risk of dying from heart disease and an overall shorter life expectancy than young men with normal cholesterol levels."[14]

Attempts to prevent heart disease need to begin in childhood. Knowledgeable parents can serve as role models who practice, rather than just talk about, healthy behaviors. Active parents should be the strongest influence, but they are not the only influence. Schools need to offer quality physical education programs throughout the twelve years of precollege education, and communities should offer opportunities and provide facilities for active participation in games and recreational play.

Blood flow

Blood flow

Plaque

Figure 2-4 Progressive Narrowing of a Normal Coronary Artery (Atherosclerosis)

typically do not experience chest pain or chest discomfort nor do they have arm, neck, or jaw pain.[15] Those most likely to experience a silent heart attack are older people, diabetics, females, those who had a prior stroke or heart failure, and nonwhites. The absence of chest pain, a hallmark of heart attacks, can more than double the risk of dying probably because these people wait longer before seeking medical treatment. Three to four million Americans experience cardiac **ischemia** without knowing it. Ischemia (reduced blood flow) occurs as the result of arterial disease or arterial spasms that restrict blood flow to any part of the body, including the heart.[1] Silent ischemia can and does initiate heart attacks without prior warning. However, the typical heart attack is obvious, and the symptoms are pronounced. See Just the Facts: Heart Attack: The Warning Signs.

~ *Just the Facts* ~

Heart Attack: The Warning Signs

The Warning Signs

- Uncomfortable pressure, fullness, a squeezing sensation as if a band were being tightened around the chest, pain in the center of the chest lasting longer than 10 minutes
- Pain that spreads to the shoulders, arms, or neck
- The above warning signs accompanied by dizziness, fainting, sweating, nausea, and shortness of breath

What to Do If These Signs Appear

If you have chest discomfort lasting more than 10 minutes:

- Do not deny what may be occurring
- Call the emergency service or have a friend or family member drive you to the nearest hospital that has 24-hour emergency cardiac care
- Know in advance which hospitals have such service
- Prominently display in your home the telephone number of the emergency rescue service and also carry a copy with you

~ *Just the Facts* ~

Stroke: The Warning Signs

The American Heart Association suggests that people be familiar with the following warning signs:

- Temporary loss of speech or difficulty in speaking or understanding speech
- Unexplained dizziness, unsteadiness, or sudden falls
- Temporary dimness or loss of vision, particularly in one eye
- Sudden, temporary weakness or numbness of the face, arm, and leg on one side of the body
- Occurrence of a series of minor strokes, or transient ischemic attacks (TIAs)

Strokes caused by hemorrhages result in a 50 percent mortality rate. Victims die from the pressure imposed by blood leaking into the brain. Those who survive this type of stroke are likely to recover more of their normal functions than are those whose strokes were caused by a blood clot. The blood that spills in and on the brain during a hemorrhagic stroke produces pressure that gradually abates as the blood is absorbed by the body. Function is regained as the pressure relents.

On many occasions a stroke is preceded by warning signs and signals days, weeks, or months before a major stroke. These must be recognized and then acted on so that prompt medical and lifestyle interventions may be instituted to prevent or delay a stroke.

Preventing a stroke is similar to preventing coronary heart disease. Both involve blood pressure and cholesterol control, smoking cessation, weight management, exercise, and proper nutrition. See Just the Facts: Stroke: The Warning Signs, which identifies the major warning signs.

Stroke (Brain Attack)

The majority of strokes (cerebrovascular accidents, or brain attacks) follow the same sequence of events that results in coronary heart disease. A stroke is essentially the result of diseased blood vessels that supply the brain. It shares the same risk factors as coronary heart disease, and it takes years to develop.

Strokes are caused by a **thrombus** (a clot that forms and occludes an artery supplying the brain) or an **embolus** (a clot that forms elsewhere in the body and fragments, dislodges, and is transported to one of the cerebral blood vessels that is too small for its passage). **Cerebral hemorrhage** (the bursting of a blood vessel in the brain caused by trauma, arterial brittleness, or aneurysm) is also a cause of stroke. An **aneurysm** is a weak spot in an artery that forms a balloonlike pouch that can rupture. It may be a congenital defect or the result of uncontrolled or poorly controlled hypertension.

Between 70 and 80 percent of all strokes are due to a thrombus or an embolus. Brain cells once supplied by these blood vessels die and do not regenerate. As a result, the functional losses that occur (e.g., paralysis on one side of the body, difficulty speaking) cannot be fully recovered. That brain cells die also means that treatment will not be very effective. Many stroke victims are unable to return to a normal lifestyle unless the stroke was mild, in which case a full recovery is possible.

Risk Factors for Heart Disease

The major risk factors for heart disease are increasing age, male gender, heredity, and race.[1] While these risk factors cannot be changed, their impact on heart disease can be reduced by a heart-healthy lifestyle. Tobacco smoke, high blood cholesterol, high blood pressure, physical inactivity, obesity and overweight, and diabetes mellitus are major risk factors that can be modified by a heart-healthy lifestyle and medication if needed. Other contributing risk factors include an individual's response to stress, hormonal factors, birth control pills, and excessive alcohol consumption. See figure 2-5 for the major risk factors.

Risk factors that cannot be changed

Increasing age   Male gender   Heredity

Risk factors that can be changed

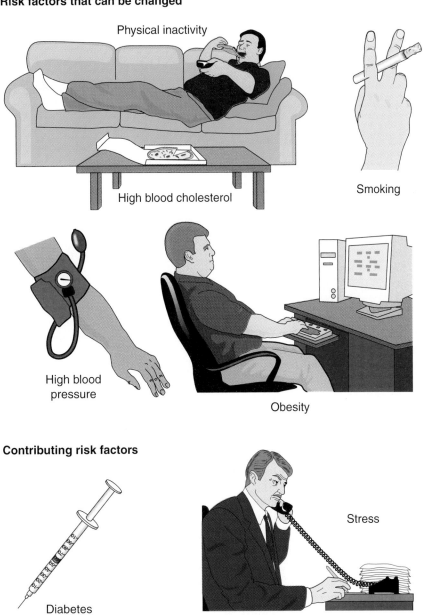

Physical inactivity

High blood cholesterol

Smoking

High blood pressure

Obesity

Contributing risk factors

Stress

Diabetes

Figure 2-5 Cardiovascular Disease Risk Factors

These risk factors account for the majority of cardiovascular disease in the United States. However, there are many other factors that can be involved, some backed by a sound and growing body of evidence. These include high serum homocysteine, lipoprotein (a), high blood fibrinogen, and high blood insulin levels. Other possible risk factors, supported by inconclusive evidence, include short stature, baldness, ear lobe creases, high serum uric acid level, and others. A few of the more important of these risk factors are covered later in this chapter.

Major Risk Factors That Cannot Be Changed

Age

Approximately 55 percent of heart attacks occur in people 65 years of age or older. This age group accounts for more than 80 percent of fatal heart attacks.[1]

Male Gender

Until recently, the incidence of coronary heart disease among women was largely unexplored. Men have been the primary subjects in coronary heart disease and risk factor studies because of the high incidence of both among men. However, coronary heart disease is also the leading cause of death and disability among women, accounting for almost 250,000 deaths annually.[1] Women have less heart disease than men, particularly before menopause. See Wellness Across the Generations: Women and Coronary Disease: Pre- and Postmenopause.

An alarming trend is the increased incidence of heart attacks in premenopausal women who have been smoking cigarettes long enough for it to affect their health, especially when combined with oral contraceptive use.

Heredity and Race

According to the American Heart Association, "A tendency toward heart disease or atherosclerosis appears to be hereditary, so children of parents with cardiovascular disease are more likely to develop it themselves."[1] A history of first-degree male relatives (father, grandfather, and brothers) who have coronary heart disease or who died of coronary heart disease before the age of 55 or first-degree female relatives (mother, grandmother, and sisters) who have coronary heart disease or who died of coronary heart disease before the age of 65 indicates a strong familial tendency.[17] If the family history is positive, the modifiable risk factors must be controlled. Some minority groups have a higher rate of heart disease than would be expected. For ex-

Wellness Across the Generations
Women and Coronary Heart Disease: Pre- and Postmenopause

Heart attacks are relatively rare among premenopausal women because of the production and presence of estrogen (the female sex hormone responsible for the development of secondary sexual characteristics and the various phases of the menstrual cycle and essential for bone formation). Estrogen is also protective in that it lowers LDL cholesterol (the harmful form), raises HDL cholesterol (the protective form), and may increase blood flow to the heart.

During and after menopause, the production of estrogen decreases and eventually stops, and the protection from heart disease diminishes. Women tend to develop coronary heart disease about ten years later than men. By age 65 the risk for men and women equalizes.[16]

To maintain a lower risk after menopause women should consider estrogen replacement therapy (ERT), because this form of therapy can cut the risk of coronary heart disease in half. ERT is particularly beneficial for women who have had a previous heart attack or for those at high risk because of cigarette smoking, high blood pressure, high cholesterol, obesity, or physical inactivity. However, ERT may not be appropriate for all postmenopausal women because it increases the risk for breast cancer.

Women should make the decision regarding ERT replacement in consultation with their physicians who are aware of their heart disease risk and who know their family histories of breast cancer.

ample, African Americans have a high incidence of hypertension. One in three African-American adults is hypertensive compared to one in four adults in the general public. They also experience higher rates of morbidity (illness) and mortality (death) from consequences of hypertension such as strokes and kidney failure.[14] Other minority groups—Mexican Americans, Native Americans, Native Hawaiians, and some Asian Americans—have high rates of heart disease primarily due to rampant obesity and one of its major consequences, diabetes.[1]

Although age, male gender, heredity, and race are major risks not under our direct control, we can modify their effects by living a wellness lifestyle. Abstaining from tobacco products; exercising regularly; controlling blood pressure, cholesterol, and body weight; managing stress; and maintaining a social support system can lessen the impact of these unchangeable risk factors.

Major Risk Factors That Can Be Changed

Cholesterol

Cholesterol is a steroid that is an essential structural component of neural tissue; it is used in the construction of cell walls and for the manufacture of hormones and bile (for the digestion and absorption of fats). A certain amount of cholesterol is required for good health, but high levels in the blood are associated with heart attacks and strokes.

The National Heart, Lung, and Blood Institute suggests that Americans reduce cholesterol consumption to less than 200 milligrams per day (200 mg/day), that fat intake may be increased to a maximum of 35 percent of the total calories consumed, and that saturated fat plus trans fats be reduced to no more than 6 percent of the total calories. (See Just the Facts: New Guidelines for Fat and Cholesterol.) Many authorities are convinced that limiting total fat and saturated fat is more important than being overly restrictive of cholesterol.

Data from 1987 to 1992 indicate that total fat consumption in the United States decreased by 6 percent, whereas saturated fat intake decreased by 11 percent. This parallels the decline in consumption of animal flesh and animal products.[18] Although this is a small step in the right direction, the dietary intake of saturated fat remains too high, at 12 percent of total calories.[19] Many authorities recommend that saturated fat consumption make up no more than 8 percent of total calories. In addition, the newest dietary fat recommendations emphasize monounsaturated fats (heart-healthy fats) to approximately 12 percent of total fat intake accompanied by an increase in omega-3 fatty acids from fish. Omega-3 fats are the most polyunsaturated of the fats, and they are also heart-healthy. These two fats lower total cholesterol and low density lipoproteins.[20]

Americans have made substantial progress in reducing cholesterol consumption. The average cholesterol consumed by men and women respectively in 1960 was 704 mg/day and 493 mg/day.[21] By 1994, cholesterol intake had dropped to 376 mg/day for men and 259 mg/day for women.

Cholesterol is consumed in the diet (exogenous, or dietary cholesterol), but it is also manufactured by the

Just the Facts

New Guidelines for Fat and Cholesterol

The National Cholesterol Education Program through the auspices of the National Heart, Lung, and Blood Institute released its new recommendations for detecting and lowering high cholesterol in adults. This revision, which occurred in May, 2001, represents the first major change since 1993. Table 2-2, later in this chapter, shows the new values and categories of risk. Some selected highlights recommended by a panel of twenty-seven experts appear here.

1. Physicians are strongly encouraged to pay more attention to the "metabolic syndrome," representative of a significant risk for heart disease. This syndrome is a combination of excessive abdominal fat, high blood pressure, high blood glucose, elevated triglycerides, and low HDL cholesterol.
2. HDL cholesterol is considered a major risk if it is below 40 mg/dL, instead of the previous 35 mg/dL.
3. Dietary intake of cholesterol should be less than 200 mg/day, instead of the previous 300 mg/day.
4. There should be more aggressive treatment of triglycerides.
5. Less than 7 percent of the calories should come from saturated fat, instead of the previous 8 percent.
6. Dietary fat may be increased to 35 percent of the total daily calories instead of the previous 30 percent provided that the majority of these come from monounsaturated and polyunsaturated sources.
7. The new recommendations strongly urge the necessity of attaining and maintaining normal body weight as well as consistent participation in physical activity.

body from saturated fats (endogenous). Cholesterol synthesis in the body would occur even if a cholesterol-free diet were consumed. The liver manufacturers about 70 percent of endogenous cholesterol with the remainder being synthesized in the intestinal and arterial walls. The total amount synthesized varies between 500 and 2000 mg/day.[22]

If you add the typical dietary intake of 259 to 376 mg/day to this total, you can see that the body must process, use, or remove considerable amounts of cholesterol to prevent it from accumulating and clogging the arteries. The liver alone produces enough cholesterol to meet the body's needs. Therefore, consuming cholesterol is not necessary to maintain health. Table 2-1 lists some common foods that contain cholesterol and saturated fat.

Table 2-1 Sources of Dietary Cholesterol and Saturated Fat

	Cholesterol (mg)*	Saturated Fat (g)**		Cholesterol (mg)*	Saturated Fat (g)**
Meats (3 oz.)			**Seafood (3 oz.)**		
Beef liver	372	2.5	Squid	153	.4
Veal	86	4.0	Oily fish	59	1.2
Pork	80	3.2	Lean fish	59	.3
Lean beef	56	2.4	Shrimp (6 large)	48	.2
Chicken (dark meat)	82	2.7	Clams (6 large)	36	.3
Chicken (white meat)	76	1.3	Lobster	46.4	.08
Egg	274	1.7	**Other items of interest**		
Dairy products (1 cup; cheese, 1 oz.)			Pork brains (3 oz.)	2,169	1.8
Ice cream	59	8.9	Beef kidney (3 oz.)	683	3.8
Whole milk	33	5.1	Beef hot dog (1)	75	9.9
Butter (1 tsp.)	31	7.1	Prime ribs of beef (3 oz.)	66.5	5.3
Yogurt (low fat)	11	1.8	Doughnut	36	4.0
Cheddar	30	6.0	Milk chocolate	0	16.3
American	27	5.6	Green or yellow vegetable or fruit	0	Trace
Camembert	20	4.3	Peanut butter (1 tbsp.)	0	1.5
Parmesan	8	2.0	Angel food cake	0	1.96
Oils (1 tbsp.)			Skim milk (1 cup)	4	.3
			Cheese pizza (3 oz.)	6	.8
Coconut	0	11.8	Buttermilk (1 cup)	9	1.3
Palm	0	6.7	Ice milk, soft (1 cup)	13	2.9
Olive	0	1.8	Turkey, white meat (3 oz.)	59	.9
Corn	0	1.7			
Safflower	0	1.2			

*There are 1000 mg in a gram.

**There are 28 g in an ounce and 454 g in a pound.

A number of population studies during the last twenty years have indicated a positive relationship between serum cholesterol (the level of cholesterol circulating in the blood) and the development of coronary heart disease. The National Heart, Lung, and Blood Institute reviewed this evidence and concluded that high circulating levels of serum cholesterol cause heart disease.

Values of serum cholesterol above 200 milligrams per deciliter (mg/dl) of blood are higher than the average risk. Table 2-2 shows the values of risk associated with total cholesterol (TC), LDL and HDL cholesterol (to be discussed shortly), and another serum lipid (blood fat), the triglycerides.

An important collaborative study involving twelve research centers throughout the United States provided clinical evidence implicating cholesterol as a culprit in coronary heart disease.[23] Half of a group of 3806 subjects was given a cholesterol-lowering drug, and the other half was given a placebo (a substance that looked like the drug but had no medicinal properties). The subjects were followed for approximately 7.4 years, at which time the data indicated that the drug group reduced their cholesterol levels by 13 percent, suffered 19 percent fewer heart attacks, and experienced 24 percent fewer fatal heart attacks. The incidence of coronary bypass surgery and angina were also significantly reduced. The researchers concluded that each 1 percent reduction in cholesterol level results in a 2 percent reduction in the risk of coronary heart disease.

A later follow-up of this study indicated that the reduction in coronary heart disease is probably closer to 3 percent for every 1 percent that cholesterol is lowered.[24] The strategies for lowering cholesterol in the blood are presented in Real-World Wellness: Strategies for Lowering Cholesterol.

The Cholesterol Carriers. The amount of cholesterol circulating in the blood accounts for only part of the total cholesterol in the body. Unlike sugar and salt, cholesterol does not dissolve in the blood, so it is

Table 2-2 Risk Profile—Lipid and Lipoprotein Concentrations

Total Cholesterol	Category of Risk
< 200 mg/dl[a]	Desirable
200–239 mg/dl	Borderline
≥ 240 mg/dl[b]	High

LDL Cholesterol	Category of Risk
< 100 mg/dl	Optimal
100–129 mg/dl	Near optimal/above optimal
130–159 mg/dl	Borderline high
160–189 mg/dl	High
≥ 190 mg/dl	Very high

HDL Cholesterol	Category of Risk
≤ 40 mg/dl[c]	Increased risk
≥ 60 mg/dl	Heart protective

Triglycerides	Category of Risk
< 150 mg/dl	Normal
150–199 mg/dl	Borderline high
200–499 mg/dl	High
≥ 500 mg/dl	Very high

[a]< is less than

[b]≥ is equal to or greater than

[c]≤ is equal to or less than

Adapted from "Revised Cholesterol Guidelines" July, 2001, *Harvard Heart Letter* 11(11):6–7.

Real-World Wellness

Strategies for Lowering Cholesterol

My doctor told me that my cholesterol level is too high. How can I lower it to reduce my risk of having a heart attack or stroke?

First, establish a realistic goal, such as about how much you think you can lower your cholesterol. Second, identify the lifestyle changes that can lower cholesterol. Third, attempt to do all of the following that apply to you:

- Reduce your fat consumption to less than 30 percent of total calories (25 percent would be better).

- Reduce your saturated fat consumption to less than 10 percent of total calories (8 percent would be better).

- Reduce your dietary cholesterol to less than 300 mg/day (less than 200 mg/day would be better).

- Lose weight if you are overweight.

- Stop smoking cigarettes and/or stop using other tobacco products.

- Increase your consumption of soluble fiber, found in fruits, vegetables, and grains.

- Do aerobic exercise at least three to four times per week for at least 30 minutes each time.

If these strategies fail to normalize your cholesterol level in six months, you may have to consider taking cholesterol-lowering drugs.

transported by protein packages, which facilitate its solubility. These transporters are the lipoproteins manufactured by the body. They include the chylomicrons, very low-density lipoprotein (VLDL), intermediate-density lipoprotein (IDL), low-density lipoprotein (LDL), and high-density lipoprotein (HDL). Dietary cholesterol enters the body from the digestive system attached to the chylomicrons. The chylomicrons shrink as they give up their cholesterol to the cells of the body. The fragments that remain are removed by the liver and used to manufacture and secrete VLDLs, triglyceride-rich lipoproteins. The triglycerides represent 99 percent of the stored fats in the body. The VLDLs are degraded as their cargo of triglycerides is either used by the cells for energy or stored in adipose cells. The VLDL remnants may be removed by the liver or converted to LDLs (figure 2-6).

LDLs are the primary transporters of cholesterol and the most capable of producing atherosclerosis. Michael S. Brown and Joseph L. Goldstein won a 1985 Nobel Prize in medicine and physiology for discovering that the liver and the cells of the body have receptor sites that bind LDLs, removing them from circulation. The liver contains 50 to 75 percent of these sites; the remainder are in other cells of the body. When LDL concentrations are excessive, the liver sites become saturated, and further removal of them from the blood is significantly impeded. As a result, plasma levels of cholesterol rise, leading to the formation and development of atherosclerotic plaque.

The development of atherosclerosis in the coronary arteries is complex. The *lipid oxidation theory* represents the latest thinking of the scientific community regarding the formation of plaque and therefore the growth and progress of atherosclerosis. This theory proposes that the initial event in the atherosclerotic process is an injury (lesion) that occurs to the inner lining of the arteries. Such injuries occur because of prolonged exposure to tobacco smoke, high blood pressure, elevated LDL cholesterol, diabetes mellitus, high amounts of serum homocysteine, and viral and bacterial infections.[3] These injuries, which occur at multiple sites, allow LDL

Figure 2-6 Cholesterol Carriers

HealthQuest Activities

• The *Heart Attack Risk* and *Cardiovascular Exploration* activities in the Cardiovascular Health Module allow you to assess your risk for cardiovascular disease. In the first of these activities, *Heart Attack Risk*, answer the questions about your health history, behavioral practices, and knowledge about heart disease. *HealthQuest* will then provide the correct answers and point out any health risks indicated by your responses. In the *Cardiovascular Exploration* section, fill out all of the items and then click on the Show Me! button to find out your overall risk. You can get more specific feedback on each risk factor by clicking on the underlined words.

cholesterol to infiltrate under the artery lining, where they become oxidized (come in contact with oxygen). Oxidized LDLs become toxic and trigger the body's immune system to destroy them. The process of destroying oxidized LDLs contributes to the formation of plaque.

Generally, two to three decades after the atherosclerotic process begins, plaque has progressed to the point that one or more arteries become so narrowed that a blood clot or spasm occurs, shutting off blood supply to a portion of the heart muscle. The result is a heart attack. See figure 2-7 for an illustration of this process.

Heart attacks are rare when LDL values in the blood are below 100 mg/dl. A national panel of experts has developed guidelines for safe and unsafe levels of LDL, and these appear in table 2-2. A high circulating level of LDL cholesterol is positively related to cardiovascular disease. Weight loss, a diet low in saturated fat and total fat, exercise, and medication (if needed) will lower LDL levels in the blood.

HDLs are involved in reverse transport; they accept cholesterol from the blood and tissues and transfer it to VLDLs and LDLs for transport to the liver, where it can be degraded, disposed of, or recycled. HDLs protect the arteries from atherosclerosis by clearing cholesterol from the blood. Cardiovascular health depends greatly on low levels of total cholesterol and LDLs and a high level of HDLs. Cigarette smoking, diabetes, elevated triglyceride levels, and anabolic steroids lower HDL, whereas physical exercise, weight loss, and moderate alcohol consumption raise it.

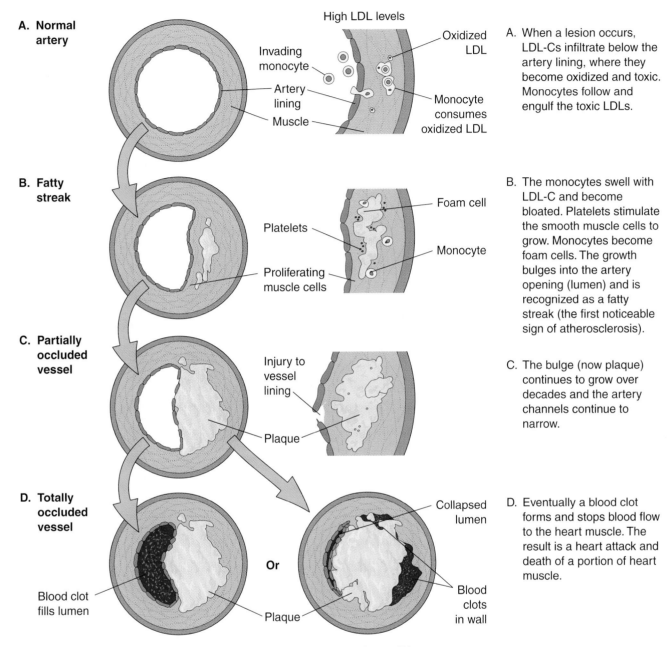

Figure 2-7 Progression of Atherosclerosis and Coronary Artery Disease

Moderate alcohol consumption (no more than two drinks per day for males and no more than one drink per day for females) increases HDL cholesterol. However, recent evidence has shown that three to four alcoholic drinks per week is sufficient to modestly raise HDL cholesterol. Caution should be exercised regarding alcohol intake because the health hazards associated with it far outweigh its few advantages. Alcohol consumption, even in moderate amounts, is not an acceptable way to raise HDL unless prescribed by a physician who is well aware of the patient's health and family history. An alcoholic drink is defined as a 5-ounce glass of wine or a 12-ounce beer or 1½ ounces of 80-proof spirits. However, alcohol is a depressant that impairs judgment and removes inhibitions so that people under its influence behave in ways they ordinarily would not while sober. Excessive alcohol intake is three drinks or more per day. Health is compromised at consumption levels above two drinks per day. The risks increase for heart disease, blood pressure, cirrhosis of the liver, breast cancer, and osteoporosis; also, the immune system weakens, red blood cell production slows down, and the brain is adversely affected. (See Chapter 10 for a more complete discussion of the effects of alcohol.)

Table 2-2 presents the current guidelines for HDL cholesterol levels in the blood. The higher the HDL, the greater the protection from cardiovascular disease. The average value for men is 45 mg/dl, and for women it is 55 mg/dl.[25] This biological difference in HDL levels between genders partly explains the lower incidence of heart disease in premenopausal women as compared with men. After menopause, HDL levels in women begin to decrease, as does their protection provided by this subfraction of cholesterol. The ratio between total cholesterol (TC) and HDL (TC/HDL) should also be considered when the risk is interpreted. This ratio is determined by dividing TC by HDL (table 2-3).[25]

Another blood fat, the serum triglycerides, is involved in the development and progression of atherosclerosis. Normal serum triglycerides range from 50 mg/dl to 150 mg/dl. Table 2-2 identifies the risk associated with various serum triglyceride levels.

High serum triglycerides usually coexist with low HDL cholesterol, a proven risk factor for cardiovascular disease. Teasing out the independent effect of serum triglyceride levels has been difficult. But recent evidence has shown that high levels are a modest independent risk factor for heart disease and a reliable predictor when coupled with low HDL cholesterol.[26] Serum triglycerides greater than 190 mg/dl increase blood viscosity (blood thickness), resulting in sluggish blood flow. Viscous blood is more difficult to circulate, so oxygen and nutrients are not delivered as efficiently to the body's tissues, and these include the heart muscle.[3]

Table 2-2 shows the relative risk posed by high serum triglycerides. Levels below 150 mg/dl are in the normal category, but evidence suggests that an optimal level is below 100 mg/dl.[27]

A number of studies have shown that sedentary people with high triglycerides can reduce serum triglycerides substantially when they participate in moderately intense aerobic exercise for 45 minutes 4 days per week.[28] Physically fit people metabolize serum triglycerides more effectively than do sedentary people and are able to clear these triglycerides from the blood more rapidly after a high-fat meal.[27]

Other strategies for lowering serum triglycerides include weight loss; reductions in dietary sugar, fat, and alcohol; and the substitution of fish for meat a couple of times during the week. Increasing fish consumption, as long as it is not fried, lowers the dietary intake of calories and saturated fat and increases the intake of omega-3 fatty acids, which tend to lower serum triglycerides.

Blood pressure

Blood pressure, recorded in millimeters of mercury (mmHg), is the force exerted against the walls of the arteries as blood travels through the circulatory system. Pressure is created when the heart contracts and

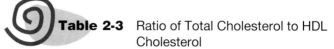

Table 2-3   Ratio of Total Cholesterol to HDL Cholesterol

Risk	Men	Women
Very low (one-half average)	<3.4	<3.3
Low risk	4.0	3.8
Average risk	5.0	4.5
Moderate risk (two times average)	9.5	7.0
High risk (three times average)	>23	>11

Keeping your blood pressure under control helps keep your heart healthy.

pumps blood into the arteries. The arterioles (smallest arteries) offer resistance to blood flow, and if the resistance is persistently high, the pressure rises and remains high. The medical term for high blood pressure is **hypertension.**

Hypertension is a silent disease that has no characteristic signs or symptoms, so blood pressure should be checked periodically. Blood pressure can be measured quickly with a sphygmomanometer. A cuff is wrapped around the upper arm and inflated with enough air to compress the artery, temporarily stopping blood flow. A stethoscope is placed on the artery below the cuff so that the sound of blood coursing through the artery can be heard when the air in the cuff is released. The first sound represents the systolic pressure (the maximum pressure of blood flow when the heart contracts), and the last sound heard is the diastolic pressure (the minimum pressure of blood flow between heart beats). A typical pressure for young adults is 120/80. Pressures of 140/90 or greater are considered to be hypertensive.[1] The lower limit of normal is 100/60. From a health perspective, having a low to normal blood pressure and maintaining it as long as possible is advantageous.

Table 2-4 Classification of Blood Pressure for Adults Age 18 Years and Older

Category	Systolic (mmHg)	Diastolic (mmHg)
Normal	<130	<85
High normal	130–139	85–89
Hypertension		
Stage 1 (mild)	140–159	90–99
Stage 2 (moderate)	160–179	100–109
Stage 3 (severe)	180–209	110–119
Stage 4 (very severe)	≥210	≥120

Standards for classifying blood pressure in adults appear in table 2-4. This table represents the latest thinking among medical researchers about the stages of blood pressure values. All hypertensive values in the table represent an increased risk for cardiovascular and kidney disease. The higher the blood pressure, the greater the risk. The lower the blood pressure (within normal range), the better. For example, a 2 mmHg decrease in systolic blood pressure is estimated to reduce the risk of mortality from stroke by 6 percent and from coronary heart disease by 4 percent.[29] Recent evidence indicates that an increase in systolic blood pressure (SBP) accompanied by a decrease in the diastolic blood pressure (DBP) doubles the risk of dying from cardiovascular disease.[17] This combination seems to be more dangerous than when both pressures increase. The DBP decreases when the large arteries stiffen.

The difference between the SBP and DBP is called the "pulse pressure" (SBD minus DBP).[30] The SBP increases because age and poor lifestyle habits cause the arteries to lose their resilience. At the same time, the DBP decreases because the stiff arteries aren't as responsive to blood flow between heartbeats. A pulse pressure of 60 mmHg or more is associated with the development and progression of atherosclerosis.

Approximately 50 million American adults and children have high blood pressure, and 35,130 people die of its complications annually.[1] The cause of high blood pressure is not known in 90 to 95 percent of the cases. This is referred to as *essential hypertension. Essential* is a medical term that means "of unknown origin or cause." Essential hypertension cannot be cured, but it can be controlled. The other 5 to 10 percent of the cases of hypertension have a specific cause. If the cause can be determined and eliminated, blood pressure will return to normal.

The heart is adversely affected by uncontrolled or undiagnosed hypertension of long duration. Pumping blood for years against high resistance in the arteries increases the workload of the heart, and it becomes enlarged in response to the strain. The heart receives inadequate rest because the resistance to blood flow is consistently high, and this produces overly stretched muscle fibers. They progressively lose the ability to rebound. The result is that they contract less forcefully. At this point the heart loses its efficiency and weakens. If intervention does not occur early, congestive heart failure is inevitable. Hypertension also damages the arteries and accelerates atherosclerosis.

Hypertension is the most important risk factor for brain attacks (strokes) as well as a major risk for heart disease. More than 500,000 brain attacks occur every year. Certain segments of the population are at higher risk, such as African Americans, who have more than a 60 percent greater risk of death and disability from stroke than do whites; this is a direct result of pervasive hypertension.[31] Stroke mortality is highest in African-American females born before 1950 and in African-American males born after 1950.

Treatment for Hypertension. Treatment for hypertension may include all or some of the following: weight loss, salt and alcohol restriction, calcium and potassium supplementation, voluntary relaxation techniques, exercise, and medication. Excess body weight increases the work of the heart because it must meet the nutrient demands of the extra tissue.

High salt intake increases the blood pressure in those who are salt sensitive. Estimates indicate that at least 30 percent of Americans are salt sensitive, but the actual number is probably higher. Salt is an acquired taste that can be modified. Curbing salt consumption while blood pressure is still normal cannot hurt and it may help.

Some calcium-deficient hypertensive people may normalize their blood pressure by taking calcium supplements. However, calcium supplementation does not work for all calcium-deficient hypertensive people, and it does not work for hypertensive people who are not calcium deficient.

Yoga, meditation, hypnotherapy, biofeedback, and other relaxation techniques can lower the pressure of hypertensive people. They can also reduce the pressure of normotensive people (those with normal blood pressure).[32] Meditating hypertensive people lowered their systolic pressure by 11 points and their diastolic pressure by 6 points more than did people in a control group counseled on the importance of losing excess weight, exercising regularly, cutting salt consumption, and drinking less alcohol.

Many people drink alcohol because it relaxes them, but ingestion of more than 2 ounces of alcohol per day raises blood pressure in some people. The same precautions regarding the use of alcohol and HDL cholesterol apply for hypertension.

Wellness On the Web Behavior Change Activities

What's Your Risk for Heart Disease?
In the battle to maintain a healthy heart, you have a powerful ally. The American Heart Association (AHA) is dedicated to educating and informing you on how to fight heart disease and stroke. Go to the OLC at www.mhhe.com/anspaugh5e, select Chapter 2, and complete the AHA's interactive risk assessment titled "What's Your Risk?" This assessment will show you what factors place you at greater risk for heart disease and allow you to take charge of your health by making more healthful lifestyle choices. Complete the 16 items and then click on the Submit button for your results. Which of your risk factors cannot be changed? Which can you change?

What Questions Should I Ask My Physician?
Often we tend to think of doctors as all-knowing gurus who can tell us everything we need to live a healthy life. The fact is, your relationship with your physician is a partnership—and for best results, you need to know what to ask when you visit your doctor. The American Heart Association reminds you that, after making healthful lifestyle changes, your second-best friend in the fight against heart disease and stroke is your doctor. For help in formulating questions for this vital partner in your health care, go to the OLC at www.mhhe.com/anspaugh5e, select Chapter 2, and read the AHA's 10 questions you should ask your doctor at your next checkup in the section titled "Ask Your Doctor." Help your physician help you live a healthier life!

The American College of Sports Medicine (ACSM) has developed a position paper on the relationship between exercise and hypertension.[33] Some of the more important conclusions follow:

1. Endurance exercises can reduce both systolic and diastolic pressures by 10 points each in people with mild essential hypertension (with systolic pressures between 140 and 180 mmHg and diastolic pressures between 90 and 105 mmHg).
2. Moderately intense endurance exercises lower the blood pressure as much as or more than vigorous exercise.
3. Endurance exercise training delays or prevents the onset of hypertension in people at high risk.
4. By itself, resistive or strength training does not seem to lower the blood pressure unless it is accompanied by aerobic training and is done in a circuit (circuit training is explained in Chapter 4).

5. Physically fit hypertensive people have a lower mortality rate than do physically unfit normotensive people.

The mechanisms through which exercise lowers blood pressure in hypertensive individuals are not fully understood. The probable mechanisms include the following:

1. Exercise contributes to weight loss, which in turn lowers blood pressure.
2. Aerobic training reduces resistance to blood flow in the arteries and at rest, lowering the force required to circulate blood.
3. Many hypertensive people have elevated levels of hormones that constrict blood vessels. Exercise metabolizes these, which results in less resistance to blood flow.
4. Exercise training sensitizes the cells to insulin, so less circulates in the blood. The kidneys respond by excreting sodium, which reduces the blood pressure.

Medications that control blood pressure have been developed. However, they have side effects that include weakness, leg cramps, stuffy nose, occasional diarrhea, heartburn, drowsiness, anemia, depression, headaches, joint pain, dizziness, impotence, and skin rash. The side effects are unique to the drugs being used to control blood pressure. Despite these side effects, many people find it easier to take the medicine than to make the difficult lifestyle changes that lower blood pressure. However, the effort to control blood pressure with medication should not negate the importance of controlling lifestyle factors that contribute to hypertension. Medicine and lifestyle efforts are not mutually exclusive—each contributes to blood pressure management.

Cigarette smoking/tobacco use

Many medical authorities consider cigarette smoking the most harmful of the preventable risk factors associated with chronic illness and premature death.[34] Cigarette smoking is responsible for one of every five deaths annually in the United States.[35] It contributes to approximately 420,000 premature, preventable deaths from cardiovascular and pulmonary diseases. About 90 percent of lung cancer, 80 percent of emphysema, 75 percent of bronchitis, and 30 percent of coronary heart disease is attributable to smoking. In 1987, lung cancer became the leading cause of cancer death among women, replacing breast cancer. In 1997, 66,000 women died of lung cancer compared to 44,000 who died of breast cancer.

Harmful Products in Cigarettes.   Nicotine; carbon monoxide; and other poisonous gases, tars, and chemical additives for taste and flavor are the hazardous products in cigarettes. Carbon monoxide and nicotine have a devastating effect on the heart and blood vessels. Nicotine is an addictive stimulant that increases the resting heart rate, blood pressure, and metabolism. For this reason, it should be reclassified as a drug and placed under the jurisdiction of the Food and Drug Administration (FDA).

A brief summary of nicotine's effects on the cardiovascular system is found in Just the Facts: Nicotine. Carbon monoxide, a poisonous gas that is a by-product of the combustion of tobacco products, displaces oxygen in the blood because it has a greater attraction to hemoglobin. The diminished oxygen-carrying capacity of the blood is partly responsible for the shortness of breath that smokers experience with mild physical exertion.

Cigarettes and other tobacco products are not regulated by the FDA because tobacco is not classified as a food or drug. The tobacco industry is under no mandate to disclose the nature and type of chemicals added to tobacco products. Some of these additives are harmful. The public has a right to know, but the tobacco industry has successfully resisted attempts by government agencies and consumer groups to force disclosure.

The harmful effects of cigarette smoking are insidious and take time to appear. The medical profession measures the damage from smoking in pack years. Smoking one pack of cigarettes per day for fifteen years is equal to 15 pack years (15 years × 1 pack per day = 15 pack years). Two packs per day for fifteen years is equal to 30 pack years (15 × 2 = 30). Medical problems become evident after 25 to 30 pack years.

The Challenge of Quitting. To quit the tobacco habit, you have to simultaneously break the addiction to nicotine and the psychological dependence on smoking. This involves changing behavior and effectively dealing with the social and situational stimuli that promote the desire to smoke. One-third of current cigarette smokers attempt to stop smoking every year but less than 10 percent of them succeed.[36] Most quitters made four to ten unsuccessful attempts and tried several stop smoking methods before finally succeeding. Quitting the smoking habit is a formidable challenge. However, 50 percent of active smokers have managed to stop smoking in the last fifty years. While exceedingly difficult, it can be done if one finds the right motivation. Since 1964, more men than women have quit, more whites than African Americans, and more non-Hispanics than Hispanics. More elderly people and more educated people also have higher quit rates.[37]

Complicating the effort to quit, particularly among young women, is the fear of gaining weight. Approximately 65 percent of those who quit do gain weight, but the physiological adaptations that occur may only

Just the Facts

Nicotine

Nicotine is a powerful stimulant that:

- Increases LDL and lowers HDL levels
- Causes the platelets to aggregate, increasing the probability of arterial spasms
- Increases the oxygen requirement of cardiac muscle
- Constricts blood vessels
- Produces cardiac dysrhythmias (irregular heart beat)
- Is a causative agent in the 30% of coronary heart disease deaths related to smoking
- Increases the viscosity of the blood

account for a 7- to 8-pound weight gain. The physiological mechanisms responsible are probably associated with a slowing of metabolism, a slight increase in appetite, and slower transit time of food in the digestive system so that more is absorbed by the body. Weight gain beyond 8 pounds is probably caused by altered eating patterns rather than physiology. Food smells and tastes better when a person is not smoking. Food may substitute for a cigarette, especially during social activities. It may provide some of the oral gratification previously obtained from smoking, and it may relieve tension. Weight gain can be avoided by eating sensibly and exercising moderately and frequently.

As a group, smokers are approximately 7 percent thinner than nonsmokers, but smokers tend to distribute more fat in the abdominal area.[38] The waist-to-hip ratio (WHR) is greater in smokers even though they are thinner. This fat distribution predisposes smokers to coronary heart disease, diabetes, stroke, and some forms of cancer.

Passive Smoking and Smokeless Tobacco. Involuntary or passive smoking (inhaling the smoke of others) is associated with premature disease and death. Estimates indicate that 38,000 to 43,000 nonsmokers who are regularly exposed to environmental smoke die annually from smoking-related causes.[39] The majority of these (35,000 to 40,000) die from heart disease, and 3000 die from lung cancer. There is a dose-response effect. The more the nonsmoker is exposed to environmental smoke, the greater his or her risk for premature morbidity (illness) and mortality (death).

Children of smoking parents are more likely to experience a higher incidence of influenza, colds, bronchitis, asthma, and pneumonia. The impact of passive smoking on them can last a lifetime and may range from delayed physical and intellectual development to the hazards associated with prolonged exposure to carcinogenic substances.

An alarming trend is the escalating sale of smokeless tobacco products. Chewing tobacco and dipping snuff have become popular among high school and college men. The World Health Organization (WHO) has described the growing use of smokeless tobacco as a new threat to society. Nicotine is an addictive drug regardless of the method of delivery, and its effects are similar whether it is inhaled, as in smoking, or absorbed through the tissues of the oral cavity, as in dipping and chewing. The incidence of oral cancer may be 50 times higher among long-term users of smokeless tobacco products than among nonusers. Smokeless tobacco is addictive and deadly, and its use is rising among adolescent males.

Cigar sales in the country had been flat for twenty-five years until 1994, when sales began to increase as the result of a marketing campaign by the magazine *Cigar Aficionado*, cigar invitation-only dinners, and celebrity endorsements of cigar smoking, characterizing it as sophisticated and glamorous. Cigar smoking is no longer looked upon as the sole dominion of males; many women have taken up the habit. Cigar sales increased from 3.4 billion in 1993 to 5.1 billion in 1997.[40]

Cigars were not specifically included in the 1984 law that required tobacco companies to place labels on packages of cigarettes warning that they were hazardous to health. As a result, cigars carry no such warning label. This does not mean that cigar smoking is not harmful to health. See Just the Facts: Cigar Smoking: A Hazard to Health for the facts on cigar smoking.

Physical inactivity

Physical inactivity has been officially recognized as a major risk factor for cardiovascular disease by the American Heart Association.[1] The upgrading of physical inactivity, which appeared in the AHA's 1993 report, reflects the importance of participating in physical activities regularly. The AHA made the upgrade because the weight of the evidence that has been accumulating in the last few decades shows that exercise produces many important health benefits. This is good news for those who have been physically active, and it may motivate some sedentary people to become active.

Physical inactivity (hypokinesis) is debilitating to the human body. A couple of weeks of bed rest or chair rest produce muscle atrophy, bone demineralization, and decreases in aerobic capacity and maximum breathing capacity. Your body was constructed for and thrives on physical exertion.

Just the Facts

Cigar Smoking: A Hazard to Health

A common assumption is that cigar smoking is not as hazardous as cigarette smoking, because people usually don't inhale cigar smoke. The facts regarding the dangers of cigar smoking are:

- Cigars contain nicotine, carbon monoxide, tars, and poisonous gases.
- Nicotine reaches the brain by being absorbed through the lining of the mouth rather than from the lungs, but the effect is the same. See Just the Facts: Nicotine for a summary of nicotine's harmful effects on the heart and blood vessels.
- Most of the same cancer-producing substances found in cigarettes are also present in cigars.
- Overall cancer deaths are 34 percent higher for men who smoke cigars than for men who do not.
- Cigar smokers have 4 to 10 times more risk of dying from mouth and throat cancers than do nonsmokers.

Two major reviews have shown that physical inactivity poses a significant risk for developing heart disease. In one review, the researchers critiqued forty-three studies and concluded that physical inactivity increased the risk for coronary heart disease by 1.5 to 2.4 times.[41] The risk associated with physical inactivity is similar to that of the other major risk factors. According to the Centers for Disease Control and Prevention, the need for regular exercise by the general public should be promoted as vigorously as efforts to control blood pressure, lower cholesterol, and stop smoking. A later review by another team of researchers concluded that inactive people have a 90 percent greater risk for developing coronary heart disease than do active people.[42]

With few exceptions, the results of later studies are consistent with the results of these two reviews. Some of the more recent studies have indicated a dose-response relationship between level of physical activity and cardiovascular disease.[43] This means that (1) men at high risk who regularly participate in light- to moderate-intensity physical activity expending about 1500 calories per week will likely lower their risk for coronary heart disease by about 25 percent to 50 percent, and (2) men who engage regularly in more intense physical activity (above the moderate level) lower their risk for coronary heart disease by 60 to 70 percent and experience greater longevity.

Several studies examined the effect on coronary heart disease of level of physical fitness rather than of total numbers of calories expended per week in physical activity. These studies corroborated the results of the calorie expenditure studies that physically fit people are less inclined to develop coronary heart disease than are unfit people.[44]

In summary, people actively engaged in leisure-time or occupational physical activity as well as those who participate in physical activities for the purpose of developing fitness are at a lower risk of death from cardiovascular disease and all-cause mortality. Other major studies have supported the view that people who regularly engage in physical activities of moderate intensity have significantly fewer heart attacks and experience fewer deaths from all causes than do people who exercise little or not at all. Moderate activity was described as the equivalent of walking 1 to 2 miles per day for a total of 5 to 10 miles per week at a speed of 3 to 4 MPH. The greatest health benefits were gained by those who expended 1500 to 2000 calories per week (15 to 20 miles of walking) in physical activity. A total of 17,000 men were followed for more than thirty years. Those who regularly walked, climbed stairs, or participated in sports activities decreased their risk from all causes of mortality. Those who expended a minimum of 500 calories per week (5 miles of walking or its equivalent) to a maximum of 3500 calories per week (35 miles of walking or its equivalent) experienced a progressive increase in longevity.

Investigators at the Cooper Institute for Aerobics Research[45] studied the relationship between physical fitness and mortality from all causes. The uniqueness of this study was twofold: first, the researchers measured the physical fitness levels of all subjects by treadmill testing, and second, more than 3000 of the 13,344 subjects were women. Because of their lower risk for cardiovascular disease, women have essentially been neglected as subjects in heart disease studies.

The results of this study indicated that a low physical fitness level increased the risk for both men and women of death from cardiovascular disease, cancer, and all other forms of disease. The difference in all-cause mortality was greatest between those in the moderately fit category and those in the low-fit category. The difference between the moderately fit and the highly fit was insignificant. For people who exercise regularly, the risk of dying from a heart attack is 35 to 55 percent less than it is for sedentary people.[46]

A study using only women as subjects investigated the physical fitness benefits versus the health benefits of three levels of walking intensity.[47] One group walked at 5 MPH, a second group walked at 4 MPH, and a third group walked at 3 MPH. The results showed that physical fitness improved on a predictable dose-response basis. The fastest walkers improved the most and the slowest walkers improved the least, but the cardiovascular risk was reduced equally among the three groups. Low-level exercise was as effective as the highest level in promoting cardiovascular health. Exercise for health does not have to be as strenuous as exercise for physical fitness.

The American College of Sports Medicine and the Centers for Disease Control and Prevention reacted to the results of these studies by jointly issuing a recommendation for exercise for Americans. The new guideline states that "every U.S. adult should accumulate 30 minutes or more of moderate intensity physical activity on most, preferably all, days of the week."[48] This is a minimum guideline for exercise and was not intended to replace previous recommendations regarding more vigorous exercise for the purpose of improving physical fitness. Instead, the recommendation is directed at that 60 percent of our population who are sedentary or marginally active. Health professionals hope that the recommendation will motivate physically inactive and underactive Americans to participate in a more active lifestyle.

The term *physical activity* refers to any physical movement that results in energy expenditure. Physical activity includes but is not limited to walking, climbing stairs, mowing the lawn (using a riding mower does not count), raking leaves without a blower, mopping and vacuuming floors, washing and waxing the car (by hand), dancing, and playing with children and grandchildren. Moderate intensity physical activity can be achieved by walking 3 to 4 miles per hour or through any other activity that burns as many calories as walking at those speeds.

People who consistently exercise above the moderate level not only receive the health benefits but also develop a higher level of physical fitness. Those who exercise in accordance with the guidelines gain about the same health benefits as those who are more physically active, but they will not attain the same degree of physical fitness. That 60 percent of the population inclined to ignore the advice to exercise regularly can become part of the estimated 250,000 premature deaths per year attributed to a **sedentary** lifestyle.[4]

The health and longevity returns from exercise and a physically active lifestyle are significant. Estimates indicate that longevity is increased by 1 minute for every minute spent walking and by 2 minutes for every minute spent jogging.[49] The potential for improving the health status of Americans through appropriate lifestyle behaviors is evident from estimates indicating that 60 percent of deaths are premature and approximately 50 to 60 percent of all illness and disabilities are preventable.[50]

Obesity

Obesity strains the heart and coexists with many of the modifiable risk factors that promote cardiovascular disease. Obese people who have no other risk factors are still more likely to develop heart disease or stroke. Obesity contributes to approximately 300,000 deaths annually in the United States.[34] Not only is obesity associated with an increased risk for heart disease, but the manner in which fat is distributed in the body might also accentuate the risk.[34] Fat that accumulates in the upper half of the body (referred to as *visceral* or *central abdominal obesity*) is likely to be accompanied by high triglycerides, low HDL cholesterol, insulin resistance, and hypertension. This cluster of factors is called *syndrome X,* and it is associated with a significant increase in the likelihood of developing cardiovascular disease.

Obese people can lower their risk with a modest weight loss of 5 to 10 percent. This is a realistic, attainable goal. But the risk remains lower only if the loss of weight is maintained. Approximately 95 percent of people who lose weight regain it in a few years. Although calorie restriction is the primary method for losing weight, regular exercise is the most effective method for maintaining the loss. Diet and exercise are not mutually exclusive; instead, they compliment each other, and both are important players in weight management.

Diabetes mellitus

Diabetes mellitus is a metabolic disorder in which the body cannot make use of sugar (glucose) as a fuel. The hormone insulin must be produced and secreted into the bloodstream so that blood sugar can be transported into the cells. The cells have receptor sites to which insulin attaches, making the cell amenable to the entrance of sugar.

In type 1 diabetes, no insulin is produced, and so it must be injected daily. Type 1, insulin-dependent diabetes mellitus (IDDM), usually occurs early in life. Type 2, or non–insulin-dependent diabetes mellitus (NIDDM), occurs in middle-aged, overweight, sedentary adults. Excessive weight is a factor because it increases cellular resistance to insulin so that more insulin than normal is required to effect the passage of sugar from the blood to the cells. In contrast, exercise decreases insulin resistance, making cellular membranes more permeable to sugar. About 90 percent of diabetes mellitus is of the type 2 variety. Data indicate that at least 75 percent of new cases of type 2 diabetes can be prevented through regular exercise and maintaining normal weight.[51]

Diabetes mellitus has numerous long-range complications. These primarily involve degenerative disorders of the blood vessels and nerves. Diabetics who die prematurely are usually the victims of cardiovascular lesions and accelerated atherosclerosis. The incidence of heart attacks and strokes is higher among diabetics than nondiabetics. Diabetes increases the risk of coronary artery disease by 2 to 3 times the normal rate in men and 3 to 7 times the normal rate in women.[34]

The arteries supplying the kidneys, eyes, and legs are particularly susceptible to atherosclerosis. Kidney failure is one of the long-term complications of diabetes. Diabetes is also the leading cause of blindness in U.S. adults. Impaired delivery of blood to the legs may lead to gangrene, necessitating amputation of the affected tissues. In addition to circulatory problems, degenerative lesions in the nervous system may result, leading to multiple diseases that result in dysfunction of the brain, spinal cord, and peripheral nerves.[52] Unfortunately, medical science has been unable to identify the biological mechanisms responsible for these long-term vascular and neural complications. However, these complications can be mitigated by leading a balanced, well-regulated life, thereby keeping diabetes under control. Control includes dietary manipulation, exercise, weight control, rest, and medication if needed.

The landmark Physician's Health Study was the first major effort to show that exercise reduced the risk of developing type 2 diabetes. The physicians participating in the study who exercised vigorously five or more times per week had a 42 percent greater reduction in the incidence of type 2 diabetes than did those who exercised less than one time per week. The reduction in risk was particularly pronounced among those at greatest risk: the obese. The researchers concluded that at least 24 percent of cases of type 2 diabetes were related to sedentary living. Even high-risk men (those who were overweight and had a parental history of diabetes) benefited from regular exercise. Every 500 calories burned per week in leisure-time physical activity reduced the risk of type 2 diabetes by 6 percent.[53]

Data collected from more than 70,000 women subjects ages 40 to 65 years indicated that those who participated in moderate exercise on a regular basis lowered their risk of developing type 2 diabetes compared to women who did not exercise regularly.[54] Accumulating evidence shows that the effect of exercise on type 2 diabetes prevention applies to both men and women.

Stress

Stress is difficult to define and quantify. Authorities agree that distress, or chronic stress, produces a complex array of physiological changes in the body. Together, these physiological events are called the *fight or flight response.* The hormones released by the body during these events produce the stress response. This includes (1) increases in heart rate, breathing rate, blood pressure; (2) the tendency for blood platelets to

Nurturing Your Spirituality

Can Stress and Depression Make You Sick?

A convincing body of evidence suggests that chronic anger, anxiety, loneliness, or depression can be catastrophic for people with coronary artery disease.[55] At the same time, emerging evidence shows that these same mood states and feelings in healthy people may increase the likelihood of developing heart disease in the future.

Scientists are beginning to unravel the connection between mood states and heart disease. Consistently high levels of stress hormones circulating in the bloodstream suppress the immune system by interfering with the normal repair and maintenance functions of the body. This increases one's vulnerability to infections and disease. Continuing high levels of cortisol and norepinephrine stimulate a prolonged fight or flight response that can eventually lead to wear and tear on the heart and arteries. Frequent and prolonged periods of stress increase blood pressure, and that usually leads to injuries of the artery walls. These injuries are the first step in the development and ultimate progression of atherosclerosis.[56] Data indicate that exaggerated responses to stress may be a triggering mechanism for heart attack and stroke.

Depression (prolonged sadness beyond a reasonable length of time) also stimulates the production of stress hormones. Depression that occurs later in life increases the risk of coronary heart disease in two ways: (1) by reducing blood flow to the heart in those whose blood vessels are narrowed and (2) by causing heart rhythm disturbances.[57]

Scientists have much to learn about the relationship between the heart and mind. Physicians are beginning to acknowledge that depression is a significant factor in producing cardiovascular complications for those who already have heart disease. The good news is that depression is treatable. Mild depression responds to regular exercise and voluntary relaxation techniques, both of which reduce the production of stress hormones. On the other hand, severe depression requires psychological counseling and medication plus regular exercise and relaxation training. Eighty percent of people with severe depression respond to treatment.

Regular exercise promotes relaxation, reduces the response to stress, enhances emotional well-being, and lowers cardiac reactivity (high heart rate, blood pressure, and resistance to blood flow). Cardiac reactivity occurs when modest stressors produce physiological responses by the heart and circulatory system that are out of proportion to the stressor. If these occur frequently, the development of atherosclerosis may well be the result.

Exercise acts as a safety valve that enables people to "let off steam" in a constructive way. Jogging, swimming, cycling, weight training, racquetball, and other physical activities focus our energies in worthwhile pursuits that rid the body of stress products that have accumulated. Exercise training, a physiological stressor, helps build tolerance to psychological and emotional stressors. In other words, the "physiological toughness" developed through exercise training enables us to cope more effectively with other types of stressors.[58]

Do stress and depression cause heart attacks? The answer is a qualified "yes." We should have a more definitive answer after a few more years of research.

aggregate (clump together); (3) blood sugar rushing to the muscles to provide more energy; and (4) the activation of the immune system. The stress response represents a significant strain on the body.

Stressors (events or situations that cause stress) may be acute or chronic. Acute stressors are situational and temporary. Taking a midterm exam or making an oral presentation are examples of events that provoke acute stress. When such an event is over, the body returns, within a short time, to its prior state of balance and harmony. However, chronic stress (characterized by prolonged elevations of stress hormones and a general feeling of uneasiness that permeates one's life) presents a much more serious problem. Constant worry about work, finances, or relationships or persistent feelings of anger and isolation are examples of chronic stress. Is chronic stress a causative agent in the development of chronic diseases in general and heart disease specifically? See Nurturing Your Spirituality: Can Stress and Depression Make You Sick?

Preventing and Reversing Heart Disease

Preventing heart disease is much preferred to treating it after the fact. Prevention includes regular exercise, maintenance of optimal body weight, sound nutritional practices, abstinence from tobacco products, nonuse of alcohol (or use in moderation), and abstinence from drugs. Dealing with stress in constructive ways, removing oneself as much as possible from destructive and disease-producing environmental conditions, and having periodic medical examinations are other aspects of prevention. It is much better physically, psychologically, and economically to make the effort to enhance health now than to reject or ignore health promotion principles and treat disease later. It is never too late to change behavior. Even patients with coronary artery disease can benefit from lifestyle changes.

Until recently, medical thinking indicated that established atherosclerotic plaques in the coronary arteries

Stress-relieving activities, such as meditation, soothe the spirit and may even lower your risk of heart disease and other chronic illnesses. How do you manage stress?

were there to stay. Progression of the disease seemed inevitable unless medical corrective procedures were employed. But evidence has surfaced indicating that reversal of the disease is possible with appropriate lifestyle behaviors.

Dean Ornish showed that comprehensive behavior changes are required to reverse established coronary artery disease. Ornish devised a program that included a vegetarian diet in which only 6.8 percent of the calories came from fat; 4.4 hours of moderate aerobic exercise per week; stress-management techniques consisting of stretching exercises, practicing of breathing techniques, meditation, progressive relaxation, and the use of imagery; smoking cessation; and attendance at regular group support meetings. The subjects in this study were evaluated against a control group who received "usual and customary" care.[59]

At the end of the first year, 82 percent of the subjects in the Ornish program showed regression of atherosclerosis compared with only 10 percent of the usual care group. Over the following four years, the Ornish subjects showed further regression, whereas the usual care group experienced progression of atherosclerosis.[60]

Other investigators have examined the effect of less stringent interventions than those advocated by the Ornish program on the regression of atherosclerosis. These attempts have been less successful than the Ornish program but more successful than the usual care program.

The main criticism of the Ornish program was that lifelong compliance would be difficult. Twenty-nine percent of the study participants dropped out during the last four years of the program. It is not easy to permanently change bad habits, but the hard work associated with following a low-fat diet, exercising consistently at a moderately intense level, and giving up smoking can make people with coronary artery disease feel better and may allow them to avoid surgery.

Refer to Assessment Activity 2-1 at the end of this chapter. Respond to each of the risk questions about factors to determine your risk status.

Other Possible Risk Factors

Iron-Enriched Blood

In 1992 a study completed in Finland found that men with high levels of iron (as measured by serum ferritin) also had a high probability of incurring heart problems. Since then, a number of studies completed in the United States have failed to confirm the high iron–high heart disease connection. These American studies found the opposite. Women with high iron levels were found to have half the heart disease risk as women with low iron stores, and men in the high iron group were 20 percent less likely to die of heart disease than were men with the lowest levels.[61] The rationale is that low iron levels lead to a reduction in oxygen-carrying hemoglobin so that less oxygen is transported to the tissues. It is possible that the decrease in oxygen transport to the cells, including the cells of the heart, is responsible for the heart problems that occur with greater frequency in those who are iron deficient.

Now that you are aware of the major risk factors for heart disease, refer to Assessment Activities 2-1 and 2-2 to test your risk and your knowledge. Be as accurate as possible when providing the necessary information for Activity 2-1. Read the case study (Assessment 2-2) and respond to all of the questions.

Homocysteine

Homocysteine is an amino acid (a building block of protein) derived from methionine metabolism.[34] Methionine is one of the essential amino acids that must be obtained through the diet protein foods. Homocysteine is carried through the bloodstream, and under normal conditions, it is broken down into two other amino acids. When that breakdown does not occur, homocysteine levels rise to present a risk for heart disease. Several studies, including the Physician's Health Study and the Framingham Heart Study, showed that the probability of having a heart attack increases to 3 times the normal level in subjects with the highest homocysteine levels. This puts homocysteine on par with the other major risk factors for coronary artery disease.[62]

Homocysteine is measured in *micromoles*, which are based on molecular weight. The normal range is 4 to 15 micromoles per deciliter of blood. Heart attacks are more likely to occur to those whose levels are above 15.[63]

Homocysteine contributes to heart disease probably by damaging the inner lining of the arteries. The damage initiates the abnormal growth of smooth muscle cells, which in turn promotes the development and progression of atherosclerosis. It also promotes blood platelet aggregation that can lead to the formation of blood clots.

The good news is that homocysteine levels can be controlled with diet. The B vitamins (folic acid or folate, B_6, and B_{12}) are needed to split homocysteine into other amino acids. Folate is the most important of the three, but evidence indicates that optimal benefits occur when all three are available in appropriate amounts. The recommended daily amounts for these vitamins are 400 micrograms of folate, 6 micrograms of B_{12}, and 2 milligrams of B_6.

Lipoprotein (a) or Lp (a)

Lipoprotein (a) represents a group of particles that resemble LDL-C (the bad form of cholesterol). A high circulating level of Lp (a) in the blood may increase the risk for coronary artery disease and stroke, and although study results are not yet conclusive, they appear to be heading in that direction.[17] Many scientists believe that high levels of Lp (a) promote the formation of blood clots and increase the ability of LDL-C to form plaque (the material that blocks arteries).

Lp (a) levels above 30 milligrams per deciliter of blood are considered high. Some medical researchers believe that high values of Lp (a) may be as dangerous to the heart as low levels of HDL-C (the good form of cholesterol).[64] Lp (a) levels are determined primarily by one's genetic composition. Healthy behaviors such as consuming a low fat diet, regular exercise, and so on seem to have little effect on Lp (a). Thus far, the only successful treatments for reducing Lp (a) are large doses of niacin, a water-soluable vitamin, and possibly estrogen supplementation for postmenopausal women.[17] People with high levels of Lp (a) should concentrate on lowering LDL-C and total cholesterol, raising HDL, and keeping the other heart disease risk factors under control.

High Sensitivity C-Reactive Protein (hs-CRP)

C-reactive protein has been used as a diagnostic test for inflammatory rheumatoid conditions. Scientists have improved this test in the last few years by making it more sensitive to inflammation in the body. The new and improved version, high sensitivity C-reactive protein (hs-CRP) can identify inflammation earlier and at lower levels than its predecessor. Atherosclerosis, the underlying cause of 80 percent of coronary heart disease, is a low-level inflammatory process. The newer, more sensitive test shows promise as a diagnostic tool for detecting atherosclerosis early so that an intervention program can be developed and put in place early in the process.

More than 28,000 postmenopausal women free of cardiovascular disease were tested for inflammation, homocysteine level, and seven different lipid or lipoprotein risk factors.[17] The subjects were followed for three years. During that time some of them experienced one or more cardiovascular events. They were compared to age-matched subjects who had not had a cardiovascular event. The most accurate predictor of a potential event was hs-CRP. The study director stated that hs-CRP was statistically twice as strong a predictor of risk for cardiovascular problems than LDL cholesterol, the current gold standard. If these results are confirmed by other studies, this test will become a routine part of a medical exam.

Fibrinogin

An elevated fibrinogin level in the blood is positively correlated with heart disease and stroke. Fibrinogin adds to the viscosity (thickness or stickiness) of the blood and it enhances the formation of blood clots.[34] High fibrinogin levels are more common in men than women, smokers than nonsmokers, in those physically inactive compared to those who are active, and in those with high serum triglycerides compared to those with low levels.

Medical Contributions

Diagnostic Techniques

Diagnosing cardiovascular disease is becoming more sophisticated. Diagnosis begins with a medical examination and patient history. This procedure may be supplemented with a variety of tests that may confirm or refute the physician's suspicions of the presence of cardiovascular disease. Graded exercise tests (GXTs) using a motor-driven treadmill with the patient hooked to an electrocardiogram (ECG) have gained popularity in the last ten years or so. Such noninvasive tests use surface electrodes on the chest that are sensitive to the electrical actions of the heart. Mechanical abnormalities of the heart produce abnormal electrical impulses displayed on the ECG strip. These are read and interpreted by the physician.

The treadmill "road tests" the heart as it works progressively harder to meet the increasing oxygen requirement as the exercise protocol becomes more physically demanding. This test is more accurate for men than women. The gender difference in response to the treadmill test is not completely understood, but it is believed that women's breasts and extra fat tissue interfere with the reception of electrical impulses by the chest electrodes.

In some cases a thallium treadmill test is required because it is more sensitive; however, it is also much more expensive. This involves the injection of radioactive thallium during the final minute of the treadmill test. Thallium is accepted, or taken up, by normal heart muscle but not by ischemic heart muscle. The absorption or nonabsorption of thallium can be seen on a television monitor. The thallium stress test increases diagnostic sensitivity to cardiovascular disease to approximately 90 percent.

Echocardiography is a safe, noninvasive technique that uses sound waves to determine the size of the heart, the thickness of the walls, and the function of the heart's valves. *Cardiac catheterization* is an invasive technique in which a slender tube is threaded from a blood vessel in an arm or leg into the coronary arteries. A liquid contrast dye that can be seen on X-ray film is injected into the coronary arteries. X-ray films are taken throughout the procedure to locate where and how severely the coronary arteries are narrowed.

Medical Treatment

A variety of drugs are used in cardiovascular therapies. These drugs lower blood pressure and cholesterol, minimize the likelihood of blood clotting, and dissolve clots during a heart attack.

Plain aspirin is proving to be an effective drug in the fight against heart disease. Low-dose (one-fourth of a regular aspirin) aspirin therapy consisting of a single daily dose for those who have heart disease reduces the risk of having another heart attack or dying from a subsequent attack. Low-dose aspirin therapy is more effective when supplemented with a "booster" dose of one whole aspirin on the first and fifteenth of each month. Also, regular aspirin use may prevent a first heart attack from occurring in apparently healthy people, but no one should take aspirin or any other drug without first consulting a physician.[65]

Surgical techniques have also affected the treatment of cardiovascular disease. *Coronary artery bypass surgery* is designed to shunt blood around an area of blockage by removing a leg vein and sewing one end of a leg vein into the aorta and the other end into a coronary artery below the blockage, thereby restoring blood flow to the heart muscle (figure 2-8).

The internal mammary arteries also are used for bypass grafts. Many authorities consider these to be the ideal grafts. There are two internal mammary arteries, but the one in the left side of the chest is preferable because it is nearer to the coronary arteries. Many surgeons would rather not use both arteries in the same patient because the diminished flow of blood to the chest impairs healing of the surgical wound. Also, fashioning bypass grafts out of these arteries is time-consuming precision surgery, and there are only two of them and they don't reach all parts of the heart. The advantage is that 95 percent of them remain open ten years after surgery.

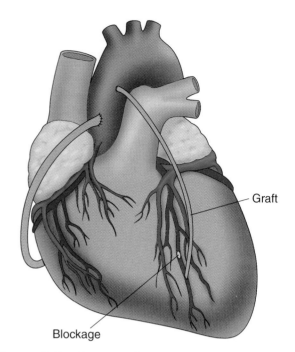

Figure 2-8 Coronary Bypass Graft

Balloon angioplasty uses a catheter with a doughnut-shaped balloon at the tip. The catheter is positioned at the narrow point in the artery, and the balloon is inflated, which cracks and compresses the plaque, stretches the artery wall, and widens the blood vessel to allow greater blood flow (figure 2-9). Laser angioplasty uses heat to burn away plaque if the catheter can be maneuvered into the correct position. This technology appears to be useful for patients with certain types of atherosclerotic narrowings or blockages. Coronary atherectomy, one of the newest techniques, uses a specially tipped catheter equipped with a high-speed rotary cutting blade to shave off plaque.

Catheterization techniques are also used to implant a coronary stent in a diseased artery. The stent is a flexible, metallic tube that functions like a scaffold to support the walls of diseased arteries, thus maintaining an open passage for blood flow (figure 2-10). Stents are positioned in such arteries by a catheter. When correctly positioned, a balloon inside the stent is inflated, causing the stent to expand. This action stretches the artery. Then the balloon is withdrawn, leaving the expanded stent behind to keep the blood vessel open.

This technique shows much promise, but there is a serious limitation associated with the procedure: It increases the risk of blood clots forming at the site of the stent. To counteract this risk, patients are given blood-thinning medications for two to three months following the stent's implantation, and then they are maintained on aspirin thereafter.

Artificial valves have been developed to replace defective heart valves, and these work well. In the summer

Figure 2-9 Balloon Angioplasty

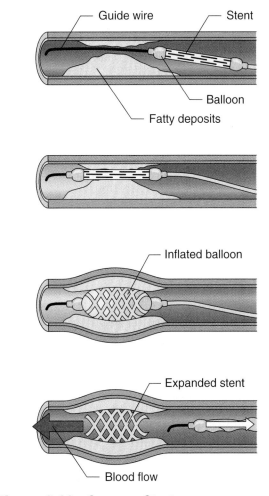

Figure 2-10 Coronary Stent

of 2001, the first successful self-contained mechanical heart was implanted in the chest of a male patient whose life expectancy was literally being measured in days. At this writing, three more patients, all of whom were extremely ill, received the same type of mechanical heart and all four patients are alive and improving. This device is considered experimental and its long-term success rate has yet to be demonstrated. However, it is a technological giant step forward compared to its predecessors, and with modifications, seems to have great potential for extending the lives of people whose hearts are so severely damaged that conventional medical treatments are ineffective.

Mechanical devices (left ventricular assist devices) have been used to aid the failing hearts of patients awaiting donor hearts. These devices take over the burden of pumping blood throughout the body and may keep patients alive for a month or more. Left ventricular assist devices suffer from the same power source problem as mechanical hearts.

Heart transplants have prolonged many lives. The outlook for patients has improved considerably because of the development and use of medicines to suppress the immune system in such patients and because of refinements in the prevention and early detection of the body's attempts to reject donor hearts. As a result, about 85 percent of transplant patients live longer than one year, and 65 percent survive for at least five years.[34] In 1968, twenty-three heart transplants were performed; in 1995, about 2350 were performed.

Candidates for transplants are those whose hearts are irreversibly damaged with disease that does not respond to conventional treatment. Without a new heart, these people will die. The main problems associated with heart transplantation are insufficient numbers of donors, the difficulty of procuring compatible donor hearts, and the constant threat of organ rejection by the recipient.

Summary

- Approximately 1.5 million heart attacks occur each year, and 500,000 of these result in death.
- The heart is two pumps in one; the pulmonary pump, which sends deoxygenated blood to the lungs, and the systemic pump, which sends oxygenated blood to all tissues of the body.
- Blood plasma is a clear, yellowish fluid that makes up about 55 percent of the blood. The remaining 45 percent consists of blood solids—red blood cells, white blood cells, and blood platelets.
- Strokes are caused by a thrombus, an embolus, or a hemorrhage.
- Coronary heart disease is a disease of the coronary blood vessels that bring nourishment and oxygen to the heart.
- Many of the risk factors for heart disease originate in childhood.
- The treatment of heart disease includes the development of appropriate lifestyle habits and medical intervention.
- The major risk factors that cannot be changed are age, male gender, and heredity.
- The major risk factors that can be changed are elevated cholesterol levels, hypertension, cigarette smoking, physical inactivity, and obesity.
- The other contributing risk factors are diabetes mellitus and stress.
- Cholesterol is a steroid that is essential for many bodily functions, but too much circulating in the blood creates a risk for cardiovascular disease.

- Low-density lipoproteins are associated with the development of atherosclerotic plaque.
- High-density lipoproteins protect the arteries from the formation of plaque.
- Blood pressure is the force exerted against the walls of the arteries as blood is pumped from the heart and travels through the circulatory system.
- *Hypertension* is the medical term for high blood pressure.
- Cigarette smoking may be the most potent of the risk factors associated with chronic illness and premature death.
- Involuntary, or passive, smoking is associated with premature disease and death.
- Obesity is a major risk factor that often coexists with many of the other risk factors for cardiovascular disease.
- Diabetes mellitus must be controlled to reduce the accompanying cardiovascular complications.
- Regular exercise significantly reduces the risk for type 2 diabetes mellitus.
- Stress predisposes a person to illness and may hasten the disease process.
- Elevated levels of homocysteine and of Lp (a) in the blood are proving to be important risk factors for heart disease.
- Medical research has made a significant contribution to reducing the incidence of heart disease through the development of sophisticated technological advances in diagnosis and treatment.

Review Questions

1. Define *pulmonary pump* and *systemic pump* and discuss the function of each.
2. Describe the advent of heart disease in the United States.
3. Identify and describe the causes of stroke.
4. What is coronary heart disease? Discuss the available treatment options.
5. What are the risk factors for heart disease and how are they categorized by the AHA?
6. What is cholesterol? LDL? HDL?
7. What is the relationship between total cholesterol and HDL?
8. What is essential hypertension?
9. What ingredients in cigarettes increase the risk for cardiovascular disease? Describe their effect on the heart and blood vessels.

10. What is the risk associated with smokeless tobacco products?
11. Defend the proposition that a moderate level of exercise improves health and increases longevity.
12. What are the cardiovascular complications of diabetes mellitus?
13. How does stress contribute to cardiovascular disease?
14. Can heart disease be prevented or at least delayed? Identify the lifestyle behaviors that may be involved in the process.
15. Can atherosclerosis be reversed? Cite evidence to support your answer.
16. What contributions has the medical profession made to decreasing the death rate from heart disease?

References

1. American Heart Association. 1998. *1999 Heart and Stroke Statistical update.* Dallas: American Heart Association.
2. Tufts University. 2000. Healthful eating habits really do protect your heart. *Tufts University Health & Nutrition Letter* 18(11): 2.
3. Squires, R. W. 2001. Coronary atherosclerosis. In *ACSM Resource Manual* (4th ed.), J. L. Roitman. Philadelphia: Lippincott Williams and Wilkins.
4. U.S. Dept. of Health and Human Services. 1996. *Physical Activity and Health: A Report of the Surgeon General.* Atlanta: U.S. Dept. of Health and Human Services, Centers for Disease Control and Prevention, National

Center for Chronic Disease Prevention and Health Promotion.

5. Kannell, W. B., et al. 1968. Epidemiology of acute myocardial infarction: The Framingham Study. *Medicine Today* 2:50.

6. Corbin, C. B., and R. P. Pangranzi. 1998. *Physical activity for children: a statement of guidelines.* NASE/AAHPERD.

7. U.S. Dept. of Health and Human Services. 2000. *Promoting Better Health for Young People Through Physical Activity and Sports.* Silver Springs, Md.: Centers for Disease Control.

8. Freedman, D. S., et al. 1999. The relation of overweight to cardiovascular risk factors among children and adolescents: the bogalusa heart study. *Pediatrics* 103:1175–1182.

9. Tufts University. 2000. More kids are getting diabetes—and more should be screened for it. *Tufts University Health & Nutrition Letter* 18(2):2.

10. U.S. Dept. of Health and Human Services. 2000. *Healthy People 2010: Understanding and Improving Health.* Washington, D.C.: U.S. Dept. of Health and Human Services, Government Printing Office.

11. Bartecchi, C. E., et al. 1994. The human cost of tobacco use. *New England Journal of Medicine* 330(13):987.

12. University of California at Berkeley. 1996. Up in smoke. *University of California at Berkeley Wellness Letter* 12(11):8.

13. Harvard Medical School. 2000. Cholesterol's effects evident in children. *Harvard Heart Letter* 10(10):7.

14. Publishers of the New England Journal of Medicine. Cholesterol concerns in the young. *HealthNews* 6(9):7.

15. Harvard Medical School. 2000. Heart attacks without chest pain: the danger is greater. *Harvard Heart Letter* 11(1):5–6.

16. Margolis, S., and S. C. Achuff. 1998. *Coronary Heart Disease.* Baltimore: The Johns Hopkins Medical Institutions.

17. Margolis, S., and G. Gerstenblith. 2001. *Coronary Heart Disease.* Baltimore: The Johns Hopkins Medical Institutions.

18. Margolis, S., and L. J. Cheskin. 1998. *Weight Control.* Baltimore: The Johns Hopkins Medical Institutions.

19. Walsh, J. 1998. Low fat, no fat, some high fat fat? Type of fat, not amount may be key. *Environmental Nutrition* 21(4):1.

20. "Heart-smart advice updated for 2000: more fat, but make it 'mono,' please." *Environmental Nutrition* 22(7):1, 4.

21. University of California at Berkeley. 1994. Fascinating facts. *University of California at Berkeley Wellness Letter* 10(6):1.

22. McArdle, W. D., F. I. Katch, and V. L. Katch. 1999. *Sports and Exercise Nutrition.* Philadelphia: Lippincott Williams and Wilkins.

23. Editors. 1984. The lipid research clinics coronary primary prevention trial results. I. Reduction in incidence of coronary heart disease. *Journal of American Medical Association* 251:351.

24. LaRosa, J. C., et al. 1990. The cholesterol facts: a summary of the evidence relating dietary facts, serum cholesterol, and coronary heart disease: a joint statement by the American Heart Association and the National Heart, Lung, and Blood Institute. *Circulation* 81:1721.

25. Steen, S. N., and G. Butterfield. 1998. Diet and nutrition. In *ACSM Resource Manual* (3rd ed.), ed. J. L. Roitman. Baltimore: Williams & Wilkins.

26. Harvard Medical School. 2000. Triglycerides and heart disease. *Harvard Heart Letter* 11(1):1–4.

27. University of California at Berkeley. 1998. The ups and downs of triglycerides. *University of California at Berkeley Wellness Letter* 14(3):4.

28. Thomas, T. R., and T. P. La Fontaine. 2001. Exercise, nutritional strategies and lipoproteins. In *ASCM Resource Manual* (4th ed.), ed. J. L. Roitman. Philadelphia: Lippincott Williams and Wilkins.

29. National High Blood Pressure Education Program. 1993. *The Fifth Report of the Joint National Committee on Detection, Evaluation and Treatment of High Blood Pressure, National Heart, Lung, and Blood Institute, National Institutes of Health,* NIH publication no. 93-1088. Bethesda, Md.: National Institutes of Health.

30. Harvard Medical School. 2001. A better way of measuring hypertension? *Harvard Health Letter* 26(4):3.

31. U.S. Dept. of Health and Human Services. 2000. *Healthy People 2010* (2nd ed.) with understanding and improving health and objectives for improving health, 2 vols. Washington, D.C.: U.S. Government Printing Office.

32. Tufts University. 1997. Meditation lowers blood pressure as well as drugs. *Tufts University Diet & Nutrition Letter* 14(111):3.

33. ACSM. 1993. Physical activity, physical fitness, and hypertension. *Medicine and Science in Sports and Exercise* 25(10):1.

34. Mooss, A., and N. F. Gordon. 2001. Conceptual basis for coronary artery disease risk factor assessment in clinical practice. In *ACSM Resource Manual* (4th ed.), ed. J. L. Roitman. Philadelphia: Lippincott Williams and Wilkins.

35. Centers for Disease Control and Prevention. 1999. Tobacco use—United States 1990–1999. *Journal of the American Medical Association* 292:2202–2204.

36. Hales, D. 2001. *An invitation to fitness and wellness.* Australia: Wadsworth.

37. Centers for Disease Control and Prevention. 1994. CDC surveillance summaries. *MMWR* 43(SS-3).

38. U.S. Dept. of Health and Human Services. 1988. *The Health Consequences of Smoking—Nicotine Addiction, a Report of the Surgeon General.* Rockville, Md.: U.S. Department of Health and Human Services.

39. American Cancer Society. 1997. *Cancer Facts and Figures—1997.* Atlanta, Ga.: American Cancer Society.

40. U.S. Dept. of Health and Human Services. 1998. *Progress Review—Tobacco, Prevention Report.* Washington, D.C.: Office of Disease Prevention and Health Promotion.

41. Powell, K. E. 1987. Physical activity and the incidence of coronary heart disease. *Annual Review of Public Health* 8:253.

42. Berlin, J. A., and G. A. Colditz. 1990. A meta-analysis of physical activity in the prevention of coronary heart disease. *American Journal of Epidemiology* 132:612.

43. Whaley, M. A., and L. A. Kaminsky. 2001. Epidemiology of physical activity, physical fitness, and selected chronic diseases. In *ACSM Resource Manual* (4th ed.), ed. J. L. Roitman. Baltimore: Lippincott, Williams and Wilkins.

44. Blair, S. N., et al. 1995. Changes in physical fitness and all-cause mortality: a prospective study of healthy and unhealthy men. *Journal of the American Medical Association* 273:1093–1098.

45. Blair, S. N., et al. 1989. Physical fitness and all-cause mortality—prospective

study of healthy men and women. *Journal of American Medical Association* 262:2395.

46. Manson, J. E., et al. 1992. The primary prevention of myocardial infarction. *New England Medical Journal* 326:1406.

47. Duncan, J. J., et al. 1995. Women walking for health and fitness. *Journal of American Medical Association* 273:402.

48. Pate, R. R., et al. 1995. Physical activity and public health. *Journal of American Medical Association* 273:402.

49. Lee, I. M., and R. S. Paffenbarger. 2000. Associations of light, moderate, and vigorous intensity physical activity with longevity: the Harvard alumni health study. *American Journal of Epidemiology* 151:293–299.

50. Pescatello, L. S., et al. 1994. Health care reform and the exercise professional. *ACSM Certified News* 4(2):1.

51. Editor. 1996. How to avoid adult onset diabetes. *Nutrition Action Health Letter* 23(7):3.

52. Campaigne, B. 2001. Exercise and diabetes mellitus. In *ACSM Resource Manual* (4th ed.), ed. J. L. Roitman. Philadelphia: Lippincott Williams and Wilkins.

53. Manson, J. E., et al. 1992. A prospective study of exercise and incidence of diabetes among U.S. male physicians. *Journal of American Medical Association* 268:63.

54. Hu, F. B., et al. 1999. Walking compared with vigorous physical activity and risk of type 2 diabetes in women: a prospective study. *Journal of the American Medical Association* 282:1433–1439.

55. Harvard Medical School. 2000. Anger and heart disease risk. *Harvard Heart Letter* 10(11):6–7.

56. Harvard University. 1998. Stress and atherosclerosis. *Harvard Health Letter* 23(4):8.

57. Harvard University. 1998. Grumpy old men: at risk for coronary disease? *Harvard Health Letter* 8(12):7.

58. Sime, W. W., and K. Hellweg. 2001. Stress and coping. In *ACSM Resource Manual* (4th ed.), ed. J. L. Roitman. Philadelphia: Lippincott Williams and Wilkins.

59. Ornish, D., et al. 1990. Can lifestyle changes reverse coronary heart disease? *The Lancet* 336:129.

60. Ornish, D., et al. 1993. Can lifestyle changes reverse atherosclerosis? Four-year results of the lifestyle heart trial. *Circulation* 88 (suppl.):2064.

61. Editors. 1997. Iron's link to heart disease. *HealthNews* 3(3):7.

62. Harvard University. 1997. Evidence mounts for heart disease marker. *Harvard Health Letter* 22(11):1.

63. Mayo Clinic. 1997. Homocysteine. *Mayo Clinic Health Letter* 15(12):7.

64. University of California at Berkeley. 1997. Ask the experts. *University of California at Berkeley Wellness Letter* 14(3):7.

65. Hennekens, C. H., M. L. Dyken, and V. Fuster. 1997. Aspirin as a therapeutic agent in cardiovascular disease—a statement for healthcare professionals from the American Heart Association. *Circulation* 96:2757.

Suggested Readings

Harvard University. 2001. Depression and heart disease. *Harvard Heart Letter* 11(8):3–5.

Discusses the differences between being depressed and actually suffering from clinical depression. Provides the major symptoms associated with clinical depression, discusses the major research that links heart disease with depression, and describes the methods by which depression is treated.

Editors of the New England Journal of Medicine. 2001. Better stroke prevention. *HealthNews* 7(4):1–2.

Discusses the causes of strokes and newer treatments that have evolved from the most recent research. Also, discusses the effects of a very old drug, aspirin, in the treatment of strokes. This article is accompanied by the comments of one of the associate editors whose medical specialty is emergency medicine.

University of California at Berkeley. 2001. A dozen ways to improve your walking workouts. *University of California at Berkeley Wellness Letter* 17(7):6.

For those who walk for heart health and other health-related reasons. Defines brisk walking and then gives twelve ways to make walking more fun and more effective.

Editors. 2001. Diabetes and heart disease: what you don't know can hurt you. *Heart Advisor* 4(3):3.

More than one-half of the diabetics in the United States are unaware that they have the disease so they are probably also unaware that diabetes is a major contributor to heart disease, stroke, kidney disease, blindness, and nerve damage. It is important to know the signs and symptoms in order to be treated early.

Editors. 2001. Strength training for heart patients. *Heart Advisor* 4(4):4–5.

Explains why strength training is important for heart patients. Discusses how heart patients can get started and then provides some tips for a successful resistance program.

Name _____ Date _____ Section _____

Assessment Activity 2-1

What's Your Heart Attack Risk?

Directions: By answering questions in the twelve items below, you can calculate your odds of having a heart attack within the next ten years. The test is based on data from four of the most extensive American studies of coronary risk. (The test is not accurate for people who already have a history of coronary disease. For definitive advice, ask your doctor.) Advice on improving your odds follows this test.

The Test

For every "yes" answer to items 1 through 9, add or subtract points as shown.

Question	Men	Women
1. Do you get little or no regular exercise?	Plus 2	Plus 6
2. Calculate your body mass index (BMI) as follows: Multiply your weight in pounds by 704. Divide the result by your height in inches. Divide that result by your height in inches again and round to the nearest whole number.		
Is your BMI from 21 to 24?	Plus 0	Plus 2
Is your BMI from 25 to 28?	Plus 2	Plus 3
Is your BMI 29 or over?	Plus 4	Plus 6
3. Do you have diabetes?	Plus 8	Plus 11
4. If you're an ex-smoker, did you quit in the past five years?	Plus 1	Plus 4
If you smoke, do you smoke fewer than 15 cigarettes a day?	Plus 2	Plus 8
Do you smoke 15 to 24 cigarettes a day?	Plus 4	Plus 15
Do you smoke more than 24 cigarettes a day?	Plus 6	Plus 18
5. Did either of your parents have a heart attack before age 60?	Plus 9	Plus 9

Question	Men	Women
6. Do you take medicine to control blood pressure? (This is a sign that your pressure was once elevated.)	Plus 1	Plus 1
7. If you are a postmeno-pausal woman, are you currently taking estrogen alone?		Minus 5
Are you currently taking estrogen plus progestin?		Minus 3
If you don't currently take estrogen, did you previously take it (with or without progestin)?		Minus 2
8. Do you take low doses of aspirin at least every other day? (A low dose is between one quarter and one whole 325-mg tablet.)	Minus 4	Minus 4
9. Do you drink alcohol in moderation? ("Moderate" drinking is 2 to 14 drinks per week. A "drink" is 12 ounces of beer, 5 ounces of wine, or 1½ ounces of liquor.)	Minus 4	Minus 4

Add up your points so far. SUBTOTAL _____ _____

Now calculate items 10 through 12, rounding to the nearest whole number.

	Men	Women
10. Multiply your systolic pressure (the higher number) by 0.14 if you are a man, by 0.15 if you are a woman.	Plus ___	Plus ___
11. Multiply your age by 0.51 if you are a man, by 0.8 if you are a woman.	Plus ___	Plus ___

12. Multiply your total cholesterol level by 0.07 if you are a man, by 0.06 if you are a woman. Multiply your HDL level by 0.25 if you are a man, by 0.3 if you are a woman. If you don't know your cholesterol levels and want to assume they're about average, you could substitute 205 for total cholesterol and 51 for HDL. Adults 20 and over should have cholesterol testing at least every 5 years.

Plus ___   Plus ___

Minus ___   Minus ___

Add up your points for items 10 through 12.   SUBTOTAL _____ _____

Add the two subtotals to get your score   TOTAL _____ _____

Probability* of Having a Heart Attack

Men			
Score	1 Year	5 Years	10 Years
0–35	<0.1%	<0.4%	<1%
36–45	0.1–0.2%	0.4–1%	1–3%
46–55	0.2–0.6%	1–3%	3–7%
56–65	0.6–2%	3–8%	7–17%
66–70	2%	8–13%	17–27%
71–75	2–4%	13–20%	27–40%
76–80	4–6%	20–30%	40–56%

Women			
Score	1 Year	5 Years	10 Years
0–60	<0.1%	<0.4%	<1%
61–70	0.1–0.2%	0.4–1%	1.3%
71–80	0.2–0.5%	1–3%	3–7%
81–85	0.5–1%	3–5%	7–12%
86–90	1%	5–8%	12–19%
91–95	1–2%	8–13%	19–29%
96–100	2–4%	13–20%	29–43%

*"Probability" indicates the percentage of people like yourself who will have a heart attack during the period cited. If your probability is 7% for the 10-year column, for example, it means that out of a random sampling of 100 people with the same score as yourself, seven will have a heart attack within a decade of today.

Name _____ Date _____ Section _____

Assessment Activity 2-2

A Case Study of Bill M.

Directions: To determine your understanding of cardiovascular health and wellness, read the following case study and answer the accompanying questions. Bill, a 38-year-old man who is 5'8" tall and weighs 205 lb, has the following history:

- His father died of a heart attack at age 48 years; his grandfather died of a heart attack at age 52 years.
- His cholesterol level is 256 mg/dl, LDL is 172 mg/dl, and HDL is 40 mg/dl.
- His blood pressure is consistently in the 150/95 range.

- He smokes one pack of cigarettes per day.
- He drinks six to eight brewed cups of coffee daily.
- He eats two eggs with bacon or sausage and buttered toast daily.
- Meat is a major part of supper; he skips lunch.
- His favorite snacks are ice cream, buttered popcorn, and salted peanuts.
- He occasionally plays tennis on Sunday afternoons.
- He owns his own business and often works 55 to 60 hours per week.

Answer the following:

What are Bill's risk factors for coronary heart disease? _____

Which of these can he control? _____

What suggestions can you give him regarding his current diet? _____

_____

What effect may a change in diet have on his coronary risk profile? _____

_____

What suggestions can you make regarding Bill's need for exercise, and how might a change in his activity level affect his coronary risk profile? _____

_____

What are the risks associated with obesity? _____

_____

3

Increasing Cardiorespiratory Endurance

 Online Learning Center

Log on to our Online Learning Center (OLC) for access to these additional resources:

- Chapter key term flashcards
- Learning objectives
- Additional goals for behavior change
- Concentration game
- Self-scoring chapter quizzes

- Additional lab activities

The OLC also offers weblinks for study and exploration of wellness topics. Access these links through **www.mhhe.com/anspaugh5e**, click on "Student Center," click on "Chapter 3," and then click on "Web Activities."

Goals for Behavior Change

- List three physical activities you normally do every week (exclusive of structured, planned exercise) and find and implement ways of making them more challenging.
- If you do not exercise regularly, list several factors that will motivate you to begin a cardiorespiratory endurance program. Begin a simple walking or other exercise program with these factors in mind.
- If you are physically active, list the main factors that will encourage you to improve the frequency, intensity, or duration of your activity. To help you stay motivated, post this list in a place where you will see it every day.
- Choose a piece of home exercise equipment that seems well suited to your exercise preferences and goals.

Key Terms

aerobic
aerobic capacity
cardiorespiratory endurance
cross-training

health-related fitness
hyperthermia
hypothermia
performance-related fitness

Objectives

After completing this chapter, you will be able to:

- Identify and define the health-related components of physical fitness.
- Discuss the principles of conditioning.
- Calculate your target heart rate for exercise by two different methods.

- Identify and discuss the health benefits of consistent participation in exercise.
- Describe the problems associated with exercise in hot and cold weather.

echnology has affected the lives of Americans by increasing productivity while simultaneously reducing and in some cases eliminating the amount of physical work for the labor force. Therefore, physical fitness for most of the population can no longer be attained on the job, and leisure hours represent the only time for its development. Dozens of physical activities, exercise regimens, sports, games, and household and other physical chores that may contribute to health enhancement and fitness development are available. These activities are sufficiently different from each other, running the gamut from low- to high-skill requirement, so that almost anyone can find one or two enjoyable, fun, and challenging activities. This chapter focuses on the principles and concepts that have evolved for developing cardiorespiratory endurance for the purposes of health enhancement and physical fitness.

The Components of Physical Fitness

According to the American College of Sports Medicine (ACSM), *physical fitness* is defined "as a set of attributes that people have or achieve that relates to the ability to perform physical activity."[1] *Physical activity* is an umbrella term defined "as bodily movement that is produced by the contraction of skeletal muscle and that substantially increases energy expenditure."[1] *Exercise* is a subset of physical activity. It is defined "as planned, structured, and repetitive bodily movement done to improve or maintain one or more components of physical fitness."[1]

Physical activity includes exercise and all other types of human movements such as mowing the lawn, raking leaves, vacuuming the floors, climbing stairs, washing the car by hand, chopping wood, shoveling snow, and so on. These activities, many of which are daily chores, may improve physical fitness for some unfit sedentary people, but when engaged in regularly, are health-enhancing for most people. Health improvement can be attained with regular participation in lower intensity physical activities whereas higher intensity physical activities that sustain an exercise target heart rate are necessary for improving physical fitness.

Most physical fitness experts have accepted the concept of performance-related and health-related fitness. **Performance-related fitness,** or sports fitness, consists of the following components: speed, power, balance, coordination, agility, and reaction time. These are essential for sports performance, but they may or may not contribute significantly to those activities performed for health enhancement (see Just the Facts: What's the Difference?).

Just the Facts

What's the Difference?

Components of Fitness

Health related
- Cardiorespiratory endurance
- Muscular strength
- Muscular endurance
- Flexibility
- Body composition

Performance related
- Speed
- Power
- Balance
- Coordination
- Agility
- Reaction time

Activities

Health related
- Walking
- Running
- Jogging
- Cycling
- Hiking
- Swimming
- Rope jumping
- Weight training
- Cross-country skiing

Performance related
- Racquetball
- Handball
- Squash
- Tennis
- Badminton
- Soccer
- Softball
- Basketball
- Football
- Water polo

Speed is velocity, or the ability to move rapidly. *Power* is the product of force and velocity and the rate at which work is performed. *Balance,* or equilibrium, is the ability to maintain a desired body position either statically or dynamically. *Coordination* is the harmonious integration of the body parts to produce smooth, fluid motion. *Agility* is the ability to change direction rapidly. *Reaction time* is the time required (usually measured in hundredths of a second) to respond to a stimulus.

The components of **health-related fitness** are cardiorespiratory endurance, muscular strength, muscular endurance, flexibility, and body composition. In this text the exercise emphasis is on health-related fitness.

Performance-related and health-related fitness, although different, clearly are not mutually exclusive. For example, competitive athletes require an abundance of the performance-related components of fitness, but the natures of their sports may also require the simultaneous development of the health-related components. Athletes who play racquetball, tennis, basketball, soccer, and handball are some that fall within this category. Conversely, the same sports are appropriate for health and fitness enthusiasts who prefer to achieve their goals through friendly competition.

However, the development and maintenance of health-related fitness do not necessarily depend on athletic ability or activities high in the performance components. Fitness for health purposes can be achieved with minimal psychomotor ability through activities such as walking, jogging, cycling, hiking, backpacking, orienteering, swimming, rope jumping, and weight training.

These are self-paced activities; that is, the exerciser selects a relatively comfortable pace that can be sustained for a minimum of 10 minutes. No competing opponent pushes the exerciser beyond his or her physiological limits.

Remember the adage "No pain, no gain"? Trying to comply with it has done more harm than good to sedentary people attempting to become physically active. The health benefits of exercise occur when exercise is somewhat uncomfortable but not painful. Only the most dedicated health enthusiasts and competitors can face exercise that constantly produces pain. Although exercise for health enhancement should stress cardiorespiratory development, the other components of fitness should not be neglected. Flexibility exercises can be a part of warm-up and cool-down procedures. Flexibility exercises may be performed three to five times per week, and the best results occur during the cool-down period following the cardiorespiratory workout.[2] Stretching is most effective at this time because muscle temperature is elevated. Warm muscles respond well to stretching, and the likelihood of muscle injury is decreased as well. Resistance/strength training plays an important role and should be an integral part of a well-rounded fitness program.

As with all components of wellness, developing and sustaining an exercise program are the responsibilities of each individual. This text provides convincing evidence of the need for regular exercise and provides guidelines for initiating a sound program or reinforcement for those currently exercising.

Cardiorespiratory Endurance

Cardiorespiratory endurance is the ability to take in, deliver, and extract oxygen for physical work, that is, the ability to persevere at a physical task at a given intensity level.[3] Cardiorespiratory endurance improves with regular participation in aerobic activities, such as speed walking, jogging, cycling, swimming, and cross-country skiing. The term **aerobic** means "with oxygen," but when applied to exercise, it refers to activities in which oxygen demand can be met continuously during performance.[4] Aerobic performance depends on a continuous and sufficient supply of oxygen to burn the carbohy-

drates and fats needed to fuel such activities. In other words, someone performing aerobically has the capacity to sustain the intensity or the energy requirement for longer than a couple of minutes,[5] a phenomenon known as *steady state*. Steady state can be achieved only during aerobic exercise, and it represents a level of exertion that feels relatively comfortable to the exerciser. It is also referred to as a *pay as you go system* in that the oxygen cost of an activity is paid in full by the body during the activity. Steady state oxygen consumption can be maintained for an average of 10 to 60 minutes during submaximal continuous exercise. This may not apply for exercise during hot and humid weather. The stress of exercising during these conditions causes a steady upward drift in oxygen consumption.[6]

Cardiorespiratory endurance is also referred to as **aerobic capacity,** or maximum oxygen consumption (VO_2 max). It is the most important component of physical fitness and is the foundation of total fitness.

The physiological changes that result from cardiorespiratory training are referred to as the *long-term* or *chronic effects of exercise*. The effects of training are measurable and predictable.

Heart Rate

A few months of aerobic training lowers the resting heart rate by 10 to 15 beats per minute (bpm).[7] It also lowers the heart rate for a given workload. For example, a slow jog may produce a heart rate of 165 beats per minute before training and 140 beats per minute after a few months of training. The trained heart is a stronger, more efficient pump capable of delivering the required blood and oxygen with fewer beats.

Stroke Volume

Stroke volume is the amount of blood that the heart can eject in one beat. Aerobic training increases the stroke volume by (1) increasing the size of the cavity of the ventricles, which results in more blood filling the heart, and (2) increasing the contractile strength of the ventricular wall, so contraction is more forceful and a greater amount of blood is ejected from the ventricles.[7] The increase in stroke volume, both at rest and during exercise, is one of the primary effects of endurance training and one of the major mechanisms responsible for improvement in aerobic fitness.

Cardiac Output

Cardiac output is the amount of blood ejected by the heart in 1 minute. Cardiac output (Q) is the product of heart rate (HR) and stroke volume (SV) ($Q = HR \times SV$). Cardiac output increases with aerobic training during maximal effort—it does not increase at rest or during submaximal exercise. Cardiac output does not change during rest or submaximal exercise because the lowered resting heart rate compensates for the increase in stroke volume. What does change is the manner in which cardiac output is achieved. This is illustrated by the following example: An untrained 25-year-old man has a resting heart rate of 72 bpm and a stroke volume of 70 ml of blood per beat. His cardiac output at rest is calculated as follows:

$$\begin{aligned} Q &= HR \times SV \\ &= 72 \times 70 \\ &= 5040 \text{ ml (5.0 L)} \end{aligned}$$

The same person after two years of aerobic training has the same cardiac output at rest, but it is achieved differently: The resting heart rate is now decreased to 55 bpm and the stroke volume is increased to 92 ml of blood per beat.

$$\begin{aligned} Q &= 55 \times 92 \\ &= 5040 \text{ ml (5.0 L)} \end{aligned}$$

The average cardiac output at rest is 4 to 6 liters of blood per minute. During maximal exertion, cardiac output reaches values of 18 to 20 liters of blood per minute for the average person but may reach as much as 40 liters per minute for large, well-conditioned athletes. What an incredible piece of work by an organ that weighs less than a pound! To put this in perspective, imagine forty 1-liter cola bottles filled with blood. This is the amount that the hearts of some highly conditioned people can pump in 1 minute. Maximal cardiac output improves with training primarily because of the resulting increase in stroke volume.[7] Maximal heart rate is essentially unaffected by training; therefore, its influence on maximal cardiac output is relatively constant. However, maximal heart rate declines with age by about 1 bpm per year after age 20. Training cannot stop the decline; it can only slow the process.

Blood Volume

Aerobic training increases total blood volume, plasma volume (the liquid portion of the blood), and the blood solids (the red blood cells, white blood cells, and blood platelets). The increase is greatest in plasma volume, so the blood becomes more liquid. The increase in the ratio of plasma volume to red blood cell volume is an adaptation to exercise that lowers the viscosity, or thickness and stickiness, of the blood. This change decreases the resistance to blood flow, allowing it to circulate more easily through the blood vessels.

Blood is automatically shunted by the body to areas of greatest need. At rest, a significant amount is sent to the digestive system and kidneys. During vigorous exercise, as much as 85 percent of the blood is sent to the

working muscles, reducing the amount sent to the digestive and urinary systems.[1]

Heart Volume

The muscles of the body respond to exercise by growing larger and stronger. As a muscular pump, the heart's volume and weight increase with endurance training.[8] Training that lowers the resting heart rate stimulates greater filling of the ventricles, whose muscle fibers respond to the increased pool of blood by stretching. This produces a recoil effect in the muscle fibers that results in a stronger contraction with more blood ejected per beat. Continued training causes the ventricles to enlarge and grow stronger, so the weight and the size of the heart increase. The hypertrophied (enlarged) heart is a normal response to endurance training that has no long-term detrimental effects. Although maintaining this effect for life is beneficial, several months of inactivity will reduce heart weight and size to pretraining levels. The atrophy (wasting away) associated with physical inactivity is inevitable.

Respiratory Responses

The chest muscles that support breathing improve in both strength and endurance with exercise.[9] Vital capacity, the amount of air that can be expired maximally following a maximal inspiration, increases slightly. A corresponding decrease occurs in "dead space" air or residual volume, the amount of air remaining in the lungs after a maximal expiration.

Training substantially increases maximal pulmonary ventilation (the amount of air moved in and out of the lungs).[9] Before training, the lungs can ventilate approximately 110 liters of air per minute. Pulmonary ventilation increases to about 135 liters of air following a few months of training. Highly trained athletes commonly ventilate 180 to 200 liters of air per minute.

Blood flow to the lungs, particularly to the upper lobes, appears to increase after training. This results in a larger and more efficient surface for the exchange of oxygen and carbon dioxide.

Metabolic Responses

Aerobic endurance training improves aerobic capacity by 5 to 25 percent in previously untrained, healthy adults. The magnitude of improvement is primarily dependent upon the initial level of physical fitness. The lower the fitness level, the greater the gain from aerobic training.[7] Rarely do improvements greater than 30 percent occur. When they do, they usually occur to those who also lose a large amount of body weight and fat.[3]

The improvement in aerobic capacity is the result of several physiological adaptations that increase the body's production of energy. First, adenosine triphosphate (ATP), the actual unit of energy for muscular contraction, is produced in greater quantities. The mitochondria, specialized organelles responsible for manufacturing ATP, respond to training by increasing in size and number to increase their output. Second, oxidative enzymes within the mitochondria that accelerate the production of ATP increase in quantity. Third, cardiac output and blood perfusion of the muscles performing the work increase. Fourth, training facilitates and increases the extraction of oxygen by the exercising muscles. These are some of the major adaptations that combine to enhance aerobic endurance.[9]

Aerobic capacity (VO_2 max) is limited by heredity and is finite. The heredity component of VO_2 max is approximately 40 percent.[10] This represents a substantial influence on a given person's potential for aerobic performance. Therefore, the sensitivity of the VO_2 max response to aerobic training is to a significant degree

dependent upon heredity. If those who inherit the genetic potential for endurance events also train diligently, they become capable of exceptionally high levels of performance. Diligent training with an average genetic potential results in average or slightly above average performance. Only a select few inherit the ability to produce world-class endurance performances. The majority of people are in the average category, but all can achieve their aerobic *potential* with training.

Aerobic capacity reaches a peak after six months to two years of steady endurance training. At this point, it levels off and remains unchanged for a number of years, even if training is intensified. However, aerobic performance continues to improve with harder training, because a higher percentage of the aerobic capacity can be maintained for a longer period. For example, six months of appropriate training may allow you to jog 3 miles at 60 percent of your aerobic capacity. Another year of harder training may allow you to run 3 miles at 85 percent of your capacity. Capacity has not changed during this time, but physiological adaptations have occurred that enable the body to function at progressively higher percentages of maximum capacity.

Aerobic capacity decreases with age. During adulthood, peak aerobic energy steadily declines by an average of about 1 percent per year between the ages of 25 and 75.[11] A significant portion of the decline is related to the lack of physical activity that accompanies aging: Those who are physically active throughout their lifetimes experience declines in aerobic capacity but not at the same rate as those who are inactive. See Wellness Across the Generations: Exercise Is for Everyone for more details about the impact of exercising on aging.

The effects of training persist as long as training continues. Training of moderate intensity may increase the VO_2 max by 10 to 20 percent. However, the VO_2 max returns to pretraining levels within a few months if training is discontinued.[8] Most of the decline occurs during the first month and slows down during the next two months. Fitness developed through years of continuous training can be lost in months if training is interrupted or discontinued. Highly conditioned athletes respond to detraining in a similar manner. In a study, subjects who suspended training for eighty-four days after ten years of active participation experienced a significant decline in aerobic capacity after three weeks of inactivity. They returned to pretraining levels in most fitness parameters by the end of the study. The exceptions to complete reversal were muscle capillary density and mitochondrial enzymes, which remained 50 percent higher than levels measured in sedentary control subjects. This study indicated that the results of inactivity are variable and affect some systems more quickly than others. Physical decline cannot be prevented with physical inactivity.

Wellness Across the Generations

Exercise Is for Everyone

The ability of the body to take in, transport, and extract oxygen for physical work and exercise declines with age. On the average, aerobic capacity declines by about 8 to 10 percent every decade after the age of 25 in both males and females. One of the major sources of this decline in the United States is the decreasing level of physical activity that tends to accompany aging. This trend toward inactivity also results in a loss of muscle weight, an increase in fat weight, and a decrease in metabolic rate, all of which contribute to the decline in aerobic capacity. Although physiological aging does lower aerobic capacity, at least 50 percent of the decline is due to "disuse atrophy" caused by inactivity.[12]

Biological aging cannot be stopped. We cannot live forever. However, exercise comes as close to an antiaging pill as anything else available. Even older people who have been sedentary for decades can benefit from aerobic exercise and weight training.

The beneficial outcomes of regular exercise for older people include an increase in energy, a favorable change in body composition (loss of fat, gain of muscle), an increase in muscular strength and endurance, an increase in metabolism, and significant improvements in cardiovascular and musculoskeletal health.[13] All of these changes translate into a higher quality of life and longevity.

Physically fit 60- and 70-year-olds have the aerobic capacity of unfit 25-year-olds.[13] This means that physically fit elderly people have the energy to live independently during their later years. The ability to perform the daily chores of living and to participate in an active lifestyle with energy to spare develops confidence that contributes to the enjoyment of life.

Three different methods for assessing your cardiorespiratory endurance are presented in the Assessments Activities. These include the Rockport Fitness Walking Test, the 1.5-Mile Run/Walk Test, and the 3-Minute Bench Step Test. Each is accompanied by norms, so you can compare your performance against the standards.

Cardiorespiratory Endurance and Wellness

Most Americans believe that exercise is good for them, but the majority cannot explain how or why. This section provides some of the answers

Consistent participation in exercise is necessary to improve health status. Sporadic exercise does not promote physical fitness or contribute to health enhancement. Infrequent participation increases the risk of sudden death during the time of exercise.[14] Physical inactivity is a major risk for coronary heart disease. The risk is approximately equal to that imposed by cigarette smoking, high blood pressure, and elevated serum cholesterol. Sixty percent of adult Americans are inactive or marginally active. The number of physically inactive people exceeds the combined total of those who smoke, are hypertensive, or have high serum cholesterol.[14] Based on these numbers, promoting regular exercise for the general public should be an important priority of public health policy.

Coronary heart disease is rarely responsible for sudden cardiac death during or after exercise among people under the age of 30. Congenital heart defects or other cardiac abnormalities, such as faulty valves, enlarged hearts, and heart muscle disease, are the usual culprits for this age group. Most exertional deaths occur among older Americans and are due to coronary heart disease. A study by Harvard medical researchers found that heavy physical exertion, such as shoveling snow, gardening, walking fast, jogging, playing softball, and playing tennis, could trigger a heart attack.[15] For the physically unfit, the risk of incurring a heart attack during and in the first hour after strenuous exertion increased by 107 times. The risk for physically fit people increased only 2.7 times. These data applied equally to men and women.

The danger attributed to physical exertion is greatly diminished in people who exercise regularly. The benefits they receive from physical training far outweigh the minimal risk associated with one bout of strenuous exercise. A similar study conducted at the same time in Germany found amazingly similar results.[16]

One and one-half million heart attacks occur every year in the United States. The Harvard researchers concluded that 75,000 of these are exertional and they usually occur after strenuous exercise. Most of these heart attacks occur among those who are physically inactive and at high risk.[15] See Just the Facts: Exercise-Related Problems for some tips on reducing the hazards associated with regular exercise. Some selected health benefits of regular exercise are listed in table 3-1. If these benefits could be distilled and sold in pill form, the American public would line up to pay any reasonable price to attain them. And yet all of these benefits are readily

Just the Facts

Exercise-Related Problems

Many health, fitness, and cosmetic benefits occur to those who exercise on a regular basis. Although they are outweighed by the benefits, risks are associated with such behavior. Despite precautions, injuries occasionally occur. Beginning exercisers are particularly susceptible to injury because of their lack of knowledge about training coupled with their misguided attempts to achieve their goals too quickly. The following suggestions should result in safer workouts:

1. Dress according to the weather: shorts, t-shirt, mesh baseball-type cap in warm weather; layers of light clothing, hat, gloves, ear protection, and windbreaker in cold weather.

2. Wear appropriate shoes for the activity in which you participate: jogging shoes, walking shoes, aerobic shoes, or cross-trainers. In general, exercise shoes should be one-half to three-quarters of an inch longer than your longest toe. There should also be room enough for the toes to spread out. The soles of most exercise shoes consist of three layers. The outer sole that contacts the floor or ground should be made of hard rubber. The next layer is the midsole, which protects the midfoot and toes. The last layer is made of a thick, spongy substance that absorbs most of the shock when the foot strikes the surface.

3. Warm up and cool down properly before and after exercise.

4. Exercise within your capacity—it should feel a little uncomfortable but not painful. According to the American College of Sports Medicine (ACSM), the initial stage of an exercise program should last a minimum of four weeks at a low intensity (50 to 60 percent of the maximal heart rate or HR_{max}). Each exercise session should last for 15 to 20 minutes during the first week and increase to 25 to 30 minutes during the fourth week. At this point, the exerciser is ready to increase the intensity, frequency, and duration of each session.

5. While following these simple guidelines reduces the possibility of incurring pain or injury, beginning exercisers may experience, as a result of overuse, shin splints, side stitch, blisters, chafing, muscle cramps, muscle soreness, Achilles tendon injuries, and lower-back pain.

   a. Muscle soreness following exercise usually occurs among beginners who have yet to adapt to physical exertion or to those at any level of fitness who exceed their physical capabilities. Following the ACSM guidelines reduces exposure to muscle pain.

   b. Side stitches occur primarily among walkers and joggers. They consist of severe pain in the upper right quadrant of the abdomen. Side stitches may be caused by reduced blood flow to the diaphragm (a large, dome-shaped muscle that separates the abdominal cavity from the chest cavity), or they may be due to the collection of gas in the intestines. In either case, deep breathing and direct pressure applied with both hands at the site of the pain may provide relief. Sometimes, stopping the activity for a few minutes is required for the pain to subside.

   c. A common injury occurring among beginners is shin splints. Shin splints produce a burning pain that radiates along the inner surface of the large bones of the lower leg. These are nagging, painful injuries better prevented than treated. The causes of shin splints include training demands that exceed a person's capacity to perform. High-impact activities such as jogging or aerobics to music, poor-quality exercise shoes, hard exercise surfaces, and walking or jogging on hilly surfaces are other contributing causes. Treatment includes applications of ice, rest, wrapping or taping the affected shin, and placing heel lifts in the shoes.

available to anyone willing to commit the time and effort. While millions of people are exercising, 60 percent of the adult population is not.

Principles of Conditioning

Becoming familiar with the principles of exercise is necessary to maximize the results of a physical fitness program. Your objectives can be met through the appropriate manipulation of intensity, frequency, duration, overload, progression, and specificity. Setting of objectives, warm-up, cooldown, and careful selection of activity are important elements that add to the enjoyment and effectiveness of exercise.

Intensity

Intensity refers to the degree of vigorousness of a single session of exercise. In 1995, The American College of Sports Medicine (ACSM) and the Centers for Disease Control and Prevention (CDC) developed and promoted

Table 3-1   Health-Related Benefits Associated with Regular Aerobic Exercise

Reduces the risk of cardiovascular disease

- Increases HDL cholesterol
- Decreases LDL cholesterol
- Favorably changes the ratios between total cholesterol and HDL-C and between LDL-C and HDL-C
- Decreases triglyceride levels
- Promotes relaxation; relieves stress and tension
- Decreases body fat and favorably changes body composition
- Reduces blood pressure, especially if it is high
- Makes blood platelets less sticky
- Decreases the incidence of cardiac dysrhythmias
- Increases myocardial efficiency
    1. Lowers resting heart rate
    2. Increases stroke volume
- Increases oxygen-carrying capacity of the blood
- Reduces the risk of colon cancer and breast cancer

Helps control diabetes

- Makes cells less resistant to insulin
- Reduces body fat

Develops stronger bones less susceptible to injury

Promotes joint stability

- Increases muscular strength
- Increases strength of the ligaments, tendons, cartilage, and connective tissue

Contributes to fewer lower-back problems

Acts as a stimulus for other lifestyle changes

Improves self-concept

---

the following recommendation for exercise: Every U.S. adult should accumulate 30 minutes or more of moderately intense physical activity on most and preferably all days of the week.[17] The recommendation refers to *physical activity* rather than *exercise*. This is an umbrella term that includes many types of physical exertion, including structured exercise. *Moderate intensity* refers to walking at a 3 to 4 mile per hour pace (15 to 20 minutes per mile) or engaging in any activity that burns a similar number of calories at a similar rate. The 30 minutes of activity can be split up into two or three bouts of 10 to 15 minutes each throughout the day. Table 3-2 provides a summary of the ACSM-CDC exercise principles and their application to the enhancement of health and physical fitness.

The recommendation for health enhancement is a minimum guideline designed to motivate and recruit that 60 percent of the population not physically active. It is not intended to lower the standard for those who currently exercise at a higher level or whose primary goal is the development of physical fitness. Programs designed primarily to improve health may not improve or may minimally improve physical fitness. It takes higher-intensity exercise to significantly improve physical fitness. Those who exercise for physical fitness purposes also derive health benefits in a two-for-one deal. It takes a slightly higher level of training to achieve both.

HR_{max} can be measured by a physical work capacity test on a treadmill or cycle ergometer. Because most people do not have access to such tests, HR_{max} can be estimated by subtracting age from 220. A 20-year-old person has an estimated HR_{max} of 200 beats per

minute (220 − 20 = 200). This formula predicts rather than measures HR_{max}; therefore, a measurement error of approximately plus or minus 10 to 12 beats per minute is associated with its use.

After the HR_{max} has been determined, the target for exercise may be calculated. The easiest method for determining the target zone for exercise is to use the percentage of HR_{max} recommended by ACSM (see the example that follows). The target zone for exercise provides the desirable heart rate for the development of physical fitness. For the 20-year-old person whose HR_{max} is 200 beats per minute, the target zone for exercise is calculated as follows:

$$\begin{array}{r} 200 \text{ (estimated } HR_{max}) \\ \underline{\times\, 0.55} \text{ (55\% of } HR_{max}) \\ 110 \text{ (lower-limit target HR)} \end{array}$$

$$\begin{array}{r} 200 \text{ (estimated } HR_{max}) \\ \underline{\times\, 0.90} \text{ (90\% of } HR_{max} \\ 180 \text{ (upper-limit target HR)} \end{array}$$

This 20-year-old person should exercise at a heart rate range between 110 and 180 beats per minute, depending on objectives and level of fitness. A 20-year-old person who is sedentary, and possibly overweight, should exercise at the lowest percentage of HR_{max} (55%). A same age subject who is at an average physical fitness level should exercise at 70 to 75% of the HR_{max}, and a 20-year-old person who is fit should exercise at 80 to 90% of the HR_{max}. The target for a person who has an average level of fitness is 140 to 150 beats per minute for exercise. The training effect occurs at heart rate levels below the maximum.

Table 3-2 Summary of Exercise Principles for the Development of Physical Fitness and Health

	Exercise Goals	
Exercise Principles	**To Develop and Improve Level of Physical Fitness (1998 Guidelines)**	**To Develop and Improve Health Status (1995 Guidelines)**
Intensity	• 55/65 to 90% of HR_{max} • 55 to 64% of HR_{max} for sedentary beginners • 40/50 to 85% of the cardiac reserve or 40/50 to 85% of the VO_2 reserve*	• Moderate (walking 3 to 4 MPH)
Frequency	• 3–5 days per week	• Most, preferably all, days of the week
Duration (time)	• 20–60 minutes at 60 to 90% of HR_{max} • 200–300 calories per exercise session	• 30 minutes or more
Overload	• Should not exceed 10% of the previous workout	• NA**
Progression	• Based on physiological readiness • According to the schedule of overload	• NA
Specificity	• For competitors training for maximal performance	• NA

*The VO_2 reserve is VO_2 max minus VO_2 rest.

**not applicable

Another method for calculating exercise heart rate, the Karvonen formula, considers fitness level and resting heart rate. The training heart rate is calculated with this formula by using a percentage of the heart rate reserve (cardiac reserve), the difference between the HR_{max} and the resting heart rate. The best way to determine the resting heart rate for this method is to count your pulse rate for fifteen seconds while in the sitting position immediately after waking in the morning. You should repeat this for four to five consecutive days and average the readings for a relatively accurate representation of your resting heart rate. Next, you should estimate your level of fitness based on your exercise habits and select a category from table 3-3 to determine the appropriate exercise intensity level. If you cannot decide which category is the most appropriate, take one of the fitness tests at the end of this chapter. Your performance on these should place you in a category that reflects your physical fitness level.

The Karvonen formula is

$$THR = (MHR - RHR) \times TI\% + RHR$$

where *THR* is the training heart rate, or the heart rate that should be maintained during exercise, *MHR* is the maximum heart rate, *RHR* is the resting heart rate, and

Table 3-3 Guidelines for Selecting Exercise Intensity Level

Fitness Level	Intensity Level (%)
Low	60
Fair	65
Average	70
Good	75
Excellent	80–90

TI% is the training intensity (see table 3-3). Therefore the exercise heart rate for a 25-year-old with a resting heart rate of 75 beats per minute and an average fitness level is calculated as follows:

$$\begin{array}{r} 220 \\ \underline{- 25} \\ 195 \end{array} \ (HR_{max})$$

$$\begin{aligned} THR &= (195 - 75) \times 0.70 + 75 \\ &= 120 \times 0.70 + 75 \\ &= 84 + 75 \\ &= 159 \end{aligned}$$

The training heart rate for this 25-year-old subject is 159 beats per minute. Assessment Activity 3-4 will enable you to determine your target heart rate for exercise.

Learning to take the pulse rate quickly and accurately is necessary to monitor exercise intensity by heart rate. Two of the most commonly used sites for taking the pulse rate are the radial artery on the thumb side of the wrist and the carotid artery at the side of the neck (figure 3-1A and 3-1B). Use the first two fingers of your preferred hand to palpate the pulse. At the wrist, the pulse is located at the base of the thumb when the hand is held palm up. To find the carotid pulse, slide your fingers downward at the angle of the jaw below the earlobe to the side of the neck. You apply only enough pressure to feel the pulse, particularly at the carotid artery. Excessive pressure at this point stimulates specialized receptors that automatically slow the heart rate, leading to an underestimation of the rate achieved during exercise. The wrist is the preferred site for the *palpation* (examination by touch or feel) of the pulse rate. Palpate the carotid pulse if you cannot feel your pulse at the wrist.

Locate and count the pulse rate immediately after exercise stops. Count the beats for ten seconds and multiply by 6 to get beats per minute. Regardless of which site you use, be consistent in its application. Some practice is required to locate the pulse quickly and count it accurately.

Another method for monitoring the intensity of exercise is to rate your subjective perception of the effort. On some days, exercise seems easier than normal, and on other days it may seem more difficult, therefore it is important to adjust the intensity according to the perception of the effort. According to ACSM, "the appropriate exercise intensity is one that is safe, is compatible with a long-term active lifestyle for that individual, and achieves the desired caloric output given the time constraints for the exercise session."[1]

The "Talk Test" is a simple subjective estimate that clearly demonstrates whether the individual is exercising too intensely. The intensity is excessive when the exerciser is unable to carry on a conversation without gasping for breath between each word or two. The remedy for such an occurrence is simple—*slow down the pace.*

Frequency

The *frequency* of exercise refers to the number of days of participation each week. The 1990 ACSM guidelines for improving physical fitness recommend that exercise be pursued three to five days per week for optimal results. Fewer than three days is an inadequate stimulus for developing fitness, and conversely, more than five days per week represents a point of diminishing returns from exercise and increases the likelihood of injury.

(a)

(b)

Figure 3-1 Sites for Taking a Pulse

The two sites for measuring pulse: (a) location for taking a pulse at the neck (carotid artery); (b) location for taking a pulse at the wrist (radial artery).

Those who are exercising for health reasons and following the 1995 guidelines are advised to engage in physical activities on most, preferably all, days of the week.

You can overdo exercise—too much results in staleness or overtraining. The signs of overtraining include the following:

- A feeling of chronic fatigue and listlessness
- Inability to make further fitness gains or regression of the level of fitness
- Sudden loss of weight
- An increase of 5 beats per minute in the resting heart rate
- Loss of enthusiasm for working out
- An increase in the risk for injury
- The occurrence of irritability, anger, and depression

Treatment requires that you cut back on training or stop completely for one to two weeks. When you resume exercise, it must be of lower intensity, frequency, and duration. You must rebuild and regain fitness gradually. Prevention is the best treatment for overtraining because people for whom exercise is a way of life are reluctant to discontinue training, even temporarily, for fear that they will lose their fitness edge. Convincing them that continuing to exercise is the worst possible action is extremely difficult.

Time (Duration)

Duration refers to the length of each exercise session. Intensity and duration are inversely related—the more intense the exercise, the shorter its duration. Some fitness experts employ the acronym "FIT Principle" as a means for people to remember the first three principles of exercise: F = frequency; I = intensity; and T = time/duration. Intensity is the most important consideration for the

Wellness On the Web
Behavior Change Activities

Why Exercise?

How do experts define physical fitness? There's no general agreement, but most authorities endorse the concept of performance-related and health-related fitness. Like all aspects of wellness, you are responsible for developing an exercise program and sticking with it. Taking this step is much easier when you understand the importance of exercise as an integral part of a quality life-style. Stephen Seiler, Ph.D, is an endurance sport enthusiast and exercise physiologist who has a strong interest in the physiology of performance and in the role of exercise as "preventive medicine." To enhance your understanding of exercise physiology as it relates to wellness, read Dr. Seiler's articles at **www.mhhe.com/anspaugh5e**. Select "Student Center," "Chapter 3," "Wellness on the Web." Scroll down the list of topics and read more about a specific area of exercise physiology as it relates to your wellness and fitness goals.

The Key to Your Heart

When we say someone is "heartless," we're speaking figuratively, not literally. From the moment we're conceived until we draw our last breath, our heart works tirelessly to fuel the processes that give us life. In an average lifetime, the heart beats more than two and a half billion times without stopping to rest. Throughout history, this life-sustaining power has created an aura of mystery around the heart. Modern science has removed much of the mystery, but we continue to be fascinated and curious about this vital human organ. To explore the heart in detail, go to **http://sln.fi.edu/biosci/biosci.html**. In "The Heart: An Online Exploration," you'll discover the complexities of the heart's development and structure. You'll have the opportunity to follow the blood as it circulates through the blood vessels and the various body systems. Most important, you'll learn how to keep your heart healthy and how to monitor your heart's health.

development of physical fitness. But reducing the intensity somewhat while increasing the frequency and duration is the safest and most beneficial method for novice exercisers to attain physical fitness and health enhancement. In 1990, the ACSM recommended 20 to 60 minutes of continuous or noncontinuous aerobic activity. The 1995 guidelines suggest the accumulation of 30 minutes or more of physical activity per day.[17]

Another way to monitor duration is to calculate the number of calories expended per exercise session. The

ACSM recommends that, if you expend 300 calories per exercise session, you should exercise three times per week; if you expend only 200 calories per exercise session, you should exercise four times per week. These guidelines are sufficient for health benefits to accrue, but for fitness purposes, they should be viewed as a minimal level of exercise. (Table 8-5 in Chapter 8 discusses the way to determine how long you need to engage in the activities of your choice to achieve these goals.)

Progression, Overload, and Specificity

As people attain a level of fitness that meets their needs and when further improvement is not desired, the program switches from developing fitness to maintaining it. At this point the principles of overload and progression may be set aside, but both are necessary for the improvement phase of fitness. *Overload* involves subjecting the body to unaccustomed stress. Challenging the body to periodically accept a slightly increased level of work forces it to adapt by attaining a higher level of fitness. Deciding when to impose each new challenge involves the principle of progression. The workload is increased only when the exerciser is ready to accept a new challenge. For aerobic exercise, target heart rate or perceived exertion may be used to establish criteria for scheduling the progression. For example, if you jog, swim, or cycle a certain distance, the exercise heart rate will decrease over time as your body adapts to training. When the exercise heart rate drops to a predetermined level or the effort required becomes comfortable, you should adjust the pace or distance to return to the original target zone. However, the new physical challenge should not exceed the current amount of exercise by more than 10 percent. This should ensure that the new workload is not excessive.

The principle of *specificity* of training suggests that the body adapts according to the specific type of stress placed on it. The muscles involved in any activity are the ones that adapt, and they do so in the specific way in which they are used. For example, jogging prepares one for jogging but is poor preparation for cycling. Cycling does not prepare one for swimming. Although these activities stress the cardiorespiratory system, they are sufficiently different in that there is little fitness carryover among them.

The principle of specificity is particularly important for competitive athletes. Competitors attempt to maximize the returns from their training effort; therefore, runners must train by running, swimmers must swim, and cyclists must cycle. The focus is on maximal improvement in one activity so that the body is trained in a specific manner. This locks athletes into regimented training programs, but noncompetitors who exercise for health and physical fitness reasons are not under such constraints. They can vary activities and prevent the boredom of participating in the same activity day after day, week after week. Cycling, jogging, swimming, racquetball, cross-country skiing, weight training, and other activities may be used in any combination or order for the development of physical fitness. This is the essence of **cross-training**. Not only does cross-training relieve boredom, it may reduce the incidence of injury because it does not stress the same muscles in the same way during every workout.

Cross-training has many advantages and is an excellent technique for attaining the health benefits of exercise. Variety, the major attraction of cross-training, can also be a disadvantage, however. By participating in many different activities, you seldom become proficient in any one. However, if the objective is physical fitness or health enhancement, proficiency is incidental.

Identifying goals provides some direction for the activities selected and the way the principles of exercise are to be manipulated to increase the probability of success. Only one or two major goals should be selected, and these should be as specific as possible so that an effective exercise program may be devised. Activities, objectives, and exercise principles must match.

When you have identified the objectives and know what you wish to achieve from the exercise program, identify the means for sustaining the program. The resolve to exercise is shakiest during the early stages of the program, usually because people push untrained bodies beyond their limits. This results in sore muscles, stiffness, and possible injury. Consequently, the dropout rate is highest in the beginning of any exercise program. The irony is that the greatest return for the effort is attained during this phase. Some tips for sustaining that effort are presented in Just the Facts: Motivational Tips.

Other Exercise Considerations

Warming Up for Exercise

Warming up prepares the body for physical action. The process involves physical activities that gradually heat the muscles and elevate the heart rate. A brisk walk, slow jog, jogging or hopping in place, rope jumping, and selected calisthenics will raise the heart rate and increase muscle temperature. A person should break out in a sweat during the warm-up. This indicates that heart rate and body temperature have increased to some extent and the person is ready for more vigorous activity. The warm-up should last 5 to 10 minutes.

Just the Facts

Motivational Tips

Follow these tips to stay motivated to exercise:

- Exercise with a friend. Make sure both of you have compatible goals and are similar in fitness level. Friends can help each other sustain a program, particularly during busy times when the temptation is high to push exercise out of an already crowded schedule.
- Exercise with a group. Exchange ideas and literature about exercise with group members.
- Elicit the support of friends and family. Their support is a powerful source of reinforcement.
- Associate with other exercisers. They represent an enthusiastic, positive, and informative group—and their values are contagious.
- Join an exercise class or a fitness club. This gives you a place to go and meet people who want to exercise.
- Keep a progress chart. This will give you an objective account of your improvement.
- Exercise to music. Music makes the effort appear easier.
- Set a definite time and place to exercise. This is particularly important during the early days of the program. Schedule exercise as you would any other activity of importance and then commit to the schedule.
- Participate in a variety of activities. Cross-training is excellent for the person who exercises for health or recreation.
- Do not become obsessive about exercise. Skipping exercise is not a good practice normally, but skipping is appropriate at times. Do not exercise when you are sick or overtired. Do not feel guilty about missing exercise for a day or two. Resume exercise as soon as you can.

Increasing the heart rate gradually during the warm-up is most important. This allows the circulatory system to adjust to the load. If the heart rate elevates suddenly, circulation cannot adjust rapidly enough to meet the oxygen and nutrient demands of the heart muscle. The effects of this lag time are abolished in about 2 minutes, but increasing the heart rate quickly can be hazardous even during those 2 minutes, particularly for those with compromised circulation. Even the healthy heart may be affected by eliminating the gradual phase of warm-up. One study showed that every one of forty-four healthy male subjects, ages 21 to 52 years, had normal electrocardiogram (ECG) responses to running on a treadmill when they were allowed a warm-up consisting of 2 minutes of easy jogging. However, 70 percent of the group developed abnormal ECG responses to the same exercise when they were not allowed to warm up.[18]

Warm-up may be specifically tailored to the activity to be performed. For example, joggers may warm up by slowly jogging the first 0.5 to 0.75 mile, gradually speeding up to the desired pace. Cyclists, swimmers, cross-country skiers, and rope skippers may use the same approach.

Passive warm-up techniques, such as massage, sauna baths, steam baths, hot showers, hot towels, and heating pads, should not be used as substitutes for an active warm-up. These techniques may precede an active warm-up if a person feels stiff and sore from the previous workout.

Stretching exercises may be performed after the warm-up is completed. At this point, muscle temperature is elevated so that stretching is more effective and muscle, tendon, and joint injuries are less likely to occur. Stretching is most effective during the cooldown following the workout because (1) muscles are heated and receptive to stretching, and (2) muscles that have contracted repeatedly during exercise need to be stretched. Figures 5-1 through 5-8 in Chapter 5 illustrate some typical stretching exercises that may be used before and after the workout period.

Cooling Down from Exercise

The cooldown is as important as the warm-up. Cooldown should last 8 to 10 minutes and consist of two phases. The first phase involves approximately 5 minutes of walking or other light activities to prevent blood from pooling in the muscles that have been working. Light activity causes rhythmic contractions of the muscles, which in turn act as a stimulus to circulate blood from the muscles to the heart for redistribution throughout the body. This boost to circulation following exercise, often referred to as the *muscle pump,* is essential for recovery and shares some of the burden of circulation with the heart. The muscle pump effect does not occur if a period of inactivity follows exercise. An inactive cooldown forces the heart to work at a high rate to compensate for the reduced volume of blood returning to it because of blood pooling in the muscles. The exerciser runs the risk of dizziness, fainting, and more serious consequences associated with diminished blood flow to vital organs.

Light physical activity after exercise also speeds the removal of lactic acid that has accumulated in the mus-

cles. *Lactic acid* is a fatiguing metabolite resulting from the incomplete breakdown of sugar. It is produced by exercise of high intensity or of long duration.

The second phase of cooldown should focus on the stretching exercises performed during the warm-up. Most participants find that stretching after exercise is more comfortable and more effective because the muscles are heated and more elastic.

Type of Activity

Many activities contribute to one or more components of health-related physical fitness. Activity selections should be based on objectives, skill level, availability of equipment, facilities, instruction, climate, and interest. Any rhythmic, continuous aerobic activity that uses large muscle groups and can be performed for an extended period is suitable for the attainment of health and fitness.

The President's Council on Physical Fitness and Sports (PCPFS) enlisted the aid of seven experts to evaluate fourteen popular physical activities for their contribution to physical fitness and general well-being. Although this assessment occurred several years ago, the ratings are as valid today as when they were originally conceived. A summary of these appears in table 3-4.

Selected sports have also been evaluated for their contribution to the health-related components of physical fitness. These appear in table 3-5. Lifetime sports (such as tennis, badminton, and racquetball) are more conducive to fitness development than are team sports (such as volleyball, soccer, softball, and basketball) because fewer players are needed. Ideally, fitness should be developed and maintained primarily through self-paced activities (for example, jogging, cycling, walking, and swimming), but the challenge inherent in sports may be necessary to sustain motivation for some people. Lifetime sports are challenging and fun, and they offer variety. However, fitness attained from these activities depends on skill level and a willingness to exert maximal effort in competition. The orthopedic demands of these activities may be greater than a sedentary beginner can tolerate. Quick stops and starts, bursts of high-intensity activity, sudden changes of direction, and rapid twists and turns place a great deal of stress on the musculoskeletal system. The physically fit can handle the aerobic and musculoskeletal requirements of active sports, but attempting to "play yourself into shape" is a mistake. With knowledge of the principles of exercise, warm-up, cooldown, and the contributions of various physical activities to physical fitness, you can design an exercise program using Assessment Activity 3-5. See Real-World Wellness: Choosing Fitness Equipment for the Home for helpful advice on exercising at home.

Table 3-4 Rating Fourteen Sports and Exercises

Exercise	Cardio-respiratory Endurance (Stamina)	Muscular Endurance	Muscular Strength	Flexibility	Balance	General Well-Being				Total
						Weight Control	Muscle Definition	Digestion	Sleep	
Jogging	21*	20	17	9	17	21	14	13	16	148
Bicycling	19	18	16	9	18	20	15	12	15	142
Swimming	21	20	14	15	12	15	14	13	16	140
Skating (ice or roller)	18	17	15	13	20	17	14	11	15	140
Handball/squash	19	18	15	16	17	19	11	13	12	140
Skiing—nordic	19	19	15	14	16	17	12	12	15	139
Skiing—alpine	16	18	15	14	21	15	14	9	12	134
Basketball	19	17	15	13	16	19	13	10	12	134
Tennis	16	16	14	14	16	16	13	12	11	128
Calisthenics	10	13	16	19	15	12	18	11	12	126
Walking	13	14	11	7	8	13	11	11	14	102
Golf**	8	8	9	9	8	6	6	7	6	67
Softball	6	8	7	9	7	7	5	8	7	64
Bowling	5	5	5	7	6	5	5	7	6	51

*The ratings are on a scale of 0 to 3; thus a rating of 21 is the maximum score that can be achieved (a score by 3 of all seven panelists). Ratings were made on the following basis: frequency, four times per week minimal; duration, 30 to 60 minutes per session.

**The rating was made on the basis of using a golf cart or caddy. If you walk the course and carry your clubs, the values improve.

Table 3-5 Rating Selected Sports

Sport	Cardiorespiratory Endurance	Muscular Strength/Endurance		Flexibility	Body Composition
		Upper	Lower		
Badminton	M-H*	L	M-H	L	M-H
Football (touch)	L-M	L-M	M	L	L-M
Ice hockey	H	M	H	L	H
Racquetball	H	M	H	M	H
Rugby	H	M-H	H	M	H
Soccer	H	L	H	M	H
Volleyball	M	M	M	L-M	M
Wrestling	H	H	H	M-H	H

*H, high; M, medium; L, low. The values in this table are estimates that vary according to the skill and motivation of the participants.

Environmental Conditions

People work and exercise in a variety of environmental conditions. Hot and cold weather produce unique problems for people who function outdoors. Their safety and comfort depend on their knowledge of the ways the body reacts to physical activity in different climatic conditions.

Heat is produced in the body as a by-product of metabolism. Physical activities significantly increase metabolism, generating more heat than normal. Heat must be dissipated efficiently, or heat may build up,

Real-World Wellness

Choosing Fitness Equipment for the Home

I'm a working mother with two young children. My only chance to exercise is at home after the children have been put to bed. I'm most interested in purchasing a good piece of cardio equipment that will burn calories and increase my energy level. What advice can you give me for selecting such equipment?

Here are some helpful hints:

1. Some of the most effective cardio equipment includes motor-driven treadmills, stationary exercise bikes, stationary rowers, stair climbers, cross-country skiing machines, videotape aerobic workouts (with or without stepping benches), and jump ropes.

2. Selecting the right piece of equipment is important. Many well-intentioned home exercisers become bored with the equipment they purchase or find that it is not meeting their needs, so they quit exercising.

3. Try out a piece of equipment before buying it. Make sure it feels comfortable, is easy to use, and is the right size for you.

4. Give equipment the three-week test: Before making your purchase, borrow or rent the piece of equipment and use it three to five times per week for three weeks. At the end of three weeks, you should know whether you enjoy it well enough to use it regularly and whether it will meet your needs and goals. The best equipment in the world is useless unless you use it regularly.

5. Check the construction of equipment to make sure that it is sturdy. The machine should not rock or wobble, and it should perform smoothly.

6. Equipment made of lightweight sheet metal or with many plastic parts may not withstand regular use.

7. Do not buy the least expensive machine. Think of this purchase as a long-term investment. Usually a middle-of-the line product will do very well. These carry a ninety-day warranty for parts, and the warranty may be extended to also include service.

8. Shop at a reputable sports equipment store that has a knowledgeable sales staff who can answer your questions and help you make the appropriate choice.

9. Make sure that the store will deliver and set up the equipment.

10. If marketing and promotional claims made for the equipment sound too good to be true, they probably are.

resulting in **hyperthermia**, abnormally high body temperature that can cause illness or even death. *Heat exhaustion* is also a serious condition but not an imminent threat to life. It is characterized by dizziness, fainting, rapid pulse, and cool skin. Treatment includes immediate cessation of activity. The victim should be moved to a cool, shady place, placed in a reclining position, and given cool fluids to drink.

Heat stroke is a medical emergency and a threat to life. It is the most severe of the heat-induced illnesses. The symptoms include a high temperature (106° F or higher) and dry skin caused by the cessation of sweating. These symptoms are accompanied by delirium, convulsions, or loss of consciousness. The early warning signs include chills, nausea, headache, and general weakness. Victims of heat stroke should be rushed immediately to the nearest hospital for treatment.

Mechanisms of Heat Loss

Heat is lost from the body by conduction, convection, radiation, and evaporation of sweat. Conduction, convection, and radiation are mechanisms responsible for heat loss *and* heat gain. These three depend on the difference between the temperature of the body and that of the environment. These mechanisms do not function alone to effect heat loss or gain.

Conduction occurs when direct physical contact is made between objects of which one is cooler than the other. The greater the difference in temperature between the objects, the greater the transfer of heat. An example is entering an air-conditioned room from outdoors on a summer day and sitting in a cool leather chair. Heat is lost through contact with the cooler chair.

Conductive heat loss occurs even more rapidly in water.[5] Water is not an insulator but a conductor. It absorbs several thousand times more heat than does air at the same temperature. Air is an excellent insulator but a poor conductor. This is the reason that sitting at poolside is more comfortable than sitting in the pool, even if the temperatures of air and water are equal.

Heat loss or gain by *convection* occurs when a gas or water moves across the skin. Heat is transferred from the body to the environment more effectively if a breeze is blowing. Convective heat loss in water is increased when a person is swimming rather than floating because of the increased movement of the water across the body. The same principle applies to running outdoors because of the air flow over the body.

Humans, animals, and inanimate objects constantly transmit heat by electromagnetic waves to cooler objects in the environment. This heat loss through *radiation* occurs without physical contact between objects. Heat is transferred on a temperature gradient from warmer objects to cooler ones.

Heat loss by radiation is effective when the air temperature (ambient temperature) is well below skin temperature. This is one of the main reasons that outdoor exercise in cool weather is better tolerated than the same exercise in hot weather. Temperatures in the upper 80s and 90s often result in heat gain by radiation.

Evaporation of sweat is the main method of heat loss during exercise, and this process is most effective when the humidity is low. High humidity significantly impairs the evaporative process because the air is saturated and cannot accept much moisture. If both temperature and humidity are high, losing heat is difficult by any of these processes. Under these conditions, adjusting the intensity and duration of exercise or moving indoors, where the climate can be controlled, may be beneficial.

Heat loss by evaporation occurs only when the sweat on the surface of the skin is vaporized—that is, converted to a gas. The conversion of liquid to a gas at the skin level requires heat supplied by the body. As liquid sweat absorbs heat from the skin, it changes to a gaseous vapor carried away by the surrounding air, resulting in the removal of heat generated from exercise. Small amounts of evaporative sweat remove large quantities of heat. For example, each pint of sweat that evaporates removes approximately 280 calories of heat. Beads of sweat that roll off the body do not contribute to the cooling process—only sweat that evaporates does.

Exercise in hot and humid conditions forces the body to divert more blood than usual from the working muscles to the skin in an effort to carry the heat accumulating in the deeper recesses to the outer shell. The result is that the exercising muscles are deprived of a full complement of blood and cannot work as long or as hard. Exercise is therefore more difficult in hot and humid weather.

Heat loss by evaporation is seriously impeded when a person wears nonporous garments, such as rubberized and plastic exercise suits. These garments encourage sweating, but their nonporous nature does not allow sweat to evaporate. This practice is dangerous because it may easily result in heat buildup and *dehydration* (excessive water loss), leading to heat-stress illnesses. You should dress for hot-weather exercise by wearing shorts and a porous top. A mesh, baseball-type cap is optional. It is effective in blocking the absorption of radiant heat if you exercise in the middle of the day because the sun's rays are vertical. You do not need to wear a cap when exercising in the cooler times of the day or if the sun is not shining.

Guidelines for Exercise in the Heat

Guidelines for exercising in heat and humidity have been developed for road races, but these guidelines can be ap-

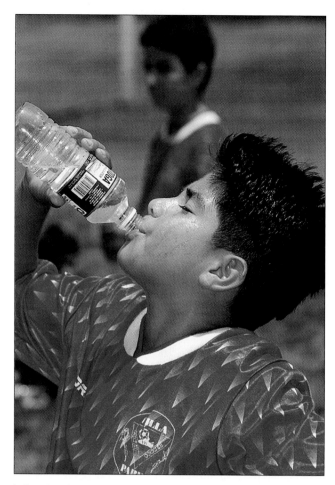

In hot, humid weather, drinking water and wearing loose clothing help prevent hyperthermia and heat stress illnesses.

plied to any strenuous physical activity performed outdoors during warm weather. Ambient conditions are considered safe when the temperature is below 70° F and the humidity is below 60 percent. Caution should be used and people sensitive to heat and humidity should reconsider exercising when the temperature is greater than 80° F or the humidity is over 60 percent. People who are trained and heat acclimated can continue to exercise in these conditions, but they should be aware of the potential hazards and take precautions to prevent heat illness.

The keys to exercising without incident in hot weather are acclimating to the heat and maintaining the body's normal fluid level. The main consequence of dehydration (excessive fluid loss) is a reduction in blood volume. This results in sluggish circulation that decreases the delivery of oxygen to the exercising muscles. Lowered blood volume results in less blood that can be sent to the skin to remove the heat generated by exercise. If too much of the blood volume is lost, sweating stops and the body temperature rises, leading to heat stress illness. Heat illness is a serious problem that can be avoided by following these guidelines designed to preserve the body's fluid level:

- Estimating water loss:
  - Weigh yourself nude before and after exercise.
  - Towel off sweat completely after exercise and then weigh yourself.
  - Each pound of weight loss represents about 1 pint of fluid loss. Be sure to drink that and more after exercise. See Just the Facts: Fluid Consumption Before, During, and After Exercise.
- Other considerations:
  - Modify the exercise program by (1) working out during cooler times of day, (2) choosing shady routes where water is available, (3) slowing the pace or shortening the duration of exercise on particularly oppressive days, and (4) wearing light, loose, porous clothing to facilitate the evaporation of sweat.
  - Never take salt tablets. They are stomach irritants, they attract fluid to the gut, they sometimes pass through the digestive system undissolved, and they may perforate the stomach lining.
  - Exercise must be prolonged, produce profuse sweating, and occur over a number of consecutive days to reduce potassium stores. For the average bout of exercise, you do not need to worry about depleting potassium or make a special effort to replace it. The daily consumption of fresh fruits and vegetables, as suggested by the food pyramid, is all that is needed (see Chapter 6).
  - Remember to use a sunscreen lotion when the weather is sunny or hazy. Be sure that the sunscreen you select has a sun-protection factor (SPF) of at least 15, and apply it liberally over exposed skin.

Guidelines for Exercise in the Cold

Problems related to exercise in cold weather include frostbite and **hypothermia** (abnormally low body temperature). *Frostbite* can lead to permanent damage or loss of a body part from gangrene. This can be prevented by adequately protecting exposed areas, such as fingers, nose, ears, facial skin, and toes. Gloves, preferably mittens or thick socks, should be worn to protect the fingers, hands, and wrists. Blood vessels in the scalp do not constrict effectively, so a significant amount of heat is lost if a head covering is not worn. A stocking-type hat is the best head covering because it can be pulled down to protect the ears. In very cold or windy weather, use surgical or ski masks and scarves to keep facial skin warm and to moisten and warm inhaled air. All exposed or poorly protected flesh is vulnerable to frostbite when the temperature is low and the wind-chill high. Air temperature plus wind speed equals the

Just the Facts

Fluid Consumption Before, During, and After Exercise

The American College of Sports Medicine[19] has issued the following recommendations about fluid consumption:

1. Make a special effort to drink plenty of fluid every day so that you will be fully hydrated prior to exercise.
2. For exercise lasting 60 minutes or less:
   - Drink a minimum of 1 pint (2 cups) of water about two hours prior to exercise.
   - Start drinking soon after exercise begins and continue drinking at regular intervals in an effort to replace the fluid lost from sweating.
   - Drink cool fluids (59° F to 72° F) flavored for palatability, because cool fluids do not interfere with stomach emptying, they do not cause stomach cramping, and they absorb some of the body's internal heat.
3. For intense exercise lasting 60 minutes or more:
   - Drink fluids that contain a small amount of carbohydrates (sugar: glucose, sucrose; starch: maltodextrin) and sodium on a regular basis.
   - Regularly ingest carbohydrates to maintain blood glucose level and delay fatigue.
   - Ingest sodium in very small amounts (0.5 to 0.75 gram per liter of fluid) to enhance taste and promote fluid retention.
   - After the workout, continue drinking the same beverage until your thirst is satisfied and then drink some more.
4. Most exercisers are reluctant drinkers during workouts and do not drink enough to match the fluid they lose through sweating, but they should make a conscious effort to get enough fluid during exercise.
5. The general rule after exercise is to drink until you satisfy your thirst and then drink some more. The thirst mechanism of humans is a poor index of the body's need for fluid.
6. Water is an acceptable drink, but it may blunt the thirst drive before rehydration is complete. Therefore, find a tasty beverage that is noncarbonated, non-alcoholic, and caffeine free to drink after exercise. Homemade lemonade, fruit juices cut in half with water to reduce the concentration of sugar, and commercial sports drinks fit the bill nicely.[13]

windchill index. This value will help you know how to dress appropriately for outdoor exercise.

People often experience a hacking cough for a minute or two after physical exertion in cold weather. This is a normal response and should not cause alarm. Very cold, dry air may not be fully moistened when it is inhaled rapidly and in large volumes during exercise, so the lining of the throat dries out. When exercise is discontinued, the respiratory rate slows and the volume of inhaled air decreases, allowing enough time for the body to fully moisturize it. Coughing stops within a couple of minutes as the linings are remoistened.

Hypothermia is the most severe of the problems associated with outdoor activity in cold weather. Hypothermia occurs when body heat is lost faster than it can be produced. This can be a life-threatening situation.

Exercise in cold weather requires insulating layers of clothing to preserve normal body heat. Without this protection, body heat is quickly lost because of the large temperature gradient between the skin and environment. A layer or two of insulating clothing can be discarded if you get too hot.

Hypothermia can occur even if the air temperature is above freezing.[20] The rate of heat loss for any temperature is influenced by wind velocity. Wind velocity increases the amount of cold air molecules that come in contact with the skin. The more cold molecules, the more effective the heat loss. The speed of walking, jogging, or cycling into the wind must be added to the speed of the wind to properly evaluate the impact of windchill.

You should wear enough clothing to stay warm but not so much as to induce profuse sweating. Knowing how much clothing to wear comes from experience exercising in different environmental conditions. Clothing that becomes wet with sweat loses its insulating qualities. It becomes a conductor of heat, moving heat from the body quickly and potentially endangering the exerciser.

If you exercise or work outdoors in cold weather, you may want to wear polypropylene undergarments. Polypropylene is designed to whisk perspiration away from the skin so that evaporative cooling does not rob heat from the body. You should wear a warm outer garment, preferably made of wool, over this material, If it is windy, wear a breathable windbreaker as the third, outer layer.

If you follow the guidelines for activity in hot and cold weather, you can usually participate comfortably all year long. Other hazards associated with outdoor exercise are discussed in Real-World Wellness: Exercising Safely in an Urban Environment.

Real-World **Wellness**

Exercising Safely in an Urban Environment

I live in a large city and like to jog outdoors in my neighborhood. How can I limit the risks associated with exercising in the heart of the city?

You can start by becoming familiar with the risks to avoid or lessen their impact. Some of the major hazards follow:

1. Traffic volume is one of the primary risks associated with jogging in a large city. This risk can be reduced by wearing reflective clothing, jogging during daylight hours, and jogging on the sidewalks rather than the streets. The best way to handle the problem is to find a nearby park or outdoor running track.

2. A second risk comes from air pollution, primarily carbon monoxide and ozone. The Centers for Disease Control and Prevention has identified outdoor exercisers as one group at high risk for the effects of ozone, carbon monoxide, and other air pollutants. Rapid, deep breathing during exercise results in inhaling more pollutants more deeply into the lungs. Some studies have shown that 30 minutes of jogging during heavy traffic conditions increased carbon monoxide levels in the blood to the equivalent of smoking half a pack of cigarettes.

   Carbon monoxide interferes with the delivery of oxygen to the body's tissues and, when inhaled in high quantities, can cause illness and death. Carbon monoxide emissions from cars, trucks, and buses are most prevalent during rush hours, so avoid jogging on busy streets during these times.

   Ozone causes lung inflammation and injury. The long-term effects of exercising in high ozone conditions are not known. Ozone tends to accumulate in the atmosphere after 10:00 A.M. It is heaviest during bright, sunny days because it is produced by the photochemical reaction of sunlight with hydrocarbons and nitrogen dioxide from motor vehicle exhaust.

   Jogging before the rush hour begins will (1) help control your exposure to motor vehicle emissions and (2) allow you to exercise prior to the buildup of ozone in the atmosphere.

3. Joggers and other outdoor exercisers can be targets for crime. Carry no visible money or valuables, such as watches or jewelry. Carry an I.D. tag with your name and the telephone number of a family member or friend in case you are involved in an accident. Do not carry addresses, yours or your family's, in case you are mugged.

Summary

- *Physical fitness* is defined in terms of performance-related and health-related fitness.
- Cardiorespiratory endurance is the most important component of health-related fitness.
- The long-term effects of physical training include modifications in heart rate, stroke volume, cardiac output, blood volume, heart volume, respiration, and metabolism.
- Aerobic capacity is finite, improves by 5 to 25 percent with training, and decreases with aging; this decrease is slower in those who are physically fit.
- The training effect is lost in stages if exercise is interrupted or discontinued.
- Exercise affects cholesterol levels, blood pressure, and triglyceride levels, may reduce the risks of diabetes mellitus and stress, and is an alternative method for quitting use of tobacco products.
- The principles of exercise can be manipulated to meet any exercise objective.
- Exercising by varying the activities per exercise session or during exercise sessions is cross-training.
- The heat generated by exercise is lost from the body by conduction, convection, radiation, and evaporation.
- Evaporation of sweat is the major mechanism for ridding the body of heat that develops during exercise.
- Hypothermia is the most severe problem associated with exercise in cold weather.

Review Questions

1. What are the physiological changes that occur from regular participation in aerobic exercise?
2. What are the health benefits that occur from regular participation in aerobic training?
3. Name and define the physiological changes that occur with exercise training.
4. Identify and define the principles of physical conditioning.
5. Define *cross-training* and give some examples.
6. Why should you warm up before exercise?
7. Identify and define the mechanisms of heat loss. Which of these is most important during exercise and why?
8. Describe fluid replacement before, during, and after exercise.

References

1. ACSM. 2000. *ACSM's Guidelines for Exercise Testing and Prescription* (6th ed.). Philadelphia: Lippincott Williams and Wilkins.
2. ACSM. 1998. The recommended quantity and quality of exercise for developing and maintaining cardiorespiratory and muscular fitness and flexibility in healthy adults. *Medicine and Science in Sports and Exercise* 30(6):975.
3. Holly, R. G., and J. D. Shaffrath. 2001. Cardiorespiratory endurance. In *ACSM's Resource Manual* (4th ed.), ed. J. L. Roitman. Philadelphia: Lippincott Williams and Wilkins.
4. McArdle, W. D., F. I. Katch, and V. L. Katch. 1999. *Sports and Exercise Nutrition*. Philadelphia: Lippincott Williams and Wilkins.
5. Foss, M. L., and S. J. Keteyian. 1998. *Fox's Physiological Basis for Exercise and Sport*. Boston: WCB/McGraw-Hill.
6. Demaree, S. R., S. K. Powers, and J. M. Lawler. 2001. Fundamentals of exercise metabolism. In *ACSM's Resource Manual* (4th ed.), ed. J. L. Roitman. Philadelphia: Lippincott Williams and Wilkins.
7. Franklin, B. A., and J. L. Roitman. 2001. Cardiorespiratory adaptations to exercise. In *ACSM's Resource Manual* (4th ed.), ed. J. L. Roitman. Philadelphia: Lippincott Williams and Wilkins.
8. Coyle, E. F. 2001. Detraining and retention of adaptations induced by endurance training. In *ACSM's Resource Manual* (4th ed.), ed. J. L. Roitman. Philadelphia: Lippincott Williams and Wilkins.
9. Powers, S. K., and E. T. Howley. 2001. *Exercise Physiology*. Boston: McGraw-Hill.
10. Blair, S. N., et al. 1995. Changes in physical fitness and all-cause mortality. *Journal of the American Medical Association* 273:1093.
11. Williams, M. A. 2001. Human development and aging. In *ACSM's Resource Manual* (4th ed.), ed. J. L. Roit-
man. Philadelphia: Lippincott Williams and Wilkins.
12. U.S. Dept. of Health and Human Services. 1996. *Physical Activity and Health: A Report of the Surgeon General*. Atlanta: U.S. Dept. of Health and Human Services, Centers for Disease Control and Prevention, National Center for Chronic Disease Prevention and Health Promotion.
13. Nieman, D. C. 1999. *Exercise Testing and Prescription*. Mountain View, Calif.: Mayfield Publishing Co.
14. Beckham, S. 2001. Emergency procedures and exercise safety. In *ACSM's Resource Manual* (4th ed.), ed. J. L. Roitman. Philadelphia: Lippincott Williams and Wilkins.
15. Mittleman, M. A., et al. 1993. Triggering of acute myocardial infarction by heavy physical exertion. *New England Journal of Medicine* 329(23):1677.
16. Willich, S. N., et al. 1993. Physical exertion as a trigger of acute myocardial

infarction. *New England Journal of Medicine* 329(23):1684.

17. Pate, R. R., et al. 1995. Physical activity and public health. A recommendation from the Centers for Disease Control and Prevention and the American College of Sports Medicine. *Journal of the American Medical Association* 273:402.

18. Barnard, R. J., et al. 1973. Cardiovascular responses to sudden strenuous exercise—heart rate, blood pressure, and ECG. *Journal of Applied Physiology* 34:833.

19. American College of Sports Medicine. 1996. Position paper on exercise and fluid replacement. *Medicine and Science in Sports and Exercise* 28:1.

20. Bernard, T. E. 2001. Environmental considerations: heat and cold. In *ACSM's Resource Manual* (4th ed.), ed. J. L. Roitman. Philadelphia: Lippincott Williams and Wilkins.

Suggested Readings

University of California at Berkeley. 2001. A dozen ways to improve your walking workouts. *University of California at Berkeley Wellness Letter* 17(17):6.

Walking is the easiest, safest, and cheapest way to become and stay fit. This article discusses and defines "brisk walking" and then presents twelve practical ways to increase the intensity of walking. Almost anyone interested in walking for fitness can incorporate at least some of these in his or her workout.

Harvard University. 2001. Walking and gardening beneficial for heart disease patients. *Harvard Heart Letter* 11(8):6–7.

The information in this article came from the British Regional Heart Study. The data suggested that moderate exercise performed on a regular basis was more effective in lowering cardiovascular risks than most medicines. The study concluded that doctors should prescribe forty minutes of daily walking, and patients should fill this prescription as willingly as they fill their prescriptions for medicine.

Harvard University. 2000. Vigorous activity lowers diabetes risk. *Harvard Heart Letter* 10(5):6–7.

Participation in vigorous physical activities provides more protection against diabetes than mild or moderate forms of exercise. Activities such as jogging, running, cycling, swimming, tennis, and aerobic dance are some of many that fall into the vigorous category.

Liebman, B., and D. Schardt. 2001. Diet and health—ten megatrends. *Nutrition Action Health Letter* 28(1):1–13.

Discusses ten major trends having substantial effects on the U.S. population. One of these trends is the declining amount of physical activity in the United States that has led to a 10-pound weight gain each decade. The authors concluded that "physical activity is as close as we've come to a magic bullet to improve health."

Welk, G. J., and S. M. Blair. 2000. Physical activity protects against the health risks of obesity. *President's Council on Physical Fitness and Sports Research Digest* 3(13):1–8.

Defines and discusses the reasons for rising obesity in the United States. It delineates the role of exercise and discusses some of the major epidemiological studies that have examined the relationship between the two. Exercise has a protective effect against obesity and the mechanisms by which this occurs are explained.

Assessment Activity 3-1

The Rockport Fitness Walking Test

Directions: This walking test estimates aerobic capacity based on the variables of age, gender, time required to walk 1 mile, and the heart rate achieved at the end of the test. The guidelines for taking the test are as follows:

1. Count your heart rate for 15 seconds and multiply by 4 to get beats per minute.
2. The course should be flat and measured, preferably a 440-yard track.
3. Use a stopwatch or a watch with a second hand.
4. Warm up for 5 to 10 minutes before taking the test. Preparation for the test should include a 0.25-mile walk followed by the stretching exercises.
5. During the test, walk at a brisk pace, covering 1 mile as rapidly as possible.
6. Take your pulse rate immediately after the test. Mark this rate on the chart on the following pages that is appropriate for your age and gender.
7. Draw a vertical line through your time and a horizontal line through your heart rate. The point where the lines intersect determines your fitness level.

Rockport provides a series of twenty-week walking-for-fitness programs based on the results of the walking test. These may be obtained for a nominal fee ($1 at this writing) by sending a request to Rockport Fitness Walking Test, 72 Howe Street, Marlboro, Massachusetts, 01752.

The charts on the following pages are designed to tell you how fit you are compared with other individuals of your age and gender. For example, if your coordinates place you in the "above average" section of the chart, you are in better shape than the average person in your category.

The charts are based on weights of 170 lbs. for men and 125 lbs. for women. If you weigh substantially more, your relative cardiovascular fitness level will be slightly overestimated. If you weigh substantially less, your relative cardiovascular fitness level will be slightly underestimated.

Men

20- to 29-year-old men

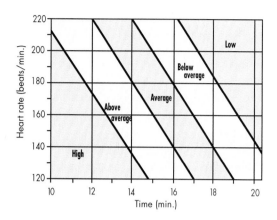

30- to 39-year-old men

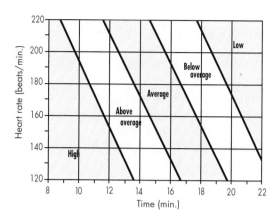

40- to 49-year-old men

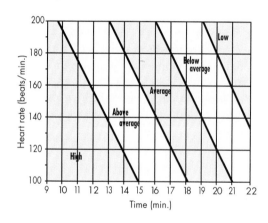

50- to 59-year-old men

60-year-old and older men

Women

20- to 29-year-old women

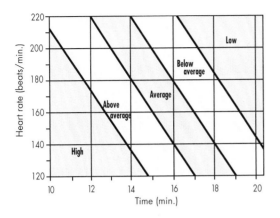

30- to 39-year-old women

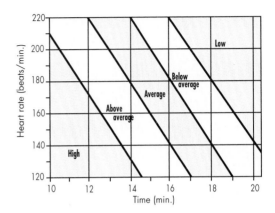

40- to 49-year-old women

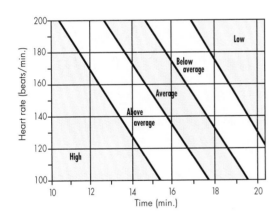

50- to 59-year-old women

60-year-old and older women

Name _____ **Date** _____ **Section** _____

Assessment Activity 3-2

The 1.5-Mile Run/Walk Test

Directions: Select a measured course, preferably a running track, so that the starting and finishing points are at the same location for ease of timing and recording. Cover the distance as rapidly as possible to attain a realistic estimate of fitness level. You will perform better if you take the opportunity to practice running the course first so that you can learn how to pace yourself.

If you cannot run the entire distance, walk until you recover enough to continue running again. Allow a 5- to 10-minute warm-up before the test and an equal amount of time for cooling down after the test. Use the following charts to compare your performance with the norm.

Aerobic Physical Fitness Classification

Men

Fitness Category	13–19 Yrs.	20–29 Yrs.	30–39 Yrs.	40–49 Yrs.
Very poor	>15:31*	>16:01	>16:31	>17:31
Poor	12:11–15:30	14:01–16:00	14:46–16:30	15:36–17:30
Fair	10:49–12:10	12:01–14:00	12:31–14:45	13:01–15:35
Good	9:41–10:48	10:46–12:00	11:01–12:30	11:31–13:00
Excellent	8:37–9:40	9:45–10:45	10:00–11:00	10:30–11:30
Superior	<8:37	<9:45	<10:00	<10:30

*>, greater than; <, less than

Women

Fitness Category	13–19 Yrs.	20–29 Yrs.	30–39 Yrs.	40–49 Yrs.
Very poor	>18:31*	>19:01	>19:31	>20:31
Poor	16:55–18:30	18:31–19:00	19:01–19:30	19:31–20:00
Fair	14:31–16:54	15:55–18:30	16:31–19:00	17:31–19:30
Good	12:30–14:30	13:31–15:54	14:31–16:30	15:56–17:30
Excellent	11:50–12:29	12:30–13:30	13:00–14:30	13:45–15:55
Superior	<11:50	<12:30	<13:00	<13:45

Assessment Activity 3-3

The 3-Minute Bench Step Test

Directions: The equipment needed includes a sturdy 12-inch-high bench; a metronome; a stopwatch; and, if possible, a stethoscope. The metronome should be set at 96 beats per minute for a total of 24 cycles. One cycle consists of four steps as follows: up left foot, up right foot, down left foot, down right foot.

Step up and down in time with each beat of the metronome for 3 full minutes. At the end of the 3 min-utes, sit down on the bench immediately. Start the pulse count within the first 5 seconds and continue for 1 full minute. Do not count for 15 seconds and multiply by 4, because the heart rate will be higher than the actual minute heart rate. The 1-minute postexercise heart rate is the score for the test. Refer to the following chart for scoring.

Postexercise 1-Minute Heart Rate (Beats per Minute)

Fitness Category	18–25 Yrs.		26–35 Yrs.		36–45 Yrs.	
	Men	**Women**	**Men**	**Women**	**Men**	**Women**
Excellent	70–78*	72–83	73–79	72–86	72–81	74–87
Good	82–88	88–97	83–88	91–97	86–94	93–101
Above average	91–97	100–106	91–97	103–110	98–102	104–109
Average	101–104	110–116	101–106	112–118	105–111	111–117
Below average	107–114	118–124	109–116	121–127	113–118	120–127
Poor	118–126	128–137	119–126	129–135	120–128	130–138
Very poor	131–164	141–155	130–164	141–154	132–168	143–152

*Count the pulse for 1 full minute after 3 minutes of stepping at 24 cycles/min. on a 12-inch bench.

Name _____ **Date** _____ **Section** _____

Assessment Activity 3-4

Calculating Target Heart Rate

Directions: Use the Karvonen method to determine your target heart rate for exercise by filling in the following chart.

Karvonen formula: $THR = (HR_{max} - RHR)$
$\times TI\% + RHR$

Key
THR = target heart rate
HR_{max} = maximum heart rate (HR_{max} = 220 – age)
RHR = resting heart rate
TI% = training intensity

Example
- A 23-year-old man in good condition (0.75 training intensity from table 3-3)
- RHR = 66 bpm (beats per minute)

- $HR_{max} = 220 - 23 = 197$ bpm
- THR = *164 bpm*

$THR = (197 - 66) \times .075 + 66 = 131 \times 0.75 + 66$
$= 164$ bpm

Your target heart rate:
$HR_{max} = 220 - AGE =$

$THR = (HR_{max} - RHR) \times TI\% + RHR$

$THR = (\rule{1.5cm}{0.4pt} - \rule{1.5cm}{0.4pt}) \times \rule{1cm}{0.4pt} + \rule{1cm}{0.4pt}$

$= \rule{1.5cm}{0.4pt} \times \rule{1cm}{0.4pt} + \rule{1cm}{0.4pt}$

$= \rule{1.5cm}{0.4pt} + \rule{1cm}{0.4pt}$

$= \rule{1.5cm}{0.4pt}$ bpm

Name _____ **Date** _____ **Section** _____

Assessment Activity 3-5

Design an Exercise Program

Directions: Design an exercise program for yourself. First, identify your goals (weight loss, health enhancement, improving your level of physical fitness, stress reduction, etc.) and second, respond accordingly to each of the following five items.

1. Activity or activities: _____

2. Frequency of exercise: _____

3. Intensity of exercise: _____

4. Duration of exercise: _____

5. Activity schedule: Place the activity or activities in the following weekly calendar with the suggested amount of time devoted to each activity.

Sunday	Monday	Tuesday	Wednesday	Thursday	Friday	Saturday

4

Building Muscular Strength and Endurance

 Online Learning Center

Log on to our Online Learning Center (OLC) for access to these additional resources:

- Chapter key term flashcards
- Learning objectives
- Additional goals for behavior change
- Concentration game
- Self-scoring chapter quizzes

- Additional lab activities

The OLC also offers weblinks for study and exploration of wellness topics. Access these links through **www.mhhe.com/ anspaugh5e**, click on "Student Center," click on "Chapter 4," and then click on "Web Activities."

Goals for Behavior Change

- Begin a strength-training program or improve the one in which you already participate.
- Supply your close family members with at least five health-related reasons they should participate in resistance training.
- Identify the parts of your body where you would like to make the greatest physical change and explain why.
- Identify some of the tasks or sports that you perform daily, weekly, or monthly that would be easier to do if you increased your strength.

Key Terms

anaerobic
atrophy
circuit resistance training (CRT)
concentric contraction
eccentric contraction
hypertrophy

isokinetic
isometric
isotonic
muscular endurance
muscular strength
variable resistance

Objectives

After completing this chapter, you will be able to do the following:

- Explain the benefits of resistance training for older people.
- Define the different types of muscle contraction.
- Identify the various systems of dynamic and static exercise training.
- Describe the limitations of isometric exercise training.
- Explain the advantages and disadvantages of circuit resistance training.

- Define each of the principles of resistance training.
- Explain the differences in strength between men and women.
- Describe the short- and long-term effects of anabolic steroid use.
- Describe the health benefits of resistance training.
- Describe the progressive resistance technique that increases muscle endurance.

vidence has been steadily mounting of the growing importance of muscular development for health enhancement, fitness, and aesthetic purposes. The muscular system improves through resistive forms of exercises, such as weight training and calisthenics. Resistive exercises complement aerobic forms of exercise, because each uniquely contributes to health, physical fitness, and personal appearance. Both types of exercise are required for a well-rounded conditioning program, and together they produce optimum results.

Aerobic exercises, which improve cardiorespiratory function and enhance health status in many ways, were presented in Chapter 3. Resistance exercises also contribute to physiological and psychological health. Many experts are convinced that resistance training is the only type of exercise capable of slowing, and possibly reversing, declines in muscle mass, bone density, and strength. Not long ago, these negative changes were considered to be the result of the aging process.[1] But today, the evidence clearly indicates that a significant percentage of age-related losses are the result of *disuse atrophy.*[2] Disuse atrophy explains the loss of muscle mass and strength because of a sedentary lifestyle personified by low-level muscle stimulation well below the threshold for developing and maintaining muscle mass.[3]

The body contains more than 600 muscles, and 65 percent of these are located above the waist. All muscles, regardless of location, respond to the physiological law of use and disuse. "Use it or lose it" is an axiom that applies to all human beings during every phase of the life cycle. Americans tend to become more sedentary as they age. The declining stimulation results in a progressive shrinking and weakening of the muscles.

With few exceptions—notably cross-country skiing, rowing, and swimming—aerobic activities provide limited stimulation of upper body musculature. Sedentary living neglects the muscular system entirely and accelerates the loss of muscle tissue and body strength. The need for resistance training was illustrated in a study of runners during a ten-year period. Runners who did no resistance training suffered muscle **atrophy** in their upper bodies while maintaining muscle size in their legs.[4] Their arms, which received little stimulation from jogging, decreased in circumference.

Jogging is unable to stimulate the arms at or above the threshold needed for muscular development or maintenance, but the addition of resistive exercises can. This is an example of how the two types of training complement each other.

The Health Benefits of Resistance Training

Irrefutable evidence proves that strength training produces unique health benefits for people of all ages as well as for those with various types of infirmities. The American College of Sports Medicine, The American Heart Association, and the Surgeon General's *Report on Physical Activity and Health* have all proclaimed and strongly supported the need for strength training for health enhancement and for improving quality of life. Strength training increases muscle mass and decreases the fat content of the body. The implications for weight loss and management are enormous, because muscle tissue is more metabolically active than is fat tissue. This means that the body burns more calories under any condition, including rest.[5]

An improvement in strength reduces the exerciser's heart rate and blood pressure while he or she is lifting weights. The practical application of these responses is that there is less stress on the heart when people lift or move moderately heavy objects in everyday life.[6] Heavy resistance training and circuit weight training have the potential to produce a high enough volume of work to improve cardiorespiratory endurance by as much as 5 to 10 percent.[7]

Resistance training increases the strength and endurance of the antigravity muscles, improving posture and producing less stress on the lower back.[8] Stronger, more stable joints are better able to withstand physical stress or trauma.

Strength training also enables one to perform the functions of daily life with less effort. Stronger muscles allow people to perform functional tasks that become more difficult as people age, such as getting in and out of a car, in and out of a bathtub, or up from an easy chair and climbing stairs. Dynamic forms of resistance training have a high degree of transferability to everyday activities.[9]

An increase in leg strength helps those who have osteoarthritis (wear and tear arthritis) because stronger muscles absorb a greater share of the physical stress at joints. In effect, stronger muscles spare the joint structures from some of the weight-bearing activity. Rheumatologists (physicians who specialize in the diagnosis and treatment of arthritic conditions) often recommend weight training to their patients because it alleviates symptoms and strengthens the muscles, tendons, and ligaments that surround the joints.[1]

An improvement in leg strength also leads to better balance and decreases the likelihood of falling, which reduces the chances that a fracture might occur.[6,9] Osteoporosis is a disease characterized by the deterioration of the skeletal system. Bone mineral content decreases so that the bones become fragile and susceptible to fracture. Women are more prone to osteoporosis, but men are also affected as they age. People can protect the skeletal system by eating a nutritious diet and by participating regularly in weight-bearing and resistive exercise. Resistive exercises are versatile, having the capacity to stress all of the joints and the bones that articulate with them, and they produce lateral forces that increase the thickness and density of bones, so they have the potential to prevent osteoporosis.

The results brought about by resistance exercises allow people to live independently and with dignity as they age. Evidence indicates that Americans are living longer, and many will live with physical and functional limitations.[10] Illnesses occur with greater frequency and severity as we age, but much of the disability associated with aging is not due entirely to the aging process. Many authorities attribute at least 50 percent of these changes to "disuse atrophy."[11] Our typically sedentary lifestyles, more prevalent among the aging population than among any other group of Americans, are responsible for a significant number of these illnesses. Those who stimulate their muscles regularly, regardless of their age, do not experience the type of physical deterioration observed in those who are physically inactive. Recent research indicates that physical inactivity is responsible for the majority of age-related muscle loss.[1,12]

Strength training also produces an impressive array of psychological and emotional benefits, which include improvements in self-esteem and self-confidence.[5,13] It helps to improve the mood of mildly to moderately depressed individuals. Resistive exercise programs improve reaction time and may contribute to more restful sleep. Just the Facts: The Benefits of Resistance Training provides a summary of the positive outcomes that can be achieved through resistance training. Also see Wellness Across the Generations: Strength Training for Older Adults.

Many cardiac patients participate in strength development exercise. Substantial benefits may be gained at minimal risk.[14] Improving upper and lower body strength allows cardiac patients to perform everyday lifting activities with less effort and greater movement efficiency. Also, strength training may have a positive impact on cardiorespiratory endurance, hypertension, blood fat levels, and psychological well-being.

Anaerobic Exercise

Strength development exercises are **anaerobic**. *Anaerobic* literally means "without oxygen," and when applied to exercise, it refers to high-intensity physical activities in which oxygen demand is above the level that can be supplied during performance. Short-term sup

Just the Facts

The Benefits of Resistance Training

Resistance training produces the following positive results:

- Increases muscle mass and decreases fat mass
- Increases strength and muscle endurance
- Increases basal metabolic rate (BMR)
- Develops the antigravity muscles (abdominal, lower back, hips, front and back of the thighs, both calves)
- Increases bone density (resulting in less risk of bone fracture)
- Improves dynamic balance (resulting in less risk of falling)
- Improves mobility, such as that necessary for walking and stair-climbing
- Improves reaction time
- Contributes to more restful sleep
- Helps to elevate the mood of mildly to moderately depressed people
- Improves body image, self-esteem, and self-confidence
- Improves the effectiveness of insulin in older adults
- Aids in weight loss and weight management
- May increase HDL cholesterol (the protective form)

plies of fuel stored in the muscles provide the energy for anaerobic activities. As a result, these can only be sustained for several seconds. Sprinting 100 yards, lifting a heavy weight, and running up two or three flights of stairs are some examples of anaerobic activities.

Muscular Strength

Muscular strength is the maximum force that a muscle or muscle group can exert in a single contraction. It is best developed by some form of progressive resistance exercise, such as weight training with free weights (barbells and dumbbells) or single or multistation machine weights.

Muscular strength is developed best through high-intensity exercise. Lifting heavier loads a few times to fatigue produces larger gains than does lifting lighter loads many times to fatigue. Weight trainers speak of the amount of work accomplished during the workout in terms of exercise repetitions and sets and in terms of the percentage of 1 repetition maximum (1 RM) for

Wellness Across the Generations

Strength Training for Older Adults

One of the realities of aging is muscle atrophy (decrease in size), resulting in a loss of strength, power, balance, and coordination. However, scientists have shown that a substantial amount of muscle loss is due to lack of appropriate physical activity rather than to the aging process. Engaging regularly in resistance exercises can build muscle, maintain muscle, and limit the loss of muscle tissue.

Inactive people can expect to lose approximately 50 percent of their muscle mass between 20 and 90 years of age.[15] This loss is accompanied by a 30 percent reduction in strength between 50 and 70 years of age. Data from the ongoing Framingham Study showed that 40 percent of female subjects 55 to 64 years of age, 45 percent of female subjects 65 to 74 years of age, and 65 percent of female subjects 74 to 85 years of age were unable to lift 10 pounds. The loss of muscle strength is most pronounced after age 70. Data show that muscle strength declines by approximately 15 percent per decade during the 60s and 70s and to 30 percent per decade thereafter.[15,16]

Because of this limitation, everyday functions taken for granted by the young become physical challenges, including opening bottle caps and jar lids, carrying groceries, and climbing stairs. If muscle atrophy progresses unabated, walking without assistance becomes difficult if not impossible, and the likelihood of falling increases.

The good news is that the muscles of older people respond to training in much the same way as the muscles of young adults. Older people may make greater gains because of their initial level of debility (weakness). Studies have shown that the elderly can double or even triple their strength level in as little as three to four months of strength training.[15] Strength training also seems to have profound anabolic (muscle-building) effects in elderly people.

each exercise. A *repetition* is one complete lift of an exercise beginning with the starting position, moving the weight through a full range of motion, and returning to the starting position. Doing this ten times in a continuous fashion is referred to as *10 repetitions* or *10 reps,* and these 10 reps represent 1 *set* of that exercise. Repeating the entire sequence two more times completes *3 sets* of the exercise. One RM represents the heaviest load that can be lifted one time. Ten RM is a lighter load that can be lifted ten times but not eleven. In other words, maximum fatigue occurs on repetition number 10, thereby preventing repetition number 11.

Select a weight that is 80 to 90 percent of 1 RM if strength development is the primary goal. If you are a beginner, be extremely careful in establishing 1 RM for each exercise, because your musculoskeletal system is not trained to handle such loads. It is recommended that beginners skip the 1 RM method of weight selection and instead, through trial and error, find a weight that can be lifted for at least but not more than 8 to 10 reps. One RM for each exercise may be safely established after six weeks of training.

Muscle Contraction and Resistance Training

Muscle contraction is either static or dynamic. *Static contractions* (isometric) occur when muscles exert force but do not move (shorten or lengthen). *Dynamic contractions* (isotonic and isokinetic) involve muscle contractions that are either *concentric* (muscle shortening) or *eccentric* (muscle lengthening).[17] See figure 4-1 for an illustration of each.

Some of the exercises commonly used to develop the major muscle groups of the body are shown in figures 4-2 to 4-17. The anatomical charts in figures 4-18 and 4-19 show the location of the muscles stressed in each exercise. These exercises are demonstrated on exercise machines and free weights, methods that are relatively equivalent and work the same muscle groups.

See Assessment Activity 4-1 for a method of determining your strength based on body weight and gender.

Static Training (Isometrics)

Isometric contractions (in which muscle length is constant) occur when muscles produce tension but do not shorten, because the resistance is beyond the contractile force that can be generated by the exercising muscles. Examples of isometric contractions are pushing against a wall, pushing sideways or upward against a door jamb, and loading a weight machine with poundage beyond one's capacity to lift. See figure 4-20 for an illustration.

Optimal strength development from isometric contractions occurs with 5 to 10 sets of 6-second contractions at 100 percent of maximum force.

Isometric exercises are effective for developing strength, but this approach has some important limitations. The most serious of these is a higher than

(a)

(b)

Figure 4-1 Contractions

The two types of contractions: (a) a concentric contraction; (b) an eccentric contraction.

(a)

(b)

Figure 4-2 Biceps Curl

(a) Start with your arms extended, palms up. (b) Flex both arms, slowly move the weight through a full range of motion, and return to the starting position. The prime mover is the biceps brachii.

(a)

(b)

Figure 4-3 Biceps Curl (Free Weights)

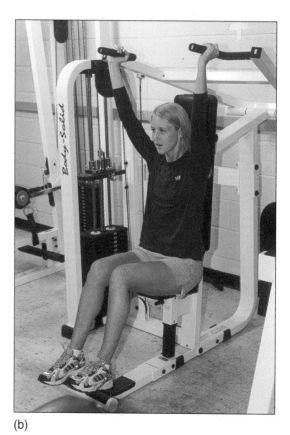

(a)

(b)

Figure 4-4 Overhead Press

(a) Sit upright with your hands approximately shoulder width apart. (b) Slowly press the bar upward until your arms are fully extended, and lower to the starting position. Avoid an excessive arch in your lower back. The prime movers are the triceps and deltoid muscles.

(a)

(b)

Figure 4-5 Overhead Press (Free Weights)

(a)

(b)

Figure 4-6 Bench Press

(a) Lie on your back with your knees bent and your feet flat on the bench to prevent arching your back. (b) Slowly press the bar forward, fully extending your arms, and return to the starting position. The prime movers are the pectoralis major, triceps, and deltoid muscles.

(a)

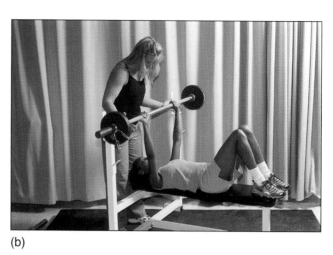

(b)

Figure 4-7 Bench Press (Free Weights)

(a)

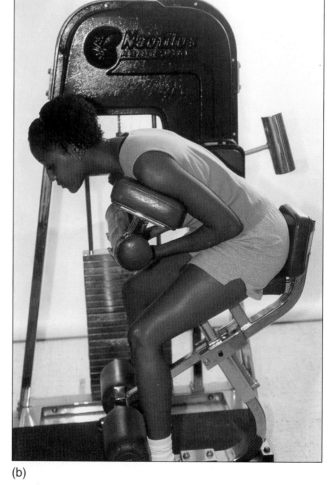

(b)

Figure 4-8 Abdominal Crunch

(a) Sit upright with your chest against the pads, hands folded across your stomach. (b) Slowly press forward through a full range of motion, and return to the starting position. The prime mover is the rectus abdominis muscle.

(a)

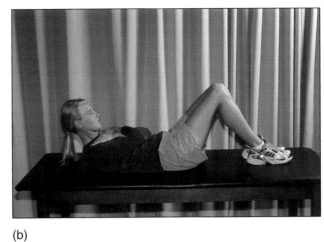

(b)

Figure 4-9 Abdominal Crunch (Mat Exercise)

(a)

(b)

Figure 4-10 Lower Back Extension

(a) Place your thighs and back against the pads. (b) Slowly press backward until your back is fully extended, and return to the starting position. The prime movers are the erector spine and gluteus maximus muscles.

(a)

(b)

Figure 4-11 Back Extension (Mat Exercise)

(a)

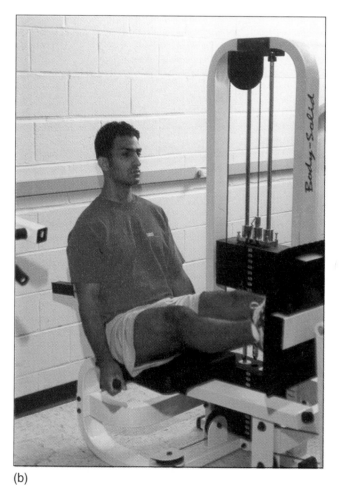

(b)

Figure 4-12 Leg Press

(a) Adjust the seat so that your legs are bent at approximately 90 degrees. (b) Slowly extend your legs fully, and return to the starting position. The prime movers are the quadriceps and gluteus maximus muscles.

(a)

(b)

Figure 4-13 Half-Squat (Free Weights)

expected rise in exercise arterial blood pressure and an increased workload on the heart throughout the entire contraction.[17] All-out straining isometric contractions should not be performed by people with heart and vascular disease. A second limitation is that strength developed isometrically is joint-angle specific. Maximum strength development occurs at the angle of contraction, with a training carryover of approximately 20 degrees in either direction from that angle.[18] To develop strength throughout the muscle's range of motion, you must perform isometric contractions in at least three different points in the range of motion.

Because muscles cannot overcome the resistance in isometric training, measuring improvement is difficult, constituting another limitation of this system. Improvements in strength can be measured if exercisers have access to specialized equipment, such as dynamometers and tensiometers, that record the amount of force ap-

plied. Motivation for exercise is difficult to sustain without feedback.

Research indicates that isometric exercise systems are as effective as dynamic exercise systems for developing strength. The question is not which system is better but which system best satisfies the intended use for the newly acquired strength. The transferability of strength to occupational and leisure pursuits is relevant.

Strength developed in the muscles is highly specific to the manner in which the muscles are trained. Muscles trained isometrically perform best when stressed isometrically; muscles trained dynamically perform best when stressed dynamically. There is some transfer of isometric training to everyday life. Carrying groceries, a baby, or any object in a fixed position or pushing and pulling objects requires isometric strength, but most movements are dynamic, and transfer is more widely applicable from dynamic systems of training.

(a)   (b)

Figure 4-14 Hamstring Curl

(a) Lie face down with your lower legs under the pads. (b) Curl the weight approximately 90 degrees, and return to the starting position. The prime mover is the hamstring muscle group.

(a)   (b)

Figure 4-15 Hamstring Curl (Free Weights)

Dynamic Exercise

Dynamic exercises include **isotonic** (equal tension), variable resistance, free weights, and **isokinetic** (equal speed) exercises.

Isotonic training

Isotonic muscle contractions occur when muscles shorten and move the bones to which they are attached, resulting in movement around the joints. Isotonic movements consist of concentric and eccentric muscle contractions. The **concentric contraction** occurs when a muscle shortens as it develops the tension to overcome an external resistance. The **eccentric contraction** occurs when the muscle lengthens and the weight (resistance) is slowly returned to the starting position. When muscles contract eccentrically, they are resisting the force of

gravity as they lengthen so that the weight is not allowed to free-fall. In general, muscles can produce about 40 percent more tension eccentrically than concentrically.[8,17] But no advantage exists for training programs that emphasize eccentric contractions. Research indicates that conventional isotonic programs develop as much strength and produce less of the delayed muscle soreness associated with eccentric contractions.

Isotonic exercises produce delayed muscle soreness twenty-four to forty-eight hours after a workout. Eccentric contractions cause microscopic damage to muscle fibers, their connective tissue, and the cell membranes.[19] Soreness occurs because the damaged tissues swell and apply pressure on the nerves. Delayed muscle soreness is more common among beginning exercisers, exercisers who attempt to overload too quickly, and those who change from one activity to another.

(a)

(b)

Figure 4-16 Chest Press

(a) Keep your upper arms parallel to the floor, bend your elbows at 90 degrees, and place your hands on the handles.
(b) Slowly push the bars until your elbows are pointing forward, and return to the starting position. The prime movers are the pectoralis major and deltoid muscles.

(a)

(b)

Figure 4-17 Lateral Supine Raises (Free Weights)

Stretching exercises, light workouts, or complete rest may be required to alleviate muscle soreness. Prevention is the best treatment. Prevention involves allowing enough time to adjust to a new routine (at least one month), overloading the muscles in small increments (not trying to do too much too fast), and exercising within capacity. Because muscle soreness may last forty-eight hours, those who use isotonic exercise systems are advised to exercise no more than every other day. This schedule ensures that the next bout of exercise will occur after soreness has abated.

Variable resistance training

Variable resistance exercise equipment was developed because isotonic exercises do not maximally stress mus-

cles throughout their full range of motion. The maximum weight lifted isotonically is limited to the weakest point in the musculoskeletal leverage system. The weight appears lighter at some points in the joint movement and heavier at others. In reality, the weight is constant and the human bony leverage system changes.

Variable resistance equipment is designed to provide maximum resistance through the full range of motion. Universal Gym equipment accomplishes this by altering the lifter's leverage. Decreasing the leverage increases the resistance at points in the movement where the muscles are strongest. Nautilus equipment uses a system of cams to decrease musculoskeletal leverage, which in turn increases lifting resistance. Variable resistance training challenges people to exert more force throughout the range of motion, which should result in

Figure 4-18 Selected Muscles of the Body—Front View

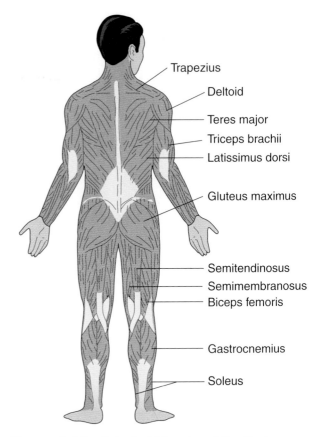

Figure 4-19 Selected Muscles of the Body—Rear View

greater returns. Whether variable resistance weight training is more effective than conventional weight training is yet to be resolved. Evidence indicates that it is as good and may be better, even though it varies the resistance imprecisely.[20]

Free-weight training

Isotonic training with free weights continues to be an appropriate method of strength development. Free-weight training provides many advantages. For athletes, it yields some flexibility in strength development because the movements are not confined to a track. Exercises can be selected or improvised to simulate the movements required by specific sports, allowing the development of the muscles that will be used in competition. Concurrently, ancillary musculature that plays a supporting or stabilizing role for the major muscles is also stimulated and developed.

For noncompetitors, free weights have several advantages. The equipment is inexpensive and versatile. A starter set of free weights typically costs less than $150. Free weights do not require much space, so the workout can occur in the home.

The main limitation of free-weight exercise is that this system does not provide maximum resistance throughout the full range of motion. A second limitation is the need for one or two spotters to assist with exercises such as the bench press and half-squats.

Isokinetic training

Isokinetic resistance training involves dynamic movements performed on exercise devices that produce maximum resistance throughout the full range of motion. The movement speed is preselected by the exerciser and remains constant throughout the movement. Isokinetic exercise theoretically improves on traditional and variable-resistance dynamic systems.[13] Isokinetic devices adjust the resistance to accommodate the force applied by the exerciser. The greater the application of force, the greater the resistance to movement supplied by the device while the speed of movement is held at a constant rate. Maximum force applied through the full range of motion is countered with maximum resistance at all joint angles. This activates the greatest number of motor units and should produce greater gains in strength than other dynamic systems of exercise.

Just the Facts

Muscle Fiber Types

In humans, it appears that the total number of muscle fibers and the fiber type are set genetically and that both are fully established at birth. Research indicates that the total number of muscle fibers probably cannot be increased and the fiber type cannot be changed. If this theory is accurate, then the increases in muscle size resulting from training must be caused by hypertrophy (increase in size) of the existing fibers. Muscle hyperplasia (an increase in the number of muscle fibers) has been shown to occur in several species of animals through heavy resistance exercise. Muscle hyperplasia has not been verified in humans, but the possibility cannot be ruled out.

Muscles consist of three types of fibers: (1) type I or slow-twitch oxidative fibers (SO); (2) type IIa or fast-twitch, oxidative glycloytic fibers (FOG); and (3) type IIb or fast-twitch glycloytic fibers (FG). Each fiber type can be identified by its speed of contraction and the primary energy source that it uses. Slow-twitch oxidative fibers rely on the aerobic or oxygen system. These fibers are responsible for exercise and activities of an aerobic or endurance nature. The fast-twitch oxidative, glycloytic fibers (type IIa) contract faster than the type I fibers and are capable of using oxygen but not as efficiently as type I fibers. These fibers support exercises that require both aerobic and anaerobic energy. The fast-twitch glycloytic fibers (type IIb) have the fastest contractile speed of the three and support high-intensity anaerobic exercises.[21]

Most scientists believe that muscle fiber types do not crossover; that is, type I fibers remain slow twitch and type II fibers remain fast twitch. However, there is evidence that has led to controversy regarding muscle fiber resistance to change. While it appears that muscle fiber types are set genetically, there is an indication in some of the data that prolonged exercise training can alter fiber type.[21] More research is needed before the impact of heavy training on muscle fiber type can be fully evaluated.

The ratio of slow-twitch to fast-twitch muscle fibers can be determined by examining under a powerful microscope muscle biopsies from selected sites in the body. The muscle composition of world-class aerobic athletes (distance runners, cyclists, cross-country skiers) is predominately slow-twitch, whereas the muscle composition of the world-class power or anaerobic event athletes (shot-putters, sprinters, power and Olympic weight lifters) is primarily fast-twitch. Knowing the ratio of fiber type could be important for these competitors, but it is relatively unimportant when one exercises for health reasons. Sedentary people have about 50 percent type I fibers distributed relatively evenly throughout the body's major muscle groups.[21] Health enthusiasts can participate in a variety of activities with some degree of success and satisfaction regardless of fiber type.

Circuit Resistance Training

Circuit resistance training (CRT) is effective for people who wish to develop several fitness dimensions simultaneously. Muscular strength and endurance, changes in body composition, and improvement in cardiorespiratory endurance can be attained together.

A circuit usually consists of eight to fifteen exercise stations. The weight selected for each exercise station should equal 40 to 60 percent of 1 RM.[20,22] The exerciser does as many repetitions as possible for 15 to 30 seconds at each station. The rest interval between exercise stations should equal the exercise time spent at each station. The circuit is repeated two to three times for a total elapsed time of 30 to 50 minutes per workout. As fitness improves, overload can be applied by (1) increasing the amount of weight at each station, (2) increasing the amount of exercise time at each station (up to 30 seconds), (3) decreasing the amount of rest between stations, or (4) any combination of these.

The CRT system is challenging, versatile, and fun. Exercise stations can be rearranged, exercises that develop similar muscle groups can be substituted for each other, and the order in which the circuit is traversed can be changed. Because relatively light weights are used, the likelihood of injury is reduced. Circuits can be set up in small spaces. Machine weights are ideal for CRT because of the speed with which resistances can be changed, but free weights are adaptable to this system as well. The main limitation of CRT is that optimal gains in strength or cardiorespiratory endurance are difficult to achieve. Strength is most efficiently developed through lifting heavy weights combined with a substantial rest period between sets. Cardiorespiratory endurance can best be achieved through rhythmic and continuous activities, such as jogging, cycling, cross-country skiing, and rowing, performed for a minimum of 20 minutes per workout. An example of a circuit is presented in Just the Facts: Circuit Resistance Training.

Figure 4-20 Isometric Contraction

An isometric contraction is a static contraction against an immovable object.

~ Just the Facts ~

Circuit Resistance Training

The following is an example of a circuit. You should warm up before CRT and finish the workout with a cooldown.

Station 1	Leg presses or half-squats	15–30 secs.
Station 2	Bench presses	15–30 secs.
Station 3	Back hyperextensions	15–30 secs.
Station 4	Biceps curls	15–30 secs.
Station 5	Overhead presses	15–30 secs.
Station 6	Sit-ups or abdominal crunches	15–30 secs.
Station 7	Push-ups	15–30 secs.
Station 8	Lateral raises	15–30 secs.
Station 9	Hamstring curls	15–30 secs.
Station 10	Pull-ups	15–30 secs.

Muscular Endurance

Muscular endurance is the application of repeated muscular force against a submaximal resistance. Inflating a tire with a bicycle pump, walking up five flights of stairs, lifting a weight 20 times, and doing 50 sit-ups are some examples of activities that develop muscular endurance. It is developed by many repetitions against resistances that are considerably less than maximum.

Research has shown that the greatest effect on muscle endurance occurs with submaximal loads that can be lifted 20 or more times.[22] Programs that emphasize low resistance and high repetitions produce limited improvement, if any, in *strength*. The primary stimulus of these programs is on the body's ability to supply blood and oxygen to the working muscles for them to contract on a repeated basis. Endurance exercises increase muscle capillarization and muscle myoglobin. An increase in muscle capillaries allows the muscles to accept more blood. The increase in oxygen carried by the capillaries is transferred to a greater quantity of myoglobin, which delivers it to the muscles. As with other types of isotonic resistance training programs, muscle endurance exercises should be performed no more than every other day.

Isometric or static muscle endurance is the ability to sustain or hold a submaximal contraction for a time.[8] Examples are carrying objects, such as groceries and other packages; pushing or pulling objects, such as a lawn mower; and carrying children.

Assessment Activity 4-2 presents a method of determining your muscular endurance. Assessment Activity 4-3 measures abdominal muscle endurance, and Assessment Activity 4-4 measures muscular strength and endurance with calisthenics.

Principles of Resistance Training

The principles of exercise—intensity, duration, frequency, overload, progression, and specificity—apply to resistance training as well as aerobic training. These principles were established over many years through research and experience. The current set of guidelines recommended for average healthy adults was published in 1998 by the American College of Sports Medicine (ACSM):[4]

> A minimum of eight to ten exercises involving the major muscle groups should be performed two to three days per week. A minimum of 1 set of 8 to 12 RM or to near fatigue should be completed by most participants; however, for older and more frail persons (approximately 50 to 60 years of age and above), 10 to 15 repetitions may be more appropriate.

These recommendations are minimum standards for weight training and are designed to motivate sedentary nonathletic adults to try this form of exercise. According to ACSM, more sets, heavier weights, and exercising three times per week produce greater results, but the additional time and effort required for more sets, heavier weights, and greater frequency probably exceed the interest of this population. Although this may be true, healthy American adults should be encouraged to exercise above these minimum recommendations.

Intensity

Intensity refers to the amount of weight used for a given exercise. It is probably the most important variable in resistance training, and it is the most important stimulus associated with the development of strength and muscle endurance.[22]

For muscular development and health enhancement, the intensity of resistance training may be set by selecting a weight (through trial and error) that can be lifted at least 8 times but no more than 12 times. This weight is probably 75 to 85 percent of a maximal effort.[22]

The intensity level for resistance exercise varies according to the training system used. Optimal strength development through isometrics involves maximal contractions, 5 to 10 sets with a total contraction time of 30 to 60 seconds. Optimal strength development through dynamic systems of exercise should include 3 to 5 sets of 4 RM to 6 RM per set, with at least 2 minutes' rest between sets, and this should be performed three times per week.[8] If muscle endurance is the primary goal, the workout should consist of 3 to 5 sets of 15 RM to 25 RM per set, with approximately 1 minute's rest between sets, performed three times per week.

There is a preferred order of exercise associated with resistance training. Large muscle exercises (half-squat, bench press, etc.) should precede small muscle exercises (biceps curl, triceps extension, etc.) because research has shown that by first exercising the larger muscles the intensity of the workout can be increased.[20,22] The rationale supporting larger to smaller muscle groups is that exercises requiring the most muscle mass should be stressed while the exerciser is fresh. If the reverse order was followed, the smaller muscle groups would be fatigued, limiting their contribution to larger muscle exercises and thereby reducing the intensity of the workout.

Duration (Time)

The duration or length of each exercise session is dependent upon the number of exercises, repetitions, and sets, the amount of rest between sets, and the time available to the performer. The ACSM estimates that

its minimum guidelines require about 20 minutes to complete. Conventional resistance programs (3 sets, 10 to 12 exercises, 8 to 12 reps) take about 50 minutes. Serious bodybuilding requires two to four hours in advanced weight training systems, six days per week. Availability of time and individual goals will dictate the length of workout.

Frequency

Frequency refers to the number of training sessions per week. Dynamic resistance exercises (isotonic and isokinetic) should be performed every other day (seven training sessions every two weeks) or three times per week (six training sessions every two weeks). Near-maximum gains in strength for novice weight trainers occur with these exercise frequencies.

Isometrics can be performed every day because muscle soreness does not result. However, for physiological and psychological reasons, you should designate two to three days of rest throughout the week. Evidence indicates that alternate day isometric training is 80 percent as effective as daily training.[20] However, daily training using maximal voluntary isometric contractions produces the best results.

Overload and Progression

The principle behind strength increase is straightforward—the muscles must be subjected periodically to greater resistance as they adapt to the previous resistance. This overload principle applies to all muscles regardless of the system of training.

Overload may be applied by progressively increasing the amount of weight lifted or the number of repetitions performed or by decreasing rest time between sets. An increase in the number of repetitions leads to increases in muscle endurance, an increase in the amount of weight lifted leads to an increase in muscle strength, and a decrease in rest time increases muscular and aerobic endurance.

The principle of progression relates to the application of overload. It dictates how much and when an increase in resistance, reps, or sets or a decrease in rest time should occur. For example, the application of overload in a strength development program featuring 6 RM is accomplished by increasing the load when the exerciser can perform more than six reps on more than one occasion. The added weight reduces the number of reps that can be performed. Continued training improves strength and increases the number of reps. Once again, when the exerciser can perform more than six reps on more than one occasion, the weight is increased. This cycle is repeated for as long as strength development is the goal.

Specificity

The principle of specificity reflects the body's response to exercise. The type of training dictates the type of muscle development. Training programs that emphasize high resistance and low repetitions increase muscle strength and size. The gains are the result of muscle **hypertrophy,** an increase in the diameter of muscle fibers, and the recruitment of more motor units.

Training programs that emphasize low resistance and a high number of repetitions develop muscle endurance. The high volume of work increases the blood and oxygen supply to the muscles by increasing capillary density and muscle myoglobin concentration.

The effectiveness of resistance training programs is based on the knowledgeable use of principles that guide such programs. However, other factors contribute to program effectiveness. These are found in Real-World Wellness: Other Important Considerations for Resistance Training.

Ergogenic Aids

Ergogenic aids are substances, techniques, or treatments that theoretically improve physical performance in addition to the effects of normal training. This discussion on ergogenic aids will be limited to a few of those reputed to accelerate muscle and strength development.

Many athletes and nonathletes take supplements of various types to accelerate muscle development. This short summary of a few of the many ergogenic aids suffices to show that some of these have performance-enhancing qualities, but many do not.

Protein Supplementation

The adult requirement for protein is 0.8 gram (g) per kilogram (1 kg = 2.2 lbs.) of body weight. Research has shown that resistance training may push this requirement to 1.6 to 1.8 g/kg of body weight.[23] Values such as these are easily obtained with the typical American diet, particularly for active people who tend to consume more calories than does the average adult. Protein in excess of these values has resulted in no further gains in strength, power, or muscle size.[24]

Vitamins and Minerals

Physical performance is adversely affected by vitamin and mineral deficiencies. Those who have deficiencies can supplement their diets with the missing element or elements. However, the performance of well-nourished, physically active people is not improved through vitamin and mineral supplementation.

Creatine

Many, but not all, studies show that supplementing with creatine may enhance performance in short-term, high-intensity activities such as resistance training. Creatine is a nitrogen-containing organic compound found in meat, poultry, and fish.[25] In addition to dietary creatine, the body synthesizes creatine in the liver, kidneys, and pancreas from nonessential amino acids. A third source is supplemental creatine monohydrate, which comes in powder, tablet, or liquid form. Creatine monohydrate supplementation increases skeletal muscle creatine content for most people. It is particularly advantageous for strict vegetarians who eat no animal flesh and have low dietary levels as a result. Creatine monohydrate supplementation promotes faster recovery from repetitive high-intensity exercises so that users can perform a higher than normal volume of work.[8]

Evidence indicates that creatine supplementation is safe in the short-term, but long-term data are lacking. It does not benefit the casual exerciser.

Ginseng

This herb has been used for centuries as a cure-all and energizer. Theoretically, it improves physical performance by combating fatigue. No credible scientific evidence supports this contention.

Chromium Picolinate

This mineral is purported to build muscle and promote weight loss. Deficiencies of chromium in the United States are rare. No good scientific evidence exists that chromium picolinate supplementation has the capacity to build muscle or enhance weight loss, but evidence indicates that it might be harmful to human cells.

Real-World Wellness

Other Important Considerations for Resistance Training

In addition to the principles of resistance exercise, what factors should I consider to ensure the effectiveness and safety of my resistance training program?

Here are some other important factors for novice weight trainers:

- *Order of exercises:* Many people believe that large muscle exercises should precede small muscle exercises. This format allows one to train at a higher intensity level. Large muscle exercises such as half-squats or leg presses should be performed prior to hamstring curls; bench presses should precede triceps extensions. If small muscle group exercises precede large muscle exercises, fatigue (preexhaustion) is carried over to the large muscle exercises, which limits their effectiveness.

   Novice exercisers should not exercise the same muscles in consecutive exercises, because they are likely then to be less tolerant to the preexhaustion phenomenon that occurs from the buildup of lactic acid resulting from the previous exercise.

- *Rest intervals between sets:* The rest period depends upon the goals of training. For example, if the goal is strength development, the rest period between sets should be 2 to 3 minutes. If body building is the goal, the rest period should be 1 minute or less. If circuit training is the system used, the rest period between exercises should be 15 to 30 seconds.

- *Speed of movement:* For the general public, speed of movement should be relatively slow and controlled. It

should take 2 to 3 seconds for the concentric contraction and the same amount of time for the eccentric concentration.

- *Multiple sets versus single sets:* Although 1 set of each exercise performed two to three days per week increases strength, it is a minimal effort. Doing 2 to 3 sets three times per week is better.

- *Breathing patterns:* Most important, never hold your breath during physical exertion because this produces an extraordinary rise in blood pressure. Breathe rhythmically during exertion. The suggested pattern of breathing during weight training is to exhale during concentric contractions, while muscles are shortening, and to inhale during eccentric contractions, while muscles are lengthening and returning weights to starting positions.

- *Spotting:* Spotters are needed for certain exercises performed with free weights. These include multijoint exercises, in which weights must be returned to a rack on completion, and exercises during which weights need to be properly positioned. Half-squats and bench presses are examples of exercises requiring assistance.

- *Safety:* The chances of sustaining an injury from resistance training are relatively small, but as with all physical activities, the chance exists. Safety is enhanced by employing correct lifting techniques, making use of spotters, breathing properly, maintaining equipment in good working order, and wearing proper exercise clothing.

- *Full range of motion:* To develop strength throughout the full range of motion, exercising muscles must produce force through complete flexion and extension. Be careful not to hyperextend or overextend, which can result in injury.

Anabolic-Androgenic Steroids

Anabolic-androgenic steroids are hormones. Their anabolic properties contribute to muscle enlargement, while their androgenic properties produce masculinizing effects. They build muscle mass and strength, and as a result, they improve, in some people's estimation, physical appearance and physical performance.

Anabolic steroid use by nonathletes is on the rise. This is particularly true for young men. A nationwide survey of 3403 male high school seniors indicated that 6.6 percent of this group were current users or had previously been users of steroids and that 25 percent of the current users showed signs of dependency.[26] According to this report, the improvement in physical appearance reputed to occur with steroid use accompanied by peer approval of those physical

changes functioned as a powerful reinforcer for continued use.

Heavy steroid users were more likely than light users to take two or more steroids simultaneously and more apt to take these drugs by injection rather than in pill form. Injection as a method of delivery is highly characteristic of drugs that involve addiction. The steroid "hook" is insidious and powerful: 30 percent of the heavy users stated that they would not discontinue steroid use if steroids were proved to cause liver cancer, 31 percent would not stop if they proved to cause heart attacks, and 39 percent would not stop if they proved to cause infertility.[27]

Although definitive evidence of the long-term effects of steroid use is not available, the potential for long-term harm is certainly real. Predicting how and when the effects of steroids will be manifested is impossible because people respond differently to these drugs as a result of differences in body chemistry. The steroid effect is complicated further by the fact that black market preparations contain additives, and some preparations are contaminated. The potential for harm is readily discernible; 80 to 90 percent of steroids used are purchased through the black market. Table 4-1 presents some of the known and possible effects of steroid use.

Keeping a Daily Training Log

Beginning weight trainers should keep a daily log of their training activities. The advantages of keeping such a record far outweigh the minimal amount of bother, time, and effort required to make the entries during the workout. Each entry should be recorded during the rest period between sets.

The advantages of maintaining a daily training log include the following:

- You will always know which exercises you performed and the amount of weight used for each.
- You will always know the number of repetitions and sets that you performed of each exercise.
- The training log provides an objective account of your improvement. You can compare the amount of weight you are currently lifting with the amount at the beginning of your training.
- The training log provides an accurate history.
- The training log is a motivating device that provides objective feedback of performance improvement.

A sample training log is shown in figure 4-21. A blank training log is given in Assessment Activity 4-5 for you to use to document your resistance training program. It will be helpful to make additional copies of this training log.

Table 4-1 Overview of Anabolic Steroid Effects

Effects Supported by Strong Evidence

In Males and Females

Stunted growth when taken before puberty	Deepening of the voice (in women)
Coronary artery disease	Menstrual irregularities (in women)
Low HDL cholesterol	
Sterility, low sperm count (in men)	Development of facial and body hair (in women)
Liver tumors and liver disease	Decreased breast size (in women)
Death	Clitoris enlargement (in women)
Acne	
Water retention	Fetal damage (when taken during pregnancy)
Oily, thickened skin	
Male-pattern baldness (in women)	

Possible Effects

In Males and Females

Diarrhea	Bone pains
Muscle cramps	Impotence (in men)
Breast development (in men)	Sexual problems
Aggressive behavior	High blood pressure
Headache	Kidney disease
Nausea	Depression

Adapted from Nieman, D. C. 1999. *Exercise Testing and Prescription.* Mountain View, Calif.: Mayfield Publishing Co.

Name ___Cathy Smith___   Starting date ___Jan. 1, 1999___

Program objectives ___To gain strength and muscle definition___

Exercise	Jan. 1			Jan. 3			Jan. 5			Jan. 7			Jan. 9			Jan. 11			Jan. 13		
	Resis. (lbs.)	Reps	Sets	Resis. (lbs.)	Reps	Sets	Resis. (lbs.)	Reps	Sets	Resis. (lbs.)	Reps	Sets	Resis. (lbs.)	Reps	Sets	Resis. (lbs.)	Reps	Sets	Resis. (lbs.)	Reps	Sets
1. Bench press	60	10	3																		
2. Biceps curl	25	10	3																		
3. Back extension	80	10	3																		
4. Leg press	150	10	3																		
5. Hamstring curl	30	10	3																		
6. Chest press	30	10	3																		
7. Abdominal crunch	—	25	3																		
8. Overhead press	35	10	3																		

Figure 4-21 Sample Training Log

Resistance (abbreviated as *Resis.*) refers to the amount of weight (in pounds) lifted or pressed. *Reps* (for *repetitions*) is the number of times the weight is lifted or pressed. *Sets* are the groups of reps.

Summary

- The physiological law of use and disuse applies to all human beings during all phases of the life cycle.
- The muscular systems of older adults are trainable and respond to resistance training with an increase in strength and muscle size.
- Muscular strength is the maximum force that a muscle or muscle group can exert in a single contraction.
- Dynamic exercises consist of concentric and eccentric muscle contractions.
- Isotonic exercises are dynamic in that muscles shorten and lengthen, producing movement around a joint.
- Variable resistance exercise equipment is designed to provide maximum resistance throughout the full range of motion.

- Circuit resistance training is a versatile system that allows a person to develop several fitness dimensions simultaneously.
- The principles of exercise—intensity, duration, frequency, overload, progression, and specificity—apply to resistance training. These can be manipulated to meet all muscle development objectives.
- The average man can generate 30 to 50 percent more force than the average woman.
- Anabolic steroids are performance-enhancing drugs that are harmful and illegal.
- Research in the last decade has shown that resistance training contributes to wellness in a variety of ways.
- Muscle endurance is the ability to apply repeated muscular force.

Review Questions

1. Define *muscular strength* and *muscular endurance.*
2. What are the differences among isometric, isotonic, isokinetic, and variable resistance exercises?
3. What are concentric and eccentric contractions?
4. What are the health benefits of participating in resistance exercise?

5. How do you account for the strength differences between men and women?
6. Name and define the principles of conditioning as they relate to resistance training.
7. What are the health consequences and physical performance benefits of steroid use?

References

1. Harvard University. 1998. Stay stronger longer with weight training. *Harvard Health Letter* 23(12):1.
2. Dudley, G. A., and L. L. Ploutz-Snyder. 2001. Deconditioning and bed rest: musculoskeletal response. In *ACSM's Resource Manual* (4th ed.), ed. J. L. Roitman. Philadelphia: Lippincott Williams and Wilkins.
3. Powers, S. K., and E. T. Howley. 2001. *Exercise Physiology.* Boston: McGraw-Hill.
4. American College of Sports Medicine. 1998. The recommended quantity and quality of exercise for developing and maintaining cardiorespiratory and muscular fitness, and flexibility in healthy adults. *Medicine and Science in Sports and Exercise* 30(6):975.
5. Bryant, C. X., and J. A. Peterson. 1998. Strength for women through the stages of life. *Fitness Management* 14(7):36.
6. Bryant, C. X., J. A. Peterson, and B. A. Franklin. 1998. Fountain of youth. *Fitness Management* 14(10):44.
7. Kraemer, W. J., J. S. Volek, and S. J. Fleck. 2001. Chronic musculoskeletal adaptations to resistance training. In *ACSM's Resource Manual* (4th ed.),

   ed. J. L. Roitman. Philadelphia: Lippincott Williams and Wilkins.
8. Nieman, D. C. 1999. *Exercise Testing and Prescription: A Health-Related Approach,* Mountain View, Calif.: Mayfield Publishing Co.
9. Spain, C. G., and B. D. Franks. 2001. Healthy people 2010: physical activity and fitness. *PCPFS Research Digest* 3(13):1–16.
10. Modifica, M. 1998. Exercise and aging. *Fitness Management* 14(10):48.
11. U.S. Dept. of Health and Human Services. 1996. *Physical Activity and Health: A Report of the Surgeon General.* Atlanta, Ga.: U.S. Dept. of Health and Human Services, Centers for Disease and Prevention, National Center for Chronic Disease Prevention and Health Promotion.
12. Davis, A., et al. 1998. Strength, physical activity, and body mass index: relationship to performance-based measure and activities of daily living among older Japanese women in Hawaii. *Journal of the American Geriatrics Society* 46:274.
13. American College of Sports Medicine. 2000. *ACSM's Guidelines for Exercise*

    Testing and Prescription (6th ed.). Philadelphia: Lippincott Williams and Wilkins.
14. Faigenbaum, A. D., and Y. Beniamini. 1997. The evaluation of muscular strength in cardiac patients. *ACSM Certified News* 7(2):1.
15. American College of Sports Medicine. 1998. Exercise and physical activity for older adults. *Medicine and Science in Sports and Exercise* 30(6):992.
16. Muscling up: better health through greater strength. 2000. *Health After 50* 12(10):4–5.
17. Bryant, C. X., J. A. Peterson, and J. E. Graves. 2001. Muscular strength and endurance. In *ACSM's Resource Manual* (4th ed.), ed. J. L. Roitman. Philadelphia: Lippincott Williams and Wilkins.
18. Graves, J. E., M. L. Pollock, and C. X. Bryant. 2001. Assessment of muscular strength and endurance. In *ACSM's Resource Manual* (4th ed.), ed. J. L. Roitman. Philadelphia: Lippincott Williams and Wilkins.
19. Foss, M. L., and S. J. Keteyian. 1998. *Fox's Physiological Basis for Exercise and Sport.* Boston: WCB/McGraw-Hill.

20. Fleck, S. J., and W. J. Kraemer. 1997. *Designing resistance training programs.* Champaign, Ill.: Human Kinetics.
21. Humphrey, R. 2001. Musculosketal anatomy. In *ACSM's Resource Manual* (4th ed.), ed. J. L. Roitman. Philadelphia: Lippincott Williams and Wilkins.
22. Kraemer, W. J., and J. A. Bush. 2001. Factors affecting the acute neuromuscular responses to resistance exercise. In *ACSM's Resource Manual* (4th ed.), ed. J. L. Roitman. Philadelphia: Lippincott Williams and Wilkins.
23. Williams, M. H. 1998. *Nutrition for Health, Fitness, and Sport.* Dubuque, Iowa: WCB/McGraw-Hill.
24. Williams, M. H. 1998. Nutritional ergogenics and sports performances. *PCPFS Research Digest* 3(20):1–8.
25. McArdle, W. D., F. I. Katch, and V. L. Katch 1999. *Sports and Exercise Nutrition.* Philadelphia: Lippincott Williams and Wilkins.
26. Yesalis, C. E., and M. S. Bahrke. 1995. Anabolic-androgenic steroids: current issues. *Sports Medicine* 19:326–340.
27. Yesalis, C. E., S. P. Courson, and J. Wright. 1993. History of anabolic steroid use in sport and exercise. *Anabolic Steroids in Sport and Exercise.* Champaign, Ill: Human Kinetics.

Selected Readings

Kutz, M. 2000, Creatine effects on performers and health. *Fitness Management* 16(6):48–51.

Discusses what is known about creatine, its benefits, and the precautions that a potential user should observe. It brings the reader up-to-date on creatine, and the material is presented primarily in nonscientific language.

Editors. Muscle fights weight gain. 2001. *Environmental Nutrition* 24(4):3

Aging is only one factor involved in the reduction in resting metabolism. A loss of cell mass, two-thirds of which comes from muscle tissue, is responsible for the reduction. But a new study indicates that weight training can speed up metabolism by rebuilding lost muscle mass.

Editors. Strength training for heart patients. 2001. *Heart Advisors* 4(4):4–5.

Recovering heart attack and bypass patients are now encouraged to participate in weight training to lessen the strain associated with everyday activities and to nullify the consequences of aging. This article provides information on how, why, and when, and it is written for a novice.

Editors. Muscling up: better health through greater strength. 2000. *The Johns Hopkins Medical Letter Health After 50* 12(10):4–5.

Discusses and makes the case that strength training is an equal partner with aerobic endurance training for all people but particularly for older people. Discusses the health benefits that can be received from strength training.

Tufts University. 2000. More people lifting weights—and getting injured. *Tufts University Health & Nutrition Letter* 18(9):1,8.

More people are lifting, therefore, there are more injuries. But this does not have to occur because weight training is safe if practitioners adhere to some simple rules and practices. This article discusses some of the ways to make strength training safer.

Name _____ Date _____ Section _____

Assessment Activity 4-1

Calculation of Strength (Selected Muscle Groups)

Directions: The calculation of strength by this method is expressed as the ratio of strength to body weight. The amount of weight accomplished for each lift is converted to a proportion of your body weight and is determined in the following manner:

1. Find your 1 RM for each of the following exercises: biceps curl (two arm), overhead press, bench press, half-squat or leg press, and hamstring curl.
2. Divide your 1 RM for each exercise by your body weight. For example, a 130-lb. woman performs a 1 RM bench press of 80 lbs. Her score is 80 ÷ 130 = 0.61. Turn to the chart for an interpretation of her score. Look under the Bench Press column and note

that her score of 0.61 is in the Average category. In this example, the woman has the following results on the five lifts: biceps curl = 0.28 (fair), standing press = 0.26 (fair), bench press = 0.61 (average), half-squat or leg press = 1.35 (good), and hamstring curl = 0.52 (good). These data are plotted in the first strength profile chart.

3. When you have computed a score for each of your lifts, turn to the strength profile charts. Plot your data in the blank chart provided.
4. Refer to figures 4-1 through 4-16 for a refresher on how to do these exercises.

Strength/Body Weight Ratio

Women

Biceps Curl	Overhead Press	Bench Press	Half-Squat or Leg Press	Hamstring Curl	Strength Category
0.45 and above	0.50 and above	0.85 and above	1.45 and above	0.55 and above	Excellent
0.38–0.44	0.42–0.49	0.70–0.84	1.30–1.44	0.50–0.54	Good
0.32–0.37	0.32–0.41	0.60–0.69	1.00–1.29	0.40–0.49	Average
0.25–0.31	0.25–0.31	0.50–0.59	0.80–0.99	0.30–0.39	Fair
0.24 and below	0.24 and below	0.49 and below	0.79 and below	0.29 and below	Poor

Men

Biceps Curl	Overhead Press	Bench Press	Half-Squat or Leg Press	Hamstring Curl	Strength Category
0.65 and above	1.0 and above	1.30 and above	1.85 and above	0.65 and above	Excellent
0.55–0.64	0.90–0.99	1.15–1.29	1.65–1.84	0.55–0.64	Good
0.45–0.54	0.75–0.89	1.00–1.14	1.30–1.64	0.45–0.54	Average
0.35–0.44	0.60–0.74	0.85–0.99	1.00–1.29	0.35–0.44	Fair
0.34 and below	0.59 and below	0.84 and below	Less than 1.0	0.34 and below	Poor

Strength Profile Charts

Example

Your Data

	Biceps Curl	Overhead Press	Bench Press	Half-Squat or Leg Press	Hamstring Curl
Excellent					
Good					
Average					
Fair					
Poor					

Name _____ **Date** _____ **Section** _____

Assessment Activity 4-2

Muscular Endurance

Directions: Through trial and error, select a weight that you can use while performing 20 RM for each of the following exercises: bench press, leg extension or half-squat, biceps curl, and hamstring curl. For example, a male subject weighing 150 lbs. can perform 20 RM of 100 lbs. in the bench press. The score for this exercise is computed as follows:

$$\frac{100 \text{ lbs. (20 RM)}}{150 \text{ lbs.}} = 0.67 \text{ or } 67\%$$

Now look at the chart under Bench Press and observe that a score of 67% is average. Perform each of the four exercises (20 RM) and calculate the muscle endurance scores following the example.

Muscle Endurance: Body Weight Ratio 20 RM

Men

Bench Press	Leg Extension or Half-Squat	Biceps Curl	Hamstring Curl	Strength Category
≥76%*	≥166%	≥50%	≥40%	Excellent
70%–75%	150%–165%	43%–49%	33%–39%	Good
60%–69%	133%–149%	37%–42%	27%–32%	Average
50%–59%	116%–132%	30%–36%	20%–26%	Fair
<50%	<116%	<30%	<20%	Poor

Women

Bench Press	Leg Extension or Half-Squat	Biceps Curl	Hamstring Curl	Strength Category
≥50%	≥115%	≥32%	≥38%	Excellent
42%–49%	100%–114%	23%–31%	31%–37%	Good
35%–41%	88%–99%	15%–22%	23%–30%	Average
27%–34%	77%–87%	12%–14%	15%–22%	Fair
<27%	<77%	<12%	<15%	Poor

*≥, equal to or greater than; <, less than.

Assessment Activity 4-3

Abdominal Muscular Endurance—the Canadian Trunk Strength Test

Directions: The Canadian trunk strength test is an alternative to the conventional sit-up test to measure abdominal muscular endurance. It is not necessary or desirable to raise the trunk more than 30 degrees. Sit-ups beyond 30 degrees cause the abdomen to contract isometrically, so the hip flexors supply the power to raise the trunk above this level. The Canadian trunk strength test is performed in the following manner:

1. Lie on your back with knees bent 90 degrees.
2. Extend your arms so that the fingertips of both hands touch a strip of tape perpendicular to the body on each side.
3. Place two additional strips of tape parallel to the first two strips, 8 cm apart.

4. Curl up, sliding your fingertips along the mat until they touch the second set of tape strips, and then return to the starting position.
5. The curl up is slow, controlled, and continuous with a cadence of 20 curl ups/min. (3 secs./curl up).
6. A metronome provides the speed of movement. It is set at 40 beats/min. (curl up on one beat, down on the second).
7. Perform as many curl ups as you can up to a maximum of 75 without missing a beat. See figure 4-22 for a demonstration of the Canadian trunk strength test and then turn to the chart for an interpretation of your score.

Standards for the Canadian Trunk Strength Test

	Number Completed					
	Men—Age			Women—Age		
Strength Category	**<35**	**35–44**	**>45**	**<35**	**35–44**	**>45**
Excellent	60	50	40	50	40	30
Good	45	40	25	40	25	15
Marginal	30	25	15	25	15	10
Needs work	15	10	5	10	6	4

(a)

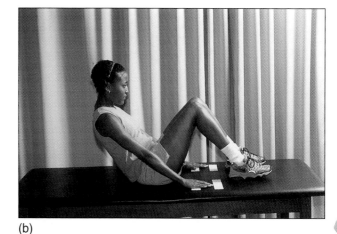

(b)

Figure 4-22 Canadian Trunk Strength Test

Name _____ Date _____ Section _____

Assessment Activity 4-4

Assessing Muscular Strength and Endurance with Selected Calisthenic Exercises

Directions: The tests making up this assessment require minimal equipment and are easy to administer.

Chin-ups: Grasp an overhead horizontal bar, hands shoulder-width apart, palms facing your body. On the upstroke your chin must go above the bar, and your arms must extend fully on the downstroke. Your legs must remain extended throughout the exercise and should not be used to thrust your body upward (figure 4-23).

Flexed-arm hang: Perform this exercise if you cannot do chin-ups. Have someone assist you to the exercise position with your chin above the bar, palms facing away from your body. A stopwatch is started as soon as you assume this position and is stopped if you tilt your head back to keep your chin above the bar, if your chin touches the bar, or if your chin drops below the bar. Record the time to the nearest whole second (figure 4-24).

(a)

(b)

Figure 4-23 Chin-Ups

Push-ups: Assume a prone position (face down) with your arms extended, hands on the floor under your shoulders. Keep your back and legs straight and your feet together. The person counting the push-ups should place a fist under your chest. Bend your elbows, lowering your chest until contact is made with the counter's fist, and then return to the starting position by straightening your arms. Repeat as many times as possible without resting to a maximum score of 46 push-ups (figure 4-25).

Modified push-ups: Perform this exercise if you cannot do the standard push-up. The modified version is performed in the same manner as the standard push-up except that you support your body weight with your hands and knees. Do as many as you can without rest to a maximum of 24 (figure 4-26).

Figure 4-24 Flexed-Arm Hang

(a)

(b)

Figure 4-25 Push-Ups

(a)

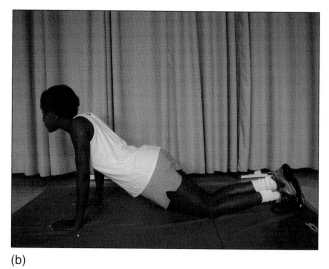
(b)

Figure 4-26   Modified Push-Ups

Muscular Strength and Endurance Standards

Chin-Ups	Flexed-Arm Hang (secs.)	Push-Ups	Modified Push-Ups	Strength Category
20 or more	30 or more	40 or more	24 or more	Excellent
15–19	24–29	32–39	14–23	Good
10–14	15–23	27–31	8–13	Average
6–9	9–14	20–26	2–7	Fair
5 or less	8 or less	19 or less	1 or less	Poor

Assessment Activity 4-5

Resistance Training Log

Directions: Keep a record of your resistance fitness activities on the form provided. Make copies of this form for repeated uses.

Daily Training Log

Name _____ Starting date _____

Program objectives _____

Exercise	Date:			Date:			Date:			Date:			Date:			Date:		
	Resis.* (lbs.)	Reps	Sets	Resis. (lbs.)	Reps	Sets	Resis. (lbs.)	Reps	Sets	Resis. (lbs.)	Reps	Sets	Resis. (lbs.)	Reps	Sets	Resis. (lbs.)	Reps	Sets

*Resis., resistance; reps, repetitions.

5

Improving Flexibility

Online Learning Center

Log on to our Online Learning Center (OLC) for access to these additional resources:

- Chapter key term flashcards
- Learning objectives
- Additional goals for behavior change
- Concentration game
- Self-scoring chapter quizzes

- Additional lab activities

The OLC also offers weblinks for study and exploration of wellness topics. Access these links through **www.mhhe.com/anspaugh5e**, click on "Student Center," click on "Chapter 5," and then click on "Web Activities."

Goals for Behavior Change

- Begin participating regularly in a stretching program to improve flexibility.
- Identify some of the tasks or sports that you perform regularly for which being more flexible would be helpful.
- Practice correct lifting techniques when moving heavy objects.
- Modify your work or study area to lower the risk of neck and back pain.
- Try two safe ergogenic aids and analyze their effectiveness.

Key Terms

ballistic stretching
flexibility
goniometer
proprioceptive
  neuromuscular facilitation
  (PNF)

static stretching
stretch reflex

Objectives

After completing this chapter, you will be able to do the following:

- Define *flexibility*.
- Identify factors affecting flexibility.
- Distinguish among static, ballistic, and proprioceptive neuromuscular facilitation stretching.
- Assess and prescribe a personal flexibility program.

- Discuss the high incidence of neck pain, upper-back pain, and lower-back pain in the United States.
- Demonstrate proper lifting techniques for prevention of lower-back injury.

We do haffa (sp) yoga (includes pur +
Yastanga yoga)

Flexibility and Wellness

Flexibility programs are planned, deliberate, and regularly performed sets of exercises designed to progressively increase the range of motion of a joint or series of joints.[1] Flexibility is an important component of health-related physical fitness but one that is often neglected even though it requires a minimal investment in time, effort, and equipment.

Factors that limit joint movement include (1) the bony structure of the joints (the skeleton is established by heredity, but it can be harmed by trauma, disease, calcium deposits, etc.); (2) the amount of tissue (muscle and fat) around and adjacent to the joint; (3) the elasticity of muscles, tendons, and connective tissue; and (4) the skin (scar tissue from surgery or a laceration over a joint may limit movement). Other factors that influence flexibility are age, gender, and level and type of physical activity. Young people are more flexible than adults because tendons lose their elasticity with age. However, inactivity may play a greater role than the aging process in the loss of flexibility because muscles and other soft tissues lose elasticity when not used. Active individuals are usually more flexible than inactive people.[2] Women tend to be more flexible than men because the hormones that permit women's tissue to stretch during the childbirth process facilitate all body stretching.[3] The range of motion for most movements begins to decline in the mid-20s for men and women.[2] (Complete Assessment Activities 5-1 through 5-4 at the end of this chapter to determine your flexibility.)

Joint flexibility is important for several reasons. Inflexible muscles around the joints limit range of movement, eventually inhibiting activities of daily life. This phenomenon is most frequently seen in older people who have difficulty reaching down to tie their shoes or bending over to get a drink of water from a fountain. Lack of flexibility in the shoulders can affect performance of normal duties, such as changing an overhead light bulb or removing a can of vegetables from a cupboard.[4] Tight muscles may also contribute to joint deterioration by subjecting the bones to excessive pressure, causing pain and abnormalities in joint lubrication. Regular flexibility exercises can improve body posture. Flexibility exercises following aerobic activity reduce muscle soreness.[4]

According to the American College of Sports Medicine (ACSM), stretching exercises may prevent injuries.[5] The supporting data come primarily from observational studies, which are not as definitive as randomized, controlled clinical trials. But, even though scientific evidence does not strongly support flexibility training for injury prevention, sports medicine specialists advocate its use.[6] Based upon the available evidence as well as experience, flexibility exercises help to maintain a full range of joint motion.

~~ *Just the Facts* ~~

Benefits of Flexibility Training

Here are some of the positive outcomes of flexibility training:

- Reduction of stress and tension
- Muscle relaxation
- Improved fitness, posture, and symmetry
- Relief of muscle cramps
- Relief of muscle soreness
- Prevention of injury
- Reduced frequency of injury
- Return to full range of motion after an injury

Maintenance of flexibility is most important for the prevention of lower-back pain.[7] For example, a sedentary lifestyle characterized by sitting for long periods leads to a loss of flexibility and increases the likelihood of lower-back injury. Flexibility of the hamstring muscles (a group of muscles in the back of the thighs) and the lower-back muscles contributes to good posture. Posture is also improved by the development of strong abdominal muscles and the maintenance of normal body weight. Extra body weight, particularly that which accumulates around the abdominal area, throws the body out of balance and applies a forward force on the lower (lumbar) spinal area, which places extra stress on the lower back.[8]

The benefits of flexibility training are summarized in Just the Facts: Benefits of Flexibility Training. See also Nurturing Your Spirituality: The Ancient Arts of Tai Chi and Yoga.

Developing a Flexibility Program

Flexibility can be improved by exercises that promote the elasticity of the soft tissues. Figures 5-1 through 5-8 demonstrate exercises that can maintain and improve the flexibility of the major body sites. These 10-minute exercises can be done every day, both before and after exercise, and also on days of rest from exercise.

When to Stretch

Stretching exercises can be included in the warm-up prior to exercise and in the cooldown following exercise and done on nonexercise days. Stretching prior to working out should occur only after the muscles have

Nurturing Your Spirituality

The Ancient Arts of Tai Chi and Yoga

Medical health care training and delivery have been gradually adopting a more holistic view of treating patients. This holistic view recognizes the role of spirituality in the healing process. Johns Hopkins Medical School currently offers an elective course for its medical students on spirituality and healing.[9] The National Institutes of Health has awarded grants to a small number of medical schools to develop and promote courses on this subject.

At the same time that spirituality is making a medical comeback, Americans are searching for ways to alleviate stress, promote relaxation, and enhance health. Two physical arts that blend spirituality and health, tai chi and yoga, are gaining popularity.

Tai chi originated as a self-defense art, but it has evolved into a religious ritual, relaxation technique, and exercise program for people of all ages, including the elderly. Tai chi features slow, balanced, low-impact movements that may reduce stress and improve flexibility, balance, and strength.[10] It requires concentration, controlled breathing, and balance while body weight is shifted as a person transitions from one movement to another. It is often referred to as *movement meditation*, because it promotes muscle relaxation through movement.

The potential benefits of tai chi include the following:

- Improved flexibility
- Physical therapy, because it may assist in recovery from injury
- Improved balance and coordination
- Improved strength, particularly of the lower body (buttocks, thighs, and calves)
- Improved posture
- Increased ability to relax
- Possible slight reduction in the resting blood pressure.

It takes years to become adept at tai chi, but several movements and positions can be learned with a few weeks of instruction.

Yoga originated in India about 6000 years ago. There are several types, but hatha yoga seems to be most popular among Americans. Hatha yoga features a system of exercises that promote physical fitness and mental well-being.[11]

Yoga is a Sanskrit word that means "union." Its practitioners strive for total union in experience, a union of physical, mental, and spiritual states. Achieving this union results in a calm, relaxed, tranquil attitude.

Research indicates that yoga's meditative characteristics may prevent or at least decrease the severity of psychosomatic illness. Psychosomatic illnesses are mind-body maladies. They are caused by negative mental states and attitudes that produce changes in body physiology that result in disease. Some common psychosomatic diseases are tension headaches, ulcers, asthma, stress, essential hypertension, impotence, back pain, and menstrual problems.

Master practitioners can, at will, influence bodily responses controlled by the autonomic nervous system, such as breathing rate, heart rate, and blood pressure. But it takes years of practice to achieve this level of control.

The exercises and body positions featured in yoga promote mobility and flexibility, but some of these positions are potentially unsafe. It is important to learn from an experienced instructor to minimize mistakes.

Practiced regularly, yoga may lower resting blood pressure, relieve mild depression, and contribute to strength and balance. Anecdotal evidence (evidence that comes from personal reports) also indicates that practitioners experience more energy and feel calmer and more focused.[11]

been warmed up with 5 to 10 minutes of such cardiovascular activities as brisk walking, slow jogging, riding a stationary bike, or similar activity.[6,12] A gradual warm-up increases heart rate slowly and raises the temperature of muscles, tendons, and ligaments by increasing blood flow to these structures. Stretching after a warm-up is safer and more productive than stretching before: Stretching cold muscles increases the probability of incurring a soft tissue injury.[13] Warm up prior to stretching for approximately 10 minutes on the days of rest between workouts.

The highest payback from stretching comes at the end of an aerobic or resistive workout. During this time, the muscles are thoroughly warmed and capable of stretching maximally and safely. Also, the muscles that have been contracting and shortening vigorously and continuously during the workout should be systematically stretched and lengthened after the workout.

Types of Stretching

Muscles must contract for movement to occur. The contracting muscles are called *agonists* and are the prime movers. For an agonist to contract, shorten, and produce movement, a reciprocal lengthening of its *antagonist* must occur. For example, when the biceps muscle of the upper arm contracts, its opposite, the triceps muscle, must relax and lengthen. In this case the biceps is the agonist and the triceps is the antagonist, but the triceps becomes the agonist for movements that require it to contract, making the biceps the antagonist. Understanding these concepts is necessary to understanding stretching techniques.

Static stretching involves slowly moving to desired positions, holding them for 15 to 30 seconds, and then slowly releasing them. This method of stretching does not activate the **stretch reflex** (automatic or reflexive contraction of a muscle being stretched), so the muscle is essentially stretched without opposition.

The stretch reflex consists of two proprioceptors: the muscle spindle and the Golgi tendon organ.[12] A *proprioceptor* is a sensory organ found in muscles, joints, and tendons that provides information regarding bodily movement and position. The *muscle spindle* is a receptor sensitive to changes in muscle length. The *Golgi tendon organ* is a receptor that is also sensitive to changes in muscle length but additionally responds to increases in muscle tension.[12]

Stretching the muscles also stretches their muscle spindles, which send volley sensory impulses, informing

(a)

(b)

(c)

Figure 5-1 Neck Stretches

Slowly bend your neck from side to side and to the front. Do not do head circles, because these require hyperextension (excessive extension) of the cervical (neck) area of the spinal column, which produces potentially harmful compression of the intervertebral disks.

(a)

(b)

Figure 5-2 Shoulder Stretch

(a) gently pull your right arm behind your head and hold for 15 to 30 seconds. (b) repeat with the other arm.

Figure 5-3 Chest and Shoulder Stretch

Stretch your arms to full extension with both palms on the floor and press your chest down to the floor. Hold 15 to 30 seconds and slowly release.

the brain that the muscles are being subjected to stretch. Impulses are sent back to the muscles, which cause them to contract reflexively, thus resisting the stretch. But if a muscle is stretched statically and the position is held for at least 6 seconds, the Golgi tendon organ responds to the change in length and tension by sending a volley of signals of its own to the brain via the spinal cord. Unlike the signals from the muscle spindle, those initiated by the Golgi tendon organ cause the antagonist muscle (the muscle being stretched) to relax reflexively. This protective mechanism allows the muscle to stretch through relaxation as the Golgi tendon organ nullifies or overrides the signals of the muscle spindle. Thus, stretching positions held for at least 6 seconds and preferably for 15 to 30 seconds allow muscles to lengthen and stretch with minimal chance of injury.

Static stretching should produce a feeling of mild discomfort but not pain. Static stretching (see figures 5-1 to 5-8) results in little or no muscle soreness, has a low incidence of injury, requires little energy, and can be done alone. For these reasons, static stretching is the preferred system for increasing flexibility.

These guidelines should be followed for safe and effective static stretching:[6]

- Warm up for a few minutes before stretching by walking, slow jogging, doing light calisthenics, or doing some similar activity.
- Stretch to the point of mild discomfort.
- Do not stretch to the point of pain.
- Hold each stretch for 10 to 30 seconds minimum.
- Do not hold your breath during a stretch; breathe rhythmically and continuously.

(a)

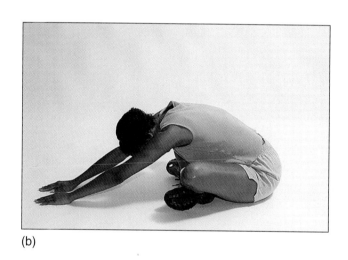
(b)

Figure 5-4 Back Stretch

(a) cross your legs and lean forward, extending your arms to the front. (b) hold for 15 to 30 seconds and slowly release.

(a)

(b)

Figure 5-5 Groin Stretch

(a) place the soles of your feet together and lean forward. Hold 15 to 30 seconds. (b) variation: push down gently on both knees and hold for 15 to 30 seconds.

Figure 5-6 Quadriceps Stretch

Lie on your side as shown. Bend the knee of your top leg, grasp your ankle with your free hand, and slowly pull your heel toward your buttocks until you feel the stretch in the muscles in the front of your thigh. Hold 15 to 30 seconds, roll over to the other side, and repeat with your other leg.

Figure 5-7 Hamstring Stretch

Place the sole of your left foot against the thigh of your extended right leg. Lean forward without bending the knee of your extended leg. Hold for 15 to 30 seconds and repeat with your other leg.

- Move slowly from position to position.
- Perform each stretch at least four times.
- Stretch after the workout; this produces the greatest benefit because the muscles are warm and more amenable to stretching.
- Perform stretching exercises five to six times per week.

Deliberate attempts to improve flexibility should occur throughout the life cycle. See Wellness Across the Generations: Flexibility Guidelines for Children and Older Adults for more specific information.

Proprioceptive neuromuscular facilitation (PNF) is another effective and acceptable stretching technique. It is more complex than most methods of stretching, but

Wellness On the Web Behavior Change Activities

Go for the Stretch . . . and Then Some

Flexibility affects both your health and wellness. It is defined as the range of motion of a given joint. If you think flexibility is related to the muscles only, then you are mistaken. While muscle flexibility is important, the actual ligaments that attach muscle to muscle and tendons that attach bone to bone are just as, if not more, important.

If you are not flexible, you have a higher risk for joint and muscle injury.

Each joint in the body must be tested for flexibility separately. To learn how to test your major joints for flexibility, go to **www.mhhe.com/anspaugh5e**. Click on Student Center, then Chapter 5, then Wellness on the Web, and then Activity 1.

Ready, Set, Stretch!

Flexibility is an important part of your exercise program, yet it's often a neglected part. How often have you gone through your routine and then decided to skip stretching because you're tired or ready to get home? Being flexible will help you function better throughout the day and make you feel good.

Keeping your muscles and ligaments flexible is important because tight muscles can cause chronic pain. For example, sitting all day can cause tight hip flexors and loose gluteal muscles. This muscular imbalance can make the joint weaker as parts of the bone surface bear more weight than they should. And, what about your back? In many cases, back pain is caused by tight hamstrings which cause the hips and pelvis to rotate back, flattening the lower back and causing back problems.

Other benefits of stretching include:

- Reduced potential for injury
- Improved performance
- Reduced soreness and lower back pain
- Increased blood flow to the body
- Improved coordination
- Keeping you active and mobile as you age
- It feels good!

To learn more about stretching, and about some of the tools you can use in a stretching routine, go to **www.mhhe.com/anspaugh5e**, click on Student Center, then Chapter 5, then Wellness on the Web, and then Activity 2.

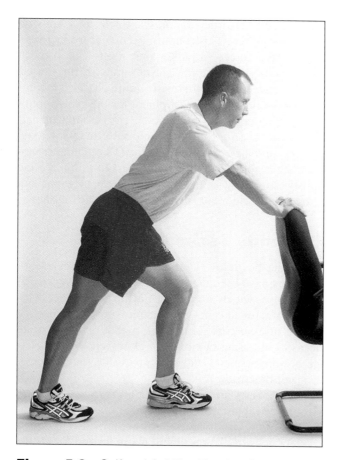

Figure 5-8 Calf and Achilles Tendon Stretch

Assume the position shown. Be sure the heel of your extended leg remains in contact with the floor and both feet are pointed straight ahead. Slowly move your hips forward until you feel the stretch in the calf of your extended leg. Hold 15 to 30 seconds and repeat with your other leg.

Wellness Across the Generations

Flexibility Guidelines for Children and Older Adults

Flexibility peaks in the mid- to late 20s for men and women and declines thereafter in people who are not actively engaged in physical activities that include planned exercises for the purpose of maintaining or increasing range of motion. Evidence indicates that flexibility can be increased in healthy older adults who participate in aerobic activities supplemented with stretching exercises.[2] Physical activities such as walking and aerobic dance coupled with stretching exercises increase the range of motion of older adults.

Recommendations for improving the flexibility of children are somewhat different. Because children are more flexible than adults, 5- to 9-year olds need less time devoted to flexibility exercises than do older adults.[15] However, some formal stretching is required, and activities such as tumbling and climbing are suggested. For older children, ages 10 through 12, the amount of time spent on improving flexibility should be greater than that of younger children but less than that of adults. Children, especially boys, begin to lose flexibility at this age, so regular stretching exercises and physical activities, such as tumbling, that promote flexibility are recommended.

It is important to establish the habit of regularly stretching the muscles, tendons, and joints throughout one's lifetime. Stretching becomes even more important as we become older.

it is the most effective.[5,12,14] By combining slow passive movements (the force for passive movement is supplied by a partner) with maximal voluntary isometric contractions, you can bypass the stretch reflex stimulation that accompanies changes in muscle and tendon length.

All variations of PNF stretching require a partner and some combination of passive stretching and isometric contractions. Two of the common PNF methods, contract-relax (CR) and slow reversal-hold-relax (SRHR), are presented in figures 5-9 and 5-10. For comparison, both figures exemplify stretching the hamstring group (muscles in the back of the thigh). The hamstrings are the antagonist muscle group, and the quadriceps muscles (muscles in the front of the thigh) are the agonists. For example, the CR method is performed as follows (figure 5-9):

A partner gently pushes the upraised leg in the direction of arrow *A*. This movement passively stretches the antagonist (hamstrings).

The subject follows this with a 6-second maximal contraction of the agonist (quadriceps).

This is followed by another passive stretch of the hamstrings.

This is repeated twice with a few seconds of rest between sequences.

The SRHR method is performed in the following manner (figure 5-10):

A partner gently pushes the upraised leg in the direction of arrow *A*.

The subject then performs a 6-second maximal voluntary isometric contraction (MVIC) of the antagonists (hamstrings) against resistance supplied by the partner.

- The subject follows this with a 6-second maximal contraction of the agonists (quadriceps).
- This is followed by another passive stretch of the hamstrings.

This sequence is repeated twice with a few seconds of rest between exercises.

Although PNF appears to be the most effective stretching method for enhancing flexibility, it has some limitations. It requires a partner; it produces more pain and muscle stiffness; it requires more time; and it increases the risk of injury, particularly when used by novices.

Ballistic stretching uses dynamic movements or repetitive bouncing motions to stretch muscles. Each time a muscle is stretched in this manner, the muscle spindle (one of two receptors that make up the stretch reflex) located in that muscle is also stretched. It responds by sending a volley of signals to the central ner-

vous system that order the muscle to contract, thus resisting the stretch. This is not only counterproductive—the muscle is forced to pull against itself—but also can lead to injury because the elastic limits of the muscle may be exceeded. Ballistic stretching is not recommended for flexibility development for the general public. Many competitive athletes—performers participating in track and field, gymnastics, martial arts, dancing, and so on—employ ballistic stretching to improve sport-specific flexibility.[16] Years of training using ballistic stretching enables these athletes to adapt and withstand the rigors of such training in relative safety.

Flexibility Assessment

Measuring flexibility is rather difficult, and several instruments have been developed for this purpose. Probably the most widely used device is the **goniometer.** This is a protractor-like device that measures the range of motion of a specific joint. This method is an accurate means of assessing flexibility.[17] However, for the average person, assessing flexibility by using the goniometer is not practical.

Several tests are suitable for measuring flexibility when more sophisticated means cannot be used. (The directions and norms for these tests are provided in the assessment activities.) You should warm up and follow the rules for general stretching before taking the assessments.

Preventing Back and Neck Pain

All people experience tense muscles and muscle soreness in various parts of the body on an occasional basis. The neck, shoulder, and back are particularly susceptible to the types of pressures that cause pain. Sedentary lifestyles contribute to back pain; unfortunately 60 percent of Americans are sedentary or marginally active. Also contributing to neck and back pain are occupations that require workers to stand for long periods or to spend a significant amount of time sitting behind a desk, in front of a computer, or behind the wheel of an automobile. According to the Bureau of Labor Statistics, approximately 92,500 cases of occupational injuries and illnesses are due to repetitive motion. Typing or key entry; repetitive use of tools; and repetitive placing, grasping, or moving objects other than tools result in such injury.[18] Musculoskeletal problems are highly associated with these work-related physical tasks when the level of exposure is high. Performing unaccustomed physical work or engaging in unfamiliar sports also produces stress on the back and neck. Activities that require repetitive overhead reaching or extended sitting at a computer may produce pain and discomfort in the back, shoulders, and neck. The

Figure 5-9 Contract-Relax (CR) Technique

Figure 5-10 Slow Reversal-Hold-Relax (SRHR) Technique

exercises in figures 5-1 through 5-4, coupled with a few minutes of moving about, may prevent or alleviate pain in these areas of the body.

These problems can be significantly lessened if (1) employers carefully design the layout of work stations, job methods, tools, and materials to reduce exposure to the physical factors related to performing repetitive tasks, and (2) employees become aerobically fit and engage in activities to promote muscle and joint flexibility.

Lower-back pain affects 80 to 90 percent of American adults at some point in their lives.[19] It is one of the main reasons people visit their primary care physicians even though 90 percent of people affected recover within a month.

The high incidence of lower-back pain is caused by the following: excess body weight, weak abdominal muscles, weak and inflexible back muscles, weak and inflexible hamstring muscles, poor posture, cigarette smoking, lifting objects incorrectly, work- or sports-related injuries, and diseases such as osteoarthritis and osteoporosis.

Excess body weight stresses the lower back by pulling the spinal column forward. This causes an excessive amount of arch in the lower back that results in poor alignment of the spine. As a result, obese people are more susceptible to lower-back problems than are normal-weight people.

Weak abdominal muscles, weak and inflexible back muscles, and tight hamstring muscles distort upright posture and tilt the pelvis forward, which increases stress on the lower back[20] Figure 5-11 illustrates exercises that stretch the lower back and develop the abdominal muscles.

(a)

(b)

(c)

(d)

Figure 5-11 Maintaining a Healthy Back

(a) to develop the abdominal muscles, lie on your back in the position shown, and contract your abdominal muscles to force the lower back against the floor. Hold for 6 to 10 seconds. Relax and repeat 5 to 10 times.

(b) to develop the abdominal muscles, lie on your back, cross your arms over your chest, and raise your shoulder blades off the floor as shown. Return to the starting position. Repeat 5 times and work up to 25.

(c) to stretch the hamstrings, hips, and buttocks, raise one leg and extend the other. Reach up and grasp the upright leg below the calf. Alternate legs and work up to 20 repetitions with each.

(d) to develop lower abdominal muscles, keep one leg bent with that foot flat on the floor. Raise the extended leg about 6 inches off the floor, and return to the starting position. Do 10 reps and repeat with the other leg. Work up to 25 reps.

Smokers have a higher incidence of lower-back pain than do nonsmokers. Smoking appears to increase degenerative changes in the spine.

Figure 5-12 demonstrates correct and incorrect ways to lift a weight from the floor. Lifting correctly substantially lowers the risk of sustaining a lower-back injury. See Just the Facts: Tips for Preventing and Treating Back and Neck Pain.

The spinal column consists of thirty-three bones (the vertebrae) and represents the only bony connection between the upper and lower halves of the body. Although humans are born with thirty-three separate vertebrae, by adulthood five vertebrae of the sacrum fuse into one bone, and the four vertebrae of the coccyx also fuse into one bone, leaving a total of twenty-four vertebral bones. See figure 5-13, which illustrates the shape and bony structure of the vertebral column.

Located between the bones of the spine are rings of tough fibrous tissue, the disks, which act as shock absorbers, keeping the vertebrae from rubbing against

Figure 5-12   How to Lift Objects

(a) lifting an object from the floor with straight legs and a bent back places significant stress on the lower back, increasing the likelihood of injury. Notice the distance between the box being lifted and the body of the lifter. (b) lifting an object from the floor with bent legs and a straight back allows the lifter to keep the box close to the body, which places the majority of stress on the legs rather than on the lower back.

Just the Facts

Tips for Preventing and Treating Back and Neck Pain

The following behaviors may help to alleviate or prevent back and neck pain:

- If you sit, stand, or work in one place for extended periods, periodically walk around for a few minutes and do some simple stretching exercises.

- If your job requires long periods of standing, you can reduce the stress on your lower back by placing one foot and then the other on a small stool for a few minutes at a time. This rounds the spine and reduces lower-back stress. You can also shift your weight from one foot to the other.

- If you drive for long periods, sit comfortably and make sure you can easily reach the dash, pedals, and steering wheel. You can also try placing a small pillow behind your lower back. Also, stop the vehicle every two to three hours to take a short stretch break.

- Exercise regularly to develop the abdominal muscles and to stretch the back muscles.

- Stretch the back muscles and hamstrings at least three times per week.

- Maintain a healthy body weight.

- Bend at the knees while lifting objects so that your legs do most of the work.

- Do not smoke cigarettes, because they contribute to the degeneration of the spine.

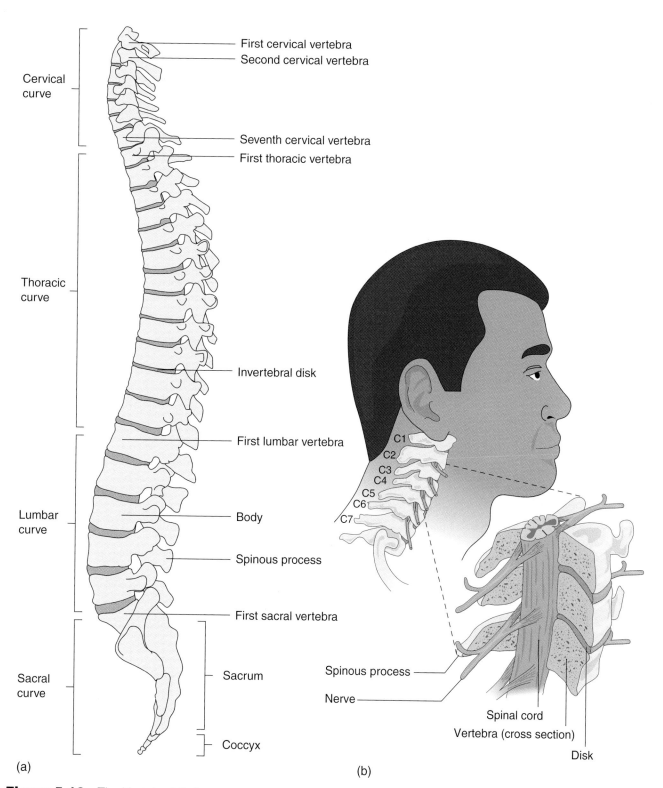

Figure 5-13 The Vertebral Column

(a) the complete column viewed from the left side. Note that the vertebrae of the sacrum are fused into one bone, and those of the coccyx have also fused into one bone. (b) the vertebrae of the cervical curve from the right side.

each other. The spinal column is S-shaped and consists of naturally occurring curves. When these curves are balanced, the body weight is evenly distributed and movement occurs fluidly. Misalignment in these regions applies substantial stress to the concave, or inner, side of the curves. The more pronounced the curves, the greater the stress because of the uneven distribution of weight on the bones and disks.

Approximately 90 percent of all back problems occur in the lumbar region (lower back) of the spine because that region carries the weight of the torso (the trunk of the human body). Fatigue causes the pelvis to tilt forward when a person is standing, increasing stress on the spinal column and its supporting structures. Wearing high-heeled shoes does the same thing.

Summary

- *Flexibility* refers to the range of motion at a joint or series of joints and is specific to each joint.
- Factors that influence flexibility of a joint are the bony structure, the amount of tissue at the joint, the skin, and the elasticity of the muscles, tendons, and ligaments at the joint.
- Flexibility is influenced by age, gender, and physical activity.
- The maintenance of flexibility of the hamstrings and lower back muscles is important in the prevention of lower-back pain.
- Normal body weight and good posture are also necessary for a healthy back.
- Ballistic stretching is counterproductive to improving joint elasticity and may contribute to injury.
- Static stretching is the recommended type of exercise. Stretches should be held for 15 to 30 seconds and repeated at least three times.

- Stretching should not be painful, only mildly uncomfortable.
- Stretching exercises can be performed daily.
- Proprioceptive neuromuscular facilitation is the most effective but most difficult form of stretching.
- Proprioceptive neuromuscular facilitation combines passive movement with isometric contractions.
- The goniometer is the most widely used device to measure flexibility.
- Lower-back pain is one of the most common reasons for visiting a physician.
- Factors associated with lower-back and neck pain include excess weight; poor posture; inactivity; fatigue; weak abdominal muscles; wearing high heels; stress; cigarette smoking; weak, inflexible back and hamstring muscles; lifting objects incorrectly; work or sports injuries; and disease.

Review Questions

1. Explain why flexibility is such an important component of health-related fitness.
2. Discuss the steps to take when developing a flexibility program.
3. What concepts are necessary to understand about stretching?
4. Distinguish among static, ballistic, and PNF stretching.
5. Discuss the guidelines that should be followed for safe and effective stretching.

6. What factors are associated with lower-back and neck problems?
7. Describe the proper lifting technique for preventing back injury.
8. Discuss the role of repetitive movements in the development of upper-back and neck pain.
9. What can an employer and an employee do to reduce the potential for repetitive motion injuries?

References

1. Alter, M. J. 1996. *Science of Flexibility.* Champaign, Ill.: Human Kinetics.
2. ACSM. 1998. Position stand on exercise and physical activity for older adults. *Medicine and Science in Sports and Exercise* 30(6):992–1008.
3. Robergs, R. A., and S. O. Roberts. 1997. *Exercise Physiology.* St. Louis: Mosby.
4. Tufts University. 1997. To stretch or not to stretch? *Tufts University Health & Nutrition Letter* 15(10):4–5.

5. ACSM. 1998. Position stand on the recommended quantity and quality of exercise for developing and maintaining cardiorespiratory and muscular fitness and flexibility in adults. *Medicine and Science in Sports and Exercise* 30(6):975–991.
6. ACSM. 2000. *ACSM's Guidelines for Exercise Testing and Prescription* (6th ed.). Philadelphia: Lippincott Williams and Wilkins.

7. McGill, S. M. 2001. Low back exercises: prescription for healthy back and recovery from injury. In *ACSM Resource Manual* (4th ed.), ed. J. L. Roitman. Philadelphia: Lippincott Williams and Wilkins.
8. Bryant, C. X., and J. A. Peterson. 1998. Treating and preventing low back pain. *Fitness Management* 14(4):52–54.
9. Johns Hopkins University. 1998. Can religion be good medicine? *The Johns Hopkins Medical Letter* 10(9):3.

10. University of California at Berkeley. 1998. Tai chi: smooth, balanced, low-impact. *University of California at Berkeley Wellness Letter* 15(2):6.

11. Harvard University. 1998. The ultimate mind-body workout. *Harvard Health Letter* 24(2):4–5.

12. Fredette, D. M. 2001. Exercise recommendations for flexibility and range of motion. In *ACSM Resource Manual* (4th ed.), ed. J. L. Roitman. Philadelphia: Lippincott Williams and Wilkins.

13. University of California at Berkeley. 1998. The home stretch. *University of California at Berkeley Wellness Letter* 15(3):4–5.

14. Nieman, D. C. 1999. *Exercise Testing and Prescription.* Mountain View, Calif.: Mayfield Publishing Co.

15. Corbin, C. B., and R. P. Pangrazi. 1998. *Physical Activity for Children: A Statement of Guidelines.* Reston, Va.: NASPE Publications.

16. Johns Hopkins University. 2001. Stretching out the benefits of exercise. *The Johns Hopkins Medical Letter Health After 50* 13(2):6–7.

17. Prentice, W. E. 1999. *Fitness and Wellness for Life.* Boston: WCB/McGraw-Hill.

18. U.S. Dept. of Health and Human Services and Office of Public Health and Science. 1998. *Healthy People 2010 Objectives: Draft for Public Comment.* Washington, D.C.: U.S. Dept. of Health and Human Services.

19. Harvard University. 1999. Fact and fiction about chiropractic. *Harvard Health Letter* 24(3):1–3.

20. Harvard University. 1998. Exercising options for a healthy back. *Harvard Health Letter* 23(11):4–5.

Suggested Readings

Perkins-Carpenter, B. 2001. Balance and stretching programs for seniors. *Fitness Management* 17(2):32–34.

Discusses the importance of balance and flexibility training for the elderly. Provides a rationale for both and presents exercises that can improve both. Also provides tips for conducting such classes to maximize results and improve the enjoyment of such participation.

Johns Hopkins University. 2001. Stretching out the benefits of exercise. *The Johns Hopkins Medical Letter Health After 50* 13(2):6–7.

Discusses the need for participating in a stretching program particularly for people over 50 years of age. Provides tips on how to stretch and discusses why we should stretch on a regular basis.

Tufts University. 2001. New twists in stretching. *Tufts University Health & Nutrition Letter* 19(3):3.

Discusses the wide range of benefits that accumulate to those who stretch regularly. Presents several common methods for stretching the major muscle groups of the body.

University of California at Berkley. 2001. A quick stretch: it can feel great. *University of California at Berkeley Wellness Letter* 17(9):6.

Discusses the role of stretching for all people but particularly for sedentary people. Provides several exercises for stretching the major muscle groups with directions on how to do the exercises.

Tufts University. 2000. To stretch or not to stretch before exercising. *Tufts University Health & Nutrition Letter* 18(10):6.

Makes the case for stretching after working out rather than before. Reports on a study that reiterates what many studies have previously shown—that stretching before exercise does not prevent injuries.

Name _____ **Date** _____ **Section** _____

Assessment Activity 5-1

Sit-and-Reach Test

The sit-and-reach test is used to measure hip flexor, lower-back, and hamstring flexibility. It is measured with a testing box that can be purchased or built. The box should be 12 inches high and have an overlap in front so that negative (minus) readings can be obtained when subjects are unable to reach their feet (the footline). For simplicity and standardization purposes, the footline is given a value of 0, with plus and minus readings given in inches.

Directions:
1. Warm up for 3 to 5 minutes before taking this test.
2. After warming up, remove your shoes and sit with both feet flat against the end board of the box with your legs fully extended and your knees locked.
3. Extend your arms forward as shown in the photo, one hand on top of the other with your fingertips perfectly even.
4. Bend forward from the waist as far as possible while sliding your hands along the scale.
5. Hold the maximum stretch for at least 1 second.
6. Perform three trials: The final score is the best of the three.
7. Lock your knees during all trials.
8. Use the following sit-and-reach test standards to interpret your score.

Trial 1: _____ inches

Trial 2: _____ inches

Trial 3: _____ inches

Sit-and-Reach Test Standards

Classification	Distance reached in inches (footline at 0)
Excellent	≥ 7*
Good	4.0–6.9
Average	0–3.9
Fair	−3.0– −0.25
Poor	≥−3.1

*≥ equal to or greater than

Name _____ **Date** _____ **Section** _____

Assessment Activity 5-2

Shoulder Flexion Test

Directions: The objective of the shoulder flexion test is to measure the deltoids and shoulder girdle. A measuring scale and straight edge are needed to perform this assessment. Begin by assuming a prone position with your arms fully extended. Your chin should remain in contact with the floor throughout the exercise.

Grasp the straight edge with both hands and raise it as high as possible from the floor. The distance from the floor to the straight edge is measured as the height in inches. Repeat this assessment three times and record the best number in inches as the final score. See the following chart for your classification.

Trial 1: _____ inches

Trial 2: _____ inches

Trial 3: _____ inches

Shoulder Flexion Test Standard*

Classification	Men	Women
Excellent	26 or above	27 or above
Good	23–25	24–26
Average	18–22	19–23
Fair	13–17	14–18
Poor	12 or below	13 or below

*All scores are in inches. Use the best of three trials as the score.

Name _____ **Date** _____ **Section** _____

Assessment Activity 5-3

Sling Test

Directions: The purpose of this test is to determine the length and flexibility of your sling muscles (the extensor muscles of the back). If you have back problems or have had back surgery, consult a physician before attempting this test. This is a test and not an exercise, so it should not be used to increase flexibility.

Begin by lying on your back on the floor and bending both knees. Pull your right leg to your chest by tightly holding your knee with both hands. Straighten out your left leg and push it to the floor without letting your right leg move away from your chest.

A tester uses a ruler to measure the distance between the floor and back of the knee. Reverse your leg position and measure.

Sling Test Standards

Classification		Standard
Excellent		Able to hold one leg firmly against the chest with the other leg flat against the floor
Average		Able to hold one knee against the chest while the other knee is bent 2 to 4 inches off the floor
Fair		Able to hold the knee firmly against the chest while the other leg is 4 to 8 inches off the floor
Poor		Unable to pull one leg firmly against the chest without pain or discomfort and/or raising the other leg off the floor significantly (more than 8 inches)

Name _____ **Date** _____ **Section** _____

Assessment Activity 5-4

Trunk Extension

Directions: The purpose of this assessment is to measure the flexibility of the abdominal and hip flexor muscles. Begin the test by lying face down on the floor. Have a partner hold your legs as shown. Grasp your hands in the lower-back area, breathe in, lift your upper body as high off the floor as possible, and hold. A tester measures the distance between floor and your chin. Repeat this two more times and record your best score. See the following chart for your classification.

Trial 1: _____ inches

Trial 2: _____ inches

Trial 3: _____ inches

Trunk Extension Assessment Standards*

Classification	Men	Women
Excellent	22	24
Good	19–21	20–23
Average	17–18	18–19
Poor	16	17

*Scores are in inches.

6

Forming a Plan for Good Nutrition

Online Learning Center

Log on to our Online Learning Center (OLC) for access to these additional resources:

- Chapter key term flashcards
- Learning objectives
- Additional goals for behavior change
- Concentration game
- Self-scoring chapter quizzes

- Additional lab activities

The OLC also offers weblinks for study and exploration of wellness topics. Access these links through **www.mhhe.com/anspaugh5e,** click on "Student Center," click on "Chapter 6," and then click on "Web Activities."

Goals for Behavior Change

- Decrease or increase your intake of the energy nutrients to meet dietary recommendations.
- Craft a nutrition profile that identifies your intake of essential nutrients and highlights your dietary strengths and shortcomings.
- Formulate a plan for implementing the *Dietary Guidelines for Americans* that addresses your dietary shortcomings.
- Identify and practice specific strategies for improving your diet.

Key Terms

amino acids
antioxidants
botanicals
calorie
complex carbohydrates
Daily Values (DVs)
Dietary Reference Intakes (DRI)
essential nutrients
fiber
folate
foodborne illness
free radicals
functional foods
Glycemic Index (GI)
hydrogenation

legumes
macronutrients
micronutrients
minerals
monounsaturated fat
nutrient density
Olestra
phytochemicals
phytomedicinals
polyunsaturated fat
Recommended Dietary Allowances (RDAs)
saturated fat
transfatty acids
vitamin supplements
vitamins

Objectives

After completing this chapter, you will be able to do the following:

- Describe the functions and purposes of the essential nutrients.
- Discuss ways to apply the *Dietary Guidelines for Americans*.
- Explain the role of nutrients that are not classified as essential, such as fiber, phytochemicals, and botanicals, but that are thought to have unique health benefits.
- Determine your RDA for protein, carbohydrates, fat, and saturated fat.

utrition has captured the interest of Americans perhaps more than any other topic related to fitness and wellness. Whether concerning antioxidants or phytochemicals, homocysteine or cholesterol, omega-3 fatty acids or trans-fatty acids, HDLs or LDLs, nutrition issues make headlines in both scientific journals and popular magazines, and everybody seems to be an expert. So much is written by so many people that it is difficult to know what and whom to believe.

This chapter presents basic concepts of the science of *nutrition*, the study of nutrients and the way the body processes them, to guide you through the maze of nutrition information. The concepts presented here are within the framework of *Dietary Guidelines for Americans* and should provide you with a basis for sound nutritional planning.

Nutrition and Health

The relationship between nutrition and health has changed dramatically during the last fifty years. The deficiency diseases of the past, such as scurvy and rickets, have been replaced by diseases of dietary excess and imbalance. Chief among such excess is the disproportionate consumption of foods high in fat, often at the expense of foods high in complex carbohydrates, fiber, and other substances conducive to good health. Americans' dietary practices contribute substantially to the burden of preventable illness and premature death and are associated with four of the ten leading causes of death.[1] Coronary heart disease, stroke, and non-insulin-dependent diabetes mellitus have long been connected to nutrition. A growing body of research has also linked cancer to nutrition. It has been estimated, for example, that about 30 percent of cancers are related to dietary factors, but a high intake of fruits and vegetables can cut cancer risk in half.[2]

Another important change in nutrition is the new attitude that previously established minimums for essential nutrients are insufficient to prevent today's major health problems. The **Dietary Reference Intakes (DRI)**, formerly known as **Recommended Dietary Allowances (RDAs)**, of essential nutrients were established to prevent deficiency diseases and to guide the consumption of the more than fifty nutrients necessary to meet the needs of nearly all healthy people in the population (see Just the Facts: RDAs, DRIs, AIs, ULs, DVs: Unscrambling Nutrition Acronyms). Now the DRIs are being revised to prevent or delay the onset of chronic diseases. The DRI for vitamin C is a good example. An intake of 60 mg of vitamin C is considered adequate to prevent the deficiency disease scurvy. Now the DRI is 90 mg for men and 75 for women. Studies today are investigating the potential additional benefits of 200 to 500 mg of vitamin C in preventing heart disease and cancer.

Also changing is the definition of *essential. Phytochemicals* (plant chemicals), *phytomedicinals* (plants with medicinal benefits), and *antioxidants* (compounds that generally prevent the oxidation of substances in food or the body) are the nutrients of the twenty-first century. A countless number of studies exploring the benefits of these nutrients may have dramatic effects on future dietary guidelines.

While the hallmark of the American diet is excess, the low intake of some foods and nutrients also causes concern. Here are a few examples that apply to persons aged 2 years and older:[1]

Only . . .

- 3 percent consume at least three daily servings of vegetables, with at least one serving being dark green or orange vegetables.
- 7 percent consume at least six daily servings of grain products with at least three being whole grains.
- 25 percent of females of childbearing age (12 to 49 years) consume enough iron.
- 28 percent consume at least two servings of fruits a day.
- 46 percent meet recommendations for calcium intake.

Fortunately, improving your diet is not difficult. You don't have to give up your favorite foods to achieve a healthy diet. For many people, cutting back on less healthful foods and making small dietary changes may profoundly affect health and wellness. It is never too late to benefit from dietary improvements. The easy availability of many healthy options makes dietary improvement a realistic goal for most Americans.

Essential Nutrients

Food is made up of six classes of nutrients including carbohydrates, fat, protein, vitamins, minerals, and water. The energy-yielding nutrients (carbohydrates, fat, and protein) are called **macronutrients** because they are required by the body in larger amounts than that of vitamins and minerals, also referred to as **micronutrients**. These nutrients are called **essential nutrients** because they cannot be made by the body and, therefore, must be supplied through the diet. Some experts list fiber as a seventh nutrient, although technically some fibers are carbohydrates and are usually listed with the carbohydrates. Carbohydrates, fat, and protein are called *energy nutrients* because they provide energy

Eating a variety of foods is the best way to ensure that your diet is nutritionally balanced. Have you tried an unfamiliar food lately?

(calories) to the body to regulate chemical processes. (See table 6-1 *Thirty-three Essential Nutrients: Daily Values for People Over 4 Years of Age and Safe Upper Limits for Selected Nutrients.*) Water and fiber are nonnutrients and are also part of a healthy diet.

Calories

Food energy is expressed in kilocalories. A **calorie** is the amount of heat required to raise the temperature of a gram of water by 1° C. A kilocalorie equals 1000 calories of heat energy. Common reference to kilocalories usually excludes the prefix *kilo*, mainly for convenience. A gram of carbohydrates provides 4 calories (kilocalories) of energy, a gram of protein also provides 4 calories, a gram of fat provides 9 calories, and a gram of alcohol (not an essential nutrient) provides 7 calories.

The recommended diet for Americans emphasizes complex carbohydrates as the main source of energy. Between 55 to 60 percent of calories should come from carbohydrates with no more than 10 percent from simple sugar. No more than 25 to 30 percent of calories should come from fat; 15 percent of calories should come from protein. The typical American diet, however, excluding alcohol, consists of 50 percent carbohydrates,

Table 6-1 Thirty-three Essential Nutrients: Daily Values for People Over 4 Years of Age and Safe Upper Limits for Selected Nutrients[3,48]

Nutrient	Unit of Measurement	Daily Value	Upper Limit*
Fat[†]	Gram	<65	
Saturated Fatty Acids[†]	Gram	<20	
Protein[†]	Gram	50	
Cholesterol[‡]	Milligram	<300	
Carbohydrate[†]	Gram	300	
Fiber	Gram	25	
Biotin	Milligram	0.3	
Calcium	Gram	1	2.5
Chloride	Milligram	3400	
Chromium	Microgram	120	
Copper	Milligram	2	
Folate	Microgram	400	1000
Iodine	Microgram	150	
Iron	Milligram	18	
Magnesium	Milligram	400	350[§]
Manganese	Milligram	2	
Molybdenum	Mirogram	75	
Niacin	Milligram	20	35
Pantothenic Acid	Milligram	10	
Phosphorus	Gram	1	4
Potassium	Milligram	3500	
Riboflavin	Milligram	1.7	
Selenium	Microgram	70	400
Sodium	Milligram	<2400	
Thiamin	Milligram	1.5	
Vitamin A	Retinol Equivalents	1000	
Vitamin B-12	Microgram	6	
Vitamin B-6	Milligram	2	100
Vitamin C	Milligram	60	2000
Vitamin D	International Units	400	2000
Vitamin E	International Units	30	1100/1500[∥]
Vitamin K	Microgram	80	
Zinc	Milligram	15	30

Daily Values (DVs) were established as a condensed system for presenting generic standards on food labels. These standards are applicable to ages 4 years old through adulthood. DVs are set at or close to the highest RDA, DRI, and/or AI standard seen in the various age and gender categories for a specific nutrient. While DVs are not to be confused with RDAs, they allow consumers to compare their intake to desirable or maximum intakes. DVs have yet to be updated to reflect the current state of knowledge. For example, the DRI for vitamin C was recently increased to 90 mg but remains at 60 mg on food labels.

*Safe upper limits have not been established for many nutrients because of insufficient research information.

[†]No RDA has been set for these nutrients except protein. Cholesterol is not classified as an essential nutrient because the body makes it on its own. The values listed are based on a 2000 calorie diet, with a caloric distribution of 30% from fat (one-third of this total from saturated fat), 60% from carbohydrate, and 10% from protein.

[‡]Based on recommendations of federal agencies.

[§]Refers to upper limit only from nonfood sources (i.e., supplements).

[∥]1100 is upper limit of synthetic vitamin E; 1500, natural vitamin E.

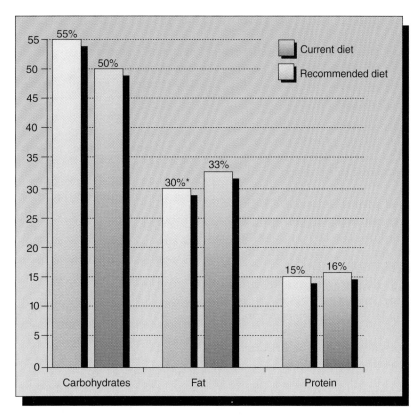

Figure 6-1 Comparison of Recommended and Actual Diets

Both diets are for Americans 20 years and older and exclude alcohol. Recommendations for carbohydrates and protein are minimums; the recommendation for fat is a maximum. Carbohydrates include sugars.
*Experts recommend a maximum of 35% fat calories if most of it is polyunsaturated and/or monounsaturated fat.

33 percent fat, and 16 percent protein[3] (figure 6-1). While significant improvements have been made Americans' diets are still high in fat calories and low in carbohydrate calories. You can tell how your calorie sources compare with dietary recommendations by completing Assessment Activities 6-3 and 6-4.

Carbohydrates

There are three types of carbohydrates: sugars, starches, and fiber. Sugar and starches provide 4 calories per gram. Fiber has no calorie value because it's not absorbed. Most of the carbohydrates are plant based. Grains, vegetables, fruits and legumes are examples. Dairy products are the only animal-based foods with significant carbohydrates.[4] The simplest form of carbohydrates is sugar, also called *monosaccharide.* Monosaccharides include glucose and fructose (fruit sugar). Fructose is the sweetest of simple sugars. Disaccharides are double sugars, meaning that they are pairs of chemically linked monosaccharides. In this group of sugars are sucrose, or table sugar; lactose, or milk sugar; and maltose, or malt sugar.

Starches, also called *polysaccharides,* are **complex carbohydrates.** Whole-grain, high-fiber starches are the preferred source of carbohydrates. A diet high in starch is likely to be lower in fat, especially saturated fat and cholesterol, lower in calories, and higher in fiber. An added benefit of starch consumption over simple sugar consumption is that it helps the body maintain a normal blood-sugar level through a slower, more even rate of digestion and glucose absorption. It takes one to four hours for the body to digest starch. This is one reason athletes involved in endurance activities, such as marathons, load up on complex carbohydrates before competition.

All carbohydrates are broken down in the intestine and converted in the liver into glucose. Glucose is blood sugar carried to cells, where it is used for energy. Glucose in excess of the body's need for energy is stored in limited amounts as glycogen in the muscles and the liver for future use; when glycogen stores are satisfied, glucose is converted to fat.

Many weight-conscious people mistakenly avoid starches, thinking that they are high in calories. Starch foods are often made fattening when they are prepared.

For example, a baked potato without additives yields a modest 90 calories. Adding fat in the form of butter, sour cream, margarine, or cheese adds substantially to the calories of a potato.

Recommended carbohydrate intake

At least 55 percent of the calories in your diet should come from carbohydrates. Many experts believe this percentage should be 60 percent or higher. An estimate of your carbohydrate intake can be determined by completing Assessment Activity 6-1.

Vegetables, fruits, and grain products are high in carbohydrates, vitamins, and minerals and generally low in fat, depending on how they are prepared and what is added to them at the table. Most Americans of all ages eat fewer than the recommended servings of these foods, even though they are associated with a lower risk of many chronic conditions.

Easy ways to add whole-grain, high-fiber carbohydrates include switching from white rice to brown rice, opting for whole-grain breads, snacking on dried fruit, and using legumes as a base for soups.

Protein

Protein is different from carbohydrates and fats in that it contains nitrogen as well as carbon, hydrogen, and oxygen. Because of their unique chemical structures, proteins contain the basic materials that help the body form muscles, bones, cartilage, skin, antibodies, some hormones, and all enzymes. Protein is also an energy nutrient yielding 4 calories per gram. As a source of energy, however, protein is inefficient because it must first be processed by the liver and kidneys. Proteins generally directly supply little of the energy the body uses.[3]

The building blocks of protein are chemical structures called **amino acids.** There are approximately twenty amino acids: Eleven can be produced in the body, and nine must be supplied by the diet.[5] The latter are called *essential amino acids.* A *complete protein* is one that contains all the essential amino acids. A *high-quality protein* is a complete protein that contains the essential amino acids in amounts proportional to the body's need for them. Meat, fish, poultry, eggs, milk, and cheese are examples of high-quality, complete protein sources.

An *incomplete protein* does not contain all the essential amino acids in the proportions needed by the body. Generally, plant protein sources are incomplete. This has important implications for *vegans,* people who limit their diets to plant sources, because protein synthesis operates on the all-or-none principle. That is, the body cannot make partial proteins, only complete ones. If an amino acid is supplied by one source in a smaller amount than is needed, the total amount of protein made from the other amino acids will be limited. It is necessary to combine protein sources from cereal and grains with legumes to obtain all essential amino acids from plant sources. The practice of combining amino acids from various plant sources is called *protein complementing.*

One plant protein source unique among sources of amino acids is **legumes.** Legumes come from plants with seed pods that split on two sides when ripe, such as black-eyed peas; chickpeas (garbanzo beans); lentils; soybeans; and black, red, white, navy, and kidney beans. Legumes are low in calories, sodium, and fat and high in fiber and minerals. They are a nutritionally dense food (see table 6-2).

The most common legume crop in the world is the soybean.[6] The protein in soy is a complete protein—the most complete you can get from plant and vegetable sources—and as good as animal protein.[7] Soybeans are high not only in protein but also in folate, omega-3 fatty acids, and minerals. Health benefits associated with the consumption of soybean products include protection against cardiovascular disease and some forms of cancer.[5] A possible reason for soy's benefits is that, by eating more soy, people consume fewer animal products. Another reason is that soy protein may

Table 6-2 Comparison of Selected Legumes

	Calories	Protein (grams)	Fat (grams)	Iron (milligrams)	Calcium (milligrams)
Soybeans	86	14	8	4	88
Lentils	100	9	<1	3	19
Kidney beans	88	8	<1	3	25
Black beans	41	8	<1	2	25
Chickpeas	82	7	1	3	40

From American Dietetic Association. 1998. Choosing Legumes: A Healthful and Versatile Food. Available online at **www.eatright.org/nfs45.html**.

change levels of certain hormones, which in turn may cause the liver to make less cholesterol. Soybeans also contain *phytoestrogens,* estrogenlike plant substances. Phytoestrogens unique to soybeans are called *isoflavones.* Isoflavones are thought to help prevent breast cancer by blocking natural estrogens.

Soy is available in a variety of foods. Tofu, soy milk, soy nuts, and soy powder, which can be mixed into smoothies, scrambled into omelets, and baked into bread, are several examples.

Recommended protein intake

For most people, the recommended dietary allowance of protein is 0.36 grams per pound of body weight, or 54 grams for a 150-pound person and 72 grams for a 200-pound person. Growing children, pregnant or lactating women, and people recovering from illness require additional protein. Older adults may also need extra protein (see Wellness Across the Generations: Older Adults May Need More Protein). You can estimate your protein intake by completing Assessment Activity 6-1.

Wellness Across the Generations

Older Adults May Need More Protein

The only three groups of people once thought to require extra protein were growing children, pregnant women, and lactating (breast-feeding) women. Now researchers think more protein may be needed by a fourth group: adults 55 years old and older. Recent studies suggest that older adults who consume the RDA of protein lose more protein than they take in. As a result, they lose muscle mass and have a reduced concentration of immunoglobulin, a substance that protects against illness. With weakened immunity, there is a greater risk of contracting a disease or of requiring more time to recover from illness or surgery. An estimated 25 percent of older adults consume less than the RDA of protein.

Based on the results of their own and other studies, researchers at highly respected Tufts University[47] advise older men and women to eat about 0.45 grams of protein per pound of body weight. That adds up to 68 grams of protein a day for someone who weighs 150 pounds and 90 grams for someone who weighs 200 pounds.

Exercise and other physical activities can change the body's need for protein (nutrition needs associated with physical activity are discussed separately in this chapter), but enough protein is usually already consumed. When more protein is consumed than is needed by the body, it is converted into energy or stored as fat. High protein intake may cause the body to excrete calcium and put excessive strain on the kidneys to excrete into the urine the excess nitrogen supplied by the protein.[5] Although the kidneys of most healthy people can handle nitrogen excess easily, diseased kidneys have more difficulty. This is why people with kidney failure are placed on low-protein diets and why people who go on high-protein diets to lose weight (see Chapter 8) are encouraged to drink large quantities of water to flush the kidneys.

Fat

Fats are oils, sterols (such as cholesterol), waxes, and other substances that are not water soluble. Fat is an essential component of all cells. Fats help synthesize and repair vital cell transport and absorb fat-soluble vitamins. Fat stored as adipose tissue provides insulation and a ready source of energy. As an energy source, fat yields 9 calories per gram.

Basic fat facts

Fat, also called *lipid,* is a compound made by chemically bonding fatty acids to glycerol to form glycerides. When three fatty acids are hooked to glycerol, the fat compound is a triglyceride. Almost 95 percent of fat stored in the body is a triglyceride, with the remaining 5 percent consisting of other glycerides and cholesterol. Scientific literature usually refers to triglycerides when it discusses fat. The fatty acids that make up triglycerides can be saturated, monounsaturated, or polyunsaturated. As an energy nutrient, fat yields 9 calories per gram regardless of its chemical make-up.

Chemically, fats are chains of carbon atoms strung together with hydrogen atoms. If a fat is a **saturated fat,** the carbon chain carries all the hydrogen atoms it can. If it is an unsaturated fat, there is room in the carbon chain for more hydrogen. If the fat is a **monounsaturated fat,** there is room for two hydrogen atoms. If the fat is a **polyunsaturated fat,** there is room for four hydrogen atoms. If it is highly polyunsaturated, there is room for many more hydrogen atoms.

Many people mistakenly assume that the word *polyunsaturated* on a food label means that the fat in the food is not saturated, but because of food-processing techniques, this assumption may be incorrect. If the words *hydrogenated* or *partially hydrogenated* are on the food label, the food contains varying amounts of saturated fat. Because fats are less stable, they are prone to spoilage. Consequently, for many foods, manufacturers use a chemical process called **hydrogenation,** in which hydrogen atoms are added to the unsaturated or polyunsaturated fats to make them more saturated and more resistant to spoilage. This process of hydrogenating food yields a new type of fat not found in nature called **transfatty acids** (see Just the Facts: How Much Transfatty Acid Is in Food?). Transfatty acids are saturated fats commonly found in margarine, fried fast foods, cookies, cakes, and many other foods made with shortening. Some scientists believe that transfatty acids, even those originating from a polyunsaturated food source, are as detrimental to health as saturated animal fat. High levels of these fats are less effective in lowering total and LDL cholesterol than are the liquid oils from which they are made. Also they seem to depress HDL cholesterol.[8]

Saturated and unsaturated fats can be differentiated by their appearance. Saturated fat is typically solid at room temperature. Lard, fat marbled in meat, and hardened grease from a skillet are good examples. Polyunsaturated fats are usually liquid at room temperature. Examples are safflower and corn oils. Solid vegetable shortenings are partially hydrogenated and have a soft consistency. Coconut oil, palm kernel oil, and palm oil are exceptions. They are vegetable oils and are liquid at room temperature, but they are among the most saturated of fats.

Fish oils are among the most unsaturated fats available. They are roughly twice as unsaturated as vegetable oils. They do not harden, even at low temperatures. Their unsaturation has created special interest in relation to heart disease. Fatty acids in cold-water seafood, such as salmon, mackerel, sardines, herring, anchovies, whitefish, bluefish, swordfish, rainbow trout, striped bass, Pacific oysters, and squid, consist of omega-3 fatty acids, thought to be effective in lowering cholesterol and triglyceride levels and reducing clot-forming rates, thereby reducing the risk of heart disease. Health experts believe omega-3s offer such protection against heart disease that one or two servings a week are recommended regardless of risk factors. For people at high risk of heart disease, the recommendation is for consumption of 10 to 15 ounces—three to five servings—of fish a week.[9]

Olestra

Olestra is a synthetic fat that has the flavor and taste of real fat but contains no calories. It cannot be digested or absorbed and, therefore, passes through the digestive system unaltered. It was approved by the Food and Drug Administration in 1998 for use in snack foods.

While consumption of Olestra in small amounts is unlikely to cause problems in healthy adults, several side effects have been reported. Olestra can cause abdominal cramps and loose stools. It also inhibits the absorption of the fat-soluble vitamins A, D, E, and K and the absorption of carotenoids, substances thought to aid the immune system in warding off some cancers, heart disease, and eye problems. To counter the effects of Olestra on the absorption of important nutrients, some snack foods are fortified with fat-soluble vitamins.

Relying on fat substitutes such as Olestra can help reduce fat in your diet. However, because a product has less fat does not mean it is also low in calories. Experts speculate that the reduction in calories associated with low-fat foods made with Olestra is unlikely to reduce obesity significantly because Olestra is not yet used in foods that contribute the most fat to our diets—high-fat meats.[3] It will be years before the true effects of fat substitutes on the American diet are known.

Cholesterol

Cholesterol, a waxy substance that is technically a steroid alcohol found only in animal foods, is probably the most researched blood lipid. High levels of cholesterol are usually included among the major risk factors for cardiovascular disease. (For information on cholesterol, see Chapter 2.)

Recommended fat intake

To many people, *fat* has negative connotations and is viewed almost as a toxin, but as stated earlier, fat is an essential nutrient. Experts recommend a diet that includes a total fat intake of no more than 30 percent of total calories. That percentage is considered a maximum. Many experts believe it is too high; other experts recommend a maximum fat intake of 35 percent as long as most of it is monounsaturated or polyunsaturated fat.[49]

The advice to consume no more than 30 to 35 percent of calories as fat does not apply to infants and toddlers below the age of 2 years. During the early stages of development, fat is critical to the development of the brain, spine, and central nervous system, so their intake of fat should not be greatly restricted.[3]

Fat intake in excess of 30 percent of total calories is consistently associated with heart disease. Saturated fat is the major dietary contributor to total blood cholesterol levels, even more than cholesterol intake. Many associations have also been made between dietary fat and certain types of cancer, notably breast, prostate, and colon cancer. Another health problem related to high fat intake is obesity. Little energy is used to transfer fat from foods to fat storage; the body requires only

Just the Facts

How Much Transfatty Acid Is in Food?

In 2000 the Food and Drug Administration submitted a proposal that requires manufacturers to include the number of grams of transfatty acids present when listing the number of grams of saturated fat on package labels.[10] If a serving of a food has 10 grams of saturated fat and 4 grams of transfatty acids, the number "14" will appear in the listing for saturated fat. A footnote saying how many of the grams are trans fat will appear at the bottom of the label.

Some time will elapse before new package labels conform to current regulations. In the meantime, it is possible to estimate the transfatty acid content of a food. To determine how much acid is in food, it is necessary to have a complete breakdown of the food's fat content. For example, a popular low-saturated fat margarine contains 10 grams of total fat, including 2 grams of saturated fat, 1.5 grams of polyunsaturated fat, and 2 grams of monounsaturated fat. Adding the amounts of these three fats and subtracting them from the total leaves about 4.5 grams unaccounted for. These grams probably represent transfatty acids. Because food labels don't always provide a complete breakdown of fat content, it is difficult to assess the amount of transfatty acids contained in a particular food. Food composition tables such as the one shown in table 6-3 and nutrition software such as those available with this text provide sufficient information to help you estimate transfatty acid content.

Table 6-3 Fat Content of Selected Foods

Food	Fat/(g)	Total†	Saturated	Monounsaturated	Polyunsaturated
			Percentage of Total Calories from Fat*		
Egg, whole, raw	5.01	64	19	25	8
Butter (pat)	11.4	100	67	31	4
Margarine, regular, hard (stick)	91.0	100	20	45	32
Cheese, cream (1 ounce)	9.9	90	57	25	3
Cheese, cheddar (1 cup)	37.5	74	47	20	2
Cheese, cottage (1 cup)	10.1	39	25	11	1
Milk, whole (1 cup)	8.2	49	30	14	2
Milk, skim (1 cup)	1.0	6	4	1	Trace‡
Frankfurter (2 ounces)	16.6	82	33	40	3
Bologna, pork (slice)	4.6	72	26	36	8
Flounder, baked (0.8 ounce)	1.9	9	Trace	Trace	Trace
Fish sticks (1 ounce)	3.4	39	10	18	10
Tuna, canned, oil-packed (3 ounces)	6.9	38	8	10	17
Tuna, canned, water-packed (3 ounces)	2.1	7	Trace	Trace	Trace
Ground beef (3 ounces)	19.2	65	25	28	3
Steak, broiled, sirloin (2 ounces)	4.89	56	24	26	2
Pork chop, broiled (3 ounces)	22.3	62	23	29	7
Chicken breast, fried, flour-coated (7 ounces)	17.4	36	10	14	8
Beans, navy (1 cup)	2.1	4	Trace	Trace	3
Potato (baked)	0.06	1	Trace	Trace	4
Potato chips (1.5 ounces)	13.0	61	16	11	31
Ice cream, vanilla, regular (1 cup)	22.5	48	28	14	2
Apple (raw, unpeeled)	0.5	6	1	Trace	2
Danish pastry	13.6	50	14	29	4

*rounded off to the nearest whole number

†includes undifferentiated fats

‡*Trace,* less than 0.9% of fat.

3 calories to store 100 calories of dietary fat as fat tissue, compared with 23 to 27 calories to digest 100 calories of carbohydrates. Fat also yields more than twice as many calories as do protein and carbohydrates.

Just how low should your fat intake be? If 30 percent is good, it might stand to reason that 20, 15, or 10 percent would be even better. Surprisingly, the answer is controversial. Research conducted by Dean Ornish has shown that a very low-fat diet (10 percent of calories from fat) combined with quitting smoking, exercising, and reducing stress can reverse atherosclerosis.[11] On the other hand, some studies have found that cutting fat intake too much may actually increase health risks.

Experts offer several explanations of why diets low in total fat may increase heart disease risk. First, low-fat diets may be associated with diets high in carbohydrates. Diets high in carbohydrates and low in fat elevate triglyceride levels and lower HDL levels. Second, low-fat diets may have a higher-than-normal ratio of saturated fat to other types of fat. Studies indicate that as long as saturated fat intake is low, the total fat content of a diet has no effect on heart disease risk. When

saturated fats are replaced with unsaturated fats, HDL cholesterol declines only moderately, and triglyceride levels remain stable.[3,11] It is possible that the important issue is not one of total fat; rather, it may be the type of fat that counts (see figure 6-2 for a comparison of dietary fats). Until the issue of quantity versus type is settled, the best advice is to reduce total fat intake to less than 30 percent and to concentrate on lowering saturated fat intake. Moderation is an important principle for fat intake just as it is for nutrition in general.

Most Americans have an excessive fat intake and are challenged to make changes in both the amount and type of fat eaten. Table 6-4 presents a quick reference of maximum fat intake for selected caloric intakes. You can estimate your personal maximum fat intake by completing Assessment Activity 6-2. You can also learn how fatty your eating habits are by completing Assessment Activity 6-5.

Saturated Fat. Experts agree that saturated fats need to be reduced in the American diet. Diets rich in saturated fats unquestionably increase the risk of heart disease and some cancers. Assessment Activity 6-2 will

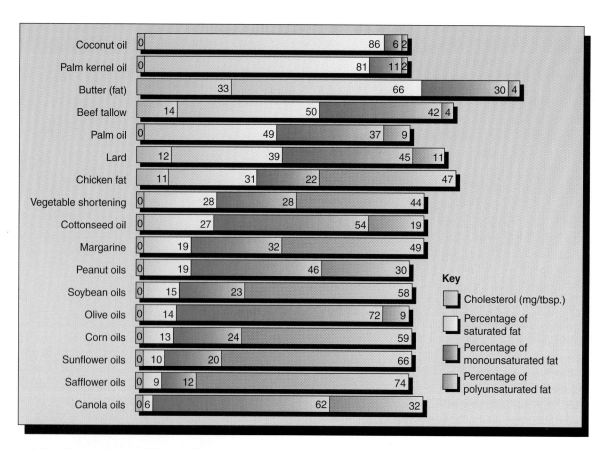

Figure 6-2 Comparison of Dietary Fats

help you estimate your maximum saturated fat intake. It is recommended that no more than 7 percent of total calories come from saturated fat.[49] This amounts to less than 8 grams per 1000 calories.

Monounsaturated Fat. Monounsaturated fats are liquid at room temperature and include olive oil, canola oil, and peanut oil. When monounsaturated fats are substituted for saturated fats, a person's blood fat profile usually improves and risk factors associated with heart disease and some forms of cancer are reduced. The recommendation for monounsaturated fats is 10 to 15 percent of total calories.[8] This amounts to 11 to 17 grams per 100 calories.

Although the diet of people in Mediterranean countries is higher in fat than that of Americans, the incidence of heart disease and stroke in those countries is much lower. The main difference is that the Mediterranean diet is high in monounsaturated fat, usually from consumption of olive oil. This has prompted some scientists to suggest that Americans adopt this pattern of eating.

Polyunsaturated Fat. There are two main types of polyunsaturated (poly) fats: omega-6 and omega-3. The omega-6s make up 90 percent of poly fats in the American diet and come primarily from plant oils, such as soybean, corn, sunflower, and safflower, and also from nuts and seeds. Omega-6 provides linoleic acid, an essential fatty acid. The omega-3s come primarily from seafood and provide linolenic acid, another essential fatty acid. The consumption of omega-6s and omega-3s is associated with cardiovascular benefits, including reduction of blood clotting, prevention of abnormal heart rhythms, and lowering of levels of total cholesterol and LDLs. Recommended intake of polyunsaturated fats is no more than 10 percent of total calories.[8] This amounts to 11 grams per 1000 calories.

Transfatty Acids. Transfatty acids start out as unsaturated fats but become like saturated fats because of the hydrogenation process. In high amounts, these fatty acids are associated with risk factors similar to those linked to saturated fats. Consumption of transfatty acids should be held to a minimum.

Vitamins

Vitamins are organic compounds (they contain carbon) that are necessary in small amounts for good health. The body can break vitamins down, but it cannot produce them, so vitamins have to be supplied in the diet. Unlike carbohydrates, fats, and proteins, vitamins yield no energy. Instead, some serve as catalysts that enable energy nutrients to be digested, absorbed, and metabolized. Some vitamins also interact with minerals. For example, vitamin C facilitates iron absorption, vitamin D improves calcium absorption, and thiamin requires the mineral magnesium to function efficiently.

Vitamins are either water soluble or fat soluble (see table 6-5). Water-soluble vitamins include vitamin C and vitamin B complex. They are present in the watery components of food, distributed in the fluid components of the body, excreted in the urine, needed in frequent small doses, and unlikely to be toxic except when taken in megadoses (very large quantities).

Fat-soluble vitamins include vitamins A, D, E, and K and are found in the fat and oily parts of food. Because they cannot be dissolved and absorbed in the bloodstream, these vitamins must be absorbed into the lymph with fat and transported in lipoproteins. When consumed in excess of the body's need, fat-soluble vitamins are stored in the liver and fat cells. Their storage makes it possible for a person to survive for months or years without consuming them. At least three of the fat-soluble vitamins (A, D, and K) may even accumulate to toxic levels. Megadoses of these vitamins should be avoided.

Table 6-4 Maximum Fat and Saturated Fat Grams for Selected Caloric Intakes*

Daily Calorie Intake	Total Fat Grams per Day		Total Saturated Fat Grams per Day	
	30% Level	**20% Level**	**10% Level**	**7% Level**
1000	33	22	11	8
1500	50	33	17	12
2000	67	44	22	16
2500	83	56	28	19
3000	100	67	33	23

*If a person on a 1500-calorie diet wants to restrict fat intake to no more than 20% of calories, the limit is 33 grams (1500 × 0.20 = 300 total fat calories; 300 ÷ 9 = 33). Saturated fat intake at the 7% level is restricted to 12 grams (1500 × 0.07 = 105 saturated fat calories; 105 ÷ 9 = 12).

Table 6-5   Vitamins: Food Sources and Wellness Benefits

Vitamins	Food Sources	Wellness Benefits
Fat-soluble vitamins		
1. Vitamin A	Liver, carrots, eggs, tomatoes, dark green and yellow-orange vegetables and some fruits	Healthy skin and mucous membranes, improved night vision, defense against infections; antioxidant benefits (from carotenoids)
2. Vitamin D	Fish oils and fortified milk; exposure to sunlight	Maintaining of blood levels of calcium and phosphorus; promotion of strong bones and teeth; possible reduction of risk of osteoporosis
3. Vitamin E	Plant oils (corn, soybean, safflower, etc.), nuts, seeds	Formation of red blood cells and use of vitamin K; antioxidant benefits
4. Vitamin K	Green vegetables, liver	Promotion of blood clotting; contribution to bone metabolism
Water-soluble vitamins		
5. Vitamin C (Ascorbic Acid)	Citrus fruits, green vegetables	Promotion of healthy gums and teeth; iron absorption; maintaining of normal connective tissues; help in wound healing; antioxidant benefits
Vitamin B complex		
6. Thiamine (B-1)	Whole grains, legumes, liver, nuts	Carbohydrate metabolism; nerve function
7. Riboflavin (B-2)	Dairy products, liver, enriched grains, spinach	Energy metabolism; production of red blood cells; improved health of skin and eyes
8. Niacin	Nuts, grains, meat, fish, tuna, mushrooms	Energy metabolism, fat synthesis, fat breakdown; lowering of cholesterol (when prescribed in large doses)
9. Pyridoxine (B-6)	Whole grains, meat, beans, nuts, fish, liver	Protein metabolism; possible immunity boost in the elderly; homocysteine metabolism
10. Pantothenic acid	Whole grains, dried beans, eggs, milk, liver	Energy metabolism; fat synthesis; production of essential body chemicals
11. Vitamin B-12	Animal foods, dairy products, seafood	Folate metabolism; nerve function; formation of red blood cells; homocysteine metabolism
12. Biotin	Cheese, egg yolks, mushrooms, grains	Glucose production; fat synthesis
13. Folate (folic acid)	Green leafy vegetables, liver, beans, grains, citrus fruits	DNA synthesis and protein metabolism; reduction of risk of certain birth defects; homocysteine metabolism

Antioxidant vitamins

Three vitamins are classified as antioxidants—vitamins C, E, and the carotenoids. **Antioxidants** are protective substances because they help neutralize the activity of free radicals. **Free radicals** are naturally produced chemicals that arise from normal cell activity. Whenever the body uses oxygen or is exposed to a toxin, such as cigarette smoke, it forms free radicals. These unstable chemicals can damage cells throughout the body. They may damage a cell's DNA in ways that lead to cancer, interact with cholesterol in the bloodstream and form oxidized LDL (see Chapter 2), cause cataracts and rheumatoid arthritis, and be a factor in the physiological changes associated with the aging

process. Excess free radical production is thought to contribute to over fifty diseases.[11] Anything that interferes with the destructive effects of free radicals offers a health advantage.

Foods can supply nutrients with antioxidant properties. Vitamins C and E, the mineral selenium, and plant pigments knows as carotenoids (including beta carotene) are well-known antioxidants. Other substances found in plants, known collectively as phytochemicals (discussed later in this chapter), may also act as antioxidants. A common cooking practice illustrates this antioxidant effect. Some foods like bananas, peaches, apples, and potatoes quickly turn brown when exposed to air. However, when such foods are dipped in lemon or orange juice, the vitamin C in the juice acts as an antioxidant and prevents browning.

Each antioxidant serves a different purpose but all of them work closely together. For example, vitamin C helps regenerate vitamin E once it has become oxidized.[11] This illustrates the importance of a diet that supplies sufficient amounts of all of the antioxidants rather than focusing exclusively on one.

Should Americans take supplements of antioxidant vitamins? Information from the research community is inconclusive. Until recently the evidence in support of vitamin supplements was so compelling that many scientists were beginning to believe that antioxidant vitamin supplements could be a highly effective, relatively inexpensive, and risk-free form of preventive medicine.

But now after some three dozen of the country's most distinguished scientists examined hundreds of studies on antioxidants and disease risk, the value of taking large doses of antioxidant supplements is still unproven.[12] It may be several years before large-scale studies provide more definitive conclusions. Even then it is unlikely that studies will ever establish a cause-and-effect relationship between antioxidants and chronic diseases. There are too many factors to consider. For example, people who eat plenty of fruits and vegetables may also lead healthy lifestyles overall. Fruits and vegetables also contain thousands of plant chemicals (phytochemicals), many beginning to show promise against disease. Consequently, some scientists advocate patience until scientific consensus is reached, and they do not recommend taking supplements at this time. Other scientists believe that thousands of Americans may die prematurely of heart disease and cancer before a consensus develops and that the ground swell of evidence, despite some inconsistencies, supports taking antioxidants now.

Presently there is only one strategy to combat disease that no scientist would dispute: Eat more produce. Fruits and vegetables are high in fiber and low in fat and contain hundreds of substances that have the potential to improve health—not just the few compounds that have been isolated and packaged as supplements. In all the research that has been done on diet, antioxidants, and disease, the strongest and most consistent pattern has been that eating a variety of fruits and vegetables produces benefits.

In preparing food for consumption remember that vitamin content is easily compromised. Improper storage; excessive cooking; and exposure to heat, light, and air may reduce the vitamin content in food.

Vitamin C

Vitamin C, also called *ascorbic acid*, is essential to the formation of collagen, a protein used to form all the connective tissues of your body. It is required in the break-

down and absorption of some amino acids and other minerals (such as iron) and in the formation of some hormones. It may also help the immune system prevent infections. As an antioxidant it may play a role in prevention of atherosclerosis and some forms of cancer.

Contrary to popular opinion, vitamin C does not prevent the common cold. Scientifically controlled studies reveal no difference in the incidence of colds among vitamin C users and nonusers. On a positive note, however, some studies suggest that large doses (about 2000 mg a day) can reduce the severity and duration of a cold's symptoms slightly. That much, however, might also cause diarrhea and kidney stones in susceptible people.[13]

The DRI of vitamin C is 90 mg for men and 75 mg for women. Smokers need more: 125 and 110 for men and women, respectively. The tolerable upper intake level is 2000 mg. Advocates of increased vitamin C often recommend intakes of 200 mg or more.[3] Still, an intake of 200 mg/day can be achieved by food intake. Megadoses (2000 mg) of vitamin C offer little benefit to the body and may be harmful. As a water-soluble vitamin, doses in excess of the body's requirement are excreted through the kidneys. In other words, the body can only absorb so much. Side effects of large doses are diarrhea and abdominal discomfort. For those who absorb excess iron, supplements of vitamin C could be dangerous. Large intakes may also produce errors in the results of some diagnostic tests (such as the hemoccult test, which tests for blood in the intestines).

Carotenoids

More than 600 carotenoids are found in nature. They give fruits and vegetables their yellow, orange, and red colors. They're also abundant in dark green vegetables. Three of the major carotenoids (alpha-carotene, beta-carotene, and beta-cryptoxanthin) can be converted by the body into vitamin A and are referred to as *provitamin A*. Until recently, beta-carotene was thought to offer the most health-protecting antioxidant effect. However, after studies showed that the incidence of lung cancer increased in smokers who took beta-carotene supplements, researchers concluded that beta-carotene was not the main protector.

One carotenoid currently being studied for its antioxidant potency is lycopene, the predominant carotenoid in the blood and in the prostate gland in males. It cannot be converted to vitamin A, but it has twice the antioxidant potency of beta-carotene. Benefits attributed to lycopene are a reduced risk of some cancers, especially those of the digestive tract and the prostate. The best source of lycopene is tomatoes. Cooked tomatoes, such as those found in sauces, are a better source than raw tomatoes and tomato juice because heat ruptures plant cell walls, releasing the carotenoid. Also, lycopene is a fat-soluble substance, so some fat, like that found in pizza and most pasta sauces, is needed for it to be absorbed.[15]

Currently, carotenoid supplements, including beta-carotene and lycopene, are not recommended. Carotenoids interact with one another, and supplemental doses of one carotenoid may impair the absorption of others. Instead, eat a variety of vegetables and fruits to get a mix of carotenoids. Five servings a day of fruits and vegetables that are mostly yellow-orange, red, or dark green are recommended. It is likely that carotenoids are more beneficial to health when they are consumed together from food than when packaged separately, as in a supplement.

Vitamin E

Vitamin E is a fat-soluble vitamin and plays a role in the formation of red blood cells and maintenance of nervous tissues, and it aids in the absorption of vitamin A. Claims that vitamin E improves the skin, heals scars, prevents stretch marks, slows the aging process, and increases fertility are more folklore than fact.

Vitamin E is a potent antioxidant that attaches to LDL cholesterol and helps prevent damage from free radicals. Large-scale studies, involving tens of thousands of participants followed for an average of four to eight years, found that those who took vitamin E supplements were significantly less likely to develop coronary heart disease than were those who did not take supplements of vitamin E. Supplemental doses of 100 to 250 IU per day for at least two years resulted in a 37 and 44 percent decrease in heart disease risk for men and women, respectively.[11] The effect of consuming vitamin E from food versus obtaining comparable levels through supplements is difficult to determine because dietary vitamin E intake rarely reaches the 100 IU per day level, the minimum amount that appears to be protective. Vitamin E is found only in small amounts in a few foods. Low-fat diets are especially scarce in vitamin E.

Although these studies are impressive, there still is not enough evidence to recommend vitamin E supplements for the general population.[16] Some experts warn of the dangers of tampering with the body's biochemistry; however, other experts recommend supplements of vitamin E because they believe it is not harmful and may be worthwhile. The people who stand to benefit the most from vitamin E supplements are those with coronary heart disease, diabetes, or high LDL cholesterol levels.[17] If you choose to take a supplement, select the natural form, rather than the synthetic, because it is absorbed more easily into the body. The label for natural vitamin E should read "d-alpha tocopherol."

Antioxidant vitamins from foods like citrus fruits may help protect young and old alike from heart disease and cancer.

Folate, Vitamin B$_6$, Vitamin B$_{12}$

Folate is a part of the vitamin B complex and combines with vitamins B$_6$ and B$_{12}$ to form parts of DNA and RNA and to make heme, the iron-containing protein in red blood cells. These three also assist in the metabolism of amino acids. The terms *folate, folic acid,* and *folacin* are sometimes used incorrectly. Folate is the form that comes from plants; folic acid is the form found most often in your body and the form added to foods and supplements; *folacin* is a collective term for these and other forms of the vitamin. Folic acid is about twice as potent as folate. Vitamins B$_6$ and B$_{12}$ are plentiful in foods, and few people, with the possible exception of strict vegetarians, need to worry about deficiencies. With advancing age, some people have trouble producing stomach acids in sufficient quantities to separate vitamin B$_{12}$ from foods. They have no trouble absorbing B$_{12}$ from supplements because it is not attached to food, so older people may also need to supplement their diets with B$_{12}$. Good sources of these vitamins are meat products, dairy products, eggs, spinach, whole-wheat bread, and breakfast cereals.

Folate, as its name implies, is found in foliage—leafy vegetables, such as lettuce and spinach. It is also found in citrus fruits, whole-grain bread, and cereals. Of the three B vitamins mentioned here, folate is the one in which Americans are most likely to fall short.

Because folate has been associated with a reduction in the chances of neurological birth defects, such as spina bifida, a woman planning a pregnancy may be advised by her physician to eat foods rich in folate and possibly to take a supplement. In an effort to reduce the incidence of these birth defects, new food fortification guidelines were established in 1998 that require food manufacturers to fortify certain grain products, such as flour, bread, and cereal, with folic acid.

Current interest in folate was sparked by studies that demonstrated that people whose blood levels were low in folic acid had high homocysteine levels. *Homocysteine* is an amino acid that plays a role in the formation of two other amino acids, cysteine and methionine. To work properly, these amino acids require three B vitamins—folate, B_6, and B_{12}. If these vitamins are in short supply, homocysteine levels might rise.[18] High homocysteine levels are thought to increase the risk of heart disease (see Chapter 2). The compound has also been implicated in several other diseases, including cancer, diabetes mellitus, and neurological disorders.

The precise mechanism for the association between homocysteine levels and heart disease isn't clear. High concentrations of homocysteine are thought to make the artery walls sticky, promoting plaque formation. Whatever the reason, one thing appears clear: High homocysteine levels are associated with low folic acid levels. In the absence of folate, along with vitamins B_6 and B_{12}, homocysteine concentrations circulate unabated. There is speculation from the scientific community that during the next several years homocysteine levels might replace cholesterol as a major risk factor of heart disease.

The best way to lower homocysteine concentrations is to consume enough B vitamins with an emphasis on folate. Megadoses of folate should be avoided to prevent the possibility of a false negative for anemia (too few blood cells) caused by a vitamin B_{12} deficiency. If you take folate supplements, tell your physician so that the appropriate tests can be ordered.

Vitamin supplements

Advertisements proclaim that vitamins provide energy, promote wellness, and prevent disease and that taking more results in more energy and better health. Consequently, many Americans take one or more **vitamin supplements** in multiple and single doses, in both natural and synthetic forms. Vitamins do facilitate energy release from carbohydrates, fats, and proteins, but they do not provide energy. It is not possible to survive on water and vitamins.

The growing interest in vitamin supplements is primarily related to the antioxidant vitamins and folate. The relationship of these vitamins to health promotion and disease prevention, discussed previously, has sparked an unprecedented trend toward supplements.

Despite this trend, however, strong definitive conclusions about supplements have not been advanced by the scientific community. The consensus among nutrition experts is that healthy adults who eat a variety of foods do not need them. These also advise that if you don't think you're getting enough vitamins in your food, taking a multivitamin pill with nutrients at recommended levels may offer some nutritional insurance, provided it is consumed in moderation and is not used as an excuse to eat a poor diet. If a supplement is needed, it is most likely to be folic acid, vitamin B_{12}, vitamin D, vitamin E, or calcium.[11] These supplements were identified because they are backed by years of supporting research and because Americans don't consume enough whole grains, fruits, and vegetables.

Although healthy people don't need vitamin supplements if they are eating a balanced diet, there are several situations[19] in which a vitamin or mineral supplement may be called for:

If you are age 65 or older, you may need supplements of vitamins B_6, B_{12}, and D because of the difficulty in absorbing these vitamins with advancing age. Women, especially those not taking estrogen, may require more calcium and vitamin D to protect against osteoporosis.

If you are dieting, consuming fewer than 1000 calories a day, you may benefit from a vitamin and mineral supplement.

If you have a disease of the digestive tract, it may interfere with normal digestion and absorption of nutrients and justify your use of vitamin and mineral supplements.

If you smoke, you may need vitamin C supplements.

If you drink excessive alcohol, you may suffer from poor nutrition and the alcohol may interfere with the absorption and metabolism of vitamins.

If you are pregnant and lactating (breast-feeding), supplements of folic acid, iron, and calcium may be recommended for you.

If you are a vegetarian who eliminates most animal products from your diet, you may need additional vitamin B_{12}. Calcium and vitamin D supplements may also be warranted if your milk intake and sun exposure are limited.

Vitamin supplements are sometimes needed by people with irregular diets or unusual lifestyles or by people following certain weight-reduction regimens or strict vegetarian diets. In addition, infants and pregnant and lactating women may need supplements. When taken as supplements, vitamins should be viewed as medicine and, therefore, should be recommended by a physician.

When shopping for supplements, it is easy to be misled by advertising hype and inaccurate labels.

Americans spend billions annually for vitamin, mineral, and herbal supplements. Much of this expenditure goes toward products with no scientifically proven health value. Consequently, it is important for consumers to be discriminating in their purchase of supplements. To that end,

- shop for supplements that carry the letters *USP* on the label. These conform to the standards set by the U.S. Pharmacopoeia.
- if you take antioxidants for their health benefits, shop by price.
- look for an expiration date that shows how long the supplement will retain its potency.
- avoid supplements that claim to have a "sustained release." The delayed release may prevent the nutrients from being absorbed.
- don't be influenced by most health store advertisements. Remember, if you need a supplement, it's most likely to be folic acid, vitamin B$_{12}$, vitamin D, vitamine E, or calcium.

Minerals

Minerals are simple but important nutrients. As inorganic compounds, they lack the complexity of vitamins, but they fulfill a variety of functions. For example, sodium and potassium affect shifts in body fluids, calcium and phosphorus contribute to the body's structure, iron is the core of hemoglobin (an oxygen-carrying compound in the blood), and iodine facilitates production of thyroxine (a hormone that influences metabolic rate).

There are twenty to thirty important nutritional minerals. Minerals should be consumed in smaller amounts than amounts of energy nutrients and water. Minerals present in the body and required in large amounts (more than 100 mg, or 0.02 teaspoon, per day) are called *major minerals* or *macrominerals*. They include, in descending order of prominence, calcium, phosphorus, potassium, sulfur, sodium, chloride, and magnesium. Major minerals contribute 60 to 80 percent of inorganic material in the human body.

Minerals required in small amounts (less than 100 mg per day) are called *trace minerals* or *microminerals*. There are more than a dozen trace minerals, the best known being iron, zinc, and iodine (see Just the Facts: Minerals).

Some minerals are similar to water-soluble vitamins in that they are readily excreted by the kidneys, do not accumulate in the body, and rarely become toxic. Others are like fat-soluble vitamins in that they are stored and are toxic if taken in excess.

Minerals are different from vitamins; they are indestructible and require no special handling during food

Just the Facts

Minerals

Here are some basic facts about minerals:

Major (Macro) Minerals
Types: calcium, phosphorus, potassium, sulfur, sodium chloride, and magnesium

Trace (Micro) Minerals
Types: iron, iodine, zinc, selenium, manganese, copper, molybdenum, cobalt, chromium, fluorine, silicon, vanadium, nickel, tin, cadmium

Minerals of Special Concern*

Calcium
Wellness benefits: contributes to bone and tooth formation, general body growth, maintenance of good muscle tone, nerve function, cell membrane function, and regulation of normal heart beat
Food sources: dairy products, dark-green vegetables, dried beans, shellfish
Deficiency signs and symptoms: bone pain and fractures, muscle cramps, osteoporosis

Iron
Wellness benefits: facilitates oxygen and carbon dioxide transport, formation of red blood cells, production of antibodies, synthesis of collagen, and use of energy
Food sources: red meat (lean), seafood, eggs, dried beans, nuts, grains, green leafy vegetables
Deficiency signs and symptoms: fatigue, weakness

Sodium†
Wellness benefits: essential for maintenance of proper acid-base balance and body fluid regulation; aids in formation of digestive secretions; assists in nerve transmission
Food sources: processed foods, meats, table salt
Deficiency signs and symptoms: rare

*Calcium and iron are of special concern because deficiencies are likely to exist, especially among women and children.
†Sodium is of concern because of potential for overconsumption.

preparation. The only precautions that need to be taken are to avoid soaking minerals out of food and throwing them away in cooking water.

Major minerals are abundant in the diet; therefore, deficiencies are highly unlikely, especially if a variety of foods is included. If a deficiency in major minerals does occur, it is most likely to be a calcium deficiency, especially among women. Four out of five women ages 9 to 19, three out of five women ages 20 to 49, and three out of four women over 50 fall below the recommended allowance for calcium.[1] The Daily Value (DV) of calcium listed on food labels is 1000 mg; adults 51 and older need 1200 mg. Here are some tips for increasing your calcium intake:

- Try to consume as much calcium as possible from food. Skim milk and low-fat dairy products are excellent sources of calcium and are also fortified with vitamin D.
- Use calcium supplements to compensate for a calcium shortfall. Getting enough calcium from food requires consuming the equivalent of a quart of milk per day. As a result, many people benefit from an over-the-counter calcium supplement.
- Calcium is best absorbed in doses of 500 mg or less taken with meals.[11] The best type of calcium supplement is calcium carbonate, available in common antacids.[20]
- Take calcium supplements with meals. Calcium is best dissolved and absorbed in stomach acids secreted during mealtime.
- Look for calcium-fortified foods. A cup of calcium-fortified orange juice, for example, contains about the same amount of calcium as a cup of milk and is absorbed more easily.
- Get the recommended intake of vitamin D. Vitamin D is necessary for the body to absorb calcium.
- If you're taking other supplements or medicines, check with your physician or pharmacist. Calcium can interfere with the absorption of iron, zinc, and certain medicines.

Of the various trace minerals, iron is the most abundant. It is also one of concern to nutritionists because certain groups are at risk of having low iron levels. These include young children and early teens; menstruating women; and people with conditions that cause internal bleeding, such as ulcers or intestinal diseases.[1]

Iron deficiency in the diet is responsible for the most prevalent form of anemia in the United States. Iron deficiency hampers the body's ability to produce *hemoglobin*, a substance needed to carry oxygen in the blood. A lack of hemoglobin can cause fatigue and weakness and can even affect behavior and intellectual function. Proper infant feeding through use of iron-fortified milk or breast-feeding is the best safeguard against iron deficiency in infants. Among adolescents and adults, iron intake can be improved by increasing consumption of iron-rich foods, such as lean red meats, fish, certain kinds of beans, dried fruits, iron-enriched cereals and whole-grain products, and foods cooked in a cast-iron skillet. For some people, especially pre-

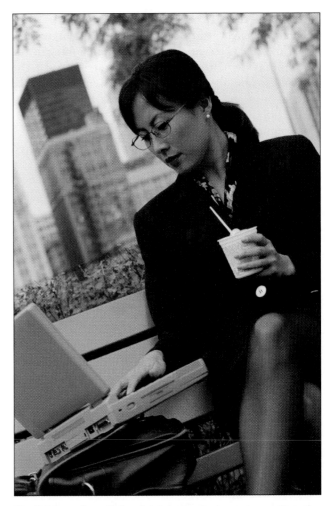

Starting your day with low-fat dairy products, such as milk and yogurt, is a good way to add calcium to your diet.

menopausal women with inconsistent diets, iron supplements may be justified. In addition, consuming foods that contain vitamin C enhances the body's ability to absorb iron.

Iron deficiency is rare among healthy men and post-menopausal women. Even strict vegetarians can get iron in sufficient amounts by consuming legumes, dark-green leafy vegetables, and fortified breads and cereals. It is possible to get too much iron. Some studies report that high iron levels may be linked to heart disease, but the jury is still out on this issue. Also, some people have a rare genetic disorder called *hemochromatosis*, which permits an unhealthy buildup of iron. Iron overload may cause liver cancer, heart disease, diabetes, sterility, or other complications.

Zinc is a trace mineral that has received widespread publicity because of its link to the common cold. Early studies reported that zinc lozenges cured the cold within hours. The results of follow-up studies, however, are mixed and suggest that earlier claims of the cold-prevention benefits of zinc may have been premature.

While zinc is essential for proper functioning of the immune system, too much can interfere with the body's use and absorption of other essential minerals, such as iron and copper. Also, excess zinc can lower HDL cholesterol.[3]

Selenium is another trace mineral that may offer unique health benefits. It is an antioxidant associated with a reduced risk of various cancers. An increase in the intake of selenium is thought to lower the chances of developing lung, colon, and other cancers. Because the results of studies of selenium as an anticancer nutrient are mixed, experts do not recommend selenium supplements at this time. Human studies are underway to determine if the health benefits of extra selenium intake can be confirmed. Fish, meats, eggs, and shellfish are good animal sources of selenium. Grains and seeds grown in soils containing selenium are good plant sources. Most adults get enough selenium in their diet.[3]

Water

Next to air, water is the substance most necessary for survival. Most everything in the body occurs in a water medium. Although people can live without vitamins and minerals for extended periods, death results within a few days without water.

Water makes up about 60 percent of the body's weight. Every cell in the body is bathed in water of the exact composition that is best for it. Even tissues that are not thought of as "watery" contain large amounts of water. For example, water makes up about 75 percent of brain and muscle tissues; bone tissue and fat tissue are about 20 percent water. As a rule, the bodies of men contain more water than do the bodies of women because men have more muscle tissue and muscle tissue holds more water than fat tissue, which is more prominent in the bodies of women.

Water performs many functions. It is vital to digestion and metabolism because it acts as a medium for chemical reactions in the body. It carries oxygen and nutrients to the cells through blood, regulates body temperature through perspiration, and lubricates the joints. It removes waste through sweat and urine, protects a fetus, and assists in respiration by moistening the lungs to facilitate intake of oxygen and excretion of carbon dioxide. It also assists with constipation relief and provides satiety, thus serving as a deterrent to the overconsumption of food.

Although most water intake comes from beverages, solid foods also make a significant contribution (see Just the Facts: Bottled Water Comes with Many Names). Most fruits and vegetables are more than 80 percent water, meats are 50 percent water, bread is 33 percent water, and butter is approximately 15 percent water.

Just the Facts

Bottled Water Comes with Many Names

If you don't like your water from the tap, you can buy purified water, spring water, mineral water, distilled water, and drinking water by the bottle, six pack, or case. Is there a difference between the various types of bottled water? There is but you almost need a dictionary to sort the differences. Here is a brief description of the common types of bottled water.[21]

- **Distilled water** comes from the stream of public water that has been boiled.
- **Drinking water** is public or municipal water, such as tap water, and comprises 25 percent of bottled water. If the water comes directly from the tap without any treatment, the label has to identify the public source it comes from. If the water has been treated, no disclosure is required.
- **Mineral water** is spring water that naturally contains at least 250 milligrams of dissolved minerals (like magnesium and calcium) per liter.
- **Purified water** has been treated with distillation, ion-exchange, reverse osmosis, or a similar process.
- **Sparkling water** is spring water that contains carbon dioxide gas (as in cola beverages).
- **Spring water** comes from underground formations beneath the earth's surface. It makes up about 75 percent of the bottled water sold in the United States. Theoretically, spring water is protected from pollution.

How much water should you drink? People are advised to drink 8 to 12 cups of fluids a day.[22] More fluids are necessary before, during, and after physical activity (see Chapter 3). To determine when and how much fluid to drink, don't rely on thirst. If you're thirsty, the body has already lost too much fluid (see Real-World Wellness: How Can You Tell If You're Getting Enough Water?).

Plain tap water is the preferred source of fluid. Tap water has an advantage over bottled water in that it often contains fluoride, an additive that impedes tooth decay. Chlorine is another additive to municipal water supplies that provides a public health safeguard by destroying bacteria. Because it is added in such small quantities, fears about chlorine causing cancer are unsubstantiated.

Under normal circumstances, too much water cannot be consumed because the body is efficient at getting rid of what it does not need. However, a sudden drinking

Real-World Wellness

How Can You Tell If You're Getting Enough Water?

Experts say that thirst is not a good indicator of when and how much water to drink. If that's the case, how can I tell if I'm drinking enough water?

The following guidelines[23] will help you determine whether to increase your fluid intake.

- Check your urine. It should be clear or pale yellow. Dark-colored urine in small amounts is a sure sign that the body's fluid needs are not being met. (Note, however, that some medicines and vitamin supplements can also cause dark urine.)

- Needing to urinate every two to four hours is a signal that your fluid intake is appropriate. Sometimes people limit fluid intake to avoid trips to the bathroom. This is a mistake. The bladder adjusts to extra fluid intake.

- If you're eating lots of protein, your kidneys need extra water to flush out the waste products of protein metabolism.

- Consume at least 8 to 12 cups of fluid each day. Water is preferred because it is absorbed faster than any other beverage. Juices, milk, and foods that are liquid at room temperature also count. Five servings of fruits and vegetables yield about 2 cups of water. Even solid foods, such as meats and bread, provide water. Alcohol and caffeinated beverages (coffee, tea, and colas) don't count because they act as diuretics and increase the need for water.

binge in a short period early in the day will not satisfy the body's needs later; the excess will be excreted by the kidneys. Water consumption should occur throughout the day.

Other Nutrients with Unique Health Benefits

In addition to the six classes of essential nutrients, many other substances in food contribute to health. Three of the most notable ones are phytochemicals, botanicals, and fiber. Interest in these substances has given rise to two recent trends: the use of **functional foods,** foods that contain substances that promote and maintain health and/or prevent disease (see Just the Facts: Functional Foods), and *chemoprevention,* the use of nutritional interventions to prevent diseases (such as cancer) by bolstering the immune system. New discoveries and recent developments in these areas have

Just the Facts

Functional Foods

The term functional foods refers to foods that provide a specific health benefit above and beyond their inherent nutritional value.[24] Functional food as a term is new but in the strict sense of its definition has been around a long time. Decades ago the food industry recognized the potential value (and profits) in adding nutrients to various foods. Milk is fortified with vitamin D, cereals are enriched with vitamins and minerals, salt is fortified with iodine, and iron is added to many breads. In a technical sense these foods meet the definition of functional foods. More recent additions to the supermarket shelves include orange juice with added calcium, grain products fortified with folate, pasta enriched with soluble fiber, eggs fortified with omega-3 fatty acids, and juices with added antioxidants.

The growing interest in functional foods has been sparked by the publicized health benefits of phytochemicals. Soy, for example, contains isoflavones that may protect against heart disease; tea contains antioxidants that may reduce the risk of cancer; cranberry juice is made up of substances that may help prevent urinary tract infections. When foods such as these are consumed primarily for their purported medicinal value, they are considered functional.

Today's supermarkets are full of functional foods and give the illusion that the grocery store almost looks like a drugstore. In some cases the benefits of functional foods are welcome. Nonmilk drinkers will likely benefit from orange juice fortified with calcium. In other cases, problems may occur. Experts don't know if juices fortified with the herb echinacea are safe or might interact adversely with other medications. The problem with functional foods, as summarized by the editor of a leading health newsletter, arises when functional foods have not been adequately tested to make sure they are safe; when the health claims are based on little or no evidence; when only a trivial amount of a beneficial ingredient is added; or when people replace healthy foods with fortified candy bars, chips, and sodas.[25]

outpaced the scientific community's ability to monitor, test, and confirm various claims. Until these claims can be validated, the public should take a wait-and-see approach. While many of the chemical compounds in food promise to promote health or prevent disease, taken indiscriminately they may do more harm than good. The exception is fiber, for which most claims are

Table 6-6 Health Benefits of Selected Phytochemicals

Phytochemical	Food Source	Possible Benefit
Allyl sulfide	Garlic, onions, leeks, chives	Decreases reproduction of tumor cells; facilitates excretion of carcinogens; blocks nitrite formation in stomach
Caffeic acid	Fruits	Facilitates excretions of carcinogens
Capsaicin	Hot peppers	Acts as an antioxidant; inhibits carcinogenesis
Coumarin	Citrus fruit, tomatoes	Prevents blood clotting; stimulates anticancer enzymes
Dithiolthione	Cruciferous vegetables	Stimulates anticancer enzymes
Phytoestrogen (isoflavones)	Soybeans, dried beans	Helps prevent breast cancer by stopping the estrogen produced by the body from entering cells
Flavonoids	Fruits, vegetables, red wine, grape juice, green tea	Acts as an antioxidant
Phenolic acids (ellagic acid, ferulic acid)	Fruits, grains, nuts	Prevents DNA damage in cells; binds to iron, which may inhibit the mineral from creating free radicals; binds to nitrites in the stomach, preventing them from being converted into nitrosamines
Indoles, isothiocynates, sulforaphane	Cruciferous vegetables	Stimulates anticancer enzymes
Limonene	Citrus fruits	Stimulates anticancer enzymes
Phytic acid	Grains	Binds to iron, which may inhibit the mineral from creating cancer-causing free radicals

backed by years of solid evidence. Some of the claims that have been studied and reported in the popular literature are highlighted here.

Phytochemicals

Phytochemicals are plant chemicals that exist naturally in all plant foods. Chemically they are not vitamins, minerals, fiber, or any of the energy nutrients. Rather they are the hundreds of thousands of active compounds found in small amounts in vegetables and fruits. Although phytochemicals have not been traditionally classified as essential nutrients, scientists believe that they might play an important role in preventing various diseases. For example, populations that consume higher amounts of fruits and vegetables have a lower risk of cancer.[3] Some phytochemicals have a structure similar to the body's natural forms of estrogen. These compounds are called *phytoestrogens* (or *plant estrogens*), and when ingested by way of the diet, they may reduce the potentially harmful effect of the more potent, naturally occurring estrogens often associated with breast and prostate cancer.[11] Although phytochemicals have largely been studied for their role in cancer prevention, researchers are exploring the relationship of phytochemicals to many other diseases, including cardiovascular disease, osteoporosis, diabetes, and hypertension.

There is a great deal of excitement in nutrition and food sciences about the potential of phytochemicals in health promotion. The reported health benefits of several phytochemicals are highlighted in table 6-6. As scientists continue to isolate, identify, and study specific plant chemicals, it is likely that the place of such chemicals in disease prevention will become more important.

Botanicals (Phytomedicinals) (Herbs)

Plants used medically are technically called **botanicals** or **phytomedicinals.** The popular literature usually refers to them as *herbs.* Herbs number in the thousands; however, few are backed by well-conducted research studies similar to those used to test over-the-counter drugs in the United States. Herbs, however, are not regulated as drugs; instead, they are classified as dietary supplements. Consequently, there is considerable debate about their effectiveness and safety. The names, food sources, and health claims of several popular herbs are presented in Just the Facts: Some Common Herbs Sold as Nutritional Supplements. Herbs are not to be confused with hormone supplements, such as melatonin, DHEA (dehydroepiandrosterone), and DMSO (dimethylsulfoxide). Unlike herbs, extracted from plants, these are synthetic compounds. The purported health benefits of these hormones have not yet been proved.

Just the Facts

Some Common Herbs Sold as Nutritional Supplements

Here are usual dosages and possible benefits and problems[26] of various herbs:

- **Bilberry** (*Vaccinium myrtillus*)

  Usual dosage: 240–480 mg dried berry extract of bilberry shrub

  Possible benefits: useful for simple diarrhea, varicose veins, hemorrhoids, glaucoma, night blindness, cataracts

- **Echinacea** (*Echinacea purpurea*)

  Usual dosage: 15–30 drops of tincture from purple coneflower extracts, up to five times a day

  Possible benefits: immune booster for colds, flus, and respiratory infections

  Potential problem: some allergic reactions reported in people with autoimmune disorders like lupus or multiple sclerosis

- **Feverfew** (*Tanacetum parthenium*)

  Usual dosage: 125 mg of dried leaf extract

  Possible benefits: prevention and treatment of migraines and associated nausea

  Potential problem: a potential allergen for people sensitive to ragweed

- **Garlic** (*Allium sativum*)

  Usual dosage: 3 cloves of dietary garlic daily or 1 tsp. dried garlic powder, or in oil or pill form

  Possible benefits: may promote antibacterial, antifungal, and antiviral activity including those associated with the common cold; may have cardiovascular benefits

  Potential problem: in excess, possible interactions with other herbs and/or medicines

- **Ginger** (*Zingiber officinale*)

  Usual dosage: 500 mg

  Possible benefits: treatment of motion sickness, nausea, indigestion

  Potential problem: may aggravate gallstones, heartburn; acts as a blood thinner

- **Glucosamine and Chondroitin** (*Glucosamine hydrochloride, chondroitin sulfate*)

  Usual dosage: 1500 mg of glucosamine and/or 1200 mg of chondroitin

  Possible benefits: may stimulate cartilage growth and relieve pain associated with arthritis and stiff joints[27,28]

  Potential problem: reduced insulin secretions

- **Ginkgo** (*Ginkgo biloba*)

  Usual dosage: 120–160 mg from leaf extract of ginkgo tree, in divided doses

  Possible benefits: may improve memory and mental functioning; acts as an antioxidant; aids blood flow to the brain and to the legs

  Potential problem: acts as a blood thinner; may cause gastrointestinal upset, headaches, allergic skin reactions

- **Ginseng** (*Panax ginsing*)

  Usual dosage: 300 mg or one-half ginseng root extract in hot water

  Possible benefits: may enhance immunity

  Potential problem: may increase blood pressure; may cause headaches and skin problems

- **Saw palmetto** (*Serenoa repens*)

  Usual dosage: 320 mg of dried fruit extract from sabal in one to two doses

  Possible benefits: may improve urinary flow in men with enlarged prostate

  Potential problem: may cause inaccurate readings on (PSA) tests

- **St. John's Wort** (*Hypericum perforatum*)

  Usual dosage: 300 mg dried leaf and flower extract

  Possible benefits: may alleviate mild to moderate depression

  Potential problem: not useful for severe depression; may cause complications with prescription antidepressants

- **Valerian** (*Valeriana officinalis*)

  Usual dosage: 400–450 mg of extract 30 minutes before bedtime

  Possible benefits: treatment for insomnia, mild anxiety, restlessness

  Potential problem: may cause complications with sedatives or antidepressants

If you decide to take an herb, here are some tips:

- Check with your physician before taking herbs, especially for serious conditions. Inform your physician of herbs you are taking, as you would for prescribed medicines. There are many potential interactions with other supplements and medicines.
- Avoid using herbs if you are pregnant or nursing.
- Check the label for the abbreviation *USP*. This means that the manufacturer has met the stringent guidelines of the United States Pharmacopoeia, ensuring the quality, strength, purity, and consistency of the product. The letters *NF,* which stands for *National Formulary,* also ensure that the product meets minimum standards. Presently, only a handful of herbs have been subjected to review using USP standards.
- Do your homework. Read about the herb; ask your pharmacist for information. There are several websites that provide helpful information:
  United States Pharmacopoeia: **www.usp.org**
  American Botanical Council: **www.herbalgram.org**
  The Herb Research Foundation: **www.herbs.org**
- Monitor your body's response. Start with a lower than recommended dose. Stop taking an herb if you have an adverse reaction.
- Don't expect miracles. Herbs take longer to work than prescribed and over-the-counter medicines.
- Take specific herbs for specific needs. Avoid taking herbs continuously.

Fiber

One advantage of a high-starch diet is that it will likely be high in fiber unless the foods are refined or highly processed.

Fiber (formerly called *roughage*) is a general term that refers to the substances in food that resist digestion. The amount of fiber in a food is determined by its plant source and the amount of processing it undergoes. In general, the more a food is processed, the more the fiber is broken down or removed and the lower its fiber content.

There are two kinds of fiber: *soluble fiber* dissolves or swells in hot water, and *insoluble fiber* does not dissolve in water. Every plant food usually contains a mixture of fiber types.

Soluble fiber

Soluble fiber appears to have several favorable effects. Because it forms gel in water, it adds bulk and thickness to the contents of the stomach and may slow emptying, thus prolonging a sense of fullness, which may help dieters control their appetites. Studies have shown that soluble fiber also lowers blood-cholesterol levels. Soluble fiber binds with certain digestive acids made from cholesterol in the liver and then escorts the acids away in the stool. The liver responds by drawing cholesterol from the blood to make more acids, which lowers blood cholesterol. According to most studies, LDL cholesterol drops when a person changes from a low-fiber diet to a high-fiber diet.[11] Diets high in carbohydrates and fiber, especially soluble fiber, improve blood-glucose control, lower insulin requirements, and decrease blood cholesterol and blood pressure in people with diabetes. Soluble fiber also slows the absorption of sugars from the small intestine, another benefit for those with type 2 (non-insulin-dependent) diabetes.[3]

Good sources of soluble fiber are fruits, vegetables, and grains. Specific fiber-rich foods are prunes, pears, oranges, apples, legumes, dried beans, cauliflower, zucchini, sweet potatoes, and oat and corn bran (table 6-7).

Insoluble fiber

Insoluble fiber adds bulk to the contents of the intestine. This speeds the transit time (time of passage) of a meal's remnants through the small and large intestines. This in turn appears to offer the following important health benefits:

- It helps prevent constipation because insoluble fiber attracts water into the digestive tract, thus softening the stool. Softer stools reduce the pressure in the lower intestine, creating less likelihood that rectal veins will swell and cause hemorrhoids.
- It stimulates muscle tone in the intestinal wall, which helps to prevent *diverticulosis,* a condition that occurs when the intestine bulges out into pockets, possibly leading to *diverticulitis,* a condition in which the pockets become infected and sometimes rupture.

Insoluble fiber may also be protective against colon cancer. A shorter transit time reduces the exposure of the intestines to cancer-causing agents in the food. Insoluble fiber also stimulates the secretion of mucus in the colon. Mucus coats the colon wall and may provide a barrier that keeps cancer-causing agents from reaching the colon's cells.

The best source of insoluble fiber is wheat bran. Other good sources are whole grains, dried beans, and peas, and most fruits and vegetables, especially those eaten with the skin. Choose foods that name one of the following ingredients first on the label's ingredient list[29] (see Just the Facts: Sample Ingredient List for a Whole-Grain Food):

- brown rice
- bulgur (cracked wheat)
- graham flour
- oatmeal
- pearl barley
- popcorn

Table 6-7 Fiber Content of Selected Foods

Food	Fiber (g)
Fruits	
Apple, with peel	4.2
Banana	3.3
Blackberries (1 cup)	9.7
Dates, chopped (1 cup)	15.5
Grapes	1.0
Orange	2.9
Peach, peeled	2.0
Pear, with skin	4.9
Prunes, dried, pitted (10)	13.5
Raisins, seedless (1 cup)	9.6
Breads	
Oatmeal (1 cup)	0.86
Pumpernickel (1 slice)	1.33
Rye (1 slice)	1.65
Wheat (1 slice)	1.40
White (1 slice)	0.68
Whole wheat (1 slice)	3.17
Cereals	
Bran Chex (2/3 cup)	5
Bran flakes (2/3 cup)	5
Cheerios (1 1/4 cup)	2
Corn flakes (1 cup)	1
Grapenuts (1 1/4 cup)	2
Life (2/3 cup)	3
Raisin Bran (1/2 cup)	4
Rice Krispies (1 cup)	Trace
Shredded Wheat (1 biscuit)	3
Vegetables	
Baked potato, with skin	4.4
Carrot	2.0
Cauliflower (1/2 cup)	1.3
Corn, canned (1/2 cup)	6.3
Garbanzo beans (1 cup)	8.6
Green beans (1 cup)	3.1
Greens (1 cup)	2.9
Lima beans (1 cup)	9.2
Navy beans (1 cup)	16.5
Tomato	2.2

- whole-grain corn
- whole oats
- whole rye
- whole wheat

Claims that insoluble fiber may actually prevent, rather than protect against, colon cancer are being debated. Regardless, there is no dispute that a high-fiber diet is strongly associated with a decreased incidence of

Just the Facts

Sample Ingredient List for a Whole-Grain Food[29]

- Ingredients: whole wheat flour, water, high fructose corn syrup, wheat gluten, soybean and/or canola oil, yeast, salt, honey.
- Note: "wheat flour," "enriched flour," and "degerminated corn meal" are not whole grains.

diverticular disease, heart disease, high blood pressure, and type 2 diabetes.[30]

If you are not accustomed to eating fiber-rich foods, gradually add them to your diet over four to six weeks, following these suggestions:[31]

- Eat whole-wheat bread rather than white bread.
- Look for whole grains, such as whole wheat, on food labels. Whole grains contain the entire seed of a plant, including the bran, germ, and endosperm. Foods "made with whole-wheat flour" are mostly refined. Wheat flour and unbleached wheat flour are not whole grain.
- Add 2 to 3 tablespoons of 100 percent bran to low-fiber foods, such as breakfast cereal, pudding, and applesauce.
- Substitute brown rice, millet, and bulgur wheat for white rice and potatoes.
- Snack on popcorn instead of potato chips (popcorn is a whole grain).
- Eat whole fruit instead of drinking juice.
- Use raspberries as a topping for ice cream and yogurt.
- Snack on an unpeeled apple or pear.
- Choose bran flakes over cornflakes.
- Top your salads and casseroles with a whole-grain cereal, such as shredded wheat.
- Eat the skin on your potato.
- Include beans in soups and vegetable salads.
- Eat oats, legumes, and fruits for insoluble fiber.

How much fiber?

Most Americans consume 14 to 15 grams of fiber per day.[3] The daily recommendation is 25 grams for a 2000-calorie diet and 30 grams for a 3000-calorie diet. Most Americans have trouble meeting this recommendation because of their heavy intake of meat products. Meat provides little or no fiber; consequently, only vegetarians are likely to get enough fiber. Eating naturally high-fiber foods, such as whole grains, fruits, vegetables, and beans, is a good way to increase fiber intake. Starting or ending the day with a high-fiber cereal is another convenient way to increase your consumption not only of fiber but also of many vitamins and minerals. Check food labels, which identify the amount of fiber per serving.

As with most other nutrients, fiber can be consumed in excess. Indiscriminate consumption of fiber may interfere with the body's ability to absorb other essential nutrients. A person who eats bulky foods but has only a small capacity may not be able to take in enough food energy or nutrients. A high intake of dietary fiber, such as 60 grams per day, also requires a high intake of water.[3]

Putting Nutrition to Work

Nutrition is a complex science and involves the study of thousands of nutrients and a countless number of possible interactions, all of which take place at the cellular level. Many of the results of nutritional practices, good or bad, take years or even decades to become apparent. Fortunately, it isn't necessary to be a biochemist to understand and follow nutritional practices that promote health and prevent the early onset of many health problems. The benchmark for developing a plan for good nutrition is the 2000 *Dietary Guidelines for Americans*.[29] These guidelines recommend that, to stay healthy, persons aged 2 years and older should follow the ABCs for good health: **A**im for fitness, **B**uild a healthy base, and **C**hoose sensibly. The ABCs provide the framework for ten specific dietary guidelines:

- **To aim for fitness**
  - aim for a healthy weight
  - be physically active each day
- **To build a healthy base**
  - let the Pyramid guide food choices
  - choose a variety of grains daily, especially whole grains
  - choose a variety of fruits and vegetables daily
  - keep food safe to eat
- **To choose sensibly**
  - choose a diet low in saturated fat and cholesterol and moderate in total fat
  - choose beverages and foods to moderate intake of sugars
  - choose and prepare foods with less salt
  - if consuming alcoholic beverages, do so in moderation

Aim for a Healthy Weight

A healthy weight is key to a long, healthy life. To be at their best, adults need to avoid gaining weight, and many need to lose weight. Being obese increases the risk for many chronic diseases. The achievement and maintenance of a desirable body weight and composi-

Wellness On the Web
Behavior Change Activities

Put "Pyramid Power" to Work for You

When you want to plan a nutritionally balanced diet, your best bet is to eat a variety of foods according to the federal government's Food Guide Pyramid. You can use the Pyramid to determine how many servings from each food group to include in your diet; it's also a great way to ensure that you consume the recommended dietary allowances (RDAs) of essential nutrients each day. To use an interactive Food Guide Pyramid, go to **www.mhhe.com/anspaugh5e**. Go to "Student Center," "Chapter 6," "Wellness on the Web," then "Activity 1." Place your mouse on any portion of the Pyramid and click to obtain a list of foods and the appropriate portions for each food group.

Diet Facts—or Fiction?

Can you lose weight on a grapefruit diet? Should you eat after 6 P.M.? Does gelatin make your nails hard? Are some vegetables and fruits negative-calorie foods? Nutrition has captured the interest of Americans more than perhaps any other aspect of fitness and wellness. Whether it's HDLs or LDLs, fat or fiber, phytochemicals or vitamins, nutritional issues make headlines in both scientific journals and popular magazines, and everyone seems to be an expert. Go to **www.mhhe.com/anspaugh5e** to discover the "Top Ten Diet Myths." Go to "Student Center," "Chapter 6," click on "Wellness on the Web," then on "Activity 2."

tion are complex issues and are treated separately in this text. For a complete discussion of the principles of balancing food intake with physical activity for evaluating and maintaining desirable body composition, refer to Chapters 7 and 8.

Be Physically Active Each Day

Aim to accumulate at least 30 minutes (adults) or 60 minutes (children) of moderate physical activity most days of the week, preferably daily. If you already get 30 minutes of physical activity daily, you can gain even more health benefits by increasing the amount of time you are physically active or by taking part in more vigorous activities. No matter what activity you choose, you can do it all at once or spread it out over two or three times during the day.

A moderate physical activity is any activity that requires about as much energy as walking 2 miles in 30 minutes. Choose activities that you enjoy and that

Figure 6-3 Food Guide Pyramid

Children, teenagers, and adults under 25 years of age should choose three servings from the milk, yogurt, and cheese group.

you can do regularly. Some people prefer activities that fit into their daily routine, like gardening or taking extra trips up and down stairs. Others prefer a regular exercise program, such as a physical activity program at their worksite. Some do both. The important thing is to be physically active every day.[29]

The benefits of exercise are discussed throughout this text; specific principles and applications of exercise and physical activity are discussed in depth in Chapters 3, 4, and 5.

Let the Food Guide Pyramid guide food choices

Variety and moderation are the essence of a healthy diet. The best way to ensure a varied and moderate diet is to use the Food Guide Pyramid as the foundation for food selection.

Variety. The Food Guide Pyramid (FGP) (figure 6-3) portrays dietary guidelines in picture form and provides a structure for dietary planning by recommending the number of servings for each food group. Variety is the cornerstone of the FGP (see Just the Facts: Variety: The Cornerstone of a Healthy Diet). The largest area of the pyramid is the base, which calls for six to eleven servings of grain products. Foods from this group

Just the Facts

Variety: The Cornerstone of a Healthy Diet

There is a plethora of studies that link a specific nutrient to good health. But the study of an isolated nutrient, when removed from its original food source, often yields misleading results and sometimes does more harm than good. For example, beta-carotene has long been reputed as a nutrient that prevents lung cancer. In a famous 1994 study, however, male smokers who took a 20 mg supplement of beta-carotene surprisingly ended up with a higher incidence of lung cancer than the placebo group. As a result, the study was stopped midstream. Researchers concluded that if beta-carotene prevents and/or delays lung cancer, it does so in combination with other foods.

The only sure way to realize the benefits of various nutrients is to eat a variety of foods. No single nutrient or food can supply all of the essential nutrients in the right proportion needed by the body. Variety is the essence of a healthy diet and may be the only practical way of making sure you're getting the full healthful effects of various nutrients.

Wellness Across the Generations

The Nutrient Gap

It has been estimated that as many as 25 percent of Americans 60 and older are malnourished. They do not suffer from nutritional diseases like scurvy or pellagra; rather, they consume insufficient amounts of key nutrients that have a direct effect on health and body function. Older adults usually expend less energy to meet the demands of their lifestyle than do their younger peers and therefore require fewer calories. This presents a dilemma because as their need for energy decreases, their need for nutrients increases or stays the same. Unfortunately, a decrease in caloric intake is usually associated with a decrease in key nutrients. There is a gap between what older adults need and what they get from food, as shown in the following chart:[32]

Nutrient	What They Need (Age 50+)	How They're Doing	Why Adults Age 50+ Need It
Calcium	1200 mg	The average intake is 400–600 mg	The capacity to absorb calcium declines with age
Folate	400 µg	Only one-fourth of older adults get 400 µg	Reducing homocysteine levels becomes more important as heart disease risks increase
Riboflavin	1.1 mg, women 1.3 mg, men	Only one-third get enough	The body's need is the same throughout adulthood
Vitamin B_6	1.5 mg, women 1.7 mg, men	50–90% don't get enough	The body's metabolism changes with age
Vitamin B_{12}	2.4 µg	20% of adults over 60 and 40% over 80 are deficient	Increased difficulty in absorbing vitamin B_{12} comes with age
Vitamin D	400 IU, ages 51–69 600 IU, 70+	The average intake is 100–125 IU	Decreased ability of skin to synthesize vitamin D from sunlight comes with age
Protein	See Wellness Across the Generations: Older Adults May Need More Protein previously in the chapter		

make up about 40 percent of the daily diet. The next largest areas of the FGP are the fruit and vegetable groups. Together, grain products, fruits, and vegetables make up nearly three-fourths of the recommended diet. The top of the pyramid allows for a smaller number of servings from meat or meat substitutes and dairy products. About 25 percent of the servings in your daily diet should come from foods in these groups. No recommendations are given for the number of servings of fats, oils, and sweets. The advice is to consume these sparingly.

As helpful as the FGP is for meal planning, it has received some criticism. One important omission is any reference to fluid intake. This is a serious oversight because most Americans do not get enough water each day (see Real-World Wellness: How Can You Tell If You're Getting Enough Water? previously in the chapter). Another criticism is of its lack of guidance for people who don't eat a typical American diet. For that reason, other food pyramids have been developed that meet the needs of alternative diets, such as those of ovolactovegetarians. One such version is presented later in this chapter (see p. 183).

The FGP identifies a range of servings for the food groups. The number of servings that fits your needs depends on your required number of calories. Your calorie requirements depend on many factors, including age, gender, height, weight, activity level, health status, and pregnancy (see Wellness Across the Generations: The Nutrient Gap). Three calorie levels along with the corresponding recommended number of servings are presented in table 6-8.

Table 6-8 Nutrition Plan for Three Calorie Levels

	Calorie Level*		
	1600	**2200**	**2800**
Grain group servings	6	9	11
Vegetable group servings	3	4	5
Fruit group servings	2	3	4
Milk group servings[†]	2–3	2–3	2–3
Meat group servings[‡]	5	6	7
Total fat (g)	53	73	93
Percent fat calories	30	30	30
Total added sugars (tsp)[§]	6	12	18

*1600 calories is appropriate for many sedentary women and some older adults; 2200 calories is appropriate for most children, teenage girls, active women, and sedentary men (women who are pregnant or breast-feeding may need more). For teenage boys, many active men, and some very active women 2800 calories is appropriate.

[†]Women who are pregnant or breast-feeding, teenagers, and young adults to age 24 need 3 servings.

[‡]Meat group amounts are in total ounces.

[§]From candy, desserts, soft drinks, and other sweets.

What Counts as a Serving?

One way to estimate serving size when food labels aren't available is to use the parts of your hand. Here is how it's done:

1 thumb = 1 ounce of cheese

1 thumb tip = 1 teaspoon of foods such as mayonnaise, peanut butter, and sugar

3 thumb tips = 1 tablespoon

1 fist = 1 cup of pasta, rice, or vegetables

1 or 2 handfuls = 1 ounce of a snack food (1 handful of small foods, such as nuts, or 2 handfuls of larger foods, such as chips and pretzels)

1 palm (minus the fingers) = 3 ounces of meat, fish, or poultry

Serving size

What counts as a serving depends on the food and how it is prepared. Sorting through serving sizes can be confusing. One ounce of a ready-to-eat cereal, for example, counts as a serving. This is equivalent to 1/2 cup of cooked cereal. One slice of bread is equivalent to one-half of a bagel. The fruit group is more confusing. One whole piece of fruit is the same as 1/2 cup of chopped fruit or 3/4 cup of fruit juice. The only sure way to determine serving size is to check food package labels. You can also refer to Just the Facts: What Counts as a Serving?

Moderation. Moderation is another important characteristic of the healthy diet. There is a place in the diet for almost any food if it is consumed prudently—the FGP doesn't label food "good" or "bad." Some foods do have a higher **nutrient density** than others, meaning they yield a higher ratio of nutrients to calories, but all foods contribute to nutrition (see Just the Facts: Nutrient Density). Moderation means exercising good judgment regarding quantity and frequency. It doesn't mean avoidance. The idea that a particular food is good or bad can be destructive to anyone trying to eat more healthfully. For example, a person with rigid attitudes who thinks that cheesecake is "bad" and then indulges in eating it might think, "I am bad, I have no willpower, and I am a weak person." The behavioral result might be a cheesecake binge, because the forbidden nature of the food makes it harder to resist. A more positive approach is to understand that cheesecake is not "bad" and that eating a slice does not make the eater a bad person.

Another reason for moderation is that even nutritionally dense foods can be consumed in excess. The interaction of the various substances in food can cause one nutrient to overpower or nullify the effects and benefits of another. The body's processes may be compromised or the nutrients in foods may interfere with the desired effects of medicines. Here are several examples of the negative effects of excessive consumption of various nutrients:

- Too much protein from animal sources may cause the body to lose extra calcium.[3]
- Botanicals such as garlic, ginger, and ginseng, when combined with vitamin E, fish oils, or blood thinning medicines (e.g., aspirin, Coumadin), may inhibit the blood-clotting mechanism of the body and cause internal bleeding.[33]
- Megadoses of vitamin A can cause birth defects.
- Megadoses of vitamin C can cause diarrhea, nausea, abdominal cramps, and headache.[3]
- Excessive intake of vitamin D causes too much calcium to move from the bones to the blood and then to the urine through which it is excreted from the body.[3]

Just the Facts

Nutrient Density

A key strategy for eating well is to select foods that offer significant amounts of nutrients but small numbers of calories. If a particular food has a high ratio of nutrients to calories, it is a nutritionally dense food. You can determine the nutrient density of food by adding the percentages of the RDA for the essential nutrients and dividing by the number of calories per serving (see the following example). The higher the score, the higher the nutrient density. The concept of nutrient density can help the health-conscious and weight-conscious person make informed choices.

Calculating the Nutrient Density of Pizza (Cheese)

Calories	354
RDA %	
Protein	28%
Vitamin A	19%
Vitamin C	20%
Thiamin	25%
Riboflavin	29%
Niacin	19%
Calcium	33%
Iron	15%
Total	**188**

Nutrient density = 53% (188 ÷ 354 × 100)

- High intake of folate may mask the symptoms of pernicious anemia, a condition associated with a vitamin B_{12} deficiency.
- Excess niacin may aggravate glucose intolerance associated with non-insulin-dependent diabetes.
- Foods high in vitamin K, such as broccoli, spinach, and turnip greens, may neutralize the effectiveness of blood-thinning medicines.
- Foods high in tyramine, such as cheese and sausage, can cause a sudden rise in blood pressure in people taking some antidepressant medicines.[34]

These examples are not meant to discourage your consumption of a particular food. Each food offers a unique contribution to health. Vitamin D, for instance, is required for calcium metabolism; however, too much of it may result in a depletion of calcium. Moderation is an important concept that applies to essential nutrients just as it applies to nutrients with bad reputations.

Choosing foods from the FGP, with an emphasis on variety and moderation, not only satisfies the body's need for essential nutrients but also helps prevent problems associated with dietary excess.

Choose a Variety of Grains Daily, Especially Whole Grains

Grain products (bread, cereal, rice, and oats) help form the foundation of a nutritious diet. They are rich in vitamins, minerals, complex carbohydrates, dietary fiber, and other substances essential for good health. The FGP recommends at least 6 servings per day, more for older children, teenagers, adult men, and active women.[29] Unrefined, "whole-grain" foods should be emphasized over refined grain products—white bread, white rice, white flour, and pasta. Refined grains are not good sources of fiber.

Meeting this dietary guideline is a formidable challenge to most Americans. For example, in planning meals Americans often think first of the entrée, which is typically a meat dish. This is usually true whether we're eating at home or dining out. The FGP challenges us to reverse this approach by thinking of plant products first.

The vegetarian alternative

The importance of a plant-based approach to eating is evidenced by the fact that a properly planned vegetarian diet is now viewed as a healthful and acceptable way of meeting all nutritional needs. Some vegetarians avoid all animal products, including dairy products, poultry, eggs, and fish. Others include eggs and milk products but exclude fish, poultry, and red meat. There are many variations of vegetarian diet. The more common types are presented in table 6-9.

With the exception of vegans, most types of vegetarians have little trouble getting all of the essential nutrients, including protein. Milk products, eggs, fish, and poultry are sources of complete, high-quality protein. *Vegans,* who eat all-plant diets, need to be discriminating in their food selections because most plants are sources of incomplete protein. One notable exception, as mentioned earlier, is soy protein. Vegans who don't consume soy products need to combine complementary foods, such as grains and legumes, to obtain all of the essential amino acids.

The nutritional problem most likely to occur in a strict vegetarian diet is a deficiency in vitamin B_{12}, which occurs naturally only in animal products. Vegans can get vitamin B_{12} by taking a supplement or consuming food fortified with B_{12}. Vitamin D is another potential problem to the vegan if he or she has limited exposure to the sun. Milk products, fortified with vitamin D, are about the only dietary source of vitamin D.

Table 6-9 Types of Vegetarians

Type	What Is Excluded from Diet	What Is Included in Diet
Vegans	All animal products	Fruits, vegetables, grains, legumes, nuts, and seeds
Lactovegetarians	Eggs, fish, poultry, and meat	Milk products and fruits, vegetables, grains, legumes, nuts, and seeds
Ovolactovegetarians	Fish, poultry, and meat	Eggs (*ova*), milk products (*lacto*), fruits, vegetables, grains, legumes, nuts, and seeds
Pescovegetarians	Poultry and meat	Fish (*pesco*), eggs, milk products, fruits, vegetables, grains, legumes, nuts, and seeds
Pollovegetarians	Red meat	Poultry (*pollo*), fish, eggs, milk products, fruits, vegetables, grains, legumes, nuts, and seeds

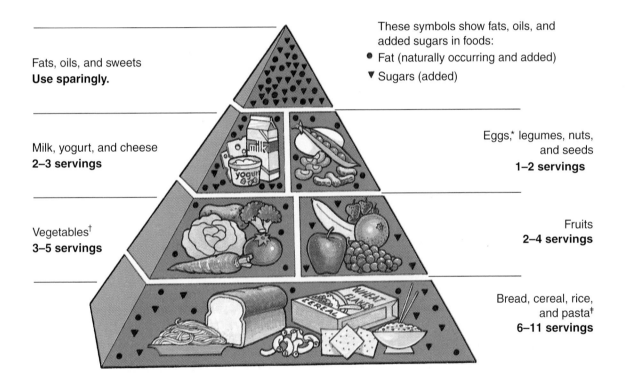

* Lactovegetarians can omit eggs from this pyramid.
† Include one dark green or leafy variety daily.
‡ One serving of a vitamin- and mineral-enriched cereal is recommended.
¶ Contains about 75 g of protein and 1650 calories.
‖ Base serving sizes on those listed for the Food Guide Pyramid.

Figure 6-4 Food Pyramid for Ovolactovegetarians‖

However, the body can produce adequate amounts of this vitamin if the skin receives sufficient exposure to sunlight. During periods of limited sunlight exposure, vegans may need to take vitamin D supplements. Other essential nutrients richly supplied by animal products and thus of concern to vegans, such as riboflavin, iron, zinc, and calcium, can be easily derived from a variety of plant sources.

Figure 6-4, a food pyramid for ovolactovegetarians, presents a helpful plan for people trying to avoid meats. The recommended number of servings of grains, fruits, vegetables, and milk products is identical to the recommended amounts in the Food Guide Pyramid. The major difference is the exclusion of meat in favor of legumes, nuts, seeds, and eggs. Lactovegetarians can omit eggs from this pyramid.

Here are some practical tips for adding fruits, vegetables, and grains to the diet that should be helpful for people opting for a meatless meal, choosing to eat vegetarian for a day, or favoring vegetarianism as a lifestyle:

- Start off the day with fruit juice.
- Add fruit to a salad.
- Serve fruit for dessert.
- Have a smoothie (blend fruit juice, ice, and a banana).
- Add fruit to cereal.
- Eat cereal as a snack.
- Eat vegetable snacks.
- Aim for a colorful plate, with dark-green, yellow, and red vegetables.
- Increase the number of vegetables in a salad by adding tomatoes, carrots, cucumbers, peppers, spinach, or broccoli.
- Eat a vegetable pizza.
- Make a soup with leftover vegetables.
- Eat an all-vegetable meal.
- Mix legumes with a salad.
- Try a new fruit or vegetable.
- Top fat-free frozen yogurt with low-fat granola and berries.
- Top salad with whole-wheat cereal.

A properly selected vegetarian diet has many health benefits (see Just the Facts: Health Benefits of a Vegetarian Diet). People who have health conditions associated with diets high in fat and saturated fat and low in folate, carotenoids, phytochemicals, and antioxidants stand to benefit from a plant-based diet.

Choose a Variety of Fruits and Vegetables Daily

Fruits and vegetables are key parts of a nutritious diet. To promote health, at least two servings of fruits and three servings of vegetables should be consumed daily. Fruits and vegetables provide essential vitamins and minerals, fiber, phytochemicals, antioxidants, and other substances good for health. They are naturally low in fat and calories are filling. Some are high in fiber, and many are quick to prepare and easy to eat.

In choosing fruits and vegetables aim for variety. Try many colors and kinds. Choose any form: fresh, frozen, canned, dried, juices. All forms provide vitamins and minerals, and all provide fiber except for most juices.

One way to cultivate a taste for a variety of vegetables and fruits (and grain products) is to acquire a taste for ethnic food. The typical diets of many other countries favor grains, fruits, and vegetables and place less

Just the Facts

Health Benefits of a Vegetarian Diet

As a group, vegetarians have lower morbidity and mortality rates from several chronic degenerative diseases than do nonvegetarians.[35] Typically, vegetarian diets are lower in fat and saturated fat and have higher concentrations of nutrients (vitamins, minerals, and phytochemicals) associated with health benefits. Here are some of the benefits of a vegetarian diet over a nonvegetarian diet:

- Lower cholesterol level
- Lower level of low-density lipoproteins
- Lower incidence of hypertension
- Fewer complications and lower mortality from type 2 diabetes mellitus
- Reduced incidence of lung, colorectal, and breast cancer
- Improved kidney function
- Reduction of coronary artery disease

emphasis on animal fats. However, watch out for the Americanization of ethnic foods. For example, the traditional Italian pasta dish comes with a tomato-based sauce containing small amounts of meat or meatballs on the side, served with crusty Italian bread or pizza with an extra-thick crust and a mere sprinkle of tomato sauce, herbs, and cheese. Americanized, the same pasta dish comes with less pasta, more creamy sauces, and more meat and is served with buttery garlic toast or pizza with a thin crust, pepperoni, sausage, olives, and extra cheese. For additional comparisons, see Just the Facts: Do You Eat Real Ethnic Food?

Keep Food Safe to Eat

Americans face a paradox: We are urged to eat more fruits, vegetables, fish, and poultry but we are warned about contamination and foodborne illness. **Foodborne illness** is a condition caused by eating food that contains harmful bacteria, toxins, parasites, viruses, or chemical contamination (see Just the Facts: Foodborne Illness: Food Sources and Symptoms). More than 33 million cases of foodborne illness occur in the United States each year, causing about 9000 deaths.[36] These illnesses are difficult to prevent because they involve different kinds of organisms infecting foods of all types grown in many parts of the world.

With the exception of hepatitis A, the organisms that cause foodborne illness are bacterial. For most of them, treatment consists of hydration and the administration of antibiotics. Other types of organisms are involved in

Just the Facts

Do You Eat Real Ethnic Food?

The typical diets of many other countries tend to contain more high-carbohydrate foods and fewer foods high in animal fats than does the common American diet. However, when ethnic foods are prepared in the United States, especially in restaurants, they are often "Americanized" by inclusion of larger portions of meat and cheese and addition of sauces. What follows are descriptions of some traditional, high-carbohydrate ethnic foods and their higher-fat Americanized versions. Which versions of these ethnic foods do you tend to eat?

Chinese

- Traditional: large bowl of steamed rice with small amounts of stir-fried vegetables, meats, and sauces as condiments
- Americanized: several stir-fried or batter-fried entrees in sauces, with a small bowl of fried rice on the side

German

- Traditional: large portions of potatoes, rye and whole-grain breads, stew with dumplings, and sauerkraut
- Americanized: fewer potatoes, less bread, more sausage and cheese

Japanese

- Traditional: large bowl of steamed rice with broth-based soups containing rice noodles, vegetables, and small amounts of meat

- Americanized: tempura (batter-fried vegetables and shrimp), teriyaki chicken, oriental chicken salad with oil-based dressing

Italian

- Traditional: large mound of pasta with tomato-based sauce containing small amounts of meat or meatballs on the side, served with crusty Italian bread or pizza with an extra-thick crust and mere sprinkle of tomato sauce, herbs, and cheese
- Americanized: less pasta, more creamy sauces, and more meat, served with buttery garlic toast or pizza with a thin crust, pepperoni, sausage, olives, and extra cheese

Mexican

- Traditional: mostly rice, beans, warmed tortillas, and lots of hot salsa and chiles
- Americanized: crispy fried tortillas, extra ground beef, added cheese, sour cream, and guacamole (avocado dip)

Middle Eastern

- Traditional: pita bread (round bread), pilaf (rice dish), hummus (chickpea dip), shaved slices of seasoned meat, diced vegetables, and yogurt-based sauces, all seasoned with garlic
- Americanized: meat kebabs, salads drenched in olive oil, less bread and pilaf

foodborne illnesses. Parasites such as *Trichinella spiralis* (found in pork and wild game) and tapeworms (found in beef, pork, and fish) also infect many people. The same is true of fungi, which produce mold spores that yield toxins such as aflatoxin.

Most foodborne illnesses can be prevented by observing some basic rules for storing, handling, and preparing food.

- Avoid cross-contamination: Do not prepare foods in an unclean sink and do not allow utensils that have come into contact with an unclean surface to touch food.
- Wash hands when first starting to handle food and after handling garbage or dirty dishes.
- Use separate cloths, sponges, and towels for washing dishes, wiping counters and tabletops, wiping hands, and drying clean dishes.
- Measure the temperature of cooked or held foods to make sure they're hot enough to destroy bacteria (see figure 6-5).

- Do not consume foods whose "use-by" dates have expired.
- Transfer leftovers from deep pots and casseroles to shallow pans before refrigeration to speed cooling (and thereby slow bacterial growth).
- Quickly freeze or refrigerate all ground meat and other perishable foods after shopping.
- Wash hands, utensils, and work areas with hot soapy water after contact with raw meat to keep bacteria from spreading. Also wash your hands after using the bathroom; diapering a child; using the telephone; handling garbage; or touching your face, your hair, or other people.
- Keep the refrigerator temperature below 40° F (37° F is optimal). Keep the freezer at or below 0° F.
- Wash whole produce. This includes melons and citrus fruits before cutting them open, to prevent the transfer of bacteria from the fruit's skin to the edible part.
- Wash or sanitize cutting boards between each use.

Just the Facts

Foodborne Illness: Food Sources and Symptoms

Here is a short list of organisms that are common culprits of foodborne illness, along with their food sources and symptoms.

Staphylococcus toxins are usually present in meats, poultry, egg products, tuna, potato and macaroni salads, and cream-filled pastries. Symptoms occur two to six hours after exposure and include diarrhea, vomiting, nausea, and abdominal cramps. Recovery normally takes place in twenty-four to thirty-six hours.

Salmonella infections are associated with eggs, poultry, meat, dairy products, seafood, and fresh produce. Symptoms usually occur within six to forty-eight hours and include nausea, vomiting, abdominal cramps, diarrhea, fever, headache, and sometimes a rash. *Salmonella* infections may be serious, even fatal, in infants, the elderly, and the sick.

Clostridium botulinum, usually referred to as *botulism,* occurs in an anaerobic environment, such as in canned goods, and affects low-acid foods like green beans, mushrooms, spinach, olives, and beef. Symptoms occur twelve to thirty-six hours after exposure and affect the central nervous system. Paralysis and death may follow. Infected food usually has an odor. Avoid canned goods that show any signs of damage.

Campylobacter jejuni contamination is linked to raw and undercooked poultry, unpasteurized milk, and untreated water. Symptoms usually occur in two to five days and include diarrhea, fever, abdominal pain, nausea, headache, and muscle pain. Infections may last seven to ten days.

E. coli O157:H7 is typically present in undercooked and raw ground beef, raw milk, lettuce, untreated water, and unpasteurized fruit juices. Symptoms include severe abdominal pain and cramping and diarrhea (first watery, then bloody).

Listeria monocytogenes is associated with soft cheeses, poultry, fish, and raw meats and vegetables. The illness causes flulike symptoms, including fever, and may progress to fatal infections of the blood and central nervous system.

Hepatitis A virus comes from contaminated fecal material from people who harvest, process, or handle food, including workers on farms, in food-processing plants, and in restaurants. Symptoms, which may not occur for several weeks, include fever, nausea, abdominal discomfort, and sometimes jaundice. The infection is usually mild, though symptoms can be severe.

- Store meat products in separate containers from fruits and vegetables.
- Flip steaks with tongs or a spatula rather than with a fork during cooking. Unlike ground beef, in which bacteria are mixed throughout the meat during the grinding process, steak harbors bacteria only on the surface. Sticking a fork into meat before it is cooked injects the interior with bacteria from the outside.
- Cook fish until it flakes with a fork.
- Put your sponge or scouring pad in the dishwasher every time you run it. Or microwave your sponge on high for thirty to sixty seconds.
- Don't store raw foods on the refrigerator shelf above ready-to-eat foods.
- Don't thaw frozen food on the kitchen counter or at room temperature. Thaw frozen food in the refrigerator or microwave.
- Don't eat hamburgers or any form of ground beef until the juices run yellow, with no trace of pink left. (The color of the meat isn't a reliable indicator of doneness. Check the juice.)
- Don't let juice from raw meat, poultry, or fish drip on your hands or any fresh foods in your grocery cart.
- Don't consume unpasteurized milk and juice or consume foods made with raw eggs.
- Don't use tasting utensils that have touched food under preparation.
- Don't grill, barbecue, broil, or pan-fry meats, poultry, or fish at extremely high temperatures. (Grills can reach temperatures in excess of 640° F. Ovens roast at a temperature of 350° F.) Cooking meats at high temperatures promotes the formation of heterocyclic amines, HCAs. HCAs are thought to be carcinogenic. Boiling, steaming, poaching, stewing, and microwaving do not produce HCAs.[37]
- Don't serve or transport cooked food on the plate used for raw meat.
- Don't store raw fish in your refrigerator for more than twenty-four hours. Raw poultry or ground beef will keep for one to two days and raw red meat for three to five.
- Reheat leftovers thoroughly to at least 165° F.[29]

Figure 6-5 How Hot Is Hot Enough?

Recommended safe cooking and storage temperatures. These food temperatures are not intended for processing, institutional, or food service preparation.

SOURCE: U.S. Department of Health and Human Services. (2000). *Nutrition and Health: Dietary Guidelines for Americans.* Washington, D.C.: U.S. Government Printing Office.

Choose a Diet That Is Low in Saturated Fat and Cholesterol and Moderate in Total Fat

Some dietary fat is needed for good health. Fats supply energy and essential fatty acids and promote absorption of the fat-soluble vitamins. Whether from plant or animal sources, fat contains more than twice the number of calories as its carbohydrate or protein equivalents. Fats are represented in the apex of the FGP; *Dietary Guidelines for Americans* calls for no servings of

Even if your weight is healthy, too many high-fat take-out dinners may mean too few fruits and vegetables.

fat because the body's need for essential fatty acids is easily satisfied by foods in the other food groups. Perhaps one of the greatest shortcomings of the American diet is the abundance of fat. Compounding this problem is that fat is usually consumed at the expense of fruits, vegetables, and grains. For many people, reducing both the amount and type of dietary fat eaten is a formidable challenge. Table 6-4 presents a quick reference of maximum fat intake for selected caloric intakes. You can estimate your personal maximum fat intake by completing Assessment Activity 6-2. You can learn how fatty your eating habits are by completing Assessment Activity 6-5.

Tips for reducing dietary fat

Here are some suggestions for reducing total dietary fat consumption, lowering saturated fat intake, and replacing saturated fats with unsaturated fats:

- Assess your fat intake. Complete the assessments at the end of this chapter along with those in *Health-Quest* to determine your fat intake. Compare your fat intake with the recommendations in table 6-4.
- Read labels and become familiar with the fat content of food. Try to identify foods that should be consumed in limited amounts; also identify foods that are low in fat (see table 6-3).
- Become familiar with sources of saturated, monounsaturated, and polyunsaturated fats (see figure 6-2).
- Check for the presence of transfatty acids by reading the fine print on food labels. Look for the words *hydrogenated* or *partially hydrogenated* to identify foods that should be consumed in limited amounts.
- Limit meat, seafood, and poultry to no more than 5 to 7 ounces per day.
- Eat chicken or turkey (without the skin) or fish instead of red meat in most meals.

- Substitute one or two meals of fish per week for red meats. Choose fish high in omega-3 fatty acids and low in saturated fat, such as Atlantic cod, haddock, salmon, shrimp, scallops, sardines, tuna, red snapper, and trout.
- Choose lean cuts of meat, trim all the visible fat, and throw away the fat that cooks out of the meat.
- Substitute meatless or low-meat main dishes for regular entrees.
- Substitute legumes for meat one or two times per week.
- Eat a vegetarian diet at least one day a week.
- Use no more than 5 to 8 teaspoons of fats and oils per day for cooking, baking, and preparing salads.
- Choose foods that contain fewer than 3 grams of fat per 100-calorie serving.
- Choose foods that contain less than 1 gram of saturated fat per 100-calorie serving.
- Use low-fat dairy products (whole milk has more than eight times the fat calories as skim milk).
- Substitute pureed fruit, such as applesauce, when cooking from a recipe that calls for cooking oil (equal substitution).
- Use soft margarine in place of hard margarine.
- Use liquid or spray margarine when possible.
- Serve dressings and condiments (for salads, potatoes, etc.) on the side. Try to cut these servings in half.
- Avoid fried foods. Substitute another cooking method (baking, grilling, broiling, or roasting) for frying.
- Eat more vegetables and fruits.
- Eat low-fat foods that have a high satiety value, such as whole grains and high-fiber foods.
- Substitute olive oil or canola oil for margarine, butter, or lard.
- Try to add diversity to your diet. Cultivate a taste for low-fat ethnic foods.
- Avoid a "forbidden fruit" approach to food selection. Any food can be enjoyed in moderation. If you consume an unusually high-fat food or meal, try to compensate with more prudent choices during the week.

Choose Beverages and Foods to Moderate Your Intake of Sugars

Sugars are carbohydrates and a source of energy (calories). Dietary carbohydrates also include the complex carbohydrates (starch) and dietary fiber. During digestion, all carbohydrates except fiber break down into sugars.[29] Americans eat sugars in many forms, and most people enjoy the taste of sugars. Some sugars are used as natural preservatives, thickeners, and baking aids in foods. Most of the simple sugar eaten by Americans has been added to foods and beverages during processing and manufacturing. A food is likely to be high in sugars if one of the following terms is listed first or second in the ingredients list on a food label: brown sugar, corn sweetener, corn syrup, fructose, fruit juice concentrate, glucose (dextrose), high-fructose corn syrup, honey, invert sugar, lactose, maltose, molasses, raw sugar, sucrose (table sugar), or syrup. Many foods contain a combination of sugars.

Nutritionists recommend that sugar consumption be limited to 10 percent of total calories. On average, Americans get 18 percent of their calories from sugar.[38]

The major health problem associated with a high sugar intake is dental caries (cavities). The main offenders are sweet and gummy foods. They stick to the teeth and supply bacteria with a steady source of carbohydrate from which to make acids that can dissolve tooth enamel. Foods that promote caries are termed *cariogenic*.

Contrary to popular belief, there is little or no evidence that high sugar intake causes hyperactivity in children, heart disease, diabetes, or obesity. If that were the case, most Americans would have all of these conditions. The major nutritional problem of a high-sugar diet occurs when sugar is substituted for more nutritionally dense foods. When this happens, the result may be insufficient vitamin and mineral intake.

Sugar Intake, Glycemic Index, and Diabetes Mellitus

The relationship between sugar intake and diabetes mellitus is being debated. In the past experts argued that if excessive sugar intake caused diabetes, then most people would have diabetes. The reality is that most Americans consume too much sugar but most of them do not develop diabetes. Another observation is that many people who develop type 1 diabetes consume no more, and sometimes less, sugar than people with normal blood sugar levels.

Currently, some health experts are exploring the relationship between blood sugar and diabetes from a different angle. It has been observed that sugar and starch cause a surge of glucose into the blood stream. The glucose, in turn, stimulates the pancreas to make insulin, the hormone that guides glucose into cells, where it is converted into energy. The **Glycemic Index (GI)** is a scale that makes food-to-food comparisons of these blood-sugar surges possible (see Just the Facts: Glycemic Index). Foods with a high GI result in quicker blood sugar surges in comparisons to foods with lower GI. Epidemiologic studies have started showing that people who eat high-GI foods are more likely to develop diabetes.[39] One theory is that the

Just the Facts

Glycemic Index (GI)

One of the hot topics in nutrition today is glycemic index. Glycemic Index (GI) is a scale that yields information about the extent to which food causes sudden blood sugar surges. Foods with a high GI cause a quick surge of blood sugar; foods with a low GI result in a slower blood sugar elevation. Health consequences are sometimes associated with foods with a high GI.

Common sense suggests foods that taste sugary have a high GI. It's not so simple. Fructose, for example, is one of the sweetest sugars but in isn't broken down into blood glucose until it reaches the liver—and even then some of it is stored as glycogen. Therefore, foods made sweet by fructose don't necessarily cause sudden, huge jumps in blood glucose levels. The same is true for sucrose (table sugar), because it's half fructose.

What does have a high GI are foods high in starch. In terms of GI, a baked potato is worse than many soft drinks. If high-GI diets are associated with diabetes (still an "if"), then starch may be more blameworthy than sugar.

What about starchy grains? If the grain is whole grain, its outer germ layer is intact and slows down the breakdown of starch into glucose—another reason to eat whole grains. The GI of white bread, for example, is nearly double that of whole wheat, pumpernickel, or oat bran bread.

SOURCE: Editors. (2001). Is sugar bad for you? *Harvard Health Letter* 26(4):1–2.

continual bombardment of blood-sugar peaks produced by high-GI foods causes the pancreas to lose its ability to respond with insulin. Exposure to blood-sugar surges may also contribute to *insulin resistance,* the inability of the cells to use insulin. As a result, excess blood sugar circulates in the bloodstream.

While there may be a relationship between the GI of food, blood sugar surges, insulin resistance, and diabetes, it is not possible to state that the intake of foods with a high GI causes diabetes. Diabetes is a complex disease; it will take considerably more time to establish cause and effect relationships.

Choose and Prepare Foods with Less Salt

Salt contains about 40 percent sodium by weight and is widely used in the preservation, processing, and preparation of foods. Sodium is an essential mineral, but it is

one that Americans consume in excess. Average daily consumption of sodium is 3900 milligrams,[11] eight times the minimum requirement of 500 milligrams (one-tenth of a teaspoon) and almost double the 2400 milligrams considered adequate.[40] The main health problems associated with consumption of too much sodium are hypertension, osteoporosis, and stomach cancer. Of the three, hypertension, discussed in Chapter 2, is the most common problem. Sodium contributes to the development of osteoporosis because it pulls calcium from bones and causes the kidneys to excrete calcium. Sodium contributes to stomach cancer because it irritates the stomach lining, causing cells to replicate themselves, increasing the odds of cancer-cell initiation.

The majority of sodium consumed is in the form of hidden salt added during the processing of food. Just how much sodium is in a processed food can be determined by reading the package label.

Taste buds cannot always judge salt content. Some foods that taste salty may be lower in salt content than foods that do not. For example, peanuts taste salty because the salt is on the surface where the taste buds immediately detect it. However, cheese contains more salt than peanuts or potato chips, and chocolate pudding contains even more salt. To cut down on salt consumption, you should do the following:

- Avoid adding salt before tasting food.
- Add little or no salt to food at the table.
- Season food with sodium-free spices, such as pepper, allspice, onion powder, garlic, mustard powder, sage, thyme, and paprika.
- Avoid smoked meats and fish.
- Cut down on canned and instant soups.
- Read labels for sodium content, especially on frozen dinners or pizza, processed meat, processed cheese, canned or dried soup, and salad dressing. When shopping for canned and processed foods, select foods with no more than 200 mg of sodium per 100 calories.
- Eat plenty of fruits and vegetables high in potassium, calcium, and magnesium. These minerals may help keep blood pressure down.

If You Drink Alcoholic Beverages, Do So in Moderation

Dietary Guidelines for Americans defines alcohol moderation as no more than one drink per day for women and no more than two drinks per day for men.[29] This limit is based on differences between men and women in both weight and metabolism. (A drink is defined as 12 ounces of beer, 5 ounces of wine, or 1.5 ounces of

80-proof spirits.) The allowance for women is smaller because women, on average, are smaller than men; they have less muscle and, therefore, less water than men (so alcohol does not get diluted as well in their bodies); and they have less of an enzyme that breaks down alcohol before it reaches the bloodstream. A maximal level of alcohol consumption has not been set for women during pregnancy, so pregnant women and women who have a high chance of becoming pregnant should not use alcohol.

From a health perspective, alcohol has both advantages and serious risks. On the one hand, it is associated with drunk-driving injuries and deaths, cirrhosis of the liver, and a host of social ills caused by alcoholism. On the other hand, when consumed in moderate amounts as recommended by the *Dietary Guidelines*, it offers protection from heart disease and stroke in some people, even more so than does abstinence. Population studies show a 30 percent reduction in coronary risk among moderate drinkers, compared with abstainers. The data are similar in men and women and in various ethnic groups.[41] People most likely to benefit from the moderate intake of alcohol are men over age 45 and women over age 55. Moderate consumption provides little, if any, health benefit for younger people.[29]

Moderate consumption of alcohol is thought to be especially beneficial for people at risk for cardiovascular disease and stroke. Several theories have been advanced to explain this benefit: Alcohol may improve blood levels of high-density lipoproteins, and it may serve as a blood thinner by inhibiting the blood-clotting mechanism often associated with atherosclerosis. Contrary to popular belief, wine does not appear to offer any advantage over other forms of alcohol.

Regardless of alcohol's potential health benefits, experts don't recommend alcohol consumption for everyone. Some people have medical, religious, and personal reasons for abstaining. People with uncontrolled hypertension, liver disease, pancreatitis, or strong family histories of addiction should avoid alcohol. The same is true for women during pregnancy. Also, some medicines may have a potentiating effect when taken with alcohol. For women there is also some concern about the link between moderate consumption of alcohol and breast cancer.[11] Remember that the health benefits associated with alcohol come from a moderate level of consumption. Alcohol consumption in excess of that recommended in *Dietary Guidelines* can cause a variety of health problems that outweigh the potential benefits. As is the case with many health issues, moderation serves as the guiding principle for alcohol consumption.

Other Nutrition Issues of Concern

Nutrition and Pregnancy

Good nutrition is crucial to a successful pregnancy, and a healthy pregnancy starts before conception. Alcohol consumption, smoking, an inadequate diet, dietary excesses of some nutrients, drug abuse, and the interactions of a host of medicines are some of the factors that may threaten a pregnancy even before conception is known or confirmed. Poor health habits throughout pregnancy, especially during the first three months, can harm the mother and developing baby. Although genetic and environmental influences introduce some risk factors beyond the mother's control, there is a considerable amount of medical advice about weight gain and the nutritional needs unique to pregnant women.

Weight gain

Adequate weight gain for a mother is one of the best predictors of pregnancy outcome. A weight gain of 25 to 35 pounds is recommended for most women and yields optimal health for both mother and fetus if pregnancy lasts at least thirty-eight weeks. To accommodate the extra demands for energy, the expectant mother needs to increase her caloric intake by about 300 calories daily, particularly after the third month of pregnancy.[3] Inadequate weight gain can lead to many problems. It is important to monitor weight throughout the pregnancy. Large fluctuations in the recommended weight-gain pattern should be brought to the attention of the health care provider.

Nutrient needs

The RDAs for many nutrients increase during pregnancy:[3]

- The protein RDA increases by 10 to 15 grams daily.
- Extra vitamin D is needed to absorb and distribute extra calcium for developing fetal bones. Approximately 20 to 30 minutes of sun exposure several times a week, a quart of vitamin D-fortified milk, or a vitamin D supplement that contains 5 μg (200 IU) should suffice.
- Because of its role in DNA synthesis, folate is a crucial nutrient during pregnancy. The DRI for folate during pregnancy increases to 600 μg per day. Folate deficiencies have been linked to some neural tube birth defects, such as spina bifida. The increased need for folate can be achieved through the diet or a prenatal vitamin and mineral supplement.

- Iron intake should double during the final six months of pregnancy to achieve the RDA of 30 milligrams per day. The extra iron is needed to synthesize the additional hemoglobin required during pregnancy and to provide iron for the developing fetus. Women often need an iron supplement if their typical iron intake is marginal. Iron deficiencies during pregnancy may threaten the health of both the baby and the mother.
- Calcium is needed during pregnancy for skeletal and tooth development of the fetus, especially during the last three months, when growth of these tissues is most prolific. The DRI for calcium is 1300 mg. A prenatal supplement usually contains 200 mg of calcium.
- The zinc RDA increases 25 percent (to 15 milligrams) during pregnancy to satisfy the requirements for growth and development of the fetus. Foods rich in protein also supply zinc. Zinc deficiencies increase the chance of a low–birth-weight baby.
- Prenatal supplements may contribute to a successful pregnancy for some women and, with the possible exception of vitamin A, provide benefits that outweigh potential risks. Because of its role in cell differentiation, megadoses of vitamin A from both supplements and dietary sources are associated with birth defects, particularly when the vitamin A is consumed during the first three months of pregnancy. It is recommended that women set their limit of vitamin A according to the RDAs.

Slight modifications of the recommended servings in the Food Guide Pyramid should satisfy women's unique nutritional needs during pregnancy. The major differences involve adding a serving of food from two food groups: the milk group and the meat group. Women who practice either ovolactovegetarianism or lactovegetarianism generally do not have difficulty meeting their nutritional needs during pregnancy. Vegans, on the other hand, must plan their diets carefully to ensure adequate amounts of protein, vitamin D, vitamin B_6, iron, calcium, zinc, and vitamin B_{12}. Vegans need to increase their intake of grains, beans, nuts, and seeds to supply the required amounts of nutrients. In addition, supplements of vitamin B_{12}, iron, and calcium along with a multipurpose prenatal supplement will probably also be necessary.[3]

Nutrition and Physical Activity

The relationship between physical activity and nutrition is obvious. The ability to engage in physical activity, whether it is low intensity and recreational or high intensity and competitive, is influenced by dietary intake. Conversely, nutritional needs change depending on the type, intensity, and duration of activity. Nutrition and athletic performance are complex subjects involving not only the science of nutrition but also the sciences of biochemistry and physiology. While a presentation of the intricacies of sports nutrition is beyond the scope of this text, the following information should help you plan to meet your nutrient needs when you participate in regular physical activities.

Type of activity and energy source

The body's use of carbohydrates, fats, and protein for energy depends on the type of activity and the level of physical fitness. For high-intensity, anaerobic activities lasting for only a minute or less, such as a 100-yard sprint, carbohydrates are the major fuel source. For aerobic activities lasting from several minutes to four or five hours, a combination of carbohydrates, fats, and protein provides fuel for work. If the activity is intense, involving 75 percent or more of maximum oxygen consumption (such as of a runner trying to achieve a personal best in a 1-mile run), carbohydrates will be in greater demand. If the activity is moderately intense, using 40 to 60 percent of maximum (such as jogging or brisk walking), fats and carbohydrates are used evenly. If the activity lasts more than a few minutes and is less intense, using less than 30 percent of maximum (such as easy walking), fat becomes a major source of energy.[42] Energy from protein is minimal during most activities because protein functions as a fuel source primarily after carbohydrate fuel is depleted, such as might occur in activities of long duration (such as long-distance running), and then its contribution accounts for only about 10 percent of the energy. In general, carbohydrates are the main fuel source for both anaerobic and high-intensity aerobic activities; fat is the main fuel source for prolonged, low-intensity exercise; and protein is a minor fuel source, primarily for endurance activities.[3]

Recommended sources of energy

The diet of a physically active person should favor carbohydrates. The body is capable of converting carbohydrates to a usable form of energy more quickly and more efficiently than it can fats or protein. As a general rule, dietary intake of carbohydrates should account for 55 to 70 percent of the energy.[42] Tables 6-10 and 6-11 present some high-carbohydrate meal options that are appropriate as preactivity meals. An increase in carbohydrate intake should be accompanied by a decrease in fat intake. Fat should account for about 15 to 30 percent of energy, depending on the percentage of carbohydrate calories; protein should provide the remaining 15 percent.

Table 6-10   Two High-Carbohydrate Preactivity* Meals

	Calories	Protein (grams)	Fat (grams)	Carbohydrate (grams)
Menu 1				
White bread, 2 slices	123	4	2	22
Peanut butter, 1 tbsp.	95	4	8	3
Grape jelly, 1 tbsp.	56	0	0	14
2% milk, 1 cup	125	8	5	12
Orange, 1 medium	60	1	0	15
Meal total:	459	17	15	66
Menu 2				
Vegetable lo mein (soft noodles with stir-fried vegetables), 2 cups	352	11	15	47
Fresh papaya, 1 cup	54	1	0	14
Herbal iced tea sweetened with honey, 12 oz.	56	0	0	13
Meal total:	462	12	15	74

*A preactivity meal should provide 1 to 4 grams of carbohydrate per kilogram of body weight, moderate amounts of protein, and small amounts of fat.

Table 6-11   Convenient Preactivity Meals

Breakfast (McDonald's)	Energy content
Hot cakes with syrup and margarine Orange juice, 2 servings English muffin (whole) with 2 tsp. margarine and 2 tsp. jam	900 cal 67% from carbohydrates (150 g)
• • •	
Cheerios, 3/4 cup Low-fat milk, 1 cup Blueberry muffin Orange juice, 1 serving	450 cal 82% from carbohydrates (92 g)
Lunch or dinner (Wendy's)	
Chili, 8-oz. portion Baked potato with sour cream and chives Chocolate Frosty, 10 oz.	900 cal 65% from carbohydrates (150 g)
• • •	
Grilled chicken sandwich Cola, 12 oz.	425 cal 65% from carbohydrates (70 g)

Protein supplement

Many physically active people, especially athletes, have the mistaken notion that intense physical activities impose a greater than usual demand for protein. This idea stems partly from the perception that, if a modest amount of a nutrient is good for you, large amounts must be even better and partly because protein is needed for the synthesis of new tissue. Both of these ideas can lead to mistaken conclusions. What athletes and others engaged in intense activities need is not extra protein but extra carbohydrates. The body's need for protein is biologically driven (see the previous discussion of recommended protein intake), and any excess in this amount is inefficiently converted to energy or stored as fat.

Two exceptions to this protein guideline occur for athletes engaged in endurance sports and athletes starting weight-training programs. The recommendations for protein range from 1.2 to 1.6 grams of protein per kilogram of body weight for the athlete.[3] This represents a two-fold increase of the RDA for protein. Experts disagree about the importance of excessive protein intake for weight training.

Vitamins and minerals

Vitamin and mineral needs of the physically active person are about the same as those of the sedentary person. People who exercise usually eat more than sedentary people do and therefore get more vitamins and minerals. Contrary to popular belief, especially among athletes, there is no need to take vitamin and mineral supplements if adequate servings of food from the FGP are consumed. The American Medical Association, the American Dietetic Association, the American Institute of Nutrition, the Food and Nutrition Board, and the

National Council Against Health Fraud have published position statements affirming that, with rare exception, there are no benefits of supplements that exceed the DRIs/RDAs.[42] Megadoses of vitamins and minerals may be counterproductive.

If a mineral deficiency occurs, it is most likely to involve iron and calcium, especially for women athletes. A deficiency of either of these minerals not only impairs athletic performance but also may lead to serious medical conditions. Dietary intake of these two minerals should be monitored regularly.

Fatty acids and activity

Most of the body's energy reserve is in its fat stores. When fat stores are broken down, fatty acids move through the bloodstream and enter muscle cells, where they are converted to energy. Well-trained muscles have a greater capacity to execute this conversion process and the ability to burn more fat. Thus, improved physical fitness causes more fat to be used for energy.[42,43] Also, the body's use of fat stores is affected by the duration of the activity. Prolonged activities (lasting more than 20 minutes) cause fat storage to be tapped for energy, particularly when the activity remains at a low-intensity level. Unlike carbohydrate stores, which are limited, an unlimited amount of fatty acids is available to sustain energy needs of low-intensity activities. Weight-conscious people interested in physical activity as a strategy for using fat, therefore, are better served by low-intensity to moderately intense activities that can be endured for a long period.

Fluid intake and activity

Consuming the right amount of fluids before, during, and after physical activity, which is addressed in Chapter 3, is crucial for the regulation of body temperature and the dissipation of heat.

Food Labels

The FDA oversees the labeling of food products other than meat and poultry. With the passage of new label laws in 1992, virtually all processed and packaged foods are required to have uniform labels. These foods include processed meat and poultry, regulated by the USDA. Guidelines for voluntary labeling of raw vegetables and fruits and fish are also available and will likely be displayed in most supermarkets.

Food labels must indicate the manufacturer and the packer or distributor, declare the quantity of contents either by net weight or by volume, and list the common name of each ingredient in descending order of prominence. Information about those nutrients most closely associated with chronic disease risk factors—the amount of total fat, saturated fat, cholesterol, sodium, sugar, dietary fiber, total carbohydrate, and protein—must also be included.

Labels are divided into two parts (figure 6-6) and present information according to generic standards called Daily Values (DVs). Daily Values are benchmarks for evaluating the nutrient content of foods. They express this content as a percentage of a 2000-calorie diet (Recommended Dietary Allowances are not used as the standards because they are age and gender specific). Information in the top part of a label will vary according to the contribution one serving of that food makes to the Daily Values listed in the bottom part of the label.

The DV standards located on the bottom panel are the same on all food labels and are based on two calorie levels: 2000 and 2500 (table 6-12). This means that total fat intake should be fewer than 65 grams for a 2000-calorie diet and fewer than 80 grams for a 2500-calorie diet. Dividing the nutrient content listed in the top panel by the DVs listed in the bottom panel yields the percent Daily Value for one serving. For example, a serving of Mac' n' Cheese contains 15 grams of fat, or 23 percent of the Daily Value of 65 g for a person on a 2000-calorie diet. With the application of simple arithmetic, you can calculate the Daily Value percents for any food with a breakdown of nutrient content.

Standard food labels are useful if daily caloric intake is approximately 2000 or 2500 calories and if the goal is to conform to minimum dietary recommendations. If your diet calls for significantly more or less of a nutrient, your DVs will differ. If that is the case, keep track of the total amount of a nutrient. For example, if you are on a 1500-calorie diet and are trying to limit fat intake to 20 percent, keep a running total of fat grams to determine when 33 g have been reached.

In the past, manufacturers often used labeling ploys to deceive consumers. Currently, the FDA has approved ten health claims that link the following foods and diseases.[44]

- calcium-rich foods and reduced risk of osteoporosis
- low-sodium foods and reduced risk of high blood pressure
- low-fat diet and reduced risk of cancer
- a diet low in saturated fat and cholesterol and reduced risk of heart disease
- high-fiber foods and reduced risk of cancer
- soluble fiber in fruits, vegetables, and grains and reduced risk of heart disease
- soluble fiber in oats and psyllium seed husk and reduced risk of heart disease
- fruit- and vegetable-rich diet and reduced risk of cancer
- folate-rich foods and reduced risk of neural tube defects
- less sugar and reduced risk of dental caries

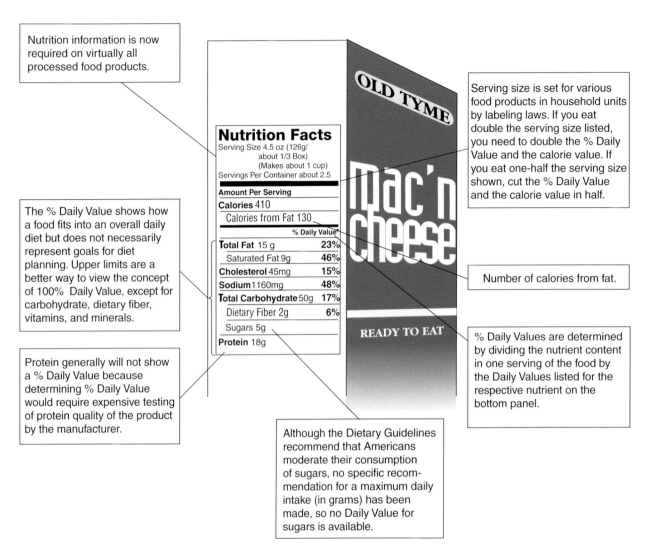

Nutrition information is now required on virtually all processed food products.

Serving size is set for various food products in household units by labeling laws. If you eat double the serving size listed, you need to double the % Daily Value and the calorie value. If you eat one-half the serving size shown, cut the % Daily Value and the calorie value in half.

The % Daily Value shows how a food fits into an overall daily diet but does not necessarily represent goals for diet planning. Upper limits are a better way to view the concept of 100% Daily Value, except for carbohydrate, dietary fiber, vitamins, and minerals.

Number of calories from fat.

Protein generally will not show a % Daily Value because determining % Daily Value would require expensive testing of protein quality of the product by the manufacturer.

% Daily Values are determined by dividing the nutrient content in one serving of the food by the Daily Values listed for the respective nutrient on the bottom panel.

Although the Dietary Guidelines recommend that Americans moderate their consumption of sugars, no specific recommendation for a maximum daily intake (in grams) has been made, so no Daily Value for sugars is available.

Nutrition Facts
Serving Size 4.5 oz (126g/ about 1/3 Box) (Makes about 1 cup)
Servings Per Container about 2.5

Amount Per Serving	
Calories 410	
Calories from Fat 130	
	% Daily Value*
Total Fat 15 g	23%
Saturated Fat 9g	46%
Cholesterol 45mg	15%
Sodium 1160mg	48%
Total Carbohydrate 50g	17%
Dietary Fiber 2g	6%
Sugars 5g	
Protein 18g	

OLD TYME
Mac'n Cheese
READY TO EAT

Figure 6-6   Food Label Showing Daily Values

Food labels provide information about those nutrients most associated with chronic disease risk factors.

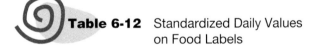

Table 6-12   Standardized Daily Values on Food Labels

	Calorie Levels	
	2000	2500
Total fat	< 65 g	< 80 g
Saturated fat	< 20 g	< 25 g
Cholesterol	< 300 mg	< 300 mg
Sodium	< 2400 mg	< 2400 mg
Total carbohydrates	300 g	375 g
Fiber	25 g	30 g

The FDA has defined commonly used words describing calories, sodium, sugar, fiber, fat, and cholesterol in food. For example, when the word *free* is highlighted on a package in reference to calories, it means that the product yields fewer than 5 calories per serving; in reference to sodium, it means the product contains fewer than 5 milligrams; and in reference to fat, it means the product contains less than 0.5 grams. When *light* or *lite* is used on a package label, it means that the product has one-third fewer calories or 50 percent less fat than a similar product. *Low calorie* foods can have no more than 40 calories per serving; *low-fat* foods can have no more than 3 grams of fat per serving. *Healthy* means that a food meets the criteria for low fat and low saturated fat, does not exceed maximum levels for sodium and cholesterol, and contains at least 10 percent Daily Value for at least one of the following: vitamins A and C, calcium, iron, protein, or fiber. The word *organic* can be used only on raw products grown without added hormones, pesticides, or synthetic fertilizers and on processed foods that contain 95 percent organic ingredients.

Freshness dates have also been defined. Phrases such as *Best Before, Better If Used Before,* or *Best If Used By* tell how long food will retain its best flavor or quality. The food is still safe to eat after the printed date, but it might become stale or change somewhat in taste or texture. The *Expiration, Use By,* or *Use Before* date, which appears on refrigerated foods, provides the deadline for consumption. A product past its expiration date is no longer of sufficient quality and should not be eaten. The *Sell By* date is usually found on highly perishable foods with a particularly short shelf life, such as meat, milk, or bread. It indicates the last day the product should appear on a supermarket shelf.

Even with the improvements in label laws, the unwitting consumer can still be misled. A brand of margarine changed its name from *Brand . . . Light* to *Brand . . . Light Taste*—manufacturers can still use light to describe taste, texture, or color. The makers of a brand of brownie mix claim that it is low fat. But the fine print says that the low-fat designation pertains only to each serving of the mix. Once an edible brownie is created by adding vegetable oil, its fat-gram content more than triples. Some foods promise fruit or other ingredients but deliver only flavor. One brand of strawberry frozen yogurt has no real strawberries despite pictures on the label of real strawberries; a brand of blueberry pancakes has no berries. Clearly, although labels have improved dramatically during the past several years, they still fall short in several areas. Deception in old labels was more obvious; today's labels challenge consumers to apply a higher level of discrimination to sort between fact and fantasy.

Changes in American Eating Patterns

Changes in the American family are mirrored in the trend toward convenience-food eating. For many families, time is a precious commodity that has a dramatic influence on how, where, when, and what people eat. Family meals at home are being replaced by a quick-stop, eat-on-the-go trend. Dining out has become a part of the quintessential American lifestyle, with nearly one-half of Americans eating away from home each day.[45] In terms of good health this is a questionable trend when considering that the more people eat out the more calories, fat, and sodium they consume.

Not only do many people eat away from home, but they also skip meals. For example, college students typically eat two meals a day and make up the difference by eating many snacks. One-fourth of adults skip breakfast, the appropriate meal to replace the carbohydrate stores used during the night's sleep.[43] It should be of little surprise, therefore, that midmorning sluggishness is a common mental and physical disposition of students and workers.

Snacking

Snacking refers to consuming food between the three main meals of the day. Most Americans have at least one snack per day, and snack foods represent one of the fastest-growing markets in the food industry. From a nutrition point of view, snacking is neither good nor bad. The three meals a day standard is based more on social custom than on physiology. The issue is not the time or frequency of eating but what is eaten. Nutritionally dense foods eaten as snacks are as good for health as they are when consumed as meals. The converse is also true; foods low in nutrient density eaten at mealtime are as worthless as when they are eaten as snacks. With the exception of foods restricted for medical reasons, all foods can contribute to a healthful diet. Problems occur when a person's diet is dominated by foods low in nutrient density. Rather than rule out snacking, consume snack foods that enhance wellness. The most direct way to improve snacking behavior is the most obvious one: Purchase and make nutritionally dense foods available (see Real-World Wellness: Snack Ideas).

From a nutritional viewpoint, the criticisms of fast-food eating are the same as those of the rest of the American diet: too much fat, too many calories, too much sodium, and not enough complex carbohydrates and fiber. The average meal of a cheeseburger, milk shake, and fries supplies about 1500 calories, 43 percent of which come from fat. Chicken and fish are as fatty as other protein sources offered by fast-food restaurants because they are breaded and fried. Frying has the same effect on potatoes. Milk shakes get most of their calories from sugars. The Food Composition Table located in the appendix of this text along with nutrition software like FoodWise provide detailed information that can be used to compare many fast-food menu items.

Eating at fast-food restaurants does not have to be a nutritionally worthless activity. Many restaurants are aware that Americans are more knowledgeable about the nutrient content of food and are demanding wholesome, safe, and nutritious foods. Consequently, there has been a trend toward more nutritious menus, including salad, pasta, and potato bars. Guided by good judgment in the choice of foods, an occasional meal at a fast-food chain does not have to compromise a well-balanced diet.

Real-World Wellness

Snack Ideas

After completing a thorough three-day dietary analysis, I was surprised to learn that the key to improving my overall nutritional profile is to make changes in my snack food choices. My meals are fairly well balanced, but my snacks are typically high in fat, high in sodium, high in sugar, and low in nutrient density. What are some examples of nutritionally dense snacks?

The following snacks are surprisingly flavorful and satisfying and will help you improve your overall nutrition:

- Fresh raw vegetables served with a cottage cheese dip
- Fresh fruit, prewashed and cut into bite-size pieces
- Fruit dipped in yogurt
- Bagels topped with reduced-fat cream cheese
- Breadsticks
- Air-popped popcorn seasoned with herbs
- Frozen fruit-juice bars
- Low-fat frozen yogurt
- Pita chips with salsa
- Pretzels
- Rye crisps or rice cakes spread with a little peanut butter or low-fat cheese
- Broth-based soup
- Cereal (low sugar, low fat)
- Shelled sunflower seeds
- Gelatin with added fruit
- English muffins
- Flour tortillas with canned chili and grated low-fat cheese
- Pita bread topped with spaghetti sauce and grated low-fat cheese
- Fruit juice with added club soda
- Hot cocoa (low sugar, low fat)
- Milkshake made with low-fat milk and frozen fruit

Prepackaged Convenience Dinners

Prepackaged convenience dinners have also become part of the American diet. Consumers spend billions of dollars a year on them, and food manufacturers are constantly turning out new lines. The challenge for health-conscious consumers is to determine which ones fit easily into a nutritious diet.

Prepackaged convenience dinners can be evaluated by applying the following criteria:

- There should be no more than and preferably fewer than 30 percent of calories from fat.
- There should be no more than 200 milligrams of sodium per 100 calories.
- They should meet at least 40 percent of the RDA for vitamins A and/or C.

Just because a dinner meets these criteria does not necessarily mean that it provides every nutrient. Some meals are likely to be deficient in some nutrients, so foods that will compensate must be added.

Planning a Nutrition Strategy for Wellness

It is not necessary to be a nutritionist to form a nutrition strategy that works for you. A nutrition plan will work only if it is personalized. Several strategies should be helpful in personalizing your nutrition plan.

Assess Your Nutrition

You should take an honest look at your eating choices and analyze your nutrition profile through Assessment Activities 6-3, 6-4, and 6-6 to determine whether you are doing the following:

- Eating a variety of foods every day from the Food Guide Pyramid
- Avoiding high-fat foods (more than the equivalent of 3 grams of fat per 100 calories)
- Including sufficient fiber in the form of whole grains, dried beans, and fresh fruits and vegetables
- Consuming 8 to 12 cups of water (8 ounces each) daily
- Consuming no more than three or four high-sugar desserts or sweets each week
- Restricting your intake of high-salt foods, such as processed meats
- Consuming no more than one or two alcoholic drinks a day and not letting drinking interfere with your appetite

Make Small Adjustments

The principle of changing health behavior is that the smaller the change, the longer it lasts (see Chapter 1). For example, rather than vowing to abstain from eating ice cream, reduce the amount or number of servings at first and substitute a low-fat brand. If your diet is heavy in salt, you can gradually substitute sodium-free seasonings. If you have a sweet tooth, you can try low-sugar snacks. If you eat for fullness, you can prepare less food or leave food on your plate. You should plan an approach that builds on the cumulative effect of many small successes.

Think of balancing your diet over a long period rather than in a day or a meal. Try to meet the dietary

Nurturing Your Spirituality

Enjoy Your Food—the Missing Dietary Guideline

The fast-paced, eat-on-the-run trend among Americans comes with a high price: Fewer and fewer people spend time preparing good, home-cooked meals, and even fewer use mealtime as a time for relaxing and social bonding. Other cultures recognize that mealtime is a key social time of the day and reflect this value in the dietary recommendations health experts offer their citizens:[46]

- In Japan, immediately following the guideline to avoid too much sodium comes the advice "Happy eating makes for a happy family life; sit down and eat together and talk; treasure family taste and home cooking."
- In Great Britain, the first guideline is "Enjoy your food."
- Korea tells its citizens to "Enjoy meals and keep harmony between diet and daily life."
- In Norway, people are told, "Food and joy equal health."
- In Vietnam, the advice is to "Serve a healthy family meal that is delicious and served with affection."

The greatest nutrition challenge for Americans may not be to reduce fat intake or cut back on sodium. It may be to construct a positive view of food and of mealtime. One highly respected nutrition publication reminds us, "Healthful eating is about more than eating the right mix of nutrients. It's also about sustaining well-being in a way that can't be measured on a blood test but that is just as important to overall health as vitamins and minerals.[46]

guidelines over several days or a week. For example, every meal does not need to contain less than 30 percent fat. Keep portions of favorite high-fat foods small, and limit other sources of fat. Check labels to get an idea of what nutrients you are consuming, but don't keep a calculator by your plate. If you eat foods from the Food Guide Pyramid, you will get all the vitamins, minerals, and protein you need.

Choose Foods for Wellness

Choosing foods for wellness means following the *Dietary Guidelines for Americans*. Your diet should

- Be low in saturated fat (maximum of 8 percent)
- Emphasize complex carbohydrates, such as bread, potatoes, and pasta
- Provide eight to twelve glasses of water throughout the day
- Provide iron and calcium
- Emphasize fresh fruits and vegetables
- Be low in sugar, salt, alcohol, and caffeine

Finally, make sure when choosing foods for wellness to enjoy what you eat (see Nurturing Your Spirituality: Enjoy Your Food—the Missing Dietary Guideline).

Summary

- The six classes of nutrients are carbohydrates, fat, protein, vitamins, minerals, and water. The nutrients that provide energy in the form of calories are carbohydrates, fat, and protein.
- The recommended diet for Americans in *Dietary Guidelines for Americans* emphasizes complex carbohydrates as the major source of energy. A diet high in complex carbohydrates is likely to be lower in fat, lower in calories, and higher in fiber.
- A complete protein is one that provides all of the amino acids in amounts proportional to the body's need for them. Protein sources from animals are complete proteins. Plant sources of complete protein, such as soy protein, come from the legume family.
- One of the greatest shortcomings of the American diet is its excessive intake of fat, especially saturated fat.
- The amount of saturated, monounsaturated, and polyunsaturated fat in foods varies considerably. Most food contains a mixture of these fats.
- The process of hydrogenation increases the saturated fat content of polyunsaturated and monounsaturated fats and yields small amounts of fat not found in nature called *transfatty acids*.
- Dietary fat intake should favor foods high in monounsaturated fats, such as olive oil, canola oil, and peanut oil.
- The consumption of antioxidant vitamins, especially in fruits and vegetables, is associated with a reduced risk of heart disease and cancer.
- Adequate folate consumption is thought to lower the concentration of homocysteine, an amino acid associated with an increased risk of heart disease.
- Two minerals of special concern are calcium and iron. Most women fall short of the RDA for calcium. People at risk for low iron levels include young children, early teens, menstruating women, and people with health conditions that cause internal bleeding.
- People are advised to drink eight to twelve cups of fluids a day. Plain tap water is the preferred fluid.

- Phytochemicals are plant chemicals found naturally in foods. They play an important role in preventing many diseases.
- Many botanicals are thought to have health benefits. Because they are considered nutritional supplements and are not regulated with the same rigor as drugs, there is debate about their effectiveness and safety. Twenty to thirty botanicals are backed by well-conducted research.
- Insoluble fiber benefits the body by adding bulk to the stool, thus speeding the transit of food through the body, which reduces the chance of developing colon cancer, and lowering blood-cholesterol levels. Soluble fiber also benefits the body by lowering blood cholesterol levels.
- A good nutritional plan is one that consists of a variety of foods from the Food Guide Pyramid.
- A food is nutrient dense when it has a high ratio of nutrients to calories.
- Variety and moderation are principles that should most influence eating habits. There is room in the diet for any food as long as it is consumed in moderation in quantity and frequency.
- *Dietary Guidelines for Americans* officially recognizes a vegetarian diet as a healthful and acceptable way of meeting all of our nutritional needs.
- The health benefits of a vegetarian diet include a lower cholesterol level; lower levels of LDLs; reduced incidence of hypertension, lung, colorectal, and breast cancer; and fewer complications from non-insulin-dependent diabetes mellitus.

- Americans consume sugar and sodium in excessive amounts. The major health issue associated with high sugar intake is dental caries; for sodium it's hypertension.
- Moderate consumption of alcohol may be beneficial for some people at risk for cardiovascular disease and stroke.
- Pregnancy imposes a greater demand for some nutrients, including protein, vitamin D, folate, iron, calcium, and zinc.
- Carbohydrates are the main source of energy for both anaerobic and high-intensity aerobic activities; fat is the main energy source for prolonged, low-intensity exercise; and protein is a minor fuel source, primarily for endurance activities.
- The risk of foodborne illness can be reduced by preventing cross-contamination of food; by washing hands, fruits, produce, and meats; and by exercising caution in the way food is prepared and stored.
- Food labels provide helpful information about nutrients associated with the common chronic health problems of Americans as well as about essential nutrients.
- The criticisms of snacking and fast-food eating are the same as those of the rest of the American diet: too much fat, sodium, and sugar; too many calories; and not enough complex carbohydrates and fiber.
- Americans are challenged not only to eat more healthfully but also to construct a positive attitude about food and mealtimes.

Review Questions

1. What is meant by "Nutritional diseases of the past have been replaced by diseases of dietary excess and imbalance"?
2. What was the rationale for revising the Recommended Dietary Allowances for essential nutrients?
3. Identify three nutrients that most Americans do not consume in sufficient amounts.
4. How many calories are supplied by carbohydrates, fat, and protein? What percent of total calories should come from each of these sources? How does Americans' intake of energy nutrients compare with dietary recommendations?
5. Why are carbohydrates the preferred source of energy?
6. What is the difference between a high-quality, complete protein and a low-quality, incomplete protein?
7. What plant sources of protein are unique in that they are considered complete proteins?
8. What are the differences between saturated, monounsaturated, and polyunsaturated fats? What are some food sources of each? What percent of fat calories should come from each type?
9. What are transfatty acids? Why should they be avoided?
10. List five dietary practices that will help lower consumption of fat, especially saturated fat.
11. What are the similarities and differences between water-soluble and fat-soluble vitamins?

12. Which vitamins are classified as antioxidants? What is the relationship between antioxidants and health?
13. What role does folate play in preventing disease?
14. Identify three situations or circumstances that would justify use of a vitamin or mineral supplement.
15. What are phytochemicals? How are they different from botanicals? How do they contribute to health?
16. What two minerals are Americans most likely to be consuming in insufficient amounts? Which segments of the population are most likely to be affected?
17. Explain why thirst is not a good indicator of how much water to drink.
18. What are the major health benefits associated with insoluble fiber? soluble fiber?
19. What is the rationale for the assertion that variety and moderation are the most important principles for a healthy diet?
20. List three negative health effects associated with the excessive intake of nutrients considered good for health when taken in recommended amounts.
21. Distinguish between the different types of vegetarianism. Which types are most likely to require some form of vitamin or mineral supplementation? What are the health benefits of a vegetarian diet?
22. Identify four nutrients that pregnant women require in larger amounts than those in the RDAs.

23. How do the intensity and duration of physical activities affect the way the body uses carbohydrates, fat, and protein for energy? What type of physical activity is most conducive to burning fat calories?
24. List six things a person can do to help prevent unnecessary exposure to foodborne illness.

25. Distinguish between the acronyms RDA, DRI, AI, UL, and DV.
26. To what does the Glycemic Index (GI) of food refer? What are the health implications of GI?
27. What are the main criticisms of snacking and fast-food eating?

References

1. U.S. Dept. of Health and Human Services. 2000. *Healthy People 2010* (2nd ed.). With *Understanding and improving health and objectives for improving health* 2 vols. Washington, D.C.: U.S. Government Printing Office.
2. Atkinson, H. 1991. Can diet prevent cancer? *HealthNews* 5(3):4.
3. Wardlaw, G. 2000. *Contemporary Nutrition: Issues and Insights.* St. Louis: McGraw-Hill.
4. Editors. 1999. Carbohydrates: what role do they play in your diet? *Mayo Clinic Health Letter* 12(2):7.
5. Consumers Union. 2001. How much protein is enough? *Consumer Reports on Health* 13(2):8–10.
6. American Dietetic Association. 1998. *Choosing legumes: a healthful and versatile food.* Available online at **www.eatright.org/nfs45.html**.
7. Mayo Foundation for Medical Education and Research. 1997. Soy—a healthful diet addition. *Mayo Clinic Health Letter* 15(5):7.
8. Editors. 2000. Chewing the fats: AHA conference prompts new look at mono's, polys, trans. *Environmental Nutrition* 23(7):1, 6.
9. Consumers Union. 2001. Fish: weighing the risks and benefits. *Consumer Reports on Health* 13(4):1, 4.
10. Tufts University. 2000. Trans fatty acids expected to appear on nutrition facts labels. *Tufts University Health & Nutrition Letter* 17(12):3.
11. Margolis, S., and L. B. Wilder. 1999. Nutrition and longevity. *The Johns Hopkins White Papers.* Baltimore: The Johns Hopkins Medical Institutions.
12. Tufts University. 2000. Should you continue taking antioxidant supplements? *Tufts University Health & Nutrition Letter* 18(4):1, 4.
13. Harvard Medical School. 2001. Vitamin C. *Harvard Health Letter* 26(6):4–5.
14. Worthington-Roberts, B., and S. R. Williams. 2000. *Nutrition Throughout the Life Cycle.* St. Louis: McGraw-Hill.
15. Forman, A., ed. 1997. As beta-carotene promises fade, focus turns to other carotenoids. *Environmental Nutrition* 20(6):1, 4.
16. Tufts University. 2001. Vitamin E supplements: the pendulum swings away. *Tufts University Health & Nutrition Letter* 19(2):1.
17. Editors. 2000. Has the vitamin E bubble burst? EN evaluates whether to supplement. *Environmental Nutrition* 23(11):1, 4.
18. Harvard Medical School. 2000. Can taking vitamins protect your brain? *Harvard Health Letter* 25(10):2–3.
19. Mayo Foundation for Medical Education and Research. 1997. Vitamin and mineral supplements—sorting out fact from fiction amid a storm of controversy. *Mayo Clinic Health Letter* supplement 15(6):1–8.
20. Tufts University. 2001. Yes, but which supplement? *Tufts University Health & Nutrition Letter: Special Supplement* 19(3):1–4.
21. Schardt, D. 2000. Water, water, everywhere. . . . *Nutrition Action Healthletter* 27(5):1–7.
22. Editors. 2001. Water, water everywhere. *HealthNews* 7(2):3.
23. Antinoro, L. 1998. Dodging dehydration: are you getting enough fluids? *Environmental Nutrition* 21(5):2.
24. Brophy, B., and D. Schardt. 1999. Functional foods. *Nutrition Action Healthletter* 26(3):1–7.
25. Blackburn, G. 1999. Functional foods: a prescription for health? The physician's perspective. *HealthNews* 5(8):1–2.
26. Klausner, A. 1998. The herbal renaissance of the 90's: what's old is new again. *Environmental Nutrition* 21(4):1, 4–5.
27. Editors. 2001. Glucosamine effective for osteoarthritis. *Environmental Nutrition* 24(3):1.
28. Editors. 2001. More good news on glucosamine. *HealthNews* 7(3):5.
29. U.S. Department of Health and Human Services. 2000. *Nutrition and Your Health: Dietary Guidelines for Americans.* Washington, D.C.: U.S. Government Printing Office.
30. Blackburn, G. 1999. The fuss over fiber: the physician's perspective. *HealthNews* 5(3):3.
31. Mayo Foundation for Medical Education and Research. 1996. Fiber—why you need more, and good ways to get it. *Mayo Clinic Health Letter* 14(8):4–5.
32. Tufts University. 1998. With age, calorie needs go down but nutrient needs go up. *Tufts University Health & Nutrition Letter* 16(10):4–5.
33. Consumers Union. 1999. Herbs and drugs: mix and mismatch. *Consumer Reports on Health* 11(7):7.
34. Neergaard, L. November 22, 1998. Consumer group warns of food-drug interactions. *The Commercial Appeal* A10.
35. Messina, V. K., & K. I. Burke. 1998. *Position of the American Dietetic Association: Vegetarian Diets.* Available online at **www.eatright.org/ada/1197.html**.
36. Zuger, A. 1997. For safety's sake; scrub your produce. *HealthNews* 3(8):3–4.
37. Gershoff, S. (ed.). 1998. If your kitchen were a restaurant, you'd fail inspection. *Tufts University Health & Nutrition Letter* 16(9):1.
38. Consumers Union. 1999. Sugar: What's the charm? *Consumer Reports on Health* 11(5):1–5.
39. Harvard Medical School. 2001. Is sugar bad for you? *Harvard Health Letter* 26(4):1–2.

40. Liebman, B. 2000. High blood pressure: the end of an epidemic? *Nutrition Action Healthletter* 27(10):1–9.
41. Klatsky, A. 1996. Sensible, safe, and beneficial alcohol drinking. *Nutri-News* (Fall):14–16.
42. Nieman, D. 1999. *Exercise Testing and Prescription—A Health Related Approach.* Mountain View, Calif.: Mayfield Publishing Co.
43. Wardlaw, G. 1999. *Perspectives in Nutrition* (4th ed.). St. Louis: WCB/McGraw-Hill.

44. Tufts University. 1999. Who's minding health claims on food? *Tufts University Health & Nutrition Letter* 17(5):1, 7.
45. Editors. 1999. Y2K: a good excuse to stock a healthful pantry. *Environmental Nutrition* 22(5):2.
46. Tufts University. 1998. The missing dietary guideline; enjoy your food. *Tufts University Health & Nutrition Letter* 16(5):3.

47. Tufts University. 1997. Older adults may not be getting enough protein. *Tufts University Health & Nutrition Letter* 14(11):2.
48. Russell, R. 2001. Vitamins & minerals: how much is too much? *Nutrition Action Health Letter* 28(5):8–11.
49. Harvard Medical School. 2001. Revised cholesterol guidelines. *Harvard Heart Letter* 11(11):6–7.

Suggested Readings

American Dietetic Association with Jean Pennington. 1999. *The Essential Guide to Nutrition & the Foods We Eat.* New York: Harper Collins Publishing.

This book provides nutrient analysis for 2500 common foods, including brand-name packaged foods and fast foods. An introductory section covers portion sizes, eating by the Food Guide Pyramid, and label reading. Using the easy-to-read tables, shoppers can compare foods for calories, fat, sodium, and more.

Busch, F. 2000. *The New Nutrition: From Antioxidants to Zucchini.* New York: John Wiley & Sons.

A complete guide to essential whole foods and supplements, including vitamins, minerals, herbs, and alternative approaches. Presents a balanced discussion of the pros and cons of traditional and nontraditional diets such as Ayurveda, macrobiotics, vegan, and The Zone. Also includes latest information on nutritional therapies for a variety of conditions, including AIDS, Alzheimer's, cancer, migraines, PMS, and osteoporosis and references to key studies, related websites, hotline numbers, "nutrition actions," and other self-assessment tools.

Eberle, S. G. 2000. *Endurance Sports Nutrition.* Champaign, Ill.: Human Kinetics.

This comprehensive resource provides detailed nutrition advice with customized, sport-specific eating plans ensuring the food choices athletes make will keep them going before, during, and after competition. Written by a registered dietician specializing in sports nutrition who is also an elite endurance athlete. Book tells readers what works—and what doesn't—in actual training and racing situations.

Griffith, H. W. 2000. *Minerals, Supplements & Vitamins: the Essential Guide.* Boise, Idaho: Fisher Books.

This book presents complicated, technical medical information in easy-to-understand terms. Learn about twenty-two minerals, twenty-six of the most popular food supplements, fourteen vitamins, and ten amino acids. The unique format of this book makes accessing information easy, quick, and enjoyable.

Raymond, C. 2000. *Student's Vegetarian Cookbook: Quick, Easy, Cheap, and Tasty Vegetarian Recipes.* Roseville, Calif.: Prima Publishing.

These recipes are designed for people with not much money and even less time. The recipes use easily obtained fresh and prepared ingredients, and each recipe gives preparation and cooking times. The book includes a blend of vegan and nonvegan dishes, as well as pointers on products and preparation for the beginning vegetarian. Includes breakfast ideas, salads, and bean dishes.

Wardlaw, G. M. 2000. *Contemporary Nutrition: Issues and Insights* (4th ed.). Dubuque, Iowa: McGraw-Hill.

This book provides in-depth, comprehensive information on all aspects of nutrition. It serves as an excellent introductory reference for the person in nutrition.

Name _____ **Date** _____ **Section** _____

Assessment Activity 6-1

Assessing Your Carbohydrate and Protein RDA

Assessing Your Carbohydrate Intake Goal

Directions: Complete the following steps to determine your goal for carbohydrate intake in grams to meet the Recommended Dietary guidelines of 55 percent of total calories from carbohydrate (including sugar and complex carbohydrate).

1. Caloric Intake
Your body weight multiplied by 15 equals caloric intake for body weight (approximate number of calories consumed daily, assuming that you are not in a weight-loss or weight-gain program):

_____ lbs. × 15 = _____ calories

2. Carbohydrate Calories
Your caloric intake multiplied by 55 percent equals recommended carbohydrate calories:

_____ calories × 55% = _____ carbohydrate calories

3. Carbohydrate (Grams)
Your recommended carbohydrate calories divided by 4 equals recommended carbohydrate in grams. Transfer this result to Assessment Activity 6-3, Part C, DV column:

_____ calories ÷ 4 = _____ g

EXAMPLE: For a person weighing 185 pounds:

Body weight:	185 lbs.
	× 15
1. Caloric intake:	2775 Kcal
	× 0.55
2. Recommended carbohydrate calories:	1526 Kcal
	÷ 4
3. Recommended carbohydrates:	382 g

This amounts to approximately 14 ounces of carbohydrate (382 ÷ 28 = 14 ounces) (28 grams = 1 ounce).

Assessing Your Protein RDA

Directions: Adults under 55 require 0.36 grams of protein per pound of body weight. Some experts recommend that people 55 years old and older consume 0.45 grams per pound. For example, a 20-year-old person who weighs 150 pounds needs 54 grams of protein: 150 × 0.36 = 54. A 60-year-old person who weighs 150 pounds needs 67.5 grams: 150 × 0.46 = 67.5.

Complete the following steps to determine your RDA for protein:

Your weight:	_____	lbs.
≥ 55 years old:	× 0.45	
< 55 years old:	× 0.36	
Protein RDA:	_____	grams

Assessment Activity 6-2

Assessing Your Maximum Fat and Saturated Fat Intakes

Assessing Your Maximum Fat Intake

Directions: Complete the following steps to determine your estimated maximum fat intake in grams to stay within the dietary guidelines of 30 percent of total calories from fat.

1. Caloric Intake
Your body weight multiplied by 15 equals caloric intake for body weight (approximate number of calories consumed daily, assuming that you are not in a weight-loss or weight-gain program):

_____ lbs. × 15 = _____ calories

2. Maximum Fat Calories
Your caloric intake multiplied by 30 percent equals maximum fat calories:

_____ calories × 0.30 = _____ calories

3. Maximum Fat (Grams)
Your maximum fat calories divided by 9 equals maximum fat in grams. Transfer this result to Assessment Activity 6-3, Part C, DV column:

_____ calories ÷ 9 = _____ g

EXAMPLE: For a person weighing 185 pounds:

Body weight:	185 lbs.
	× 15
1. Caloric intake:	2775 Kcal
	× 0.30
2. Maximum fat calories:	832.5 Kcal
	÷ 9
3. Maximum fat:	92.5 g

This amounts to approximately 3 ounces of fat (92.5 ÷ 28 = 3.3 ounces).

Assessing Your Maximum Saturated Fat Intake

Directions: Complete the following steps to determine your estimated maximum saturated fat intake in grams to stay within the dietary guidelines of 8–10 percent of total calories from fat. The more desirable 8 percent is used in this assessment.

1. Caloric Intake
Your body weight multiplied by 15 equals caloric intake for body weight (approximate number of calories consumed daily, assuming that you are not in a weight-loss or weight-gain program):

_____ lbs. × 15 = _____ calories

2. Maximum Saturated Fat Calories
Your caloric intake multiplied by 8 percent equals maximum saturated fat calories:

_____ calories × 0.08 = _____ calories

3. Maximum Saturated Fat (Grams)
Your maximum saturated fat calories divided by 9 equals maximum saturated fat in grams. Transfer this result to Assessment Activity 6-3, Part C, DV column:

_____ calories ÷ 9 = _____ g

EXAMPLE: For a person weighing 185 pounds:

Body weight:	185 lbs.
	× 15
1. Caloric intake:	2775 Kcal
	× 0.08
2. Maximum saturated fat calories:	222 Kcal
	÷ 9
3. Maximum saturated fat:	24.7 g

This amounts to less than 1 ounce of saturated fat (24.7 ÷ 28 = 0.88 ounces).

Assessment Activity 6-3

Nutrient Intake Assessment

One way to determine if you are getting sufficient quantities of the proper nutrients is to keep a record of your diet. Ideally, this record will cover a time span of at least one week. However, in this exercise you are asked to assess your dietary selections for only one day. Therefore, choose a day representative of your overall nutritional practices. (Your instructor may ask you to conduct a two- or three-day assessment. In this case photocopy additional copies of the assessment forms as needed.)

Directions: There are two options for completing this assessment: (1) use the FoodWise software that accompanies the textbook or (2) analyze your diet manually by following the instructions and completing the forms in Assessment Activities 6-3 and 6-4. Whichever option you choose, record all of the foods and beverages that you consume during one day with the exception of vitamin or mineral supplements. Be specific regarding the amount eaten, how it is cooked, and so on. List condiments and seasonings, such as mustard, ketchup, and butter, and dressings and trimmings, such as lettuce, onions, marshmallows, and sugar. The more detailed your record, the more accurate it will be and the more you will learn from it. Remember, the quality of the results is dependent on the quality of the information entered. A carefully and thoroughly prepared dietary recall will yield an accurate nutritional profile.

Instructions for Computer Analysis Using FoodWise Software Once foods have been listed, you are ready to use the FoodWise nutrition software that accompanies this text to generate your personal nutrition assessment report. Follow the instructions for installing the program on your personal computer. Enter your new User Profile information. When you have completed data entry, print and arrange the results in the following order:

1. User profile with Instant Analysis information: recommended carbohydrate, fat, protein, total caloric intake, and BMI
2. Nutrient summary of macronutrients, vitamins, minerals (ABC button)
3. Nutrient spreadsheet (Spreadsheet button)
4. Food pyramid breakdown of servings for one day (Pyramid button)

5. Bar graph showing dietary intake analysis of nutrients and percent RDA (Bar graph button for RDA analysis)
6. Pie chart comparing breakdown of carbohydrates, fat, protein with recommendations (Left pie chart button)
7. Pie chart showing breakdown of fat (Right pie chart button)
8. Major source of nutrients for those vitamins and minerals that do not meet the RDAs in #2
9. Summary paragraph describing what you learned about your dietary strengths and deficiencies and what changes are needed to improve your nutrition profile

Instructions for Conducting a Manual Nutrition Assessment Complete Parts A, B, C, and D. Then proceed to Assessment Activity 6-4.

Part A: Recording Your Nutrient Intake

1. Use the following form to record your dietary selections for one day. Photocopy extra copies of the form as needed.
2. Refer to the Food Composition Table in the appendix and record appropriate values in the spaces provided. For foods not included in the appendix, refer to package labels, if available, to determine nutritive values.
3. Add the values for each nutrient and enter the result in the total column.

Foods for One Day: List in column headings. Photocopy extra copies as needed.

Nutrients							Total
Calories							
Protein (g)							
Carbohydrate (g)							
Fat (g)							
Cholesterol (mg)							
Saturated Fat (g)							
Sodium (mg)							
Potassium (mg)							
Iron (mg)							
Vitamin A (RE)							
Vitamin C (mg)							
Thiamin (mg)							
Riboflavin (mg)							
Niacin (mg)							
Calcium (mg)							
Fiber (g)							
Folate (mg)							
Selenium (mg)							

Part B: Are You Meeting the RDA?

1. Transfer the values in the Total column in Part A to the Total column in Part B for the following nutrients.
2. Fill in the DV column with your protein RDA results from Assessment Activity 6-1.
3. Subtract the DV from your totals and indicate your status in the appropriate column. A positive value means that you are meeting the DV for that nutrient; a negative value means that you are deficient in that nutrient.
4. For nutrients with a negative value, identify several specific foods that will eliminate the deficiency. Refer to the Food Composition Table in the appendix.

Nutrient	Total	DV	Status	Food Prescription
Protein		see Assessment 6-1		
Iron		18 mg		
Vitamin A		1000 RE		
Vitamin C		60 mg		
Thiamin		1.5 mg		
Riboflavin		1.7 mg		
Niacin		20 mg		
Calcium		1 g		
Folate		400 mg		
Selenium		70 mg		

Part C: Are You Meeting the DVs?

1. Transfer the values in the total column from part A to the total column in Part C for the following nutrients. (Refer to Assessment Activities 6-1 and 6-2 for your personal DV for fat, saturated fat, and carbohydrate.)

2. Compare the DV listed with your totals. Indicate your status by subtracting the DV value from your value. Note that some values are maximum and should not be exceeded; others are goals that serve as minimums.

Nutrient	Total	DV*	Status
Fat		(maximum)†	
Saturated fat		(maximum)†	
Cholesterol		300 mg (maximum)	
Sodium		2400 mg (maximum	
Carbohydrate		(goal)‡	
Fiber		25 g (goal)	
Potassium		3500 mg (goal)	

*DV based on 2000-calorie diet.

†See Assessment Activity 6-2

‡See Assessment Activity 6-1

Part D: What Did You Learn?

Write a summary paragraph describing what you learned about your dietary strengths and deficiencies and what changes are needed to improve your nutrition profile.

_____

_____

_____

_____

_____

_____

_____

_____

_____

_____

_____

_____

Name _____ **Date** _____ **Section** _____

Assessment Activity 6-4

How Does Your Diet Compare with the Recommended Diet?

Directions: The recommended guidelines suggest that carbohydrate calories should make up at least 55 percent of the diet (including complex carbohydrates and sugar), fat calories should be less than 30 percent, and protein calories should be 15 percent. The purpose of this assessment is to compare your diet with these recommendations. First convert your caloric intake to percentages as follows.

Percent Carbohydrate Calories   Your carbohydrate intake (refer to total carbohydrate intake from Part A, Assessment Activity 6-3) multiplied by 4 equals your carbohydrate calories:

_____ g × 4 = _____ carbohydrate calories

Your carbohydrate calories divided by total calories (refer to Part A, Assessment Activity 6-3) multiplied by 100 equals percent carbohydrate calories:

_____ carbohydrate calories ÷ _____ total calories × 100 = _____%

Draw a bar on the graph to indicate percentage of carbohydrate calories.

EXAMPLE: For a person on a 2000-calorie diet who consumed 175 grams of carbohydrate:

175 × 4   = 700 carbohydrate calories
700 ÷ 2000 = 0.35
0.35 × 100 = 35%

Percent Protein Calories   Your protein intake (refer to total protein intake from Part A, Assessment Activity 6-3) multiplied by 4 equals protein calories:

_____ g × 4 = _____ protein calories

Your protein calories divided by total calories (refer to Part A, Assessment Activity 6-3) multiplied by 100 equals percent protein calories:

_____ protein calories ÷ _____ total calories × 100 = _____%

Draw a bar on the graph to indicate percentage of protein calories.

EXAMPLE: For a person on a 2000-calorie diet who consumed 100 grams of protein:

100 × 4   = 400 protein calories
400 ÷ 2000 = 0.20
0.20 × 100 = 20%

Percent Fat Calories   Your fat intake (refer to total fat intake from Part A, Assessment Activity 6-3) multiplied by 9 equals your fat calories:

_____ g × 9 = _____ fat calories

Your fat calories divided by total calories (refer to Part A, Assessment Activity 6-3) multiplied by 100 equals percent fat calories:

_____ fat calories ÷ _____ total calories × 100 = _____%

Draw a bar on the graph to indicate percentage of fat calories.

EXAMPLE: For a person on a 2000-calorie diet who consumed 100 grams of fat:

$100 \times 9 \quad = 900$ fat calories
$900 \div 2000 = 0.45$
$0.45 \times 100 \ = 45\%$

Example Profile   The following graph shows the percentages for the example as the yellow bar below the recommended amount, shown as a red bar.

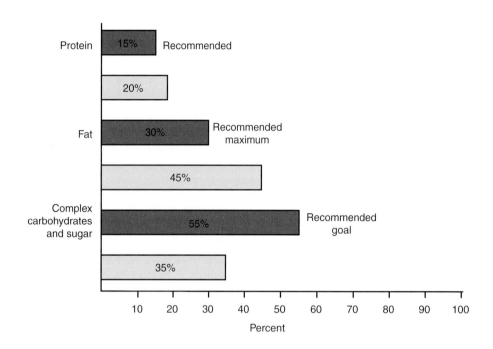

Your Profile   Complete the bars with amounts calculated for your diet:

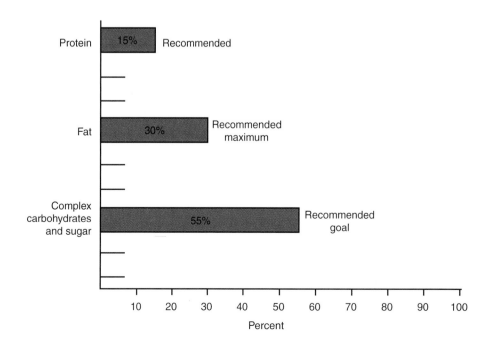

Name _____ Date _____ Section _____

Assessment Activity 6-5

Do You Have Fatty Habits?

Fat has earned a bad reputation because of the health problems it contributes to in high-fat diets. The following questionnaire will help you think about the amounts and types of fat that you generally eat. For each general type of food or food habit, circle the category that is more typical for your diet. If you never or almost never eat any items of a particular food type, skip it.

Food Type/Habit	High Fat	Medium Fat	Low Fat
Chicken	Fried with the skin	Baked, broiled, or barbecued with the skin	Baked, broiled, or barbecued without the skin
Fat present on meats	Usually	Sometimes	Never
Fat used in cooking	Butter, lard, bacon grease, chicken fat	Margarine, oil	Nonstick cooking spray or no fat used
Additions to rice, bread, potatoes, vegetables, etc.	Butter, lard, bacon grease, chicken fat, coconut oil	Margarine, oil, peanut butter	Butter-flavored granules or no fat used
Pizza toppings	Sausage, pepperoni, extra cheese, combination	Canadian bacon	Vegetables such as peppers, onions, and mushrooms
Sandwich spreads	Mayonnaise or mayonnaise-type dressing	Light mayonnaise, oil and vinegar	Mustard, fat-free mayonnaise
Milk and milk products (e.g., yogurt)	Whole-milk and whole-milk products	Low-fat milk products and milk products	Skim milk and milk products
Sandwich side orders	Chips, potato salad, macaroni salad with creamy dressing	Coleslaw, pasta salad with clear dressing	Vegetable sticks, pretzels, pickle
Salad dressings	Blue cheese, Ranch, Thousand Island, other creamy type	Oil and vinegar, clear-base dressing	Oil-free dressing, lemon juice, flavored vinegar
Typical meat portion	6–8 oz. or more	4–5 oz.	2–3 oz.
Sandwich fillings	Beef or pork hot dogs, salami, bologna, pepperoni, cheese, tuna or chicken salad	Turkey hot dogs, 85% fat-free lunch meats, corned beef, peanut butter, hummus (chickpea paste)	95% fat-free lunch meats, roast turkey, roast beef, lean ham
Ground meats	Regular ground beef, sausage meat, ground meat, ground pork (about 30% fat)	Lean ground beef, ground chuck, turkey sausage meat (20–25% fat)	Ground turkey, extra-lean ground beef, ground round (about 15% fat)
Deep-fried foods (e.g., french fries, onion rings, fish or chicken patties, egg rolls, tempura)	Eat every day	Eat once a week	Eat once a month or never
Bread for sandwiches	Croissant	Biscuit	Whole wheat, French, tortilla, pita or pocket bread, bagel, sourdough, or English muffin
Cheeses	Hard cheeses (such as cheddar, Swiss, provolone, Jack, American, processed)	Part-skim mozzarella, part-skim ricotta, low-fat cheeses	Nonfat cheese, nonfat cottage cheese, no cheese
Frozen desserts	Premium or regular ice cream	Ice milk or low-fat frozen yogurt	Sherbet, Italian water ice, nonfat frozen yogurt, frozen fruit whip

Food Type/Habit	High Fat	Medium Fat	Low Fat
Coffee lighteners	Cream, liquid or powdered creamer	Whole milk	Low-fat or skim milk
Snacks	Chips, pies, cheese and crackers, nuts, donuts, chocolate, granola bars	Muffins, toaster pastries, unbuttered commercial popcorn	Pretzels, vegetable sticks, fresh or dried fruit, air-popped popcorn, bread sticks, jelly beans, hard candy
Cookies	Chocolate coated, chocolate chip, peanut butter, filled sandwich type	Oatmeal	Ginger snaps, vanilla wafers, graham crackers, animal crackers, fruit bars
Scoring	(_____ × 2) +	(_____ × 1) +	(_____ × 0) =

Total score: _____

Once you have completed the questionnaire, count the number of circles in each column and calculate your score as follows: Multiply the number of choices in the left-hand (high-fat) column by 2 and multiply the number of choices in the middle (medium-fat) column by 1; then add these two values together. Based on your total score, rate yourself as follows:

Less than 10 = Excellent fat habits
10 to 19   = Good fat habits
20 to 30   = Fat habits needing improvement
Over 30   = Very high-fat diet

If your score is 20 or higher, try to substitute more foods from the middle (medium-fat) column or, better still, the right (low-fat) column for foods in the left-hand (high-fat) column.

Name _____ **Date** _____ **Section** _____

Assessment Activity 6-6

Eating Behaviors to Consider

Directions: Answer the following questions to reveal information about your eating habits, how you devel- oped certain tastes, and your attitude about various foods:

1. When was the last time you tried a new food? What was the food? What were the circumstances? _____

   _____

2. What new foods have you learned to eat during the past year? _____

   _____

3. Name the foods that have been on your "will not try" list (that is, foods that you will not eat under any circum-

   stances). _____

4. What special events do you celebrate in some way with food? _____

5. Where is your favorite place to eat? _____

6. If you were to go on an eating binge, what foods would you be most likely to eat? _____

   _____

7. Describe in detail your favorite meal. _____

   _____

8. Do you consider yourself a slow eater, moderately fast eater, or gulper? What do you think is responsible for

   your eating pattern? _____

   _____

9. To what extent, if any, are your eating habits related to stress? emotions?_____

   _____

10. What do you consider to be your good eating habits? poor eating habits?_____

   _____

7

Understanding Body Composition

Online Learning Center

Log on to our Online Learning Center (OLC) for access to these additional resources:

- Chapter key term flashcards
- Learning objectives
- Additional goals for behavior change
- Concentration game
- Self-scoring chapter quizzes

- Additional lab activities

The OLC also offers weblinks for study and exploration of wellness topics. Access these links through **www.mhhe.com/ anspaugh5e**, click on "Student Center," click on "Chapter 7," and then click on "Web Activities."

Goals for Behavior Change

- Use table 7-5 to calculate your body mass index and interpret your results.
- Make a commitment to either maintain your existing weight or select a healthier weight.
- Formulate a long-range plan to achieve or maintain an ideal body weight and improve your body composition.

Key Terms

amenorrheic
body composition
body mass index (BMI)

obesity
overfat
overweight

Objectives

After completing this chapter, you will be able to do the following:

- Define *body composition*.
- Define *essential fat* and *storage fat*.
- Define and differentiate between *obesity* and *overweight*.
- Discuss the health implications of regionally distributed fat.

- Discuss the limitations of height/weight tables for weight management.
- Calculate body mass index and interpret the results.
- Describe hydrostatic weighing, bioelectrical impedance, and skinfold measurements as methods for determining body composition.

he body is composed of fat mass and fat-free mass. **Body composition** is the ratio between the two. Fat-free weight includes all tissues—muscle, bone, blood, organs, fluids—exclusive of fat. Fat is found in the organs (such as the brain, heart, liver, and lungs) and adipose cells.[1] Adipose cells are fat cells located subcutaneously (beneath the skin) and surrounding various body organs. They are an insulator against heat loss and a protection for the internal organs against trauma. The majority of body fat is found in adipose cells, where it acts as a vast storage depot for energy.

A certain amount of fat is required for normal biological functions. This is referred to as *essential fat*. Essential fat is located in the bone marrow, organs, muscles, and intestines; it is a component of cell-membrane structure as well as of brain and heart tissue. The amount of essential fat in the male and female bodies differs. Essential fat constitutes 3 to 5 percent of the total weight of men and 8 to 12 percent of the total weight of women.[2]

The higher female requirement for essential fat is directly related to fertility and childbearing. Women whose body fat drops below essential requirements such as gymnasts, ballerinas, long-distance runners, and anorexics, often become **amenorrheic;** that is, they stop having a menstrual cycle. The period of infertility continues until they gain weight and their essential fat is restored. In both genders, essential fat represents a minimal threshold or lower limit for the maintenance of health.

Obesity

Obesity, or overfatness, is gender specific. For men, **obesity** is defined as body fat equal to or greater than 25 percent of total body weight, and for women, it is equal to or greater than 32 percent of total body weight.[3] These values are arbitrary because the point at which fat storage increases health risks has not been

determined. Contributing further to the confusion is the fact that methods of assessing the amount of body fat are indirect, and each contains a degree of measurement error. Another complicating factor is that all obesity is not the same. The distribution of body fat in the abdominal area is highly correlated with illness and premature death.[4] A discussion of this topic occurs later in the chapter.

Acceptable body fat percentages have been derived from young adult subjects, and these standards have been applied to all age groups—age-specific standards have yet to be determined, and it is possible that such standards will vary somewhat with age. The results of studies of young adults demonstrate that fat typically ranges from 20 to 30 percent for young females and 10 to 20 percent for young males.[1] These data have led many authorities to suggest that body fat values of 25 percent for females and 15 percent for males are acceptable.

However, more recent body fat health standards based on age and gender allow for an increase in percent body fat with age. This allowance amounts to a trade-off in risks for chronic diseases, especially for women. Low body fat among middle-aged women is associated with losses of bone mineral content, which can lead to osteoporosis and bone fractures. However, leanness or low body fat helps protect these women against heart disease. It is best for women to be lean enough to prevent heart disease yet not so lean as to risk the development of osteoporosis. This is particularly problematic for small-framed women, whose bone mineral content is already low. See tables 7-1 and 7-2 for recommended body fat percentages for women and men of different ages. These are only recommendations designed to recognize differences between males and females, and increasing age is taken into account. Whether these recommendations are accepted or rejected by the scientific community will become evident in the near future. See also Nurturing Your Spirituality: Setting Realistic Fitness and Weight-Loss Goals.

Table 7-1   Recommended Body Fat Percentages for Women

Age	Essential Fat %	Minimal Fat %	Recommended Fat %	Obese Fat %
Over 56	8–12	10–12	25–38	> 38
35–55	8–12	10–12	23–38	> 38
34 or younger	8–12	10–12	20–35	> 35

Adapted from Lohman, T. G., L. B. Houtkooper, and S. B. Going. 1997. Body composition assessment: Body fat standards and methods in the field of exercise and sports medicine. *ACSM Health Fitness Journal* 1:30.

Table 7-2 Recommended Body Fat Percentages for Men

Age	Essential Fat %	Minimal Fat %	Recommended Fat %	Obese Fat %
Over 56	3–5	5	10–25	> 28
35–55	3–5	5	10–25	> 28
34 or younger	3–5	5	8–22	> 25

Adapted from Lohman, T. G., L. B. Houtkooper, and S. B. Going. 1997. Body composition assessment: Body fat standards and methods in the field of exercise and sports medicine. *ACSM Health Fitness Journal* 1:30.

Nurturing Your Spirituality

Setting Realistic Fitness and Weight-Loss Goals

Success in any endeavor requires the establishment of long-term goals. Goals that are challenging and worthwhile but not impossible to accomplish are the keys to success. For instance, it would be unrealistic to expect to run a marathon after a few months of sporadic training or to lose 30 pounds in one month and keep it off.

A more feasible approach is to set realistic short-term goals that can be accomplished relatively easily and quickly. The accomplishment of these will provide the feedback you need to stay on track and the reinforcement to continue the program.

Attainable, realistic goals for exercise should be consistent with the American College of Sports Medicine guidelines for exercise, and realistic weight loss should not exceed 1.5 to 2 pounds per week. People often throw themselves into exercise with a vengeance, as if to wipe out years of inactivity with a frenzied few weeks of activity. The same degree of impatience surfaces with weight-loss attempts.

The following guidelines increase the likelihood of succeeding with exercise and weight loss:

1. Genetics is responsible for 25 to 40 percent of the factors that determine how aerobically fit we may become.[5] We can achieve our aerobic potential with regular exercise, but world-class endurance performances are beyond the reach of most of us. Exercise and enjoy it, be as good as you can, and be satisfied with a significant accomplishment. You should be encouraged to know that you are in the select 15 percent of the adult population who exercise regularly and vigorously.

2. Genetics is responsible for 25 to 40 percent of the factors that lead to overweight and obesity. Although this represents a substantial influence, authorities are convinced that overweight individuals inherit only the *tendency* to become overweight or obese.[6] Our physical activity patterns and eating habits determine whether genetic history becomes destiny.

3. For weight loss or physical fitness, participate in moderate physical activity (preferably low impact if you are a beginner) that builds exercise into your daily life, such as mowing the lawn, washing the car by hand, and climbing stairs instead of taking elevators, plus participate in a structured exercise program (walking, walking/jogging, cycling, swimming, aerobics, etc.). Thirty minutes or more of exercise per day, preferably five days per week, plus eating nutritious meals based on the Food Guide Pyramid, will improve physical fitness and produce sensible weight loss that can be maintained for life.

4. Avoid the inflexible pursuit of artificial aesthetic ideals and aim for reasonable goals. Don't pressure yourself to achieve your goals too rapidly. Remember, healthy eating and sensible regular exercise are for a lifetime, not just a few weeks or months. Let the bodily changes that result from this lifestyle occur slowly, and you will be able to enjoy them for a lifetime.

Taking care of your body does not result in instant health. To make real changes in your lifestyle, you must change the way you think. You must do more than nurture your body; you must nurture your mind as well.

Overweight

Overweight refers to excessive weight for height without consideration of body composition. Because the term *overweight* makes no allowances for body composition, it is a poor criterion for determining the desirability of weight loss. For example, a well-muscled person may be overweight but lean in regard to body fat. By American social standards, such body mass is healthy, aesthetically pleasing, and desirable. It is also possible for a person to be well within the norms for total body weight but **overfat**; that is, such a person carries a large proportion of body weight in the form of fat rather than lean tissue. Overfat is unhealthy and, according to American social standards, unattractive.

See Real-World Wellness: Practical Ways to Estimate Overweight and Obesity.

Regional Fat Distribution

Deposition of fat varies among people. The amount of fat and the storage sites are influenced by heredity and gender (figure 7-1). After puberty, women generally deposit fat in the buttocks, hips, breasts, and thighs. These preferential sites are largely dictated by the

---

Real-World Wellness

Practical Ways to Estimate Overweight and Obesity

What are some practical techniques I can use to determine whether I'm overweight or obese that don't require much time, a technician, or sophisticated measuring equipment?

Practical sources for measuring overweight and overfatness rely on subjective observations and other sensory information. These estimates do not quantify, in a real sense, the extent of the problem should one exist.

Our mirrors supply us with visual feedback. Stand naked in front of a full-length mirror and, as objectively as possible, observe the shape of your body, determine where fat has accumulated, and estimate the amount of muscle you have. Use a tape measure to measure the circumference of your waist and hips. Your hips should be larger than your waist. While you have the tape measure in your hands, measure the circumference of your ankle according to the directions in table 7-3. This will estimate your skeletal size or frame size. People with large frame sizes can carry more weight than can people of the same height with small frame sizes. Knowing your frame size may help you to more accurately interpret the results from the bathroom scale in conjunction with height/weight charts.

A few years ago the slogan "pinch an inch" became popular. If you can pinch an inch at various sites on the body, you are probably somewhat overweight.

The fit of your clothes will provide other clues. If your pants or dress size is increasing steadily, you are gaining weight. Conversely, if the sizes are getting smaller, you are successfully losing weight, changing your body composition, or both. If you are not consciously trying to lose weight and don't need to lose but are doing so anyway, this could be a sign of emerging disease and should be evaluated by a physician.

There is always the feedback you receive from other people. They may tell you that you appear to have either gained or lost some weight. Their perceptions may or may not be correct, but your size has led them to their conclusions.

After all is said and done, remember this: About 40 percent of men are dissatisfied with their appearance and two-thirds of young women between 13 and 19 years think they weigh too much. Millions of normal-weight Americans, particularly young women, are also attempting to lose weight.

We are preoccupied with thinness in the United States. Beauty is in the eye of the beholder, but the vision has been distorted by Madison Avenue's preoccupation with excessive leanness. We need to be realistic and understand that excessive leanness is not within the grasp of most people, nor should it be. Thinness does not always go hand in hand with robust health.

Table 7-3   Measurement of Ankles to Determine Body Frame Size

Measure the ankle at the smallest point above the two bones that protrude on each side of the ankle. The tape measure should be pulled very tightly. Read the tape measure in inches and see the table for an interpretation.

Gender	Small Frame	Medium Frame	Large Frame
Males	< 8 inches	8–9¼ inches	> 9¼ inches
Females	< 7½ inches	7½–8¾ inches	> 8¾ inches

female hormone estrogen.[6] This tendency is known as the *gynoid*, or feminine, pattern of fat deposition. Gynoid fat is not confined exclusively to women; a few men deposit fat in this configuration as well.

Because they produce little estrogen, men usually deposit minimal amounts of fat in the female pattern. Instead, they primarily store fat in the abdomen, lower back, chest, and nape of the neck. Some women store fat this way as well. After menopause, estrogen production decreases and the prevalence of android fat deposition increases.

Although the general claim is that android or upper body fat (sometimes called *central fat*) is harmful, newer evidence indicates that not all android fat is equal.[7] Intra-abdominal fat, stored deep within the abdominal cavity, carries a much higher risk than does subcutaneous abdominal fat, stored directly beneath the skin. Physical activity tends to reduce intra-abdominal fat as well as subcutaneous fat. Moderately intense physical activities, such as gardening and casual walking, may not improve one's cardiorespiratory endurance, but when coupled with modest caloric restriction, they can decrease abdominal fat.

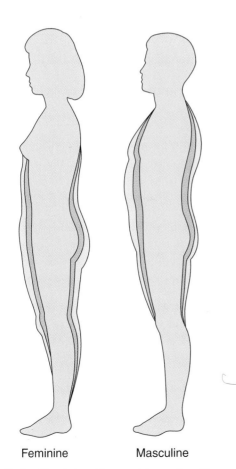

Feminine Masculine

Figure 7-1 Feminine Versus Masculine Deposition of Fat

The waist-to-hip ratio (WHR) is a simple method for determining the distribution of body fat. It requires an accurate measurement of the circumference of the waist at the narrowest point between the rib cage and the navel and of the hips at the largest circumference of the hip/buttocks region. The waist measurement is then divided by the hip measurement. The resulting value may be interpreted by comparing the WHR to the following standard:[8]

Males: A WHR greater than 0.95 indicates an excessive amount of upper body fat. Acceptable levels are less than 0.95.

Females: A WHR greater than 0.80 indicates an excessive amount of upper body fat. Acceptable levels are less than 0.80.

The WHR has been criticized for failing to recognize factors other than abdominal fat, such as skeletal size and muscle mass in the buttocks. An expert panel convened by the National Heart, Lung, and Blood Institute in 1998 concluded that a circumference measure of only the waist is more highly predictive of disease risk than is the WHR.[9] For males, a high waist circumference is greater than 40 inches, and for females it is greater than 35 inches. The power of waist circumference to predict heart disease is unaffected by height, and its predictive power is increased if combined with a body mass index greater than 25kg/m². Body mass index (BMI) is described in detail later in this chapter.

The masculine, or android, pattern of fat deposition is related to an increase in the risk for heart disease, stroke, type 2 diabetes, and some forms of cancer.[6] There are several reasons for this increased risk.

First, enzymes in abdominal adipose cells are active, so fat moves in and out easily. In sedentary people, abdominal fat enters the bloodstream and is routed directly to the liver, where it becomes the raw material for the manufacture of very low-density lipoprotein (VLDL) triglycerides. Later these are converted to low-density lipoprotein cholesterol (LDL-C), and this increases the risk for cardiovascular disease. Conversely, active people direct abdominal fat to the muscles, where it is used as fuel for physical work.

Second, abdominal fat cells are larger than other fat cells. Large fat cells are associated with blood glucose (sugar) intolerance and excessive amounts of insulin in the blood. Such an environment is conducive to the development of type 2 diabetes because the cells' receptor sites become resistant to insulin. Higher than normal amounts of insulin must be secreted to transport sugar from the blood to the cells, but excessive insulin remains in the blood. The body's cells continue to resist insulin so blood sugar also remains high. This sequence of events is characteristic of glucose intolerance or poor regulation of sugar. Over the years these factors can lead to type 2 diabetes. A person does not have to be

Wellness On the Web
Behavior Change Activities

What's Your BMI?

Body mass index (BMI) is not everyone's favorite number. Why? Because it provides an acceptable estimate of the proportion of our body weight that's composed of fat. Although knowing your BMI is more fun if you're fit, don't be discouraged if you're not there yet—use this useful measure to help you achieve your desired level of fitness. BMI is the ratio of body weight in kilograms to height in meters squared. There are several body mass index protocols, all of which represent attempts to adjust body weight to derive a height-free measure of body fat. Although BMI doesn't provide an estimate of percent body fat, it's far more useful than height/weight tables. Calculate your BMI easily and quickly by going to www.mhhe.com/anspaugh5e. Click on "Student Center," "Chapter 7," "Wellness on the Web," then "Activity 1." Type in the information requested, then click on "calculate" to view your BMI.

Is There Really an "Ideal Weight"?

Your "ideal weight," if there is such a thing, depends on a host of factors: your gender, age, height, and frame size, to name the most prominent. Instead of agonizing over outdated height and weight tables published years ago by insurance companies, turn to the experts on the internet. You can calculate your ideal weight painlessly by going to the website mentioned previously and clicking on "Activity 2." Type in the information requested, then click on "calculate," and view your ideal weight.

excessively overweight to be at risk for type 2 diabetes; it is enough that fat be concentrated in the abdominal region. This pattern of fat deposition increases the risk of developing type 2 diabetes 10 to 15 times.[8] Extra fat that accumulates in the hips (gynoid pattern) also increases the risk, but only 3 to 4 times.

Third, excessive insulin in the blood interferes with the removal of sodium by the kidneys, possibly leading to hypertension. Concurrently, the high circulating level of insulin stimulates the overproduction of epinephrine and norepinephrine, both of which raise the blood pressure. This cluster of disorders—high blood pressure, high blood sugar (glucose intolerance), high blood lipids (cholesterol and triglycerides), and abdominal obesity—has deadly consequences. Researchers refer to this combination as *syndrome X* or *metabolic syndrome*.[10]

The good news about android fat is that it is more easily removed from the body than is fat stored in the gynoid pattern. Fat stored in the feminine pattern is highly resistant to removal from its storage depots. Losing gynoid fat usually requires calorie restriction and exercise. Even the best effort may not result in the removal of enough fat from the lower half of the body to satisfy the dieter. Lower-extremity fat is stubborn and much more difficult to lose than is upper-body fat.

Methods for Measuring Body-Weight Status

Height/Weight Tables

Optimal body weight is not necessarily reflective of optimal body composition. This was illustrated by a comparison of young and middle-aged men within 5 percent of their ideal weight as determined by height, weight, and frame-size charts. Although both groups were within the ideal range, the middle-aged subjects had twice the amount of fat as the young subjects.

Height/weight tables do not measure body composition. They act as a standard for total body weight based on height and gender without regard to the composition of weight. Some of the height/weight tables also require users to know their body frame sizes. One method for determining body frame size is presented in Real World Wellness: Practical Ways to Estimate Overweight and Obesity, which appeared earlier in the chapter. These tables are poor criteria for the establishment of weight-loss recommendations.

Body Mass Index

Another method for measuring body-weight status is to calculate **body mass index (BMI)**. Body mass index is the ratio of body weight in kilograms (kg) to height in meters (m) squared (BMI = wt [kg]/ht [m²]). There are several body mass index protocols, all of which originate from height/weight measurements. These protocols represent an attempt to adjust body weight to derive a height-free measure of obesity. Although BMI does not provide an estimate of percent body fat and although BMI uses height/weight data, it is more useful than the height/weight tables[5] and it can be used to compare population groups. It also correlates fairly well (r = 0.70) with percent fat derived from underwater weighing.[6]

In June 1998, the American Heart Association added *obesity* to its list of major controllable risk factors for heart disease.[11] Obesity is now viewed as a chronic disease that represents a "dangerous epidemic" in this country. Later that same month, The National Heart, Lung, and Blood Institute (NHLBI) issued its initial clinical recommendations on obesity (see table 7-4). A panel of twenty-four experts commissioned by the NHLBI

Table 7-4 Disease Risk Based on Body Mass Index (BMI) and Waist Circumference*

Class	BMI (kg/m²)	Disease Risk Based on Waist Circumference†	
		Men ≤ 40 in.‡ Women ≤ 35 in.	Men > 40 in.‡ Women > 35 in.
Underweight	< 18.5‡		
Normal	18.5–24.9		
Overweight	25.0–29.9	Increased	High
Stages of Obesity			
I	30.0–34.9	High	Very high
II	35.0–39.9	Very high	Very high
III	> 40	Extremely high	Extremely high

*Adapted from NHLBI, 1998, "Obesity Education Initiative Expert Panel Clinical Guidelines on the Identification, Evaluation, and Treatment of Overweight and Obesity in Adults," National Heart Lung and Blood Institute, Washington D.C.

†Disease risk is for cardiovascular disease, hypertension, and type 2 diabetes.

‡Increased waist circumference may be a marker for an elevated risk even for people of normal weight.

≤ equal to or less than

> greater than

< less than

conducted an extensive review of the research literature on obesity and concluded that people with BMIs of 25.0 to 29.9 kg/m² should be classified as overweight.[12] The panel recommended that people whose BMIs fall in this category should attempt to lose weight if they have two or more weight-related risk factors for illness. These include high blood pressure, diabetes, impaired glucose tolerance, and a waist circumference of greater than 40 inches for men and greater than 35 inches for women.

People whose BMIs are 30 kg/m² and higher are considered to be obese, and the panel advises these people to make serious attempts to lose weight.[12] According to the new BMI guidelines, approximately 61 percent of Americans are currently overweight.[13] This figure was recently reported by the Centers for Disease Control and Prevention. This value reflects the increasing number of Americans who have become overweight, up 6 percent compared to the recent past.

There are two major limitations to using BMI measurements: (1) the technique is misleading for people with greater than average muscle mass because it measures overweight rather than overfat; and (2) the results are difficult for the general public to interpret, and the average person does not know how to apply BMI values to weight loss. The first limitation is easily surmounted. People with large amounts of muscle tissue should be directed to use a technique such as skinfold measurements or underwater weighing to measure their body composition.

The second limitation is more challenging. Follow these guidelines to establish and interpret BMI measurement. Calculate BMI taking care to accurately measure weight and height.

Weigh yourself in the morning after voiding and prior to breakfast. Wear light clothing and no shoes. For the height measurement, take off your shoes and stand with your back against a flat wall with your heels, buttocks, shoulders, and head against it. Have another person establish your height by using an object that has a right angle, such as a carpenter's square, a textbook, a clipboard on edge, or any other rigid item that is rectangular and has a 90-degree angle. The person doing the measuring should place the right angle against the wall and slide it down to the top of your head, mark the wall at the bottom of the right angle, and use a tape measure to measure from the mark to the floor.

The simplest way to calculate BMI is to bypass the formula and to use table 7-5. Find your height in the left column and move across to your weight in the same row. The number at the top of this column is your BMI. For example, a man who is 71 inches tall and weighs 200 pounds has a BMI of 28 kg/m². This man is in the "overweight" category. How much weight would he need to lose if he wanted to achieve a BMI of 24 kg/m²? He can easily calculate this from the table. Find the column with the desired BMI of 24 kg/m² and drop down in the table to the row with his height (71 inches). He should weigh 172 pounds to achieve a BMI of 24 kg/m². Then subtract his desired weight (172 pounds) from his current weight (200 pounds). He needs to lose 28 pounds to reach his goal. Turn to Assessment Activity 7-1 to calculate your BMI and your desired body weight.

Measurement of Body Fat

The only direct means to measure the fat content of the human body is to perform chemical analysis on cadavers. The information obtained from cadaver studies has been used to develop indirect methods for estimating fat content. Because these estimates are indirect, they contain some degree of measurement error and should be interpreted accordingly. These indirect methods are commonly used in exercise physiology laboratories and fitness and wellness centers. See Wellness Across the Generations: Body Composition of Children and Adolescents.

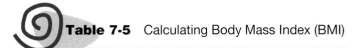

Table 7-5 Calculating Body Mass Index (BMI)

Each entry gives the body weight in pounds for a person of a given height and BMI. Pounds have been rounded off. To use the table, find the appropriate height in the far-left column. Move across the row to a given weight. The number at the top of the column is the BMI for that height and weight.

Height (Inches)	BMI (kg/m²)													
	19	20	21	22	23	24	25	26	27	28	29	30	35	40
	Body Weight (Pounds)													
58	91	96	100	105	110	115	119	124	129	134	138	143	167	191
59	94	99	104	109	114	119	124	128	133	138	143	148	173	198
60	97	102	107	112	118	123	128	133	138	143	148	153	179	204
61	100	106	111	116	122	127	132	137	143	148	153	158	185	211
62	104	109	115	120	126	131	136	142	147	153	158	164	191	218
63	107	113	118	124	130	135	141	146	152	158	163	169	197	225
64	110	116	122	128	134	140	145	151	157	163	169	174	204	232
65	114	120	126	132	138	144	150	156	162	168	174	180	210	240
66	118	124	130	136	142	148	155	161	167	173	179	186	216	247
67	121	127	134	140	146	153	159	166	172	178	185	191	223	255
68	125	131	138	144	151	158	164	171	177	184	190	197	230	262
69	128	135	142	149	155	162	169	176	182	189	196	203	236	270
70	132	139	146	153	160	167	174	181	188	195	202	207	243	278
71	136	143	150	157	165	172	179	186	193	200	208	215	230	286
72	140	147	154	162	169	177	184	191	199	206	213	221	258	294
73	144	151	159	166	174	182	189	197	204	212	219	227	265	302
74	148	155	163	171	179	186	194	202	210	218	225	233	272	311
75	152	160	168	176	184	192	200	208	216	224	232	240	279	319
76	156	164	172	180	189	197	205	213	221	230	238	246	287	328

Wellness Across the Generations
Body Composition of Children and Adolescents

The body composition of children changes during the growth process. It has been well established that obese children and adolescents have a higher probability of becoming obese adults than do normal-weight children and that dramatic changes in body fat and body composition can occur during the peripubertal years (the time before, during, and after puberty). The proportion of body fat in young children ranges from 10 to 15 percent, with boys toward the lower end and girls toward the upper.[14]

Body fat generally increases in adolescent boys and girls and continues to do so into young adulthood so that the percentage of fat in males increases to 15 to 20 percent, whereas that of females increases to 20 to 25 percent. As we age, the percentage of fat continues to increase while muscle mass decreases. By middle age, fat accumulation exceeds 25 percent of the total weight of many men and 30 percent of the total weight of many women. The reason is a growing disparity between energy intake (food consumption) and energy expenditure (level of physical activity). We become less active with age. Television, computers, automobiles, elevators, escalators, remote controls, golf carts, riding mowers, and a lack of quality physical education programs in the public schools have diminished the energy expended by American children and adults.

Skinfold measurements made on children and adolescents in the 1960s and 1970s have been compared with those made on similar subjects in the 1980s. A trend surfaced in this comparison, indicating that a systematic increase in body fat percentage had occurred during the interim.[2] For example, the incidence of obesity in the 6 to 11 age group increased from 17.6 to 27.1 percent. *The Surgeon General's Report on Physical Activity and Health* indicated that 15 to 25 percent of U.S. children are overweight.[15]

A study completed in 1992 examined the relationship between body fatness and health status among children and adolescents.[16] The risks for high blood pressure, high total and LDL cholesterol (the harmful form), and low HDL cholesterol (the protective form) were associated with body fat above 25 percent for men and 30 percent for women. These levels have subsequently been proposed as useful health standards for those between 6 and 18 years of age.

Selected Methods for Measuring Body Composition

Underwater Weighing

Underwater weighing, one of the most accurate of the measurement techniques, involves weighing subjects both on land and while completely submerged in water (figure 7-2).

Whole-body density is calculated from body volume according to Archimedes' principle of displacement. Several thousand years ago, Archimedes discovered that a body immersed in water loses an amount of weight equal to the weight of the displaced water. The loss of weight in water is directly proportional to the volume of the water displaced or the volume of the body that displaces that water. The density of bone and muscle is higher than that of water and tends to sink. The density of fat is lighter than water and tends to float. Therefore, people with more muscle mass weigh more in water than do those who have less. Formulas have been developed that use weight on land and weight in water to determine the percent of the total weight that consists of fat.

Underwater weighing has an inherent error of measurement that can be minimized when the residual volume of air (the air left in the lungs after a maximal expiration) is accurately measured. If residual air is measured, the error is approximately 2.7 percent.[17] Accuracy also depends on the subject's ability to exhale maximally on each trial and to sit still while completely submerged for six to ten seconds.

The equipment required for underwater weighing includes an autopsy scale with a capacity of approximately 9 kg (about 20 lbs.). The scale is suspended over a tank of water at least 4 feet deep. The subject sits suspended chin-deep, exhales completely, and bends forward from the waist until entirely submerged. This position is maintained for 6 to 10 seconds to allow the scale to stabilize. Five to ten trials are required, and the underwater weight is attained by averaging the three heaviest readings. The subject's net underwater weight is calculated by subtracting the weight of the seat, its supporting structure, and a weight belt (if needed) from the gross underwater weight. Percent body fat can be calculated from body density by using appropriate formulas.

(a) (b)

Figure 7-2   Underwater Weighing Apparatus

(a) subject is in the ready position for underwater weighing. (b) subject is being weighed.

Bioelectrical Impedance Analysis

Bioelectrical impedance analysis (BIA) is a relatively new and simple method of determining body composition. The equipment is portable and computerized but fairly expensive. It is safe, noninvasive, quick, and convenient to use (figure 7-3). Additionally, it does not require a high degree of technical skill, it intrudes less on the subject's privacy than other methods, and it is generally more comfortable.

The most common application of BIA employs a harmless, low-level, single-frequency electric current. This current is passed through the body of the person being measured via electrodes attached to specific sites on the right hand and foot, as shown in figure 7-3. Impedance represents resistance to the transmission of an electrical current. Impedance is least in lean body tissues because of their high water content (approximately 73 percent water). Water is an excellent conductor of electricity. Conversely, fat contains only 14 to 22 percent water and is resistant to electrical flow.[2]

A major limitation of BIA is that it does not accurately estimate fat-free mass in very lean or very fat subjects. Body fatness is generally overestimated for lean subjects and underestimated in obese subjects.

Recent advances in BIA instrumentation have improved the technique.[2] The newer instruments use multiple electrical frequencies (MFBIA), which seem to be less susceptible to the hydration status of subjects. As a result, a better estimate of lean body mass can be achieved.

Bioelectrical impedance analysis is as accurate as skinfold measurements provided potential error sources are controlled.[2,17] The main sources of error are the hydration state of the subject and the prediction equation used. Hydration is affected by eating, drinking fluids, urination, and exercise, and it significantly influences the results. Technician error is relatively minor provided standard procedures for electrode placement and body position of the subject are followed. To reduce error, the temperature of the testing room should be comfortable, and the following guidelines should be given to subjects the day before they are scheduled for testing:

- No eating or drinking within four hours of the test
- No exercise within twelve hours of the test
- No urination within thirty minutes of the test
- No alcohol consumption within forty-eight hours of the test
- No diuretic medicines within seven days of the test

Skinfold Measurements

Skinfold measurements are one of the least expensive and most economical methods of measuring body composition. The cost of skinfold calipers can be as low as

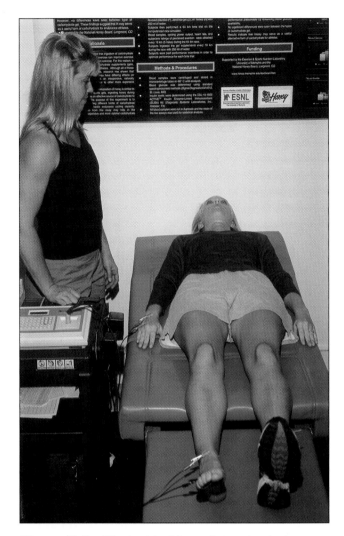

Figure 7-3 Bioelectrical Impedance Analysis

$10. Computerized models, however, can run as high as $600. The most accurate calipers maintain a constant jaw pressure of 10 g/mm^2 of jaw surface area.

The thumb and index finger are used to pinch and lift the skin and the fat beneath it. The caliper is placed beneath the pinch (figures 7-4 through 7-8). Tables 7-6 and 7-7 show how to convert the sum of millimeters of skinfold thickness to percentage of body fat. When performed by skilled technicians, skinfold measurements correlate well (.70–.90) with body density calculated from underwater weighing.[18]

As suggested by the American College of Sports Medicine, these guidelines should be followed when taking skinfold measurements.[18]

1. All measurements should be made on the right side of the body.
2. The caliper heads should be placed about 1/4 to 1/2 inch below the thumb and index finger, perpendicular to the fold, and halfway into the length of the fold.

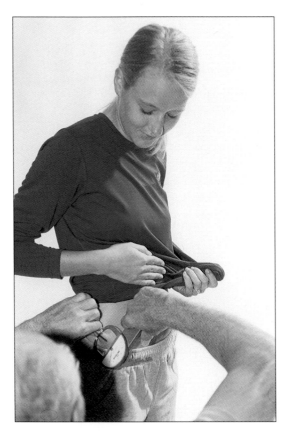

Figure 7-4 Suprailium Skinfold Measurement

Take a diagonal fold above the crest of the ilium directly below the midaxilla (armpit).

Figure 7-5 Chest Skinfold Measurement

Take a diagonal fold half the distance between the anterior axillary line and the nipple.

Figure 7-6 Thigh Skinfold Measurement

Take a vertical fold on the front of the thigh midway between the hip and the knee joint. The midpoint should be marked while the subject is seated.

Figure 7-7 Abdominal Skinfold Measurement

Take a vertical fold about 1 inch from the navel.

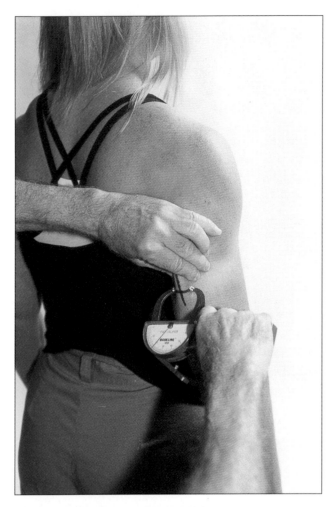

Figure 7-8 Triceps Skinfold Measurement

Take a vertical fold on the midline of the upper arm over the triceps, halfway between the acromion and olecranon processes (tip of the shoulder to the tip of the elbow). The arm should be extended and relaxed when the measurement is taken. All skinfold measurements should be taken on the right side.

3. Pinch should be held continuously while reading the caliper.
4. Wait no more than one to two seconds before reading the caliper.
5. Take duplicate measures at each site, and retest if the measures are farther than one to two millimeters (mm) apart.
6. Measure each of the sites one time, and then repeat the measurements again. This will allow time for the skinfold to return to normal before the next measurement.

Determining Desired Body Weight from Body Fat

Calculating desirable body weight is a simple procedure when the percentage of body fat is known. The following example is for a 148-pound woman whose body fat is equal to 30 percent of her total body weight, based on her skinfold measurements. She wishes to reduce her body fat to 23 percent.

Find fat weight (FW) in pounds:

$$FW \text{ (lbs.)} = \frac{\text{Body weight (BW) (lbs.)} \times \% \text{ fat}}{100}$$
$$= \frac{148 \text{ lbs.} \times 30}{100}$$
$$= \frac{4440 \text{ lbs.}}{100}$$
$$= 44.4 \text{ lbs.}$$

Find lean weight (LW) in pounds:

$$LW \text{ (lbs.)} = BW - FW$$
$$= 148 \text{ lbs.} - 44.4 \text{ lbs}$$
$$= 103.6 \text{ lbs.}$$

Find desirable body weight (DBW) in pounds:

$$DBW \text{ (lbs.)} = \frac{LW \text{ (lbs.)}}{1.0 - \% \text{ fat desired}}$$
$$= \frac{103.6 \text{ lbs.}}{1.0 - 0.23}$$
$$= \frac{103.6 \text{ lbs.}}{0.77}$$
$$= 134.5 \text{ lbs.}$$

The method for calculating desirable body weight based on percent body fat is relatively effective if the subject does the following:

- Exercises to maintain muscle tissue
- Loses no more than 1.5 pounds per week
- Is evaluated for body fatness two to three times during the weight-loss period
- Understands that indirect measurements of body fatness contain some error

Complete Assessment Activity 7-2 to determine your desirable body weight.

Air-Displacement Plethysmography

Air-displacement plethysmography is one of the more recent methods developed to measure body composition through densiometry techniques. In lieu of being

Table 7-6 Percentage of Fat Estimated for Men (Sum of Chest, Abdomen, and Thigh Skinfolds)

Sum of Skinfolds (mm)	Age to Last Year								
	Under 23	23–27	28–32	33–37	38–42	43–47	48–52	53–57	Over 57
8–10	1.3	1.8	2.3	2.9	3.4	3.9	4.5	5.0	5.5
11–13	2.2	2.8	3.3	3.9	4.4	4.9	5.5	6.0	6.5
14–16	3.2	3.8	4.3	4.8	5.4	5.9	6.4	7.0	7.5
17–19	4.2	4.7	5.3	5.8	6.3	6.9	7.4	8.0	8.5
20–22	5.1	5.7	6.2	6.8	7.3	7.9	8.4	8.9	9.5
23–25	6.1	6.6	7.2	7.7	8.3	8.8	9.4	9.9	10.5
26–28	7.0	7.6	8.1	8.7	9.2	9.8	10.3	10.9	11.4
29–31	8.0	8.5	9.1	9.6	10.2	10.7	11.3	11.8	12.4
32–34	8.9	9.4	10.0	10.5	11.1	11.6	12.2	12.8	13.3
35–37	9.8	10.4	10.9	11.5	12.0	12.6	13.1	13.7	14.3
38–40	10.7	11.3	11.8	12.4	12.9	13.5	14.1	14.6	15.2
41–43	11.6	12.2	12.7	13.3	13.8	14.4	15.0	15.5	16.1
44–46	12.5	13.1	13.6	14.2	14.7	15.3	15.9	16.4	17.0
47–49	13.4	13.9	14.5	15.1	15.6	16.2	16.8	17.3	17.9
50–52	14.3	14.8	15.4	15.9	16.5	17.1	17.6	18.2	18.8
53–55	15.1	15.7	16.2	16.8	17.4	17.9	18.5	19.1	19.7
56–58	16.0	16.5	17.1	17.7	18.2	18.8	19.4	20.0	20.5
59–61	16.9	17.4	17.9	18.5	19.1	19.7	20.2	20.8	21.4
62–64	17.6	18.2	18.8	19.4	19.9	20.5	21.1	21.7	22.2
65–67	18.5	19.0	19.6	20.2	20.8	21.3	21.9	22.5	23.1
68–70	19.3	19.9	20.4	21.0	21.6	22.2	22.7	23.3	23.9
71–73	20.1	20.7	21.2	21.8	22.4	23.0	23.6	24.1	24.7
74–76	20.9	21.5	22.0	22.6	23.2	23.8	24.4	25.0	25.5
77–79	21.7	22.2	22.8	23.4	24.0	24.6	25.2	25.8	26.3
80–82	22.4	23.0	23.6	24.2	24.8	25.4	25.9	26.5	27.1
83–85	23.2	23.8	24.4	25.0	25.5	26.1	26.7	27.3	27.9
86–88	24.0	24.5	25.1	25.7	26.3	26.9	27.5	28.1	28.7
89–91	24.7	25.3	25.9	26.5	27.1	27.6	28.2	28.8	29.4
92–94	25.4	26.0	26.6	27.2	27.8	28.4	29.0	29.6	30.2
95–97	26.1	26.7	27.3	27.9	28.5	29.1	29.7	30.3	30.9
98–100	26.9	27.4	28.0	28.6	29.2	29.8	30.4	31.0	31.6
101–103	27.5	28.1	28.7	29.3	29.9	30.5	31.1	31.7	32.3
104–106	28.2	28.8	29.4	30.0	30.6	31.2	31.8	32.4	33.0
107–109	28.9	29.5	30.1	30.7	31.3	31.9	32.5	33.1	33.7
110–112	29.6	30.2	30.8	31.4	32.0	32.6	33.2	33.8	34.4
113–115	30.2	30.8	31.4	32.0	32.6	33.2	33.8	34.5	35.1
116–118	30.9	31.5	32.1	32.7	33.3	33.9	34.5	35.1	35.7
119–121	31.5	32.1	32.7	33.3	33.9	34.5	35.1	35.7	36.4
122–124	32.1	32.7	33.3	33.9	34.5	35.1	35.8	36.4	37.0
125–127	32.7	33.3	33.9	34.5	35.1	35.8	36.4	37.0	37.6

Table 7-7 Percentage of Fat Estimated for Women (Sum of Triceps, Suprailium, and Thigh Skinfolds)

Sum of Skinfolds (mm)	Age to Last Year								
	Under 23	23–27	28–32	33–37	38–42	43–47	48–52	53–57	Over 57
23–25	9.7	9.9	10.2	10.4	10.7	10.9	11.2	11.4	11.7
26–28	11.0	11.2	11.5	11.7	12.0	12.3	12.5	12.7	13.0
29–31	12.3	12.5	12.8	13.0	13.3	13.5	13.8	14.0	14.3
32–34	13.6	13.8	14.0	14.3	14.5	14.8	15.0	15.3	15.5
35–37	14.8	15.0	15.3	15.5	15.8	16.0	16.3	16.5	16.8
38–40	16.0	16.3	16.5	16.7	17.0	17.2	17.5	17.7	18.0
41–43	17.2	17.4	17.7	17.9	18.2	18.4	18.7	18.9	19.2
44–46	18.3	18.6	18.8	19.1	19.3	19.6	19.8	20.1	20.3
47–49	19.5	19.7	20.0	20.2	20.5	20.7	21.0	21.2	21.5
50–52	20.6	20.8	21.1	21.3	21.6	21.8	22.1	22.3	22.6
53–55	21.7	21.9	22.1	22.4	22.6	22.9	23.1	23.4	23.6
56–58	22.7	23.0	23.2	23.4	23.7	23.9	24.2	24.4	24.7
59–61	23.7	24.0	24.2	24.5	24.7	25.0	25.2	25.5	25.7
62–64	24.7	25.0	25.2	25.5	25.7	26.0	26.7	26.4	26.7
65–67	25.7	25.9	26.2	26.4	26.7	26.9	27.2	27.4	27.7
68–70	26.6	26.9	27.1	27.4	27.6	27.9	28.1	28.4	28.6
71–73	27.5	27.8	28.0	28.3	28.5	28.8	29.0	29.3	29.5
74–76	28.4	28.7	28.9	29.2	29.4	29.7	29.9	30.2	30.4
77–79	29.3	29.5	29.8	30.0	30.3	30.5	30.8	31.0	31.3
80–82	30.1	30.4	30.6	30.9	31.1	31.4	31.6	31.9	32.1
83–85	30.9	31.2	31.4	31.7	31.9	32.2	32.4	32.7	32.9
86–88	31.7	32.0	32.2	32.5	32.7	32.9	33.2	33.4	33.7
89–91	32.5	32.7	33.0	33.2	33.5	33.7	33.9	34.2	34.4
92–94	33.2	33.4	33.7	33.9	34.2	34.4	34.7	34.9	35.2
95–97	33.9	34.1	34.4	34.6	34.9	35.1	35.4	35.6	35.9
98–100	34.6	34.8	35.1	35.3	35.5	35.8	36.0	36.3	36.5
101–103	35.3	35.4	35.7	35.9	36.2	36.4	36.7	36.9	37.2
104–106	35.8	36.1	36.3	36.6	36.8	37.1	37.3	37.5	37.8
107–109	36.4	36.7	36.9	37.1	37.4	37.6	37.9	38.1	38.4
110–112	37.0	37.2	37.5	37.7	38.0	38.2	38.5	38.7	38.9
113–115	37.5	37.8	38.0	38.2	38.5	38.7	39.0	39.2	39.5
116–118	38.0	38.3	38.5	38.8	39.0	39.3	39.5	39.7	40.0
119–121	38.5	38.7	39.0	39.2	39.5	39.7	40.0	40.2	40.5
122–124	39.0	39.2	39.4	39.7	39.9	40.2	40.4	40.7	40.9
125–127	39.4	39.6	39.9	40.1	40.4	40.6	40.9	41.1	41.4
128–130	39.8	40.0	40.3	40.5	40.8	41.0	41.3	41.5	41.8

submerged in water, subjects sit inside a precisely calibrated chamber, marketed commercially as the BodPod (figure 7-9), where they displace air instead of water.[19] Preliminary investigations have shown that this method of assessing body composition is highly compatible with underwater displacement. The difference in body fat measured between the two methods was a scant 0.3 percent.

The BodPod has several advantages over underwater weighing, which include: (1) the measurement only takes about five minutes, (2) the system is easy to operate, (3) the device is mobile, (4) minimal technical training is required due to the menu-driven software, and (5) it may more effectively accommodate special populations including, but not limited to, the disabled, the obese, children, elderly, and nonswimmers afraid to completely submerge in a water tank. This technique seems to have a great deal of promise. The major disadvantage is its cost—approximately $34,000.

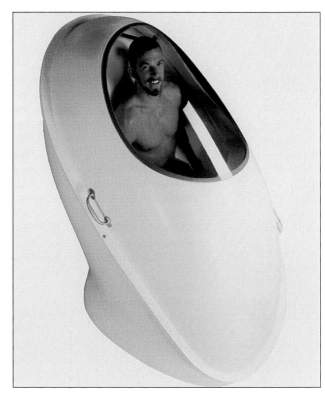

Figure 7-9

A subject prepared for air-displacement plethysmography measurement using the BodPod body composition system.

Summary

- Essential fat is necessary for normal biological function.
- Men carry 3 to 5 percent of their weight in the form of essential fat; women carry 11 to 14 percent of their weight as essential fat.
- *Obesity* is defined as overfatness.
- Men are obese when fat constitutes 25 percent or more of the body's weight, and women are obese when fat constitutes 32 percent or more of the body's weight.
- The majority of women store fat in the hips, buttocks, thighs, and breasts (gynoid fat).
- The majority of men store fat in the abdomen, lower back, chest, and nape of the neck (android fat).
- Height/weight tables are limited and poor instruments for weight-loss recommendations.
- Body mass index correlates fairly well with percent fat derived from hydrostatic weighing.
- A high body mass index correlates with hypertension, high total cholesterol, low HDL cholesterol, high serum triglycerides, and poor glucose tolerance.
- Bioelectrical impedance is a safe, quick, and relatively accurate method for assessing percent body fat.
- Skinfold measurements are one of the most economical methods of measuring body composition in terms of the cost of equipment and the time required to determine percent body fat.
- Underwater weighing is still considered the "gold standard" for measuring body composition.
- Air-displacement plethysmography is one of the newest techniques for measuring body composition, and it correlates highly with underwater weighing.

Review Questions

1. What is essential fat, and how is it distributed in men and women?
2. How would you define *obesity* and *overweight*?
3. At what level of fat deposition does obesity become a health hazard for men and women?
4. What are *gynoid obesity* and *android obesity*? Which is a greater health risk and why?
5. What are the limitations of height/weight tables for recommending weight loss?
6. What is body mass index, and how is it classified for men and women?
7. How are underwater weighing, bioelectrical impedance, and skinfold measurements used to determine percent body fat?
8. How is healthy body weight determined when the percent body fat is known?

References

1. Going S., and R. Davis. 2001. Body composition. In *ACSM's Resource Manual* (4th ed.), ed. J. L. Roitman. Philadelphia: Lippincott Williams and Wilkins.

2. Robergs, R. A., and S. O. Roberts. 2000. *Fundamental Principles of Exercise Physiology*. Boston: McGraw-Hill.

3. ACSM. 1995. *ACSM's Guidelines for Exercise Testing and Prescription*. Baltimore, Md.: Williams and Wilkins.

4. Powers, S. K., and E. T. Howley. 2001. *Exercise Physiology*. Boston: McGraw-Hill Higher Education.

5. Blair, S. N., et al. 1995. Changes in physical fitness and all-cause mortality. *Journal of the American Medical Association* 273(14):1093.

6. Grillo, C. M., and K. D. Brownell. 2001. Interventions for weight management. In *ACSM's Resource Manual* (4th ed.), ed. J. L. Roitman. Philadelphia: Lippincott Williams and Wilkins.

7. Despres, J. P. 1997. Visceral obesity, insulin resistance, and dyslipidemia: contribution of endurance exercise training to the treatment of plurimetabolic syndrome. *Exercise and Sport Sciences Reviews* 25:271.

8. Bryant, C. X., and J. A. Peterson. 1998. Determining ideal body weight. *Fitness Management* 14(7):24.

9. NHLBI. 1998. *Obesity Education Initiative Expert Panel Clinical Guidelines on the Identification, Evaluation, and Treatment of Overweight and Obesity in Adults*. National Heart, Lung, and Blood Institute. Washington, D.C.

10. Mooss, A., and N. F. Gordon. 2001. Conceptual basis for coronary artery disease risk factor assessment in clinical practice. In *ACSM's Resource Manual* (4th ed.), ed. J. L. Roitman. Philadelphia: Lippincott Williams and Wilkins.

11. Harvard University. 1998. Guidelines call more Americans overweight. *Harvard Health Letter* 23(10):7.

12. Tufts University. 1998. Should fewer calories be in your future? *Tufts University Health & Nutrition Letter* 16(6):8.

13. Tufts University. 2001. Portion distortion. *Tufts University Health & Nutrition Letter* 18(12):4–5.

14. Williams, M. A. 2001. Human development and aging. In *ACSM's Resource Manual* (4th ed.), ed. J. L. Roitman. Philadelphia: Lippincott Williams and Wilkins.

15. U.S. Dept. of Health and Human Services. 1996. *Physical Activity and Health: A Report of the Surgeon General*. Atlanta: U.S. Dept. of Health and Human Services, Centers for Disease Control and Prevention, National Center for Chronic Disease Prevention and Health Promotion.

16. Williams, D. P., et al. 1992. Body fatness and risk for elevated blood pressure, total cholesterol, and serum lipoprotein ratios in children and adolescents. *American Journal of Public Health* 82:363.

17. Nieman, D. C. 1999. *Exercise Testing and Prescription*. Mountain View, Calif.: Mayfield Publishing Co.

18. American College of Sports Medicine. 2000. *ACSM's Guidelines for Exercise Testing and Prescription*. Philadelphia: Lippincott Williams and Wilkins.

19. McCrory, M. A., et al. 1995. Evaluation of a new air displacement plethysmography for measuring human body composition. *Medicine and Science in Sports and Exercise* 27:1686–1691.

Suggested Readings

Harvard University. 2001. Weight gain and loss. *Harvard Health Letter* 26(5):1–3.

Discusses genetic influences, age, leptin, and weight-loss strategies. Additionally, it covers the use of body mass index and waist circumference as indirect measures of body fat. It includes an excellent table that facilitates the calculation of body mass index and indicates the category in which the calculated body mass index falls.

Going S., and R. Davis. 2001. Body composition. In *ACSM's Resource Manual* (4th ed.), ed. J. L. Roitman. Philadelphia: Lippincott Williams and Wilkins.

Chapter 45 in this text discusses five methods for determining weight status and body composition. Each of the methods is evaluated for effectiveness. New body fat standards are recommended for consideration by the scientific community.

McArdle, W. D., Katch, F. I., and V. L. Katch. 1999. *Sports and Exercise Nutrition*. Philadelphia: Lippincott Williams and Wilkins.

Chapter 12 in this text presents comprehensive coverage of body composition and body composition assessment. A number of the more commonly used measurements are presented in some detail.

Payne, W. A., and D. B. Hahn. 1998. *Understanding Your Health*. Boston: WCB/McGraw-Hill Higher Education.

Chapter 6 of this text contains a relatively brief presentation of body composition but one that is adequate for the novice reader. It covers the basics of body composition as well as several of the most commonly used assessment techniques.

Wardlaw, G. M. 2000. *Contemporary Nutrition: Issues and Insights* (4th ed.). Boston: McGraw-Hill Higher Education.

Chapter 9 in this text is devoted to weight control. Some of the topics in this chapter include estimating energy needs, body mass index to set a healthy weight, energy imbalance, and techniques for measuring body weight status and body fatness.

Name _____ **Date** _____ **Section** _____

Assessment Activity 7-1

Using BMI to Estimate Body-Weight Status and Calculate Desirable Body Weight

Directions: Calculate your BMI:

1. Your body weight: _____ lbs.

2. Your height: _____ in.

3. Use the nomogram in table 7-5 to calculate your BMI.

    Your BMI: _____ kg/m^2

4. Your desired BMI: _____ kg/m^2

5. Once again, use the nomogram to calculate your desired body weight. Connect your desired BMI to your height and extend the line through the weight column.

    Your desired weight: _____ lbs.

6. Subtract your desired body weight from your current body weight to determine how much weight you need to lose or gain.

    Current weight – desired weight = weight to gain or lose

    _____ lbs. – _____ lbs. = _____ lbs.

Name _____ Date _____ Section _____

Assessment Activity 7-2

Calculating Desirable Body Weight from Percent Body Fat

Directions: To find your desirable body weight, insert your current weight, percentage of body fat, and the desirable body fat that you wish to attain in the appropriate spaces. Then calculate fat weight, lean weight, and desirable body weight. Subtract desirable body weight from current weight. This figure tells you how much weight you must lose to achieve your desirable percentage of body fat.

Current weight = _____ lbs.

Current percentage of body fat = _____ %

Desirable body fat = _____ %

1. Fat weight

   $$= \frac{\text{Body weight} \times \text{Percentage of fat}}{100}$$

   = _____ lbs.

2. Lean weight

   = Body weight – Fat weight

   = _____ lbs.

3. Desirable body weight

   $$= \frac{\text{Lean weight}}{1 - \text{Percentage of fat desired}}$$

   = _____ lbs.

4. Amount of weight to lose = _____ lbs.

8

Achieving a Healthy Weight

Online Learning Center

Log on to our Online Learning Center (OLC) for access to these additional resources:

- Chapter key term flashcards
- Learning objectives
- Additional goals for behavior change
- Concentration game
- Self-scoring chapter quizzes

- Additional lab activities

The OLC also offers weblinks for study and exploration of wellness topics. Access these links through **www.mhhe.com/ anspaugh5e**, click on "Student Center," click on "Chapter 8," and then click on "Web Activities."

Goals for Behavior Change

- Compare physical characteristics of your ideal body image with your actual body image.
- Estimate caloric expenditure for your basal metabolism and physical activity level.
- Adjust your caloric intake and physical activity as necessary to achieve a healthy weight.
- Formulate a plan for achieving a healthy weight.

Key Terms

anorexia nervosa
basal metabolic rate (BMR)
binge-eating disorder
body dysmorphic disorder (BDD)
bulimia nervosa
caloric deficit
caloric expenditure
caloric intake
diet resistance
disordered eating
eating disorders

fasting
female athlete triad
hyperplasia
hypertrophy
novelty diets
overcompensatory eating
set point
thermogenic effect of food (TEF)
very low-calorie diets (VLCDs)
weight cycling

Objectives

After completing this chapter, you will be able to do the following:

- Define *obesity* and *overweight*.
- Differentiate between hypertrophic and hyperplastic development of adipose cells.
- Identify and discuss the health aspects of obesity.
- Discuss biological and behavioral causes of obesity.
- Discuss the relationship of genetics, setpoint, overeating, and physical activity to body shape, fat distribution, and obesity.
- Define, identify, and distinguish between various forms of eating disorders and disordered eating.
- Calculate the caloric cost of physical activities.
- Compare and contrast dieting and physical activity as strategies for weight management.
- Identify principles of weight management.

heoretically, achieving a healthy weight is a simple issue: A person balances **caloric intake,** calories supplied by food, with **caloric expenditure,** calories expended by physical activity and metabolism. In practice, however, people vary considerably in their responses to caloric intake and caloric expenditure. No two people have identical experiences with dieting or physical activity regimens. Some people who chronically face weight problems eat no more and sometimes less than their normal-weight peers. Conversely, some normal-weight people have voracious appetites and do not expend any more calories than their overweight peers.

How can this be explained? Are the differences due to heredity, metabolism, or errors in reporting food intake and physical activity expenditures? Although on the surface body weight appears to be a function of the basic laws of nature (caloric intake vs. caloric expenditure), in truth it is a complex issue still not fully understood by medical experts. For many people, self-improvement goals involving weight management are achievable and worthwhile. For others, formulating weight management goals means first constructing a realistic view of body image (see Nurturing Your Spirituality: Body Image Begins on the Inside). This chapter addresses some of the complexities of body weight issues and presents basic principles for achieving a healthy weight.

Americans' Obsession with Body Weight

Americans are preoccupied with their body weight. Books that offer creative but questionable advice for losing weight invariably become best sellers and add fuel to the next diet craze. The diet industry earns annual revenues of more than $50 billion by hawking far-out gadgets and gimmicks including lipo-slim briefs, which supposedly massage away cellulite; slimming insoles, shoe insoles that reportedly stimulate weight-loss

Nurturing Your Spirituality

Body Image Begins on the Inside[1]

If you are unhappy with your body image, you are not alone. More than one-half of women and more than four of ten men are dissatisfied with their overall appearance; even more people are dissatisfied with their weight. Perceptions about body image are worse for young women. Almost two-thirds of girls and young women, ages 13 to 19, think they weigh too much. One-half of American women overestimate the sizes of their bodies.

Why are so many people unhappy with their body shapes or weights? Why do people tend to focus on their physical imperfections? Why does such a large discrepancy exist between the ways people see their bodies and the ways others see them? Body image studies identify the following factors as being responsible for negative body images:

- Weight gain
- The media's preoccupation with thinness as the trademark for beauty
- Cultural pressures
- Disapproving messages from others
- Fluctuating moods
- Physical changes, such as pregnancy
- Chronic illness
- Childhood teasing
- Sexual abuse

What are the costs of an exaggerated negative body image? People who are deeply troubled about their appearance or preoccupied with selected physical "flaws" often limit their social activities; may not be assertive at work, school, or in personal relationships; may experience difficulty in forming a positive sexuality; may engage in high-risk behaviors; and often become victims of unrealistic fad diets. Extreme cases may involve a psychological disorder called *body dysmorphic disorder (BDD)*. People with this condition are so preoccupied with what they see as a disfiguring flaw that they shun social activities, including school and work.

Although self-improvement is a worthy goal for most people, when it comes to body image it is important to separate nature from nurture, heredity from environment. The challenge for many people with negative body images is to set realistic goals about what can be changed and to accept what can't be changed. Every one of us has a natural and unique size and shape. Our self-esteem depends on accepting the physical features unique to each of us. Changing what and how you think about your body can be healthier than constantly working to change your body weight and shape by diet and exercise. Having a positive body image is not just about losing weight or working with what is on the outside. It begins on the inside.

acupressure points as you walk; and aroma pens, inhalants that come in banana, green apple, and peppermint claimed to squelch hunger pangs.[2] At any given time a large percentage of women and men are on a diet, often several a year. Even children are getting the message that dieting is fashionable—a large number of elementary-aged girls are on a diet, although only 11 percent are overweight or obese.[3]

The evidence for this obsession can be found in advertisements and the news. Numerous television celebrities have engaged in special diet or weight-loss programs. Both the print and video media show countless numbers of advertisements that associate super svelte body images with almost every imaginable product. Consumers demand low-calorie versions of every consumable food, and much of this demand is motivated more by the desire to achieve an unobtainable physique than by health reasons. Consumers have been observed counting the number of calories even in a dose of laxatives. The phrase *calorie anxiety* applies to many Americans. Even health magazines and professional journals reinforce this preoccupation by featuring headlines of diet articles or diet studies on their covers. If some new diet finding is released by the scientific community, it will surely be headlined on national and local news shows and will quickly be followed by feature stories.

For some people the obsession with weight is so intense that it causes serious body-image problems; distorts their self-esteem; and eventually leads to eating disorders, such as anorexia nervosa, bulimia, and compulsive eating, three conditions almost unheard of twenty years ago. Extreme cases may involve a psychological disorder called **body dysmorphic disorder (BDD)**. BDD is defined as a preoccupation with an imagined defect in appearance.[4] If a slight flaw is present, the person's concern is markedly excessive. This preoccupation leads to compulsive checking and questioning; inappropriate surgeries; and occasionally, self-inflicted injury. These symptoms, in turn, may lead to social isolation. This preoccupation is not to be confused with the "normal" dislikes many people associate with one of their physical features. People often complain about the shape of their noses, the size of their ears, or skin blemishes. However, these dislikes do not seriously limit anyone's life. BDD goes far beyond mere dislike into the realm of distress and serious perceptual distortion.

The effects of weight obsession may be more subtle. Some people who are neither anorexic nor bulimic may develop aversive attitudes toward food, eating, and mealtime. Rather than serving as a source of pleasure and enjoyment, the eating experience becomes a constant test of willpower that rarely yields positive results. For too many people, attitudes about appearance, body weight, and food combined with the ubiquitous messages and body images promulgated by the media form a vicious cycle of guilt, denial, and unhappiness. For example, the average height and weight of a contemporary fashion model is 5 foot 9 inches and 110 pounds. In contrast, the average height and weight of an American woman is 5 foot 4 inches and 140 pounds.[5] Only 10 percent of the population genetically fits models' height and weight zone.[6] The rest of the population is left with unobtainable and unrealistic body images. The challenge for many people is to break this cycle by constructing realistic views of their bodies, establishing positive attitudes toward food, and formulating realistic strategies to address the weight problem (see Assessment Activity 8-1).

Defining the Problem

For many Americans, weight loss is a healthy goal. Losing weight often means reducing the risk of developing common chronic health problems. However, many people who are not overweight and have good body composition try to lose weight. For them, losing weight offers no health benefits and may even be harmful.

The number of people who stand to benefit from weight loss is at an all-time high. New standards established by the National Institutes of Health define a healthy weight as a BMI equal to or more than 19 and less than 25. Being overweight is defined as having a BMI of 25 or higher; obesity is defined as having a BMI of 30 or higher. By these definitions, 61 percent of U.S. adults 20 years or older are overweight, up from 55 percent of several years ago.[20] Nearly one-fourth (23 percent) of U.S. adults are obese.[3] Both of these figures are significantly higher than comparison figures for each of the previous decades since data have been collected. Adults are not the only ones overweight. Eleven percent of children, ages 6 to 19, are overweight or obese.[3] The dramatic increase in body weight has led some experts to proclaim that obesity is a chronic health condition of epidemic proportion. Obesity has been declared a disease by the National Institutes of Health (NIH); it has also been elevated to the status of a major risk factor for heart disease (see Chapter 2).

Americans are getting heavier for two reasons: too much energy going in (as food) and too little energy going out (as exercise). The majority of Americans are sedentary; at the same time they are consuming more calories than they were fifteen years ago. The average daily caloric intake is 100 to 300 calories higher for Americans today than it was five years ago.[7] This equates to a potential 30 pound weight gain in one year if compensatory adjustments in energy expenditure don't occur. Table 8-1 presents the calorie intake for men and women between the ages

Table 8-1   Average Calorie Intake*
by Selected Age and Gender

Age	Men	Women
16–19 years	3097	1958
20–29 years	3025	1957
30–39 years	2872	1883
Combined average	2998	1933

*Average calorie intake for all age groups and both genders from
2 months to over 80 years is 2200.

of 16 and 39 and reveals that men consume an average of almost 3000 calories per day, women a little over 1900 calories.[8]

Although BMI provides a basis for classifying levels of overweight and obesity, it is not without its limitations (see Chapter 7). It is also important to remember that BMIs of 25 and 30 (for overweight and obesity, respectively) are not precise points on a scale that when exceeded magically increase a person's risk for health problems. For example, although a BMI of 29.9 does not technically fall into the category of obesity, it is a small step away from the "magic number" of 30, the cutoff point for obesity. For all practical purposes, a BMI of 29.9 carries the same risk of obesity as a BMI of 30.

Health Aspects of Obesity

In declaring obesity a disease, the NIH signaled a new approach toward obesity. Medical experts no longer regard being obese as a failure of willpower. Instead, obesity is considered a chronic disease. This is a radical departure from traditional thinking. Like any other chronic disease, obesity is a complex issue with multiple causes and diverse treatments. No single cause and effect relationship has been established that accounts for the wide variance in eating and activity patterns among the obese. What we know today about obesity is the tip of the iceberg and represents a small portion of this evolving and growing medical field.

One aspect of obesity that has not changed is its medical consequences. Morbidity occurs more frequently and with greater severity and mortality occurs at an earlier age among obese people than among those of normal weight.[3] In an extensive review of the scientific literature on obesity and health, a panel of twenty-four experts summoned by the National Heart, Lung, and Blood Institute proclaimed that obesity is second only to smoking as the largest cause of preventable death in the United States.[9] The magnitude of the risk of morbidity and premature death is dependent on the degree of obesity and the distribution and location of excess fat cells. Fortunately, losing as little as 10 percent of body weight can yield significant improvement in health and self-esteem.[5] This is often referred to as a *healthier weight*. Although a person might not achieve a BMI below 25, he or she might still be healthier after a small, permanent degree of weight loss.

Obesity is highly correlated with coronary heart disease and stroke. LDL cholesterol, which contributes to the development of atherosclerosis, is associated with obesity. According to the Framingham Heart Study, a 20 percent weight loss may reduce the risk of coronary heart disease by 40 percent.[10] One-third of hypertension cases are considered a result of obesity. Many hypertensive people experience a decline in systolic and diastolic blood pressures within the first two to three weeks of a weight-loss program.[10]

Obesity is also a major risk factor for some forms of cancer; it predisposes men to cancers of the colon, rectum, and prostate and women to cancers of the ovaries, uterus, and breasts.

About 85 percent of people with type 2 diabetes are overweight. For people with a predisposition to type 2 diabetes, losing 10 pounds can reduce the chances of contracting the condition by 30 percent. For those who already have diabetes, a 5 percent weight loss can significantly improve the body's use of insulin and lower blood sugar levels.[10]

Obesity increases the risk of osteoarthritis. It intensifies symptoms in those who already have the disease.

Obesity is a prime risk factor for gallbladder disease. Obese individuals have a 3 to 7 times greater risk of gallstones, stones usually composed of cholesterol, than do normal weight people. Weight loss can reduce the risk of gallbladder disease, even though rapid weight loss temporarily increases gallstone formation.[10]

Obesity is a leading cause of sleep apnea, a condition characterized by loud snoring and brief halts in breathing (for about ten to thirty seconds at a time) during sleep. This condition is thought to be caused, in part, by the accumulation of fat tissue in the upper airway, which obstructs breathing. Sleep apnea can lead to daytime sleepiness and may also adversely affect heart function. A 10 to 15 percent weight reduction may relieve or even cure this condition.[10]

For some people, the first symptom of strain placed on the body by excess fat is shortness of breath. As fat accumulates, it crowds the space occupied by organs. Some people cannot sit comfortably because of fat accumulation in their abdomens. In a sitting position a person's lungs have limited space in which to expand.

Postsurgery complications occur more often in overweight people than in those who are not overweight. Wounds don't heal as well or as fast. Infections are more common.

In addition to suffering from medical hazards, it is not uncommon for obese people to suffer psychological stress, depression, social discrimination, and reduced income. They pay higher premiums for health insurance or are denied coverage. Obese children are often ridiculed by their normal-weight peers. Armed forces personnel are forced out of the military if they gain weight beyond an acceptable level.

The link between obesity and chronic disease is well established, but evidence has emerged indicating that the *distribution* of fat is equally important to the development of disease. Studies have confirmed that abdominal fat is associated with a higher rate of heart attack and stroke than is fat distributed around the hips and thighs (see Chapter 7). Guidelines for doctors now suggest that, in addition to calculating BMI, they should assess waist circumference. A waist measurement of more than 39 inches in men and over 34 inches in women is considered a predictor of health risks.[10] (See Just the Facts: Waist Size Matters at **www.mhhe.com/anspaugh5e** Student Center, Chapter 8, Just the Facts.)

In summary, the medical community clearly concurs that the health risks and complications of obesity are associated with premature death. This is not necessarily the case for overweight, however. A twelve-year study of 324,135 adults found overweight people as a group have a slightly higher death rate from all causes than their normal-weight peers. However, the increased risk is modest and declines by age and/or fitness levels. By age 65 the increased risk is slight, and by age 74 it disappears.[11] In long-term studies of thousands of men, those who went from being unfit to fit cut their death rate by 44 percent. According to researchers, this is true for the most overweight subjects.[12] Physical activity may not make the overweight skinny but it does make them healthier (see Just the Facts: Can You Be Fat and Fit?).

The response of medical experts to these findings has been mixed. Any increased risk of premature death, however slight, is reason enough to view excess weight as a serious health hazard. However, the dangers of overweight may have been exaggerated, and for some people, the cure may be worse than the condition. Although controversy exists about the health effects of being overweight, maintaining a physically active lifestyle is associated with good health regardless of body weight status.

Weight Loss: A New Attitude Emerges

The term *weight loss* lacks specificity, and it is often used in such a way to imply that indiscriminate weight loss—of body fluids, protein, and fat—is desirable. A more appropriate weight-related goal is to measure success by the amount of fat lost, not by weight loss.

Just the Facts

Can You Be Fat and Fit?

Overweight men as a group are less physically fit and have a higher death rate than their normal weight peers. But what about overweight men who are fit? Researchers at the Cooper Institute of Aerobics Research in Dallas, Texas, revealed some surprising results when they examined the weight and fitness levels of almost 22,000 men, ranging in age from 30 to 83. They found that being unfit, regardless of one's weight status, increased the risk of death 2.24 times beyond those in the "fit and of normal weight" reference group.[13] What surprised them the most was that fit but overweight men suffered fewer deaths by all causes than unfit but normal weight men. In other words, it is better to be physically fit and overweight than to be unfit and normal weight. In this study, fitness was defined as the equivalent of 30 minutes a day of moderate-intensity activity—briskly walking a couple miles a day at a 15-minute per mile pace.

The term *weight loss* should be replaced by the more specific term *fat-weight loss*.

Until recently, advice to overfat people was imprecise. For example, the suggestion to "cut back on calories" reinforces the misconception that diet alone can lead to fat-weight loss. Successful weight management is rarely the result of following a diet or counting calories for a specific period. Successful weight management usually requires a lifelong lifestyle change. The loss or gain of body weight, the development of fat cells, and the causes of obesity are complex issues related to the interaction of three factors—heredity, diet, and exercise.

Development of Obesity

The body consists of 30 to 40 billion adipose cells (fat cells) that provide storage space for extra energy. Adipose cells may be viewed as collapsible, thin-walled containers with unlimited storage capacities (figure 8-1). In prehistoric humans large fat stores developed when food was available in spring and summer, and this proved biologically advantageous when winters were long and harsh and food was scarce. Energy stored in fat cells could be tapped for use later. This is not the case today. Food is available year-round for most Americans and surplus fat storage is not advantageous.

Obesity occurs when adipose cells increase excessively in size (**hypertrophy**) or number (**hyperplasia**) or both. Obesity that results from an increase in the size of fat cells is hypertrophic, obesity that results

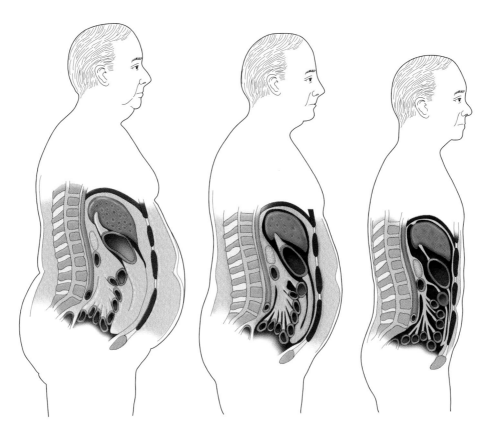

Figure 8-1 Adipose Cell Deposits

Adipose (fat) tissue can be deposited in many areas of the body. Losing fat and building lean muscle tissue boosts metabolism, reduces strain on the hips and knees, and may prevent lower-back pain.

from an increase in the number of fat cells is hyperplastic, and obesity that results from an increase in both is hypertrophic/hyperplastic.

Adipose cells follow a normal pattern of growth and development. When obesity develops in infancy or childhood (juvenile-onset obesity), more adipose cells develop, and each cell grows greatly, resulting in hypertrophic/hyperplastic obesity. When obesity develops in adulthood (adult-onset obesity), a normal number of adipose cells usually develops, but each cell contains a large amount of fat (see Just the Facts: Classification of Obesity). In extreme cases, adult-onset obesity can be both hyperplastic and hypertrophic.[14] Once developed, fat cells do not disappear in the adult state.

Adipose cells have a long lifespan. If adult obesity is both hypertrophic and hyperplastic, is it more difficult to lose weight than if adult obesity is due to hypertrophy alone? Some evidence indicates that an increased number of fat cells increases the body's reluctance to reduce fat stores. The needs of adipose cells may require that they store at least nominal amounts of fat. More fat cells would then result in more fat storage, complicating efforts to lose weight. The longer a person remains obese, the more difficult it is to correct the problem.

Just the Facts

Classification of Obesity

There are several types of obesity, each resulting from different causes:

- Juvenile-onset obesity: Caused by an increase in both the number (hyperplastic) and size (hypertrophic) of fat cells

- Adult-onset obesity: Caused primarily by an increase in size of fat cells (hypertrophic)

- Other types of obesity: Caused by endocrine and/or genetic disorders, such as hypothyroidism, brain tumors, and Turner's syndrome

Gender differences in depositing fat become noticeable during and after puberty. Men distribute fat primarily in the upper half of the body, and women tend to deposit it in the lower half. The percentage of fat in the body reaches peak values during early adolescence for boys and then declines during the remainder of adolescent growth. Girls experience a continuous increase in the percentage of fat from the onset of puberty to age 18.

From approximately 2 years of age, obese children develop a greater number of fat cells than do children of normal weight. Although it is widely believed that obese children become obese adults, only 20 percent of obese adults were obese as children.[10] The large majority of obesity is thought to be adult-onset obesity. Still, childhood obesity should not be ignored since about 40 percent of obese children and about 80 percent of obese adolescents become obese adults. (See Just the Facts: Adult Obesity: Does It Start in Childhood? at **www.mhhe.com/anspaugh5e** Student Center, Chapter 8, Just the Facts.) Significant weight gain generally begins either between ages 5 and 7 or during the teenage years.[3]

Causes of Obesity

The laws of thermodynamics state that energy cannot be destroyed; it is used for work or converted into another form. Accordingly, the progressive accumulation of stored fat in the body is the result of consumption of more calories (energy) than are expended. Food energy in excess of the body's need results in storage of fat in adipose cells (figure 8-2). This relationship is demonstrated in almost all people. Excessive caloric intake and deficient energy expenditure are responsible for most obesity. What is more difficult to explain, however, is the difference among people's responses to the laws of energy conservation and expenditure. Two people may be overfed the same number of calories and yet differ in the amount of weight gained, even if their activity levels are held constant. What accounts for these differences? The answer suggests that obesity is a complex issue, involving both biological and behavioral theories.

Biological Theories

Age, metabolism, gender, disease, heredity, and set point are biological factors that influence body weight and obesity. As people age, their amount of muscle tends to drop, and fat accounts for a greater percentage of their body weight. Metabolism also slows naturally with age. Together these changes reduce calorie needs, often adding an extra pound a year after age 35.[1] Women usually have higher fat-to-muscle ratios than men because of the influence of hormones unique to fertility and the female reproductive system. Also men typically have higher muscle-to-fat ratios than women, which increases metabolism and caloric expenditure. Diseases that affect the thyroid gland may have a dramatic impact on body weight. An overactive thyroid gland (hyperthyroidism) increases the resting metabolic

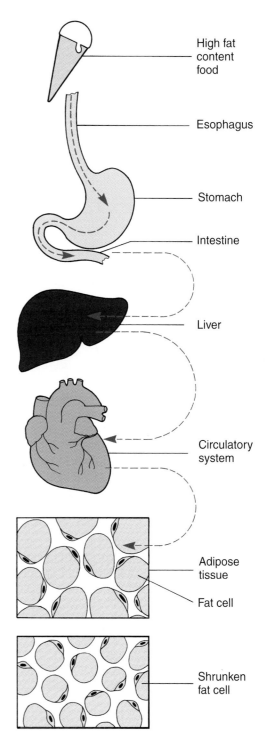

High fat content food

Esophagus

Stomach

Intestine

Liver

Circulatory system

Adipose tissue

Fat cell

Shrunken fat cell

Figure 8-2 Fat Storage

Fat can be manufactured in the body from any food and stored when caloric intake exceeds expenditure. Fat droplets travel to the liver from the stomach and intestines and then enter the circulatory system, where they are delivered to the cells and organs. Excess fats are stored in adipose tissue. When more energy is needed, fats are released from adipose cells. If the energy needs continue, the cells shrink.

rate (RMR) and may cause weight loss. Conversely, an underactive thyroid gland (hypothyroidism) lowers RMR and may lead to overweight or obesity.

Infections may also be a factor in obesity. This is not altogether unexpected because a number of chronic conditions have been connected to viral and/or bacterial infections. Atherosclerosis and ulcers are two examples. Recently, viral infections have been shown to cause obesity in animals. It is possible that future discoveries will reveal a relationship between infection and obesity in humans[19] (see Just the Facts: Viral Infections and Obesity at **www.mhhe.com/anspaugh5e** Student Center, Chapter 8, Just the Facts).

The two major biological explanations of obesity are heredity and set point. Although they are interrelated, they are discussed separately here.

Heredity

The study of obesity lends itself to the classic question of nature versus nurture, heredity versus environment. Does obesity run in families? If so, is it caused by eating habits learned from family influence or by genetic influence?

Studies of adoptees and identical twins help to reveal the influence of the genetic component on obesity. In classic longitudinal studies when researchers follow adoptees over time, they find that their body weight classification resembles their biological parents rather than their adoptive parents even though they learned and practiced the lifestyles of their adoptive parents.

Identical twins are excellent subjects for these studies because they have identical genetic makeup. Any physical differences that occur in one of a pair of identical twins can be attributed to environmental and/or lifestyle factors. Classic, longitudinal studies[15,16] of identical twins consistently reveal a strong genetic influence. When comparing height, weight, and BMI, identical twins follow similar patterns. Each member of the pair can be expected to gain the same amount of weight at approximately the same time in life. The similarity in identical twins is twice that observed in fraternal twins (twins who emanate from separate eggs that do not have identical genes).

The connection between heredity and obesity is also confirmed in studies that correlate the prevalence of childhood obesity with the prevalence of obesity in parents. Eighty percent of children born to two obese parents will themselves become obese, compared to 40 percent of children born to one obese parent and 14 percent of children born to nonobese parents.[17]

Studies support the idea that obesity and fat deposition are significantly influenced by heredity. Approximately 25 to 40 percent of the reason a person weighs a certain amount is related to inherited factors.[18]

Just the Facts

Body Shapes

According to somatotype (body type) experts, there are three classic body shapes. Most people are a combination of all three. The body shapes/body types are as follows:

Ectomorphic   **Ectomorphs** have long, thin body frames; are slender; and have a low capacity for fat storage.

Endomorphic   **Endomorphs** have rounded physical features and large frames. Of the three classic body shapes, they have the greatest capacity for fat storage.

Mesomorphic   **Mesomorphs** have muscular, athletic body frames with an ability to store fat that falls in between ectomorphs and endomorphs.

In addition to influencing body weight, heredity influences body shape. Body shape generally falls into one of three categories: ectomorph, endomorph, and mesomorph (see Just the Facts: Body Shapes). Most people are a combination of all three with a tendency to be more like one or two of them. If a person's body shape strongly favors a particular classification, the person cannot realistically hope to attain another body type. It would be more appropriate for such a person to seek changes in body composition that reduce fat weight regardless of body-shape tendencies. *Shape acceptance* is essential in constructing a realistic view of body weight.

Another factor that helps to explain the connection between heredity and obesity surfaced with the discovery of *leptin,* a hormone made in fat cells by a gene called *ob* (for its connection with obesity), often referred to as the *fat gene.* Leptin senses when fat cells are satisfied and signals the hypothalamus to suppress appetite. The hypothalamus is a part of the brain that regulates such functions as heart rate, blood pressure, body temperature, and food and water intake. Scientists hypothesize that obesity occurs for one of three reasons: (1) the gene fails to produce enough leptin, (2) the body's cells do not recognize leptin, or (3) the body develops a resistance to leptin. The prevailing theory is the hypothalamus is resistant to leptin thus denying the brain of the usual signals to suppress appetite. In the absence of this signal, appetite continues regardless of intake. This explanation prevails because leptin deficiencies are exceedingly rare.[18] It is too early to know if the leptin connection is a true medical breakthrough or another false alarm, and experts warn against the idea that leptin is the magic key for weight loss. Even if human studies confirm the connection, leptin will still be a pharmaceutical adjunct to diet and exercise, not a replacement for them.

The set point theory

The set point theory of weight control also reflects the role of genetics. Proponents of this theory suggest that the body works to maintain a certain weight. More specifically, each person has an internal **set point** for fatness, sometimes called the *adipostat,* that seems to regulate the body by adjusting hunger, appetite, food intake, and energy expenditure. Researchers have demonstrated that human and animal subjects put on low-calorie or high-calorie diets lose and gain only to a certain level. When the diet ends, food consumption increases and they return to their approximate original weight.

How the body determines its set point is not known. One hypothesis is that the body is able to adjust its energy expenditure by adjusting its metabolism. Gordon Wardlaw, well-known nutrition author, provides an analogy and explanation.[5] The analogy is to view set point as a coiled spring: the farther you stray from your usual weight, the harder the force acts to pull you back to that weight. When dieters lose weight their metabolism slows down. When weight is gained, metabolism increases.

There is physiological evidence to support the set point explanation. If energy intake is reduced, the blood concentration of thyroid hormone falls, and the metabolic rate slows. In addition, lower body weight decreases the energy cost of activity and the total energy used by muscle tissue falls because some of these tissues are also lost. In addition, the enzyme used by fat cells and muscle cells to take up fat from the bloodstream often increases its activity. Through these changes the body resists further weight loss.

If a person overeats, in the short run the metabolic rate tends to increase because total body mass increases. This causes some resistance to further weight gain. People often recognize the body's resistance to weight loss when dieting but do not think much about the resistance to weight gain after eating a big holiday meal. However, in the long run, resistance to weight gain is much less than resistance to weight loss. When a person gains weight and stays at that weight for a while, the body tends to defend the new weight.

Can a person change his or her set point? Proponents of the set point theory think that the set point does shift over time in response to behavioral factors: Eating a high-fat diet tends to raise the set point for fatness, and regular physical activity tends to lower it. This shift may be so slight and gradual as to go unnoticed for years.

Some proponents of the set point theory suggest that because some people are genetically programmed to have unwanted pounds, efforts to eliminate fat with diet, exercise, or both are doomed. The body can shut down its calorie-losing mechanism by lowering metabolism and can stimulate appetite to the point that a person must have food.

Other proponents of the set point theory argue that vigorous regular exercise brings about physiological changes in muscle that speed up metabolism and lower the set point, thereby lowering the level of fat the body will accept and defend. Exercise induces the body to stabilize at a lower body weight, precisely what dieters try to do.

Proponents of the set point theory argue that while exercise cannot negate heredity, it can modify it. Obesity need not be destiny.

Behavioral Theories

Behavioral explanations of obesity include excessive caloric intake (overeating) and lack of physical activity (hypokinesis).

Overeating

The basic laws of nature require that calories be consumed before energy can be stored as excess weight. The body cannot make energy on its own. For the obese and overweight, therefore, caloric intake is an important issue.

Do obese people eat more than normal-weight people? This has been a controversial question and researches fall into two camps regarding this issue. One camp suggests that obese people eat no more and sometimes less than normal-weight people. They maintain that blaming obesity on a lack of willpower is unfair and oversimplifies the facts. The body of the obese person is more efficient at converting calories to adipose cells for reasons beyond his or her control, such as genetic predisposition or higher set point for fatness. Stated another way, obese people may not eat more than normal-weight people; they just consume more calories than are required by their bodies.

The other camp claims that obese people do eat more than normal-weight people; the problem, they argue, is a discrepancy in reporting of food intake. In one study, obese subjects underestimated their intake by 47 percent and overestimated physical activity by 51 percent.[10] According to these researchers, the phenomenon referred to as **diet resistance,** the inability to lose weight by dieting, has little to do with innate biological factors.

Although researchers are divided on the issue of overeating, they tend to agree that the abundance of food high in fat and calories is a major factor in the prevalence of obesity in the United States. In his review of the literature on obesity—a review that included more than 300 citations from the scientific literature—Nieman wrote, "Of all the current theories attempting to explain the epidemic of obesity in most Western societies, the high dietary fat intake hypothesis is most widely accepted by experts."[17] Overweight people tend to eat a higher-fat diet than do people of normal weight. Ounce for ounce, fat yields more than double the number of calories than protein or carbohydrates do (9 calories versus 4). This energy difference partially explains the relationship between dietary fat intake and weight gain. It is not a complete explanation because, in studies that hold the total number of calories constant and in which more calories are consumed than needed, subjects eating high-fat diets tend to store more excess calories as body fat than subjects eating lower-fat diets.[21] Calories from fat appear to be more readily converted to body fat than are calories from carbohydrate and protein.

Excess carbohydrates are converted to glycogen in the liver and muscle. The body can only store a limited amount of glycogen. This is not true for fat. Fat cells are distributed throughout the body. Whereas carbohydrate storage is carefully regulated, fat storage is not, allowing a high degree of expansion. Given the sedentary lifestyles of most Americans, glycogen stores are rarely exhausted. The reality for too many people is that they burn carbohydrates and store fat.

Dietary fat also has less of a thermogenic effect than does carbohydrate or protein and can thus be easily stored as adipose tissue. The **thermogenic effect of food (TEF)** represents the amount of energy required by the body to digest, absorb, metabolize, and store nutrients. The body expends only 3 calories of energy to process 100 calories from fat compared with 25 calories to process 100 calories from carbohydrates. Between 10 percent and 15 percent of total body energy goes to support the TEF.[11] For example, after a meal containing 1000 calories, the body uses 100 to 150 calories to process the meal. The TEF helps explain why studies consistently show that, when adults and children overeat and consume high amounts of dietary fat, they tend to gain weight. Conversely, when the intake of dietary fat is low and the intake of carbohydrate and fiber is high from nutrient-dense foods, desirable body weight is more readily achieved.[17]

The high-fat theory of obesity leads to an important question: Can a person lose weight by focusing on fat calories? The answer depends on whether a reduction in fat calories is also accompanied by a reduction in total calories. Studies of the eating habits of both men and women who consume low-fat products reveal that they often compensate by consuming more calories so the use of low-fat foods becomes an excuse to eat more. The idea that people can eat as much as they want as

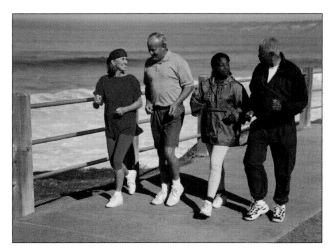

Exercising with a friend is a fun way to stay active and keep your weight in check.

long as it is fat free appears to be more fantasy than fact. Although some researchers believe that fat is the main culprit associated with obesity; other experts emphasize calories. This helps to explain why Americans are getting heavier with each passing year, even though they are consuming a lower proportion of fat. Increased consumption of low-fat foods does not alone result in weight loss. Whereas eating low-fat foods is good for health and weight control, eating them in buffet-sized portions is not.

Hypokinesis

Obesity is in large part caused by the sedentary lifestyle of most Americans. Scientific improvements have led to modern conveniences and labor saving devices that decrease the need for physical activity. Advancements in technology make it possible to bank, shop, and even complete college courses without leaving the desktop computer. Less than 1 percent of the energy for operating factories comes from muscle power. Devices such as mechanized golf carts have made leisure activities less strenuous. Each new invention fosters a receptive attitude toward a life of ease. The mechanized way is generally the most expedient way in the time-oriented American society. Exercise for fitness is now separate from other parts of life. Even when people do exercise during their leisure time, their total daily energy expenditure still falls far short of what was typical several decades ago. The average sedentary person usually expends only 300 to 800 calories a day in physical activity, most of this through informal, unplanned types of movement.[17] Some experts believe that lack of physical activity is the distinguishing factor that separates the obese from those of normal weight.

The general decline in physical activity and fitness is correlated with the rise in obesity. According to the

Surgeon General's report on physical activity and health, 60 percent of Americans are not regularly active and 25 percent are not active at all.[10] These findings are remarkably similar to the weight status of Americans (61 percent of Americans are overweight and 23 percent are obese) and suggest a powerful link between sedentary lifestyles and obesity.

When physical activity levels of overweight people are compared with normal-weight people, normal-weight people are about twice as active as their overweight peers. Obese men informally walk an average of 3.7 miles per day, whereas normal-weight men walk 6 miles; obese women walk 2 miles per day, and normal-weight women walk 4.9 miles.[17]

To state that obese people are less physically active than normal-weight people is one thing; to claim that lack of physical activity causes obesity is different. Researchers are not clear which comes first: Does obesity lead to physical inactivity or does physical inactivity lead to obesity? The cause-and-effect nature of the relationship between these two factors has yet to be determined and is complicated by the fact that energy expenditure from exercise differs very little between the obese and the normal-weight. Because of their extra weight, the obese expend more energy when they participate in physical activity. In other words, even though they exercise less, they expend more energy in the course of activity. For this reason overeating is considered by most experts to be more important than inactivity as a determinant of obesity.[17] Still there is general agreement that exercise is vital to the success of weight maintenance. In its guidelines on the treatment of obesity, the National Heart, Lung, and Blood Institute (NHLBI) notes that according to randomized, controlled trials, physical activity among overweight and obese people reduces abdominal fat "only modestly or not at all." But don't dismiss exercise. It is the number one way to prevent weight gain.[22]

Dieting and Exercise: Strategies for Weight Maintenance or Weight Loss

To maintain weight, caloric intake must be balanced by caloric expenditure. To lose weight a person has to achieve a **caloric deficit** in which the number of calories burned exceeds the number of calories consumed. This is the basic principle of weight management. It is simple and straightforward, and it includes three obvious strategies: (1) restricting caloric intake by dieting, (2) increasing caloric expenditure through physical activity, and (3) a combination of dieting and physical activity. What is not so easy to explain is how two people can respond so differently to dieting and exercise

weight-loss strategies. Complex forces, many of which are still not clearly understood, influence the success of weight-management/weight-loss efforts.

The loss of 1 pound of body fat requires a caloric deficit of 3500 calories. (The loss of 1 pound of adipose tissue yields more than 1 pound of body weight because fat storage includes some lean support tissue—muscle, connective tissues, blood supply, and other body components. A caloric deficit of 2700 calories results in a loss of 1 pound of body weight.)[14] A loss of 1 pound of body fat per week is a good goal and requires an average daily caloric deficit of 500 calories. A caloric deficit of more than 500 calories per day, unless medically supervised, borders on the extreme and is difficult to sustain over long periods. A loss of 2 pounds of body fat per week is considered a maximum goal.

Body fat loss in excess of 2 pounds per week is not practical for most people. For example, diets that promise a fat-weight loss of 10 pounds per week require a caloric deficit of 35,000 calories per week; that is an average of 7000 calories per day. For that kind of caloric deficit, a person would have to go to the extremes of fasting while running two marathons in one day. Weight loss in excess of a couple of pounds per week usually involves lean tissue weight, which should be retained, and fluid weight, which needs to be replaced to prevent health consequences ranging from dehydration to electrolyte imbalance.

A desirable long-term goal for a person needing to lose weight is 1 to 2 pounds per week until about 10 percent of excess weight is lost. The emphasis should be on a slow, steady weight loss rather than on a rapid weight loss. Once this goal is reached, the dieter should go into maintenance for about six months before attempting more weight loss.[14] For example, a 250-pound person should go into a six-month maintenance program after losing 25 pounds. This conservative approach to weight loss is likely to yield health improvements while promoting a more stable, consistent body weight.

Dieting

Statistics show that dieting is the method of choice for most Americans trying to lose weight. Although dieting usually works only temporarily, most people who fail to maintain weight loss are willing to try again. Many people seek the miraculous diet that will transform them from fat to thin, preferably with minimal effort and in the shortest time possible.

The success rate of diet-only strategies is dismal. Only 5 percent of dieters are successful in reducing to a target weight and maintaining the weight for more than five years. Typically, one-third of the weight lost during dieting is regained within the first year, and almost all weight lost is regained within three to five years.[14] Maintaining postdiet weight is one of the major failures of weight loss through dieting because dieters do not learn the habits and behaviors needed to remain at the new weight. As a result, they lose and regain weight many times in their lives. This pattern of repeated weight loss and gain, known as **weight cycling,** *yo-yo dieting,* and *seesaw approaches* to weight loss, is potentially harmful and counterproductive (see Just the Facts: Yo-Yo Dieting and Toxicity: Another Reason to Lose Weight Slowly and Keep It Off).

The consequences of weight cycling are numerous. The most immediate negative effect is rebound weight gain. Typically, weight gained after dieting includes not only the weight that was lost but additional weight as well. After years of yo-yo dieting, many dieters experience a weight gain pattern that takes on a stair-step effect, increasing in small but noticeable increments with each successive effort. In addition, the weight regained is in the form of adipose tissue, whereas the weight that was lost consisted of a mixture of adipose and muscle tissue. The result of weight cycling is not only extra weight but also extra fat weight.

Weight cycling also takes its toll on emotional well-being.[24] The more often diets fail, the more enthusiasm and confidence ebb, and the harder it becomes to make a long-term commitment to keep off extra weight.

The high recidivism rate of diet-only programs coupled with the negative effects of weight cycling seems to negate dieting as a strategy for losing weight. The reality, however, is that weight loss requires a caloric deficit, and limiting food intake is the most direct and immediate way to get results. The mistake people tend to make with most diet-only strategies is to set unrealistic goals. They want to lose too much weight and they want to lose it immediately. An ideal approach is to lose weight at the same rate as weight is gained. For most people this would involve a plan of modest dietary restrictions implemented over a period of months or years, rather than days or weeks. Weight-loss goals structured according to the guidelines mentioned are more likely to be successful.

In diet-only strategies, the caloric intake should not drop below 1200 per day in women or 1400 per day in men (see table 8-2: Daily Calorie Goals for Weight Loss).[25] Gender differences in caloric intake are due to differences in physical activity patterns, metabolism (from more or less muscle tissue), and size. Because fat is more than twice as energy dense as carbohydrates, many experts recommend concentrating on limiting fat intake rather than on counting calories. If an eating plan calls for a caloric intake below 1200 calories for women and 1400 calories for men per day, discuss it with your health care provider. You may need to take vitamin and/or mineral supplements. One last caveat to people frustrated because they can't lose weight on a

Table 8-2   Daily Calorie Goals for Weight Loss[25]

	Daily Calorie Goal	
Weight of Dieter	**Men**	**Women**
250 pounds or less	1400	1200
251–300	1600	1400
301 or more	1800	1600

1200- or 1400-calorie diet: If you can't lose weight at this caloric level, you probably don't need to lose weight. You might be better served by reexamining your reasons for losing weight.

In structuring a diet, some modification in the Food Guide Pyramid (FGP) is recommended (see Chapter 6). Figure 8-3 presents the Mayo Clinic Healthy Weight Pyramid and recommends food selections that start first with fruits and vegetables.[25] At least four servings of vegetables and at least three servings of fruit are recommended each day, but you are allowed to eat an unlimited number of servings of both. Next in ascending order is the carbohydrate group (grains, pasta, etc.) with 4 to 8 servings recommended. This represents a 33 percent reduction in the number of servings of carbohydrates in comparison with the FGP. Whole-grain, high-fiber foods are the

Mayo Clinic Healthy Weight Pyramid

Sweets — Up to 75 calories daily

Fats — 3 to 5 daily servings

Protein/dairy — 3 to 7 daily servings

Carbohydrates — 4 to 8 daily servings

Daily Physical Activity

Fruits and vegetables — Unlimited (minimum 3 or 4 servings each)

Figure 8-3 The Mayo Clinic Healthy Weight Pyramid shows you where to focus when selecting foods that help promote healthy weight. What's more, you'll never be hungry with this dining approach.

preferred source of carbohydrates. Protein and dairy foods are combined as one food category with a recommendation of 3 to 7 servings.

The Mayo Clinic Healthy Weight Pyramid emphasizes foods that promote both healthy weight and good nutrition. Hunger should not be an issue with this approach. Also, in the center of the pyramid is the recommendation to engage in physical activity on a daily basis.

Very low-calorie diets

Very low-calorie diets (VLCDs) are diets containing fewer than 800 calories a day. They are considered extreme diets (food is usually replaced with a powdered supplement) and should be viewed as a medical intervention. Typically, VLCDs are undertaken under medical supervision and administered in hospital/clinic settings for a period of three to four months and include counseling, behavior management, nutrition and dieting classes, and support groups. Often, they include an exercise program. Once the diet is completed, dieters on a VLCD gradually return to food intake.

VLCDs are usually recommended for people whose obesity is threatening to their health and who are unable to lose weight through dieting and exercise. People who have insulin-dependent diabetes mellitus, liver dis-

ease, kidney disease, or a history of heart disease are warned against this method of losing weight.

For people who can stay on them, VLCDs produce dramatic reductions in weight. Still, they are not a panacea. About 25 percent of people who start a VLCD drop out of the program. Like most extreme dieting programs, VLCDs have a high failure rate. Very low-calorie diet studies that include three- and five-year follow-ups indicate nearly total recidivism.[32] As a result, VLCD programs are worthless without careful attention paid to long-term maintenance that incorporates newly learned eating patterns.[10]

Low-fat diets

Low-fat diets are potentially effective techniques for losing weight. With its high-caloric yield and almost unlimited capacity for storage, fat is a major threat to weight maintenance. Consequently, Americans are fixated on fat-free or low-fat foods. The assumption is that, if a food is low in fat, it is also low in calories. As a result, although Americans are consuming fewer fat calories percentagewise, they are consuming more total calories from all sources and are getting heavier. (Actual fat intake remains the same as it was during the past ten years.) Percentagewise, it dropped because of an increase in total calories consumed.

Low-fat foods and overcompensatory eating

Although diet experts advocate restricting fat calories, low-fat diets have not been effective for many dieters because of **overcompensatory eating.** This occurs when the consumption of low-fat foods is accompanied by an increase in total calories. Researchers at Pennsylvania State University demonstrated this point when, on separate occasions, they gave a group of women two kinds of yogurt: One was labeled *high fat,* and one was labeled *low fat.* The ingredients were manipulated so that both kinds of yogurt had the same number of calories. A comparison group of women was given the same, but unlabeled, yogurt. Thirty minutes after consuming the yogurt, the women ate lunch. After eating the yogurt labeled *low fat,* subjects compensated by taking in more calories during lunch than they did when they consumed the yogurt labeled *high fat.* This pattern of overcompensatory eating was not observed for the comparison group who ate the unlabeled yogurt. The researchers concluded that, when the women ate yogurt labeled *low fat,* they rationalized that they could indulge more at lunch. When they didn't know what kind of yogurt they had eaten, they were more tuned in to their bodies' physical cues and naturally adjusted the amount they ate.[26]

The attitude that people can eat what they want, in unlimited quantities as long as it is fat free is wrong. Calories do count. Fat-free foods can help people lose weight if they are used properly, if they don't result in overcompensatory consumption of food, and if total calories are kept in line.

Low-fat diets and Olestra

The approval of Olestra (Olean) as a fat substitute is partly responsible for the proliferation of low-fat and fat-free foods. Many people unwittingly consume foods in large quantities thinking that, if it is fat free, it is also calorie free. A fat-free product made with Olestra may turn out to have more total calories (from carbohydrates) than a companion product made with typical ingredients, including fat. For that reason it is important to check labels. The bottom line to look for is total calories. Diets high in Olestra also carry the risk of compromising the body's use of essential nutrients, such as fat-soluble vitamins. For some people the consumption of Olestra causes various abdominal symptoms (see Chapter 6).

Portion sizes and volume eating

Managing caloric intake is made more difficult today than in years past because of not only the increased availability of food but also the way food is marketed, packaged, and delivered. In trying to get a better value

Wellness On the Web
Behavior Change Activities

Eating Disorder Alert

In today's appearance-focused culture, we're all familiar with the terms anorexia nervosa, bulimia nervosa, and binge eating. Although these eating disorders differ markedly from each other in many respects, people who have them share a common trait: an intense fear of becoming overweight. Does this describe you? Whether the answer is yes or no, go to www.mhhe.com/anspaugh5e to complete a self-test that will help you determine whether you may have an eating disorder. Click, on "Student Center," Chapter 8, "Wellness on the Web," and then "Activity 1." The questions presented involve behaviors and feelings common to persons who have eating disorders. Whatever your results, remember that you and no one else are the final judge of whether you have an eating disorder. If you think you do, you'll find help and support from a wide array of reputable sources.

Boost Your Metabolism—Naturally!

Looking for the magic key to successful weight management? Magic or not, compelling evidence points to the importance of regular exercise in weight control and weight-loss maintenance. People who lose weight and keep it off almost always exercise daily. Studies that attempt to identify predictors of successful weight maintenance point to physical activity as one of the best markers for long-term success. Walking is considered an excellent form of exercise for shedding pounds. To calculate how many calories you burned walking, go to the website mentioned previously, then select "Activity 2." Enter your weight and the duration of your walk, then select your approximate speed and click on "walk it off" to calculate your calories burned.

for the dollar, people think *bigger* and *more* are better. Food producers know this and use this approach to gain an advantage over the competition. *Supersized, all-you-can-eat, buffet-style eating,* and *a meal in a sandwich* are some of the catch phrases used to increase business. When it comes to calories, the phrases are not all hype (see Just the Facts: Restaurant Dining and Supersized Calories). The problem with large serving sizes is that we tend to eat what is served. This is true for beverages just as it is for solid food (see Just the Facts: Solids Calories vs. Liquid Calories at www.mhhe.com/anspaugh5e Student Center, Chapter 8, Just the Facts). When people are served larger portions of food, they eat more than when they are given small portions and allowed to get up for more.[27] People get accustomed to large amounts and feel cheated when served a normal portion. The challenge for many people

~ *Just the Facts* ~

Restaurant Dining and Supersized Calories

Americans are overwhelmed with supersized servings of food, especially when eating out. A medium-size baked potato served at a fast-food restaurant weights 7 ounces compared with the typical potato, which weighs 4 ounces; a medium bagel weighs 4 ounces, double the size listed in food composition tables; a medium muffin is 6 ounces, triple the size of regular muffins; a double hamburger at one popular fast-food restaurant has almost three times the number of calories as its single hamburger counterpart; a serving of BBQ ribs and fries at another national chain restaurant consists of 15 ounces of meat and seventy French fries (the FDA says a serving of fries numbers 10); a pasta serving at one popular restaurant consists of 8 cups of pasta and 6 ounces of sausage (this is equivalent to 16 servings or two days worth of carbohydrates and 2 to 3 servings of meat); and one casual dining restaurant offers a no-frills entree that weighs as much as the Manhattan *Yellow Pages*.

Exacerbating the problem of supersized portions served at restaurants is that Americans are eating out more than before. In the 1970s, Americans spent about 20 percent of their food dollar on restaurant meals. Now, that figure has nearly doubled.[28] Almost half of adults dine in a restaurant on a typical day.[29] People eat out an average of almost four times per week.[30]

These two trends, eating food in supersized portions and eating out, are recipes for creeping weight gain. The challenge for most people when eating out is to ask for small portions; another option: eat modest amounts of food and take the rest home.

Real-World Wellness

Practical Tips for Coping with Supersize Foods

My friends and I enjoy eating out and prefer fast food or casual dining restaurants. The local restaurants provide some supersize bargains that fit a college budget. My problem is that I am a volume eater—I eat what is served, usually much more than I need and certainly more than is good for my waistline. But I live on a tight budget and refuse to throw away good food. What are some strategies that will help me manage my tendency for volume eating without being wasteful?

Here are some suggestions for volume purchasing without waste:

- Eat what you need, not necessarily what is served. Take the rest home.

- Share an entree, appetizer, or dessert. This saves calories and money. (Some restaurants add a surcharge for sharing meals.)

- Start each day with a plan. Think first of your main meal and work around it. If you're planning a prime rib dinner, for example, favor vegetables and fruits for breakfast and lunch. One serving of prime rib is plenty of meat for one day.

- At a buffet, serve yourself small portions and eat slowly. Give your food time to digest. Emphasize vegetables and fruits in your food selections.

- Ask for a half order of an entree.

- Order only appetizers.

- When grocery shopping, plan ahead. Make a list of the amount or quantity of each item to buy. Stick to your list.

- If you're watching calories, learn what makes a serving. One small fistful of candy, french fries, or nuts is a serving. A portion of pasta, rice, or mashed potatoes is the size of your fist (see Chapter 6).

- Picture what you think is a reasonable serving before food is served. If more is served, take it home.

is to overcome the "I'm going to eat what I pay for" attitude. Usually this means now, rather than later.

Signs in supermarkets can also encourage people to buy more food. A consumer planning to purchase one carton of ice cream is likely to return home with two cartons if the product is priced at two for $8 instead of at $4 each. When grocers suggest purchase of a specific number of items, shoppers are more likely to buy more than the one or two they intended to buy.

Do people eat more when food is packaged in larger quantities? In trying to answer this question, researchers gave either a 1- or 2-pound bag of M&Ms plus either a "medium" or "jumbo" movie theater-sized tub of popcorn to participants. On average, participants ate 112 M&Ms from the 1-pound bag and 156 from the 2-pound bag. Likewise, the average person ate roughly half a tub of popcorn, whether it was

medium or jumbo, which held twice as much as the medium tub. The researchers concluded that people often eat about 50 percent more of pleasure-foods such as candy, chips, and popcorn when they come in bigger packages. With other foods, the increase is usually about 25 percent.[31]

Some common-sense approaches help people avoid overeating despite the gluttony of supersized portions of food. See Real-World Wellness: Practical Tips for Coping with Supersize Foods.

Popular diets

Many diets on the market are nutritionally sound, and many are not. Some are potentially hazardous, and many are based on faulty nutritional and physiological concepts. Some require that food be eaten in a certain order and severely restrict foods. Some require medical supervision. Others impose unrealistic caloric restrictions, and still others make promises based more on fantasy than facts. (You can explore a list of popular diets that includes descriptions, the type of weight loss expected, health drawbacks, and pros and cons for each diet on this text's Online Learning Center at **www.mhhe.com/anspaugh5e** Student Center, Chapter 8, Popular Diets.) The Food and Drug Administration (FDA) does not investigate every new fad diet, and many diet plans are published without the FDA's endorsement (see Just the Facts: Outlandish Weight-Loss Promises—What to Do). If a diet is published, it is usually because a publisher sees potential profits from its sales. Publishers know that the advice to "eat less fat and increase physical activity" will not sell books, but fad diets with secret ingredients or magic formulas will.

Because fad diets are unlikely to disappear, identifying some of the characteristics and marketing strategies used by diet promoters to appeal to unwitting consumers is helpful.[5] Fad diets

- Promote quick results
- Stress eating one type of food to the exclusion of others
- Emphasize gimmick approaches, such as eating food in a particular order
- Cite anecdotes and testimonials, usually involving well-known people
- Claim to be a panacea for everyone
- Often promote a secret ingredient
- Often recommend expensive supplements
- Rarely emphasize permanent changes in eating habits
- Usually show little concern for accepted principles of good nutrition (see Chapter 6)
- Are usually cynical about the evidence that comes from the scientific community

Dieting is an ineffective weight-management method. The expectation that temporary changes in eating habits will lead to permanent weight loss is unrealistic. Sensible and permanent dietary changes that depend on wise food choices are an excellent way to cut calories and a healthy way to eat. (Table 8-3 demonstrates how to reduce calories that come from fat and cholesterol by making appropriate substitutions.)

Low-carbohydrate diets

The low-carbohydrate diet is the most common form of diet.[5] Without carbohydrates the liver is forced to produce needed glucose. Once glycogen stores are used,

Just the Facts

Outlandish Weight-Loss Promises— What to Do

Quick and unrealistic weight-loss schemes that promise outlandish results are common, and the number of fad diets promoted in print and video media exceeds the FDA's capacity to check claims and promises.[2,37] One newspaper published an advertiser's claim: "Lose 40 pounds by Christmas." The date of the advertisement was November 3, about seven weeks before Christmas. This ad was an example of blatantly misleading advertising. The responsibility for demonstrating "proof" rests with authors and publishers, often motivated more by profits than by credible and reliable information. What can the average consumer do if he or she is exposed to some outrageous claims?

- First and foremost, adopt an attitude of skepticism. If it sounds too good to be true, it probably is. No one diet device or pill can work miracles. Even respectable diet programs require you to eat less and exercise more.

- Call your local chapter of the Better Business Bureau to check claims and reputation before you enlist in a program or buy a product or gadget.

- Register a complaint with the source (newspaper, magazine, television station) of the advertisement.

- If you see a suspect ad, send it to NAD, Consumer Inquiries, 845 Third Avenue, 17th floor, New York, NY 10022.

- And remember, if you don't lose weight with a particular product, don't automatically blame yourself. You may have not failed; the product may have failed you.

the body calls on protein stores for glucose. Thus, a low carbohydrate diet results in protein tissue loss. Because protein tissue is mostly water, the dieter loses weight rapidly. When a normal diet is resumed, the protein tissue is replaced along with the weight.

Popular diets that represent some variation of low carbohydrate diets include Dr. Atkins' New Diet Revolution, Protein Power, Sugar Busters, The Carbohydrate Addict's Diet, Dr. Stillman's Calories Don't Count Diet, the Scarsdale Diet, the Drinking Man's Diet, Four-Day Wonder Diet, and the Air Force Diet.[2,5] Major claims of these diets are that carbohydrates boost insulin production and insulin facilitates the body's use of carbohydrates, which is turn causes obesity (in actuality eating almost anything causes insulin production). Most of these diets provide a larger allowance for the consumption of protein and/or fats. The three major criticisms of

Table 8-3 Food Substitutions That Reduce Fat, Cholesterol, and Calories

Instead of eating . . .	Substitute . . .	To save*
1 croissant	1 plain bagel	35 calories, 10 g fat, 13 mg cholesterol
1 cup cooked egg noodles	1 cup cooked macaroni	50 mg cholesterol
1 whole egg	1 egg white	65 calories, 6 g fat, 220 mg cholesterol
1 oz. cheddar cheese	1 oz. part-skim mozzarella	35 calories, 4 g fat, 15 mg cholesterol
1 oz. cream cheese	1 oz. cottage cheese (1% fat)	74 calories, 9 g fat, 29 mg cholesterol
1 tsp. whipping cream	1 tbsp. evaporated skim milk, whipped	32 calories, 5 g fat
3.5 oz. skinless roast duck	3.5 oz. skinless roast chicken	46 calories, 7 g fat
3.5 oz. beef tenderloin, choice, untrimmed, broiled	3.5 oz. beef tenderloin, select, trimmed, broiled	75 calories, 10 g fat
3.5 oz. lamb chop, untrimmed, broiled	3.5 oz. lean leg of lamb, trimmed, broiled	219 calories, 28 g fat
3.5 oz. pork spare ribs, cooked	3.5 oz. lean pork loin, trimmed, broiled	157 calories, 17 g fat
1 oz. regular bacon, cooked	1 oz. Canadian bacon, cooked	111 calories, 12 g fat
1 oz. hard salami	1 oz. extra-lean roasted ham	75 calories, 8 g fat
1 beef frankfurter	1 chicken frankfurter	67 calories, 8 g fat
3 oz. oil-packed tuna, light	3 oz. water-packed tuna, light	60 calories, 6 g fat
1 regular-size serving french fries	1 medium-size baked potato	125 calories, 11 g fat
1 oz. oil-roasted peanuts	1 oz. roasted chestnuts	96 calories, 13 g fat
1 oz. potato chips	1 oz. thin pretzels	40 calories, 9 g fat
1 oz. corn chips	1 oz. plain air-popped popcorn	125 calories, 9 g fat
1 tbsp. sour-cream dip	1 tbsp. bottled salsa	20 calories, 3 g fat
1 glazed doughnut	1 slice angel-food cake	110 calories, 13 g fat, 21 mg cholesterol
3 chocolate sandwich cookies	3 fig bars	4 g fat
1 oz. unsweetened chocolate	3 tbsp. cocoa powder	73 calories, 13 g fat
1 cup ice cream (premium)	1 cup sorbet	320 calories, 34 g fat, 100 mg cholesterol

*The values listed are the most significant savings; smaller differences are not shown. Weights given for meats are edible portions.

these diets are that they limit the intake of many foods (fruits, vegetables, whole grains) that are good for health, they encourage the intake of foods high in fat and saturated fat, and they have a high recidivism rate. Dieters on low-carbohydrate diets are often encouraged by initial rapid weight loss but once the diet is over they almost always regain the lost pounds.

Novelty Diets

Novelty diets are the classic fad diets typically based on gimmicks. Often the gimmicks are explained with scientific terminology. A novelty diet promotes certain nutrients, foods, or combinations of foods as having unique, magical, or previously undiscovered qualities. The rationale behind some of these diets is that the dieter eats only a certain food for so long; eventually gets bored; and, theoretically, ends up by consuming fewer calories. Some low-carbohydrate diets are also novelty diets.

Novelty diets, like most other extreme diets, don't work if success is judged by weight maintenance. Once dieters reach their goal they usually regain the weight

upon resuming previous eating patterns. Some novelty diets espouse views that are misleading, even absurd. A well-known nutrition expert explains: "The most bizarre of the novelty diets proposes that 'food gets stuck in your body.' Fit for Life, the Beverly Hills Diet, and the Eat Great, Lose Weight are examples. The supposition is that food gets stuck in the intestine, putrefies, and creates toxins that invade the blood and cause disease. This is utter nonsense. Nevertheless, the same idea has been promoted in health-food books since the 1800s. Today, Fit for Life suggests that meat eaten with potatoes is not digested and that fresh fruit should be consumed only before noon. These recommendations are absurd. They are gimmicks that appear controversial but are really designed to sell books."[5]

The age-old advice of caveat emptor applies, especially to novelty diets. There is no limit in the creativity of hucksters willing to promote weight-loss products and fad diets, usually at considerable expense to the consumer. It's helpful to be reminded that if a new diet gimmick sounds too good to be true, it is.

Diet Drugs

If recent history is a good predictor of the future, American dieters can anticipate a new arsenal of drug solutions for losing weight. Drugs that suppress appetite by stimulating the satiety center in the brain have helped many dieters lose weight temporarily. Drugs marketed under the names *fen-phen* (fenfluramine) and *redux* (dexfenfluramine) during the mid-1990s quickly sold in huge quantities. The popularity of these drugs did not last long, however, because of the plethora of side effects, including death, which eventually led to their withdrawal from the marketplace. Newer-appetite suppressant drugs such as Meridia (sibutramine) offer another pharmacologic solution for dieters. Although early studies of Meridia are encouraging, the drug is not off the safety hook. Some people on this drug experience dangerous jumps in blood pressure. Because of this and other adverse effects, Meridia should be used only by people at-risk for serious weight-related health problems.[33]

Diet drugs are not intended for people who are overweight or marginally obese. Instead, they are intended for the management of severe obesity that does not respond to dieting and exercise regimens and for people whose obesity causes serious health risks that outweigh the possible risks of the medication. Unfortunately, many people are drawn to the quick-fix of a drug, and many physicians are willing to provide a prescription.

The reality is that drugs offer only a temporary solution. They do not correct the underlying cause of persistent weight gain. People who take weight-loss medications can anticipate the typical weight cycling effect of other dieting strategies with an added problem: Diet drugs are powerful medicines that tamper with the body's delicate balance of hormones and body chemicals. Except for the severely obese, long-term exposure to diet drugs creates harmful effects that may far outweigh the health benefits of fewer pounds of body weight.

Diet Supplements and Herbal Remedies

Numerous supplements and herbal versions of prescription drugs used for losing weight are available in health food stores, many drugstores, and online. Some are promoted as "fat burners" wile others act as diuretics, stimulants, and/or laxatives.

Conjugated linoleic acid (CLA) is the so-called wonder "fat burner" because it claims to develop muscle tissue and at the same time reduce fat tissue. CLA is a type of polyunsaturated fat found, in small amounts, in dairy products, beef, and other meats. It is also available as a concentrated dietary supplement. Animal studies reveal promising results. Researchers theorize that CLA works either by helping to draw fat out of the body's fat cells or by inhibiting their incorporation of additional fat, thereby redirecting food calories into muscle rather than fat cells. These results of human studies fall into two camps. One camp suggests that while CLA has not yet been proven as an effective weight loss supplement, it may be useful in helping people put on more muscle and less fat when a dieter regains lost weight.[34] The other camp acknowledges that while CLA subjects loose more fat than placebo subjects, changes in body weight are insignificant.[35] This camp of researchers also warns that a few small studies don't provide enough evidence to establish this supplement as a panacea for overweight people. While CLA looks promising, there is not enough human research to determine if long-term use is safe.

Some herbs act as diuretics (chemicals that increase urine production), so they can help people lose water weight. Examples are buchu, celery seed, dandelion, juniper, parsley, and uva ursi. Diuretics are not effective for long-term weight loss because they trigger the body's thirst reflex to replace lost fluids. The body eventually adjusts to the continued use of diuretic herbs and retains water despite them.

Some herbs are stimulants that reportedly increase metabolism and suppress appetite. Examples are ephedra (in Chinese, *ma huang*) and caffeine. Ephedra (or ephedrine) is viewed as a natural form of fen-phen. To be effective, these herbs have to be taken in such large doses that they often cause unpleasant side effects such as insomnia, irritability, jitters, and elevated blood pressure. Ephedra has shown no weight-reduction benefits for mildly overweight people who want to lose 5 to 10 pounds.[36]

Another group of herbs produce a feeling of fullness. These are mucilaginous herbs: They absorb fluids, such as might occur in the stomach at mealtime, and expand substantially. The most notable herb in this group is psyllium. Psyllium seed is sold in bulk in herb shops and is also available in drugstores as the common bulk-forming laxative Metamucil. Studies of obese women taking psyllium before meals do not report any weight-loss advantage.[36]

Hot, spicy herbs such as red pepper and mustard reportedly increase metabolism, which, in turn, causes more calories to be burned. Hot herbs also stimulate thirst. Researchers who observe weight-loss benefits from these herbs do not know if they are from the herbs' effect on metabolism or if they cause people to fill up on water and, therefore, ingest fewer calories.

The view that herbs are safe because they come from nature is misleading. When packaged in large, concentrated doses and taken as pills or supplements, they should be viewed as drugs with potential side effects.

From a medicinal point of view, a major shortcoming of herbs is that they are classified as supplements and, therefore, are not subjected to the same scientific testing as are FDA-approved drugs. Medical groups usually recommend that herbal weight-loss products be avoided, especially those containing ephedrine, until they are adequately tested.[35]

Fasting

Fasting, or complete starvation, has been practiced throughout history. Traditionally, people fasted for religious reasons. Although fasting is still used to achieve spiritual enlightenment by some people, a growing number of people fast for dubious physical reasons: to lose weight, to detoxify their bodies of impurities, and to cure everything from allergies to chronic diseases. The physical benefits of fasting have not been demonstrated in carefully planned studies. Most people who are in good health can tolerate a twenty-four-hour fast without a problem as long as they drink plenty of water. However, prolonged fasting can be harmful and even fatal.

Modified fasts that allow for fruit and vegetable juices in addition to water are generally safer. In terms of weight loss, however, fasting is not an effective strategy. Fasting is an extreme action. Like any extreme diet plan, when this one is over, the weight returns. If you are healthy and still choose to fast, don't fast for more than twenty-four hours and drink plenty of fluids. If you are taking medicines, consult your physician before fasting.[38]

Physical Activity

The optimal approach to weight loss combines mild caloric restriction with regular physical activity. A weight loss of 1 pound per week requires a caloric deficit of 3500 calories or 500 calories per day. This can be accomplished by the following:

- Reducing caloric intake by 500 calories per day.
- Reducing daily caloric intake by 250 calories and increasing daily energy expenditure 250 calories or any combination that equates to 500 calories per day.
- Increasing caloric expenditure via physical activity by 500 calories per day.

The last option may be the most difficult for people who are obese or severely overweight. Initially, they may not be able to tolerate the frequency, duration, or intensity of exercise needed to achieve this energy level. A combination of caloric restriction and moderately intense physical activity is most likely to achieve the best result.[39]

Use of calories

One of the obvious benefits of physical activity is that it burns calories. Calories are consumed according to body weight, so heavier people burn more calories per

Table 8-4 Estimated Caloric Cost of Selected Activities

Activity	Calories/Min./Lb.*
Aerobic dance (vigorous)	0.062
Basketball (vigorous, full-court)	0.097
Bathing, dressing, undressing	0.021
Bed making (and stripping)	0.031
Bicycling (13 MPH)	0.071
Canoeing (flat water, 4 MPH)	0.045
Chopping wood	0.049
Cleaning windows	0.024
Cross-country skiing (8 MPH)	0.104
Gardening	
Digging	0.062
Raking	0.034
Weeding	0.038
Golf (twosome, carrying clubs)	0.045
Handball (skilled, singles)	0.078
Horseback riding (trot)	0.052
Ironing	0.029
Jogging (5 MPH)	0.060
Laundry (taking out and hanging)	0.027
Mopping floors	0.024
Peeling potatoes	0.019
Piano playing	0.018
Rowing (vigorous)	0.097
Running (8 MPH)	0.104
Sawing wood (crosscut saw)	0.058
Shining shoes	0.017
Shoveling snow	0.052
Snowshoeing (2.5 MPH)	0.060
Soccer (vigorous)	0.097
Swimming (55 yds./min.)	0.088
Table tennis (skilled)	0.045
Tennis (beginner)	0.032
Walking (4.5 MPH)	0.048
Writing while seated	0.013

*Multiply calories/min./lb. by your body weight in pounds and then multiply that product by the number of minutes spent in the activity.

minute than do lighter people for the same activity. Table 8-4 presents the calorie consumption of some physical-fitness activities and a few common physical activities. To use it, multiply your body weight by the coefficient in the calories/min./lb. column and then multiply this value by the number of minutes spent participating in the activity. For example, to determine the calories expended by a 170-pound person who walks at 4.5 MPH for 30 minutes, do the following:

1. Multiply body weight by calories/min./lb.:

$$170 \text{ lbs.} \times 0.048 \text{ calories/min./lb.}$$
$$= 8.16 \text{ calories/min.}$$

2. Multiply calories/min. by the exercise time in minutes:

8.16 calories/min. × 30 min. = 244.8 calories

If this person performs this exercise daily, 1 pound will be lost in approximately fourteen days or 25 pounds will be lost in one year, provided caloric intake is unchanged. The annual weight loss is calculated as follows:

3500 calories/lb. ÷ 245 calories/day = 14.29 days/lb.
365 days/year ÷ 14.29 days/lb. = 25.5 lbs./year

Follow the example in Assessment Activity 8-2 and apply the directions to your situation or to a hypothetical situation.

Aerobic exercises such as walking and cycling contribute significantly to weight loss. The American College of Sports Medicine (ACSM) emphasizes consistency, adherence, and enjoyment, rather than intensity or mode of exercise when developing a weight-loss plan.[39] A good goal is one that requires an expenditure of 300 calories per day at least three times per week or 200 calories per day at least four times per week. Deconditioned people should start slowly and gradually progress according to the principles of exercise intensity, frequency, and duration discussed in Chapters 3 and 4 in this text. Complete Assessment Activity 8-4 to determine the number of minutes that you should devote to your favorite activities to burn a minimum of 300 calories.

For many people, low-intensity, long-duration physical activity, such as walking is optimal. For weight loss, all calories do not have to be expended in one exercise session. Three 15-minute walks in a day result in a substantial expenditure of energy. Any physical activity above the amount normally done in a day is a bonus for weight control. The cumulative effect of activities such as walking upstairs, mowing the lawn, and mopping floors can be combined with a structured exercise program to produce steady, safe weight loss.

Exercise stimulates metabolism

Basal metabolic rate (BMR) is the energy required to sustain life when the body is in a rested and fasted state. BMR is measured in calories and represents the energy needed to keep the heart, lungs, liver, kidneys, and all other organs functioning. More calories are used to maintain BMR than to perform any other function.

Metabolism is affected by age, gender, nervous system activity, secretions from endocrine glands, nutritional status, sleep, fever, climate, body surface area, and amount of muscle tissue. Because men have more muscle tissue than do women, their BMRs average 5 to 10 percent higher. See Assessment Activity 8-3 to learn how to estimate your BMR.

Muscle tissue stimulates metabolism. Therefore, physical activity is a key strategy for weight management. This is especially true for people as they get older (see Wellness Across the Generations: Age and Weight Gain Do Not Have to Go Together).

Wellness Across the Generations

Age and Weight Gain Do Not Have to Go Together

Weight gain is one experience people ages 25 to 65 have in common. From the time people embark on their professional careers until the time they start thinking about retirement, they often experience creeping weight gain, sometimes obesity. Often they blame the aging process. But is creeping obesity a function of biological factors that are part of the aging process, or are other factors involved? Rather than aging, it is more likely to be a higher standard of living that is responsible for such weight gain. A higher standard of living usually results in an easier, less active life. Improvements in standard of living go hand-in-hand with labor-saving devices that add convenience and save energy. Many experts believe that weight gain associated with increased age is a function of the subtle changes in metabolism caused by less muscle tissue, which is caused by less physical activity.

Metabolism is an important issue for the weight-conscious person, because 70 percent of our energy is expended to support basic life processes. Muscle tissue burns more energy at rest than does fat tissue, so changes in body composition that favor muscle tissue over fat tissue provide a calorie-burning advantage throughout the day. Conversely, changes in body composition that favor fat over muscle lower the body's metabolism and promote weight gain. Metabolism declines with age, primarily because of the physical inactivity and muscle loss that often accompany aging. The annual decrease in BMR beginning at 25 years of age, though imperceptible, has serious ramifications for weight management and accounts for a significant amount of the weight gained with age. The loss of muscle tissue is equal to 3 to 5 percent every decade after age 25. The subsequent decline in BMR produces changes in body composition. Exercise and physical activities are the keys to weight management because they increase or sustain muscle tissue, thus accelerating metabolism and using calories.

The key to weight control

Although scientifically controlled studies have not yet proven that physical activity is instrumental in losing weight, they provide compelling evidence of its importance in weight control and weight-loss maintenance. People who lose weight and keep it off almost always exercise daily. Studies that attempt to identify predictors of successful weight maintenance point to physical activity as one of the best markers for long-term success.[17] Researchers at the University of California at Davis found that 90 percent of women who had lost 20 pounds and kept it off for at least two years were avid exercisers; of the women who had regained the weight, only 35 percent were physically active. At the Baylor College of Medicine in Houston, another group of researchers put 160 obese adults on one of three year-long weight-loss programs: diet-only, exercise-only, or exercise and diet. Everyone lost weight. (The exercise and diet group lost the most.) But two years later, the exercise-only participants were the only ones to keep the weight off.[40] Other large-scale studies that follow men and women in weight-loss programs for ten years consistently show that major weight gain is much more likely to occur in people who are sedentary than in those who are physically active.[17] Ninety percent of people who lose weight and keep it off do so because they are likely to be exercising enough to burn more than 1500 calories a week.[29] Thus, although physical activity as a singular strategy has modest effects on weight loss, it is the key strategy for lifelong weight control. Stated more directly, weight maintenance gets easier when people exercise. More importantly, moderate exercise improves health and reduces risk factors associated with morbidity and mortality for the obese just as it does for normal-weight people.

Exercise intensity and fat loss

In Chapter 6 a distinction is made between the intensity and duration of exercise and the accompanying use by the body of energy nutrients. In general, carbohydrates are the main source of energy for high-intensity exercise, and fat is the main source of energy for low-intensity exercise sustained for a prolonged time. (The body instinctively spares its protein reserve except when needed for activities of exceptional duration.) The fat-burning benefit of low-intensity exercise should be a source of encouragement for people trying to shed extra fat, making exercise a viable option for most people. Walking, gardening, yard work, housework, and golfing (assuming you're walking) burn fat calories.

Does this mean that high-intensity exercises are of little value as a weight-management strategy? The answer is no, because the overall goal is to create a caloric deficit, and calories count regardless of exercise intensity. Physically demanding activities such as jogging, running, rock climbing, swimming, cycling, and aerobics burn more total calories than do low-intensity activities if participation time is held constant; they just require a higher proportion of fuel from glycogen stores than from fat. Still, both energy sources are tapped. For example, if you burn 200 calories exercising for a half hour at a low intensity, 41 percent of those calories come from fat, giving you a fat loss of 82 calories. If you exercise for the same amount of time at a high intensity, you burn 375 calories, including 90 fat calories, even though the percentage of energy supplied by fat is only 24 percent. The point of this example is not to discourage participation in low-intensity activities but only to suggest that, if you're in good health and enjoy vigorous exercise, you do not need to limit yourself to low-intensity exercise. Exercising on a consistent basis is the best strategy for managing weight, regardless of intensity level.

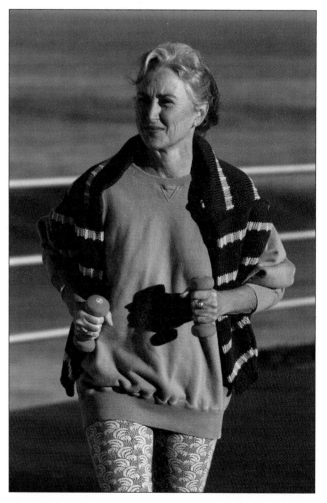

Physical activities that develop muscle can also increase your metabolism.

Regular Exercise Is the Key to Weight Management: Make It Fun

Whatever kind of exercise you do on a regular basis, it is the best strategy for weight management. If your motivation for exercise is based solely on external factors, such as losing weight or preventing disease, it is unlikely that exercise will become a permanent fixture in your lifestyle. Many experts believe that physical activity is more likely to become a lifestyle pattern if it is motivated by intrinsic factors, such as fun, pleasure, and feeling good. Losing weight is a good reason to start exercising, but you probably won't sustain exercise unless you learn to enjoy it and to value the way it makes you feel. People who are consistently physically active shift their focus from the outcome (weight loss) to the process of exercise. Regular exercisers want to work out because they like it and it makes them feel better.[41] (For tips on making exercise fun, see Nurturing Your Spirituality: Fun Is the Key to Regular Exercise for Weight Maintenance.) With this approach to exercise, even if weight loss is modest, overall health is improved.

Combining Dietary Modification and Exercise

Because caloric consumption and expenditure are involved in weight management, both should be manipulated to be effective. Combining sensible exercise and sensible changes in eating habits that can be maintained for life is the most effective approach to permanent weight management. Dieting alone can promote significant weight loss, but a substantial component of the weight loss may be lean tissue. Physical activity alone results in modest fat loss and an increase in lean body mass. Combination strategies involving both food restriction and physical activity meet the goals of weight management most effectively: These strategies improve body composition by promoting weight loss, fat loss, and lean-tissue gain.

Behavioral Effects

Some evidence suggests that obese people are more likely than normal-weight people to eat in response to external cues. A clock that says it is suppertime; media messages advertising food and beverages; and the sight, sound, and aroma of food are more apt to elicit eating behavior in the obese. This tendency is the basis of the "externality" hypothesis: If people can learn to eat in response to external cues, they can also learn to recognize cues that stimulate eating behavior, substitute other behaviors for eating, and use techniques that de-

Nurturing Your Spirituality

Fun Is the Key to Regular Exercise for Weight Maintenance

Experts have shifted the paradigm of weight management from counting calories burned in exercise to promoting movement that is social, playful, and pleasurable. If exercise is fun, if it makes you feel good about yourself, and if it provides that mini-vacation each day (a time and place where nothing else interferes), it is more likely to be incorporated permanently into daily living. As noted by one expert, "Inner joy is the key to dutiful exercise. The body fails to persist if the soul is in rebellion."[41]

Do you want to move from an occasional dreaded workout to one that you look forward to on a regular basis? Here are some tips passed on by others who once were couch potatoes:

- First, examine your likes and dislikes. Think in terms of activities that are fun for you. These may be taking a stroll in a park, working in the flower garden, skating to class, or joining a fitness club.

- Build relationships with people who share your interests and goals. Workout partners often provide incentive and encouragement for working out.

- Tell people if you notice improvements in their energy level and in appearance after exercising. Not only will they feel better but so will you, and the compliment will likely be returned at some point.

- Join a fitness club or participate in a structured fitness program that will increase your repertoire of skills and activities.

- Find a comfortable workout environment with a supportive staff.

- Vary your activities. Variety is the antidote for boredom; cross-training is the key for many longtime exercisers.

crease the amount of food eaten. As a result of this training the response to external cues should be reduced and replaced by attention to internal hunger signals. Many techniques have been developed over the past twenty years that may assist people in resisting the tendency to eat indiscriminately or to overeat. Generally, these techniques employ one or more of the following approaches:

1. *Self-monitoring:* A journal or daily log records food consumption, physical activities, and circumstances

Real-World Wellness

Behavioral Strategies for Reshaping Your Eating Habits

In Chapter 1, I learned about intervention strategies for changing behavior. In this chapter I've learned about the importance of gaining control over the tendency to overeat. How can I apply behavioral principles from Chapter 1 to my goal of curbing overeating?

Try the following strategies:

- Eat in a certain place—not in every room of your home.
- Eliminate from your immediate environment all food that can be eaten without careful preparation.
- Always eat at a carefully set place at the table and eat only one helping of planned foods.
- Prepare only enough food for one meal.
- Eat slowly.
- Chew each bite twenty-five to fifty times.
- Set down your utensils after every mouthful.
- Partway through the meal, stop and relax without eating for two to three minutes.
- Leave some food on your plate at each meal.
- Plan to eat some meals alone. (There is a tendency to overeat in social situations.)
- Eat a carefully balanced diet so that you are not deprived of a particular food element.

related to eating. In a recent study of dieters from two weeks before Thanksgiving until two weeks after New Year's, it was found that participants who were most consistent in monitoring food intake were also most successful in losing weight and keeping it off.[42]

2. *Control of precursors to eating:* The events and circumstances that elicit eating and overeating are identified.

3. *Control of eating:* Behavioral modification techniques are used to control, change, or modify specific eating behaviors. (See Real-World Wellness: Behavioral Strategies for Reshaping Your Eating Habits.)

4. *Reinforcement through the use of rewards:* Rewards tied to the achievement of behavioral goals are identified and used.

These techniques may be useful especially if they are combined with sensible food choices and exercise.

Eating Disorders and Disordered Eating

Anorexia nervosa (anorexia) and *bulimia nervosa* (bulimia) are eating disorders familiar to most Americans. More recently, *binge-eating disorder* and *female athlete triad* have emerged as health issues that require professional intervention. Full-blown anorexia and bulimia are eating disorders; binge-eating disorder and female athlete triad usually involve disordered eating patterns. The major difference between the two types of conditions is that **eating disorders** meet certain criteria as outlined by the American Psychiatric Association. **Disordered eating**, on the other hand, entails sporadic eating, poor nutrition, unnecessary dieting, or occasional bingeing and purging.[43] While each of these conditions shares some common characteristics, each also has some distinctive qualities.

Anorexia Nervosa

The chief characteristic of **anorexia nervosa** is a refusal to maintain a minimally normal weight for age and height. Refusal to eat is the hallmark of the disease, regardless of whether other practices, such as binge-purge cycles, occur. Although specific causes of anorexia have not been identified, a combination of biological, social, and psychological factors contributes to the disorder. Support for an organic influence has centered on the hypothalamus (the portion of the brain reputed to house the appetite center) and the pituitary gland (the master gland of the body). Sociocultural theories focus on the compulsion of adolescent girls to become and remain lean. This exaggerated goal manifests at a time when girls are naturally depositing fat.

Anorexia is characterized by extreme weight loss, amenorrhea (absence of a menstrual period), and a variety of psychological disorders culminating in an obsessive preoccupation with the attainment of thinness. Fortunately, most anorectics recover fully after one experience with the disease. However, the longer a person practices anorexic behaviors, the less the chance for recovery. Just the Facts: Criteria for Diagnosing Anorexia Nervosa lists the criteria that have been developed by the American Psychiatric Association for diagnosing anorexia.[44]

When confronted, anorectics typically deny the existence of a problem and the weight-loss behaviors that have resulted in their emaciated physical appearance. They also avoid medical treatment, refuse the well-intended advice of family and friends regarding professional assistance, and submit to treatment only under protest. Anorexia is a subtle disease, and anorectics become secretive in their behaviors. They are evasive, and many hide their disease in deep denial

Just the Facts

Criteria for Diagnosing Anorexia Nervosa

The American Psychiatric Association[44] has identified the following criteria for a diagnosis of anorexia nervosa:

- Weight change
  - unwillingness to maintain minimal normal body weight for the person's age and height
  - weight loss that leads to the maintenance of a body weight that is 15 percent below normal
  - failure to gain the amount of weight expected during a period of growth, resulting in a body weight that is 15 percent below normal
- Inordinate fear of gaining weight or becoming fat despite being significantly underweight
- Disturbed and unrealistic perceptions of body weight, size, or shape; feeling of being "fat" although emaciated; possible perception of one specific part of the body as "too fat"
- Absence of at least three menstrual cycles for women when they would normally be expected to occur (amenorrheic women have a normal menstrual cycle only during administration of hormone therapy)
- Rigid dieting; maintenance of rigid control in lifestyle; security found in control and order
- Rituals involving food and excessive exercise

even while undergoing treatment, making the diagnosis especially difficult.

The course of treatment for anorexia is complex, involving a coordinated effort by several health care specialists. Hospitalization is often required because anorectics may have to be fed intravenously or by some other method if they cannot or will not eat. Medications that stimulate the appetite and medications that calm the patient are usually necessary. Nutritional counseling and psychological counseling—individual, group, and family—are integral components of treatment (see Real-World Wellness: Helping a Friend Overcome an Eating Disorder). Finally, behavior modification techniques are used to help change the perceptions and lifestyle of the anorectic. At this point, no single treatment has proved to be unusually successful in the treatment of anorectic patients.

Bulimia (Bulimia Nervosa)

Bulimia nervosa is characterized by alternate cycles of binge eating and restrictive eating. Binge eating is distinguished from ordinary overeating in that it involves the consumption of a large amount of food in a relatively

Real-World Wellness

Helping a Friend Overcome an Eating Disorder

I suspect a friend of mine is struggling with an eating disorder. How can I help without making matters worse? Are there some internet resources available?

Try doing the following:
- Talk to the person alone.
- Tell the person why you are concerned.
- Be nonjudgmental; ask clarifying questions; listen carefully.
- Offer to go with the person to talk to someone.
- Encourage her or him to verbalize feelings.
- Show how much you care by asking frequently how the person is doing.
- Show an interest in the person's life outside of eating.
- Enlist the help of a counselor if you think the disorder is severe; however, eating disorders are usually not emergency situations.
- Anticipate and accept that denial and anger are part of the illness.

Avoid doing the following:
- Threaten or challenge the person.
- Give advice about weight loss.
- Get into an argument.
- Try to keep track of the person's food consumption.
- Try to force the person to eat.
- Be patronizing by being overly caring.
- Try to be a hero or rescuer; the person may resent such efforts.

Here are some internet sites that serve as good resources:
- Eating Disorders Awareness and Prevention, Inc., at www.edap.org
- National Eating Disorders Information Centre at www.nedic.on.ca
- American Dietetics Association at www.eatright.org
- The Center for Eating Disorders at www.eatingdisorder.org
- Pale Reflections Weekly Newsletter for Those with Eating Disorders at www.members.aol.com/paleref/index.html

brief time (that is, within a one- to two-hour period) and is accompanied by lack of control. Bingeing is nearly always done in private; in public, the bulimic tends to eat normal or even less than normal amounts. Unlike the occasional splurge almost everyone has, the bulimic becomes compulsive and habitual and often resorts to secretive eating. Binges are usually followed by purging, primarily by self-induced vomiting supplemented with laxatives and diuretics. Some people with this disorder may purge excess energy by *hypergymnasia* or excessive exercise. The physical ramifications of bulimia include esophageal inflammation, erosion of tooth enamel caused by repeated vomiting, and the possibility of electrolyte imbalances. Psychological ramifications include guilt, shame, self-disgust, anxiety, and depression.

The diagnostic criteria for bulimia are given in Just the Facts: Criteria for Diagnosing Bulimia.[44] These criteria specify that, to be diagnosed a bulimic, a person must vomit at least twice a week for three months. Binge-purge cycles may occur daily, weekly, or in other intervals. Bulimic behaviors range from binge eating frequently or from time-to-time, binge eating with a feeling of being unable to control food intake, severely restricting the diet between binge periods, and binge eating followed by purging. Purging in the form of laxatives, vomiting, diuretics, fasting, and excessive exercise follows in the hope that weight gain will be blunted. Because many people with bulimia engage in binge-purge practices in isolation and because bulimics are often not excessively thin, they cannot be diagnosed easily or by their appearance.

Bulimics are treated similarly to anorectics except that hospitalization is usually not required. In addition to nutritional and psychological counseling, treatment often includes antidepressive medication because bulimia is associated with clinical depression. Treatment focuses on correcting typical bulimic behaviors, such as "all-or-none" thinking: "If I'm not perfect, I'm a failure, so one slipup—one cookie—justifies a binge." Generally, psychotherapy aims primarily to help a person with self-acceptance and to be less concerned with body weight.[5]

Binge-Eating Disorder

Binge-eating disorder is similar to bulimia in two ways: (1) it involves eating large amounts of food in a short time, and (2) it is accompanied by a sense of lack of control regarding eating. It is different from bulimia in that it is not associated with compensatory behaviors, such as purging, fasting, and excessive exercise. When binge eating occurs on average at least two days a week for six months, it becomes an eating disorder. The American Psychiatric Association has identified additional criteria for this disorder.[44] (See Just the Facts: Criteria for Diagnosing Binge-Eating Disorder.)

Just the Facts

Criteria for Diagnosing Bulimia

The American Psychiatric Association[44] has identified the following criteria for a diagnosis of bulimia:

- Episodic secretive binge eating characterized by rapid consumption of large quantities of food in a short time; never overeating in front of others
- At least two eating binges per week for at least three months
- Loss of control over eating behavior while eating binges are in progress
- Frequent purging after eating; using techniques such as self-induced vomiting, laxatives, or diuretics; engaging in fasting or strict dieting; or engaging in vigorous exercise
- Constant and continual concern with body shape, size, and weight
- Erosion of teeth; swollen glands
- Purchase of syrup of ipecac

Just the Facts

Criteria for Diagnosing Binge-Eating Disorder

The American Psychiatric Association[44] has identified the following criteria for a diagnosis of binge-eating disorder:

- Recurrent episodes of eating an amount of food clearly larger than most people would eat in a similar circumstance
- Binge eating that occurs, on average, at least two days a week for six months
- A sense of lack of control over eating
- Binge eating associated with any three of the following:
  - eating large amounts of food when not feeling hungry
  - eating alone because of embarrassment over the amount of food eaten
  - eating much more rapidly than normal
  - eating far beyond comfort level
  - feeling guilty or depressed after eating

Female Athlete Triad

Female athlete triad is a condition marked by three characteristics: disordered eating, *amenorrhea* or lack of menstrual periods, and osteoporosis or low age-adjusted bone density.[5] It most often affects women athletes engaged in appearance-based, weight-based, and endurance sports. The components of the triad are interrelated. Typically the triad begins with disordered eating. Poor nutrition combined with intense training results in an energy deficit. In time, the energy deficit can cause the body to shut down the production of estrogen, which in turn can trigger amenorrhea. The lack of estrogen combined with nutritional deficiencies particularly in calcium and vitamin D may seriously compromise bone density and increase the risk of contracting osteoporosis.[43] Some young women diagnosed with female athlete triad have bones equivalent to those of 50- to 60-year-olds, making them overly susceptible to fractures during both sports and general activities. Much of the bone loss is irreversible.[5] Women with this condition should seek professional help to reduce their preoccupation with food, weight, and body fat; to regain body weight; to establish regular menstrual cycles; and to increase their consumption of food.

Underweight

A small number of people who are not anorectic or bulimic are naturally thin, and some of them are dissatisfied with their appearance. Being underweight presents as much of a cosmetic problem for affected people as obesity does for the obese person. Many underweight people find it more difficult to gain a pound than it is for obese people to lose one.

In their attempts to gain weight, many lean people consume large quantities of food, particularly those rich in calories. Unfortunately, these foods are also high in fat and sugar. This eating pattern is unhealthy for anyone, regardless of body weight. The preferred approach is to combine muscle-building exercises with three well-balanced, nutritious meals supplemented by two nutritious snacks. Increasing caloric intake by 500 calories a day should yield a weight gain of about a pound a week. In doing so, emphasize calorie-rich foods from the Food Guide Pyramid. Whole-grain cereals with nuts and raisins and dried fruits are examples. Also emphasize foods that are good sources of monounsaturated fats. Examples include olive oil and canola oil. Finally, plan an exercise program that includes resistance training. Instead of gaining fat as calories are increased, muscle weight will be added.

The amount and type of weight gain should be closely monitored. Fat stores should not be increased unless the person is extremely thin and on the verge of dipping into stores of essential fat.

Principles of Weight Management: Putting It All Together

The best approach to weight management is the most obvious: maintaining a moderate lifestyle so that excess weight is not gained. In summary, the basic principles of weight maintenance and weight loss are the following:

1. Avoid the obsession with body weight. Remember that body weight per se is not the most important issue; rather, body composition is. Modest weight gain distributed in the wrong places increases health risks. Conversely, significant weight gain in the form of muscle tissue enhances health and well-being. You should consider losing weight if it becomes excessive or if you have a family history of disease that may be worsened by excess weight.

2. The most important factor in weight maintenance is physical activity. Americans weigh more now than ever because of sedentary lifestyles. The challenge is either to sacrifice some labor-saving devices and their convenience or to consciously seek opportunities to impose extra physical demands on the body. This may mean choosing the stairs rather than the elevator or walking to class rather than driving. Participating in physical activities on a consistent basis is the best way to prevent excessive weight gain. It is also the best way to maintain weight loss over time. Almost all people who successfully lose weight and keep it off exercise daily. Exercise is the best way to overpower the body's set point for fatness.

   Exercise is just as important to the chronically obese and overweight as it is to those who are trying to lose or maintain weight. Obese people who are fit enjoy the same health benefits as normal-weight people.

   The ACSM recommends a caloric deficit of 500 calories a day to lose 1 pound in a week. This can be achieved by reducing caloric intake by 250 calories and exercising to burn 250 calories. A 250-calorie workout is equivalent to a 2.5 mile walk for most people. Remember, energy expenditure through exercise does not have to occur at one time. The effects of physical activity are cumulative and reinforce the value of activity spread throughout the day. The key issue in exercising is consistency and moderation. Plan an activity program that can be sustained one year and five years from now. People who boost their lifestyle activity are just as successful at keeping the weight off as people who participate in formal exercise programs.[29]

3. Follow the Mayo Clinic Healthy Weight Pyramid by eating nutrient-dense foods and stress consumption of fruits and vegetables. Calories from fat convert easily to fat, with only 3 percent being lost in the digestive process. By comparison, 25 percent of carbohydrate calories are lost in the process.

   Emphasize fiber in your diet. Because of fiber's high satiety value, people who eat a great deal of it usually consume fewer total calories at mealtime. An added benefit is that fiber may help block the digestion of some of the fat consumed with it. The less fat digested, the less absorbed in the bloodstream.[5]

4. Avoid volume eating. Calories count regardless of their source. The penchant to practice compensatory eating behavior may be especially common among people who choose low-fat and/or low-calorie products. People are eating food in larger quantities. Avoid buffet-style, all-you-can-eat restaurants. Practice behavioral strategies that make volume eating more difficult. And when eating low-fat or low-calorie foods, be aware of the tendency to overcompensate by eating more food. Remember, two servings of a low-fat food that contains 5 grams of fat yields 90 total fat calories and may exceed the number of fat calories in one serving of the regular, high-fat version. The tendency to overcompensate by consuming more calories also applies to beverages. Liquid calories don't have the satiety value of solid food and often result in extra calories. Drink plenty of water and substitute calorie-free beverages or limit calorie-containing beverages.

5. Set realistic goals. Don't be misled by messages and advertisements that promise huge weight loss in a short time. Weight loss per week usually should not exceed 1 to 2 pounds. The ideal approach is to lose pounds at the same rate at which they were gained. In trying to set goals, ask yourself these questions: What is the least I have weighed as an adult, for at least a year? Based on past experiences what is the most weight I can expect to lose? Then, adjust your goals upward. A good goal is to lose 10 percent of your body weight. A good weight loss goal for a 200-pound person is 20 pounds. People who focus on losing just 10 percent of their weight have the best chance of long-term success.[45] Losing these first pounds produces the biggest health gains in lower blood pressure, lower blood cholesterol, and lower blood sugar. This is especially true for people with abdominal fat.

6. Make a gradual lifestyle change. Such change represents a calm, deliberate approach rather than a frenetic "lose it now" attitude. A 200-pound person should exercise, reduce calories, and eat like a 180-pound person to become a 180-pound person. Once the weight is lost, the person must resist reverting to the habits of a 200-pound person. A diet is only successful if the weight does not return.

7. Anticipate a plateau. During the first week of a diet, weight loss comes primarily from loss of protein, glycogen, and water but little fat. As the body adjusts to a diet, fat loss increases. This adjustment takes about a week on a moderate diet and still longer when the diet is severe. Many dieters experience a plateau after about three to four weeks, not because they are suddenly cheating but because they have gained water weight while still losing body fat. If physically active, dieters may gain lean body mass and lose fat while maintaining weight. If weight loss is drastic during the early stages, it induces an adaptive response in the body that slows down metabolism. The body resists drastic change of any sort. Once its internal signals recognize a substantial reduction in caloric intake, it slows down to conserve fuel. After losing 20 to 30 pounds, expect to reach a stable plateau.

8. Avoid diet pills, special formula diets, all-you-can-eat diets, fat-burning concoctions, skin creams, and other fad diets. Some of these fads impose health risks, and others simply don't work or, if they do, their results are temporary and lead to weight cycling. The more extreme the diet, the less likely the weight loss will be permanent.

   The new generation of diet pills currently being investigated as a potential solution for the chronically obese should be viewed with caution. Even if such pills prove successful, they must be taken for life, and they may have side effects as harmful to health as the extra weight. Many experts are reluctant to endorse a lifelong pharmaceutical solution to obesity.

9. Avoid very low-calorie diets. Such diets decrease RMR up to 20 percent, making weight loss success even harder.[32] The reduction in RMR may partly account for the plateau mentioned in number 7. Diets that cut calories to under 1200 (if you're woman) or 1400 (if you're man), however, do not allow enough food to be satisfying over the long haul and are unlikely to meet the body's

needs for nutrients. Remember, if you can't lose weight at the 1200 or 1400 calorie-level, you probably don't need to.

10. Develop an eating plan that includes easily obtained foods.

11. Develop a less rigid lifestyle, one that reduces the need to consciously control what is eaten. Maintaining weight loss is the antithesis of counting every calorie. Also, it doesn't matter what time of the day calories are consumed. A calorie is a calorie regardless of the time (see Just the Facts: A Calorie is a Calorie).

12. Avoid fasting and restrictive dieting. These practices often lead to a preoccupation with food, weight, and/or dieting. Dieting should allow people to attend parties, eat at restaurants, and participate in normal activities. People erroneously assume that if they have eaten just a little bit of a "forbidden" food, they have "crossed the line." Foods are neither "good" nor "bad." Labeling them as such often promotes a denial-guilt-preoccupation cycle in which one slight deviation from a diet or food choice is interpreted as a failure: A forbidden food is eaten (denial), a sense of relief from restraint leads to a binge, the binge leads to guilt and a feeling of failure, and both denial and guilt exacerbate the preoccupation. The preoccupation leads back to denial and the cycle continues. This cycle exerts considerable pressure on the dieter. To avoid the dissonance that comes with failure, the dieter often abandons attempts to lose weight. Given moderation and discretion, almost any food can be enjoyed. Food is one of life's pleasures, so you need not avoid any one food. If it is high in fat and calories, eat a small portion. If you do not deny yourself, you might not feel compelled to cheat.

13. Avoid meal skipping. One strategy that surprises some dieters with its effectiveness is eating frequent small meals and snacks. The more often a person eats, the less hungry that person feels and the less food that person will eat.[45] Eating five to six times a day—breakfast, a midmorning snack, lunch, an afternoon snack, dinner, and a before-bed snack—might require some retraining. Keep portions small and emphasize fruits and vegetables.

   Resist the temptation to skip breakfast. People who eat a healthy breakfast generally feel less hungry throughout the day.

14. Form a buddy system or join a support group. The support and encouragement of a friend or relative are often the difference between success and failure.

∽ Just the Facts ∽

A Calorie Is a Calorie

A common misconception is that eating at night facilities weight gain. If this is true it is because of the amount of calories consumed at night, not the time. When researchers gave overweight women 70 percent of their calories either before noon or closer to dinnertime, it didn't affect their body fat. In a large survey of almost 2000 people, how much people ate in the evening had no bearing on the extent of their change in weight over ten years.[46] The body doesn't distinguish between calories consumed in the morning or at night. A calorie is a calorie.

15. If you stop smoking, don't be discouraged by subsequent weight gain. If you are a heavy smoker, you can expect on average an increase in weight of 10 pounds. That's not enough to make most smokers obese. From a health perspective, you would have to gain 100 to 150 pounds after quitting to make your health risks as high as when you smoked.[47]

16. Don't indulge yourself in self-blame for past failures. View past dieting attempts objectively as a psychologist would. Focus more on what you learned from past experiences. Most people who are successful at maintaining weight loss are not successful in their first attempt. In studies that track dieters listed in the Weight Control Registry, 90 percent of them are repeaters. In some studies, nearly 60 percent of dieters were found to have made five attempts before achieving success.[48] Rather than blaming yourself, reflect on what you learned about yourself and what worked and didn't work.

17. Finally, accept yourself. Before trying to lose weight, determine how great a risk your weight poses to your health. People at risk for chronic conditions, such as hypertension and type 2 diabetes, for example, often improve dramatically with a modest weight loss. Some people, however, are overweight despite their best efforts to reduce. For such people, striving to attain a certain weight may be futile and even damaging to health. If a person was overweight throughout childhood, chances are that person will never be thin. Be realistic and aim for a healthy weight for you, not for an actor or actress. Everyone cannot be skinny. Everyone can try to be healthy.

Summary

- Americans' obsession with body weight is evidenced by the large number of women, men, and even children trying to lose weight at any given time.
- A healthy weight is defined as a BMI of 19.0 to 24.9. Overweight occurs with a BMI of 25 or over. Obesity occurs with a BMI of 30 or over. Only 39 percent of U.S. adults meet current standards for healthy weight; 61 percent are overweight.
- Obesity is a risk factor for coronary heart disease, stroke, hypertension, LDL cholesterol, some forms of cancer, impaired glucose tolerance, osteoarthritis, gallbladder disease, and sleep apnea.
- Obesity occurs when fat cells increase excessively either in size (hypertrophy) or in number (hyperplasia). Most obesity is adult-onset and caused by hypertrophy.
- Heredity and set point are the major biological factors associated with obesity.
- The development and distribution of body fat is under substantial genetic control.
- The classic types of body shapes are ectomorph, endomorph, and mesomorph. Ectomorphs have a low capacity for fat storage; endomorphs have a large capacity for fat storage; and mesomorphs fall somewhere in between ectomorphs and endomorphs.
- Physical activity is the best way to alter the body's set point for fatness.
- Overeating and lack of physical activities are the major behavioral explanations of obesity.
- The abundance of food high in fat and calories is a major factor in the prevalence of obesity in the United States.
- Dietary fat has less of a thermogenic effect than do carbohydrate and protein and therefore is more efficiently and easily stored as fat tissue.
- The general decline in physical activity is highly correlated with the rise in obesity.
- Engaging in a physically active lifestyle is the best way to prevent weight gain.
- Approximately 70 percent of the energy liberated from food is expended to support BMR.
- Physical activity improves body composition, increases BMR, improves insulin sensitivity, and increases oxygen capacity and glycogen storage in muscles.
- Weight loss requires a caloric deficit in which food intake and exercise are manipulated so that caloric expenditure exceeds caloric intake.
- Complex forces influence the success of weight-loss efforts and help to explain why people respond so differently to similar dieting strategies.
- Low-fat diets often result in overcompensatory eating behaviors as a result of which the dieter ends up consuming more total calories.
- A desirable long-term goal for losing weight is 1 to 2 pounds per week until about 10 percent of excess weight is lost. A six-month maintenance period is suggested before more weight loss is attempted.
- Diet-only strategies should provide a loss of at least 1200 calories per day for women and 1400 for men.
- The optimal approach to weight loss combines mild caloric restriction with regular physical activity. Together these two strategies should provide a caloric deficit of 500 calories per day.
- In structuring a diet to lose weight, follow the recommendations in the Mayo Clinic Healthy Weight Pyramid. Emphasize fruits and vegetables. Observe recommended servings for carbohydrates, protein sources, and fats.
- Diet drugs are not intended for people who are overweight or only marginally obese. The harmful effects of long-term exposure to diet drugs may outweigh the health benefits of losing weight.
- Low-intensity exercises sustained for a prolonged period are effective in burning fat calories. However, regardless of intensity level, exercising on a consistent basis is the best strategy for managing weight.
- Anorexia, bulimia, binge-eating, and female athlete triad are four potentially destructive eating disorders and/or disordered eating patterns with complex causes.

Review Questions

1. What evidence exists to support the idea that Americans are obsessed with weight control?
2. In terms of BMIs, what are the definitions of *healthy weight, overweight,* and *obesity*?
3. What health problems and chronic conditions are associated with obesity?
4. What is the relationship between obesity and morbidity and mortality?
5. What are the major biological and behavioral factors that help to explain obesity?
6. What evidence can you use to support the existence of an influential role of heredity in the development of obesity?
7. What does *set point* mean in reference to body shape and body weight? What strategy is best for altering a person's set point for fatness?
8. What dieting strategies need to be emphasized in weight-loss programs?
9. Why are more Americans overweight today than in the past, especially when considering that there has been a drop in the percent of calories from fat?
10. What are the major differences between dietary recommendations in the Food Guide Pyramid and the Mayo Clinic Healthy Weight Pyramid?

11. Compare and contrast dieting and exercise as strategies for (a) losing weight and (b) maintaining or preventing weight gain.
12. What is weight cycling?
13. Why is the thermogenic effect of food an important issue in weight management?

14. What is the relationship between BMR, physical activity, and body composition?
15. What are the differences and similarities of anorexia, bulimia, binge-eating, and female athlete triad?
16. What guiding principles should be observed in planning a reasonable approach to weight loss/weight management?

References

1. Mayo Foundation for Medical Education and Research. 1998. Body image: what do you see in the mirror? Available online at www.mayohealth.org/mayo/9704/htm/body_ima.htm.
2. Liebman, B: 2000. Diet vs diet: battle of the bulge doctors. *Nutrition Action Health Letter* 27(4):9–13.
3. U.S. Department of Health and Human Services. 2000. *Health People 2010* (2nd ed.). With *Understanding and improving health and objectives for improving health,* 2 vols. Washington, D.C.: U.S. Government Printing Office.
4. Penzel, F. I. 2001. Body dysmorphic disorder: symptoms. mental help net & CMHC systems. Available online at http://mentalhelp.net/disorders/sx42.htm.
5. Wardlaw, G. M. 2000. *Contemporary Nutrition: Issues and Insights.* St. Louis: McGraw-Hill.
6. Womancomnetwork. 1998. *Imagetalk—Women's wire on body image: role models?* Available online at www.womenswire.com/image/models2.html.
7. National Center for Health Statistics. 2001. Energy and macronutrient intakes of persons ages 2 months and over in the United States. *Advanced Data from Vital and Health Statistics.* Available online at www.cdc.gov.nchs/products/pubs/pubd/ad/260-251/ad255.htm.
8. McDowell, M. A., et al. 1994. *Energy and Macro-Nutrient Intakes of Persons Ages 2 Months and Over in the United States: Third National Health and Nutrition Examination Survey, Phase I, 1988–91. Advanced Data from Vital and Health Statistics; No. 255.* Hyattsville, Md.: National Center for Health Statistics.
9. Harvard University. 1998. Guidelines call more Americans overweight. *Harvard Health Letter* 23(10):7.
10. Margolis, S., and L. J. Cheskin. 1999. *The Johns Hopkins White Papers: Weight Control.* Baltimore, Md.: The Johns Hopkins Medical Institutions.
11. Margolis, S., and L. J. Cheskin. 1998. *The Johns Hopkins White Papers: Weight Control.* Baltimore, Md.: The Johns Hopkins Medical Institutions.
12. Consumers Union. 1999. Workouts that work. *Consumer Reports* 64(2):31–34.
13. AAHPERD. 1999. Fit or fat may not fit. *Physical Activity Today* 5(1):1.
14. Wardlaw, G. M. 1999. *Perspectives in Nutrition* (4th ed.). St. Louis: WCB/McGraw-Hill.
15. Stunkard, A., et al. 1986. An adoption study of human obesity. *New England Journal of Medicine* 314:193–198.
16. Stunkard, A., et al. 1986. A twin study of human obesity. *Journal of the American Medical Association* 256:51–54.
17. Nieman, D. 1999. *Exercise Testing and Prescription—A Health Related Approach.* Mountain View, Calif.: Mayfield Publishing Co.
18. Harvard University. 2001. Weight loss and gain. *Harvard Health Letter* 26(5):1–3.
19. Crenson, M. July 28, 2000. Researchers suspect virus can spread obesity like a cold. *The Commercial Appeal* A4.
20. Tufts University. 2001. Portion distortion. *Tufts University Health & Nutrition Letter* 18(12):4–5.
21. Tufts University. 1997. On whether reduced-fat foods make reduced-fat bodies. *Tufts University Health & Nutrition Letter* 15(9):2.
22. Harvard University. 2001. Weight gain and loss. *Harvard Health Letter* 26(5):1–3.
23. Editors. 1999. Yo-yo dieting danger? *Environmental Nutrition* 22(5):3.
24. Tufts University. 1999. Yo-yo dieting less risky than you might think. *Tufts University Health & Nutrition Letter* 17(9):1.
25. Mayo Foundation for Medical Education and Research. 2001. Healthy weight: a process of changing your lifestyle habits. *Mayo Clinic Health Letter* 19(1)1–2.
26. Liebman, B. 1997. Fooled by low-fat. *Nutrition Action Health Letter* 24(3):2.
27. Tufts University. 1999. Served up with your restaurant meal: too many calories (and too few nutrients). *Tufts University Health & Nutrition Letter* 17(4):6.
28. Tufts University. 2000. Americans' weight gain: it's no mystery. *Tufts University Health & Nutrition Letter* 18(6):1.
29. Liebman, B. 1999. Ten tips for staying lean. *Nutrition Action Health Letter* 27(6):1, 3–7. Consumers Union. 1998. Top selling diets: lots of gimmicks, little solid evidence. *Consumer Reports* 63(1):60–61.
30. Harvard University. 2000. Superpower, heavyweight. *Harvard Health Letter* 25(3):6.
31. Liebman, B. 1998. Supersize foods, supersize people. *Nutrition Action Health Letter* 25(6):6.
32. ACSM. 2001. *ACSM's Resource Manual for Guidelines for Exercise Testing and Prescription* (4th ed.). Philadelphia: Lippincott Williams and Wilkins.
33. Massachusetts Medical Society. 2001. Diet drug helps keep weight off. *HealthNews* 7(2):6.
34. Schardt, D. 1999. Fat burners. *Nutrition Action Health Letter* 26(6):9–11.
35. Consumer Union. 2001. Fat-fighting fat shows promise. *Consumer Reports on Health* 13(6):7.
36. Nethealth, Inc. 1999. *Herbal therapies.* Available online at www.weightloss2000.com/herbs/herbs_06_all.htm.
37. Goldblatt, B. I. 1997. Advertisers get away with incredible weight-loss claims; how not to succumb. *Environmental Nutrition* 21(1):3.
38. Environmental Nutrition, Inc. 1997. Fasting for health offers few benefits, questionable safety. *Environmental Nutrition* 20(5):7.

39. ACSM. 2000. *ACSM's Guidelines for Exercise Testing and Prescription* (6th ed.). Philadelphia: Lippincott Williams and Wilkins.

40. Eller, D. 1997. The best way to lose weight. *Health* 11(4):34–36.

41. White, D. 1999. Inner joy is key to dutiful exercise, *the Commercial Appeal*, 160(4):C1–3.

42. Tufts University. 1998. Ever 'forget' you're trying to eat less? Write it down. *Tufts University Health & Nutrition Letter* 16(8):8.

43. Furia, J. 2001. The female athlete triad. *Medscape Orthopaedics & Sports Medicine* 3(1), Medscape, Inc., **www.medscape.com/medscape/ Orthosportsmed/journal**.

44. American Psychiatric Association. 1994. *Diagnostic and Statistical Manual of Mental Disorders* (4th ed.). Washington, D.C.: The Association.

45. Consumers Union. 2000. Secrets of successful losers. *Consumer Reports on Health* 12(1):1, 3–4.

46. Tufts University. 1999. Hungry an hour after eating Chinese food. *Tufts University Health & Nutrition Letter* 17(8):4–5.

47. Tufts University. 1996. If you want to quit smoking but fear the weight gain. *Tufts University Health & Nutrition Letter* 13(11):6–7.

48. Tufts University. 1998. What it takes to take off weight (and keep it off). *Tufts University Health & Nutrition Letter* 15(11):4–5.

Suggested Readings

Kirby, J. 1999. *Dieting for Dummies*. Chicago: The American Dietetic Association.

Written by a registered dietician who represents the American Dietetic Association, a trustworthy source of scientifically sound nutrition and food information. This book presents a way to achieve and maintain a healthy weight without starvation, fear, or failure. Packed with smart, practical insight into nutrition and weight, it provides straight answers to dieting questions. It offers no magic bullet; neither is it filled with dietary restrictions and weight loss gimmicks. Instead, it provides strategies and tips for long-term weight management success. It deciphers fact from fiction. The focus is on health, not cosmetics. This book discusses all facets of weight loss, including helpful information about eating disorders, overweight children, dietary guidelines, fat replacers, calorie-shaving substitutions, a comparison of weight-loss programs, and an exposè of diet fads and scams (including some best-selling diet books).

Margolis, S., and L. J. Cheskin. 1999. *The Johns Hopkins White Papers: Weight Control*. Baltimore, Md.: The Johns Hopkins Medical Institutions.

Designed for the lay public, this monograph presents an overview of issues related to weight loss, compares popular weight-loss methods, describes medical conditions that may cause obesity, and outlines lifestyle treatments for weight loss. This monograph is updated annually.

Nichter, M. 2001. *Fat Talk: What Girls and Their Parents Say About Dieting*. Cambridge, Mass.: Harvard University Press.

The author uses a narrative style to explore the influence of peers, family, and media on girls' sense of self. In extensive excerpts from interviews, we hear how these girls differ from those we encounter in surveys. In particular, despite widespread dissatisfaction with one aspect or another of their bodies, the girls did not diet so much as talk about dieting. "Fat talk," Nichter wryly argues, is a kind of social ritual among friends, a way of establishing solidarity. Nichter examines the issues and struggles that mothers face in bringing up healthy daughters today—and suggests how girls may be moved beyond punishing images of ideal beauty. This book presents results of a study that followed hundreds of teenaged girls for three years that revealed how girls think about their bodies, their appearance, their culture.

Nieman, D. 1999. *Exercise Testing and Prescription—A Health Related Approach*. Mountain View, Calif.: Mayfield Publishing Co.

In this text a separate chapter is devoted to the relationship of physical activity and obesity. The author provides a comprehensive review of the literature on physical activity and obesity citing more than 300 studies. Concepts, issues, and misconceptions are thoroughly discussed and documented.

Peeke, P. 2000. *Fight Fat Over Forty*. New York: Penguin Publishing.

The author is a medical doctor who thinks that most diets are science fair projects that human beings put themselves through to lose weight fast. The author maintains that everyday stress leads to the overproduction of stress hormones, which in turn boosts appetite. The prescription for weight loss and weight maintenance comes in three parts: stress-resilient nutrition, physical activity, and regrouping.

Wardlaw, G. M. 2000. *Contemporary Nutrition: Issues and Insights* (4th ed.). St. Louis: WCB/McGraw-Hill.

Comprehensive reference text on nutrition with separate chapters on dieting, weight control, and eating disorders.

Name _____ **Date** _____ **Section** _____

Assessment Activity 8-1

Assessing Your Body Image

Accepting those physical characteristics unique to you is an important first step to constructing a positive body image. In this assessment you will assess your body image from two perspectives: ideal and actual.

Directions: The following sets of bipolar adjectives relate to physical characteristics and appearance. Indicate your rating of these characteristics as follows:

1. Ideal body image: Circle the number that best represents how you would like your body to be in terms of each characteristic.
2. Actual body image: Put an X through the number that represents how you believe your body actually is in terms of each characteristic.

Body Image Characteristics

Graceful	1	2	3	4	5	6	7	8	9	10	Clumsy
Tall	1	2	3	4	5	6	7	8	9	10	Short
Slim	1	2	3	4	5	6	7	8	9	10	Fat
Large	1	2	3	4	5	6	7	8	9	10	Small
Attractive	1	2	3	4	5	6	7	8	9	10	Unattractive
Rugged	1	2	3	4	5	6	7	8	9	10	Delicate
Flabby	1	2	3	4	5	6	7	8	9	10	Muscular
Soft	1	2	3	4	5	6	7	8	9	10	Hard
Shapely	1	2	3	4	5	6	7	8	9	10	Unshapely
Weak	1	2	3	4	5	6	7	8	9	10	Strong
Well-proportioned	1	2	3	4	5	6	7	8	9	10	Poorly proportioned

Now answer the following questions:

1. Which characteristics of the ideal body image, if any, do you think can be achieved by dieting alone? by exercise alone?
2. How many of the items had a gap between the circles and the Xs?
3. On those items with a large gap, which characteristics of your actual body image can be changed?

4. What difference would it make if your body conformed to your "ideal body image"? Would it have any real influence on your relationships and your happiness?

From *Your Body Image*. Available online at www.hc-sc.gc.ca/hppb/nutrition/pube/vtlk/vitlk13.htm.

Name _____ **Date** _____ **Section** _____

Assessment Activity 8-2

Calculating Caloric Expenditure Through Exercise

Directions: This exercise illustrates the calculations used for determining weight loss through exercise. In the example in Part 1, a subject weighing 195 pounds wishes to lose 12 pounds by exercising 40 minutes per day five times per week. The form of exercise will be riding a bike at 13 MPH. Table 8-4 gives the appropriate coefficient (0.071) for this activity, and as previously mentioned there are 3500 calories in 1 pound of fat. Study this example and then apply it to the problem presented in Part 2 to answer the following questions:

- How many calories are expended per exercise session?
- How many pounds may be lost per week at this energy expenditure?
- How long will it take to lose 12 lbs.?

Part 1

1. Multiply body weight by the appropriate activity coefficient:
   195 lbs. × 0.071 = 13.8 calories/min.
   13.8 calories/min. × 40 min. = 552 calories

2. Multiply the number of calories expended per workout by the number of workouts per week:
   552 calories × 5 workouts/week = 2760 calories/week
   $$\frac{2760 \text{ calories/week}}{3500 \text{ calories/lb.}} = 0.79 \text{ lost/week}$$

3. Divide the total pounds you want to lose (12 lbs.) by the number of pounds lost per week:
   $$\frac{12 \text{ lbs.}}{0.79 \text{ lbs. lost/week}} = 15.2 \text{ weeks}$$

   This subject would lose 12 pounds in fifteen weeks by riding a bike at 13 MPH for 40 minutes per day five times per week. Your weight-loss goals can be determined in the same way.

Part 2

Now apply your knowledge of energy expenditure through exercise by solving the following problem. Jim weighs 220 pounds and wishes to lose 25 pounds by jogging at 5 MPH for 30 minutes per exercise session five days per week. Do the calculations to solve Jim's problem by following these steps:

1. Multiply body weight by the appropriate activity coefficient from table 8-4 for jogging 5 MPH.

   220 lbs. × _____ coefficient = _____ calories/min.

   _____ calories/min. × 30 min. = _____ calories

2. Multiply the number of calories expended per workout by the number of workouts per week:

   _____ calories × 5 workouts/week = _____

   _____ calories/week ÷ 3500 calories/lb. = _____ lbs. lost/week

3. Divide the total pounds to be lost by the number of pounds lost per week.

   25 lbs. ÷ _____ lbs. lost/week = _____ weeks

4. a. How many calories would Jim expend per exercise session? _____

   b. How many pounds will he lose per week at this energy expenditure? _____

   c. How many weeks will it take Jim to lose 25 pounds? _____

Name _____ **Date** _____ **Section** _____

Assessment Activity 8-3

Estimating Your Basal Metabolic Rate

Directions: Study the example in Part 1 and then calculate your personal total energy expenditure in Part 2.

Part 1
The calculations for estimating BMR use different constants for men and women. The constant for men is 1 calorie per kilogram (2.2 lbs.) per hour; for women it is 0.9 calories per kilogram per hour. These constants are referred to as the *BMR factor*. An example for a 125-pound woman follows:

1. Convert body weight in pounds to kilograms:
   125 lbs. ÷ 2.2 lbs. = 56.8 kg
2. Multiply weight in kilograms by the BMR factor:
   56.8 kg × 0.9 calories/kg/hr. = 51.1 calories/hr.
3. Multiply calories per hour by 24 hours:
   51.1 calories/hr. × 24 hrs./day = 1226.4 calories/day
4. The BMR is 1226.4 calories per day.

To determine the total daily calories expended, you need to estimate the number of calories used in muscular movement during a typical day. This is a rough approximation at best, but you should be within your range if you follow these guidelines and select the category that fits you best.

1. Sedentary—student, desk job, sitting during most of your work and leisure time: add 40–50% of the BMR.
2. Light activity—teacher, assembly-line worker, walk 2 miles regularly: Add 55–65% of the BMR.
3. Moderate activity—waitress, waiter, aerobic exercise at about 75% of maximum heart rate: Add 65–70% of the BMR.
4. Heavy activity—construction worker, aerobic exercise above 75 percent of maximum heart rate: Add 75–100% of BMR.

If our subject determines that her level of activity is in the light category, she will calculate the range of her daily total caloric expenditure as follows:

1. Multiply BMR by the level of activity:
   1226.4 calories/day × 0.55 = 674.5 calories/day
   1226.4 calories/day × 0.65 = 797.2 calories/day

2. Add BMR calories to level of activity calories to get total calories:
   a. 1226.4 + 674.5 = 1900.9 calories/day
   b. 1226.4 + 797.2 = 2023.6 calories/day

This subject's total calorie expenditure in a day falls between 1900.9 and 2023.6 calories.

Part 2
Calculate your BMR by doing the following:

1. Convert body weight (BW) in pounds in kilograms:
   _____ lbs. ÷ 2.2 = _____ kg
2. Multiply weight in kilograms by the BMR factor for your sex (male factor 1.0, female factor 0.9):
   _____ × _____ kg = _____ calories/hr.
3. Multiply calories per hour by 24 hours per day to get the number of calories burned per day:
   _____ calories/hr. × 24 = _____ calories/day
4. BMR: _____ calories/day

Determine your level of physical activity:

1. Multiply BMR by the level of activity factor:
   _____ × _____ = _____ calories/day
   _____ × _____ = _____ calories/day
2. Add the number of BMR calories to the level of activity calories to get the range of total calories expended in a day:
   _____ calories + _____ calories = _____ calories/day
   _____ calories + _____ calories = _____ calories/day

3. Total calories expended range from _____ to _____.

Name _____ **Date** _____ **Section** _____

Assessment Activity 8-4

Assessing Calorie Costs of Activities

According to the ACSM, optimal weight-loss benefits are derived from activities that burn 300 calories per activity session. The purpose of this assessment is to determine the amount of time required to expend 300 calories.

Directions: Following are listed the caloric costs for three activities (see table 8-4). Add seven activities of your choice from table 8-4 and complete the information required in each column to determine the amount of time required to burn 300 calories. An example is provided for a person weighing 180 pounds who walks at a rate of 4.5 MPH.

Activity	Caloric Cost/Min./Lb.	×	Weight	=	Calories/Min.	300 Calories/Min.	=	Recommended Workout Time
Example (180-lb. person):						$\frac{300}{8.64}$		
1. Walking	0.048	×	180	=	8.64		=	34.7 min.
Personal Assessment:						$\frac{300}{}$		
1. Walking	0.048	×		=			=	
2. Aerobic dance	0.062	×		=		$\frac{300}{}$	=	
3. Raking	0.034	×		=		$\frac{300}{}$	=	
4.		×		=		$\frac{300}{}$	=	
5.		×		=		$\frac{300}{}$	=	
6.		×		=		$\frac{300}{}$	=	
7.		×		=		$\frac{300}{}$	=	
8.		×		=		$\frac{300}{}$	=	
9.		×		=		$\frac{300}{}$	=	
10.		×		=		$\frac{300}{}$	=	

9

Coping with and Managing Stress

 Online Learning Center

Log on to our Online Learning Center (OLC) for access to these additional resources:

- Chapter key term flashcards
- Learning objectives
- Additional goals for behavior change
- Concentration game
- Self-scoring chapter quizzes

- Additional lab activities

The OLC also offers weblinks for study and exploration of wellness topics. Access these links through **www.mhhe.com/ anspaugh5e**, click on "Student Center," click on "Chapter 9," and then click on "Web Activities."

 Goals for Behavior Change

- Identify your personal sources of stress.
- View stress as holding potential for personal growth.
- Develop a time-management plan.
- Select strategies for managing stress.
- Put into action a stress-management plan.

Key Terms

coping
distress
eustress
general adaptation
  syndrome (GAS)

psychoneuroimmunology
  (PNI)
relaxation techniques
stress
stressor

Objectives

After completing this chapter, you will be able to do the following:

- Define *stress*.
- Identify potential stressors.
- Describe the various types of stress.
- Describe the stages of the general adaptation syndrome (GAS).

- Explain the body's physiological response to stress.
- List the short- and long-term health effects of stress.
- Identify strategies that effectively deal with stress.

tress profoundly affects people's lives. Everyone—students, businesspeople, parents, athletes—lives with stress. Stress is frequently viewed as an enemy. This is a misconception. Stress is often neither positive nor negative. How people deal with or react to what they perceive as stress is what determines its effect on their lives. As has been stated, "It is often said that stress is one of the most destructive elements in people's daily lives, but that is only a half truth. The way we react to stress appears to be more important than the stress itself."[1] The effects of stress can be either positive or negative. Positively used, stress can be a motivator for an improved quality of life. Viewed negatively, it can be destructive.

What is Stress?

Dr. Hans Selye was the first to define the term **stress** as the "nonspecific response of the body to any demands made upon it." It can be characterized by diverse reactions, such as muscle tension, acute anxiety, increased heart rate, hypertension, shallow breathing, giddiness, and even joy. From a positive perspective, stress is a force that generates and initiates action. Using Selye's definition, stress can accompany pleasant or unpleasant events. Selye referred to stress judged as "good" as **eustress.** This form of stress is the force that serves to initiate emotional and psychological growth. Eustress provides the experience of pleasure, adds meaning to life, and fosters an attitude that tries to find positive solutions to complex problems. Eustress can accompany a birth, graduation, the purchase of a new car, the development of a new friendship, the accomplishment of

a difficult task, and success in an area that previously produced anxiety. **Distress,** on the other hand, is stress that results in negative responses. Unchecked, negative stress can interfere with the physiological and psychological functioning of the body and may ultimately result in a disease or disability.[2]

Stress also provides humans with the ability to respond to challenges or dangers. It is vital to self-protection and also serves as a motivator that enhances human ability.

A **stressor** is any physical, psychological, or environmental event or condition that initiates the stress response (figure 9-1).

See Assessment Activity 9-2 to evaluate your own stress level in the different categories listed in figure 9-1.

What is considered a stressor for one person may not be a stressor for another. Speaking in front of a group may be stimulating for one person and terrifying for another. Some people experience extreme test anxiety and others feel confident about written assessments. Fortunately, the stress response is not a genetic trait, and because it is a response to external conditions, it is subject to personal control. A person may not avoid taking a test, but he or she can apply techniques and take precautions that lessen the effects of the stress. For example, knowing the material thoroughly and engaging in deep breathing several minutes before a test helps dissipate anxiety. To maximize quality of life, people can find positive ways of coping with stress.

A stress response can enhance and increase the level of either mental or physical performance. This response is referred to as the *inverted-U theory*.[3] Not enough stress (hypostress) may result in a poorer effort, but too

Figure 9-1 Stressors That Can Create Distress

much stress can inhibit effort. There appears to be an optimal level of stress that results in peak performance (figure 9-2). Achievement of an appropriate level of stress depends on the person and the type of task. Table 9-1 lists some of the potentially positive outcomes associated with stress. Your body is constantly attempting to maintain a physiological balance. This balance is referred to as *homeostasis*. Any event or circumstance that causes a disruption (a stressor) in your body's homeostasis requires some type of adaptive behavior. Physiologically, whether a stressor is perceived as positive or negative, the body responds with the same three-stage process. This series of changes is known as the **general adaptation syndrome (GAS).**[4] The three phases are alarm, resistance, and exhaustion (figure 9-3).

The *alarm* phase occurs when homeostasis is initially disrupted. The brain perceives a stressor and prepares the body to deal with it, a response sometimes referred to as the *fight-or-flight syndrome*. The subconscious appraisal of the stressor results in an emotional reaction. The emotional response stimulates a physical reaction associated with stress, such as the muscles becoming tense, the stomach tightening, the heart rate increasing, the mouth becoming dry, and the palms of the hands sweating.

The second stage is *resistance*. In this phase the body meets the perceived challenge through increased strength, endurance, sensory capacities, and sensory acuity. Hormonal secretions regulate the body's response to a stressor. Only after meeting and satisfying the demands of a stressful situation can the internal activities of the body return to normal. Girdano and George[5] argue that people have different levels of energy to deal with stressors. For short-term stressors, only a superficial level of energy is required, allowing deeper energy levels to be protected. Superficial levels of energy are readily accessible and easily renewable. Unfortunately, all stress cannot be resolved with superficial energy levels. When long-term or deep levels of stress are experienced, the amount of energy available is limited. If sufficient stress is experienced for an extended period, loss of adaptation can result. Although some scientists believe that energy stores may be genetically programmed, all people can replenish their energy stores through exercise, good nutrition, adequate sleep, and other positive behaviors.

When stressors become chronic or pervasive, the third phase, *exhaustion*, is reached. In exhaustion, energy stores have been depleted and rest must occur. Although weeks to years may pass before the effects of long-term stressors occur, if a person does not learn how to adequately deal with stress, exhaustion will result. At this point, stress may affect the stomach, heart, blood pressure, muscles, and joints. Fortunately, the effects of stressors can be completely or partially reversed when adequate management techniques are initiated. The earlier these management techniques are learned and used, the fewer problems result.

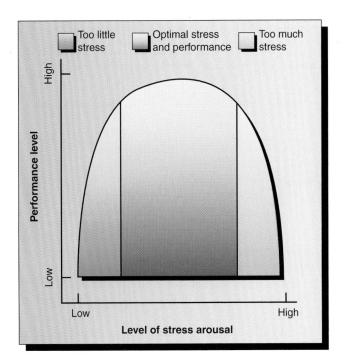

Figure 9-2 The Inverted-U Theory

Table 9-1 Positive Outcomes of Stress

Mental	Emotional	Physical
Enhanced creativity	Sense of control	High energy level
Enhanced thinking ability	Responsiveness to environment	Increased stamina
Greater goal orientation	Improved interpersonal relationships	Flexibility of muscles and joints
Enhanced motivation	Improved morale	Freedom from stress-related disease

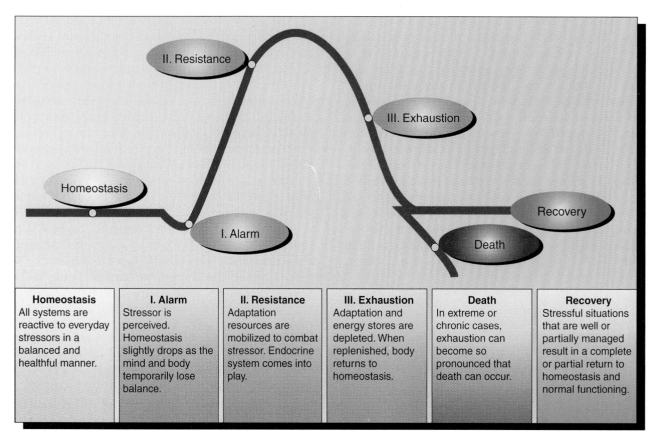

Figure 9-3 The General Adaptation Syndrome (GAS)

Homeostasis	I. Alarm	II. Resistance	III. Exhaustion	Death	Recovery
All systems are reactive to everyday stressors in a balanced and healthful manner.	Stressor is perceived. Homeostasis slightly drops as the mind and body temporarily lose balance.	Adaptation resources are mobilized to combat stressor. Endocrine system comes into play.	Adaptation and energy stores are depleted. When replenished, body returns to homeostasis.	In extreme or chronic cases, exhaustion can become so pronounced that death can occur.	Stressful situations that are well or partially managed result in a complete or partial return to homeostasis and normal functioning.

Sources of Stress and Warning Signs

Most stressful situations fall into one of three categories: (1) harm and loss, (2) threat, and (3) challenge.[6] Examples of *harm-and-loss situations* are the death of a loved one, loss of personal property, physical assault, physical injury, and severe loss of self-esteem. *Threat situations* may be real or perceived and can range from being caught in traffic to being unable to perceive an event. Threatening events tax a person's ability to deal with everyday life. Threat stressors are any stressors that result in anger, hostility, frustration, or depression. *Challenge situations* are catalysts for either growth or pain. These stressors often involve major life changes and include such events as taking a new job, leaving home, graduating from college, and getting married. Challenge events are usually perceived as being good but involve stress because they disrupt homeostasis and require considerable psychological and physical adjustment.

Being aware of the mental and physical signals associated with stress is the beginning step in learning how to manage it. Assessment Activity 9-1 will aid you in identifying some of the major stressors. By using self-assessments to monitor for signs of stress, you can avoid excessive stress. The negative results of distress are shown in table 9-2. Indicators of excessive distress include the following:

- Chronic fatigue, migraine headaches, sweating, lower-back pain, sleep disturbances, weakness, dizziness, diarrhea, and constipation
- Harder and/or longer work or study while accomplishing less, an inability to concentrate, general disorientation
- Denial that there is a problem or troubling event
- Increased incidence of illness, such as colds and flu or constant worry about illness or becoming ill; overuse of over-the-counter drugs for the purpose of self-medication
- Depression, irritability, anxiety, apathy, an overwhelming urge to cry or run and hide, and feelings of unreality
- Excessive behavior patterns, such as spending too much money, drinking, breaking the law, and developing addictions
- Accident proneness
- Signs of reclusiveness and avoidance of other people
- Emotional tension, "keyed up" feeling, easy startling, nervous laughter, anxiety, hyperkinesia, and nervous tics

Table 9-2 Negative Results of Distress

Mental	Physical	Emotional
Short-term effects		
Poor memory	Flushed face	Irritability
Inability to concentrate	Cold hands	Disorganization
Low creativity	Gas	Conflicts
Poor self-control	Rapid breathing	Mood swings
Low self-esteem	Shortness of breath	Chronic sleep problems
	Dry mouth	Acid stomach
		Overindulgence in alcohol, drugs, food
Long-term effects		
Bouts of depression	Hypertension	Overweight/underweight
Mild paranoia	Coronary disease	Drug abuse
Low tolerance for ambiguity	Ulcers	Excessive smoking
Forgetfulness	Migraine/tension headaches	Ineffective use of work/leisure time
Inability to make decisions/quick to make decisions	Strokes	Overreaction to mild work pressure
	Allergies	

HealthQuest Activities

- The *How Stressed Are You?* activity in Module 1 allows you to look at several areas of your life (including money, school, relationships, and health) and identify stress caused by events and daily hassles. You can also rate your perceived stress level for each area. Use this feature to find out which area or areas generate the highest levels of stress for you.

- The *CyberStress* activity in Module 1 simulates a stress-filled day and can be used to help you assess your reactions to daily stressors. Choose the scenario that most closely matches your scenario. For example, if you work and go to school, you should check both on the preferences screen. As you are presented with stressful situations, choose the reaction closest to how you would react. At the feedback screen, print the screen showing your score. Then evaluate your experience by answering the questions in the *What Do You Think?* section.

Factors Generating a Stress Response

As mentioned earlier, the criteria for a stressful event and the response to that event for any person are unique to the individual. Figure 9-4 provides an overview of the complexity of the stress experience and some of the many moderating effects. For instance, a dysfunctional homelife (characterized by an alcoholic parent, a difficult divorce, or extreme poverty) may contribute to a personality that is more susceptible to difficult events, such as poor grades or a failed relationship. This combination of inadequate preparation for life along with an event perceived as personal failure is likely to lead to depression, anxiety, or anger. Conversely, a person whose background has fostered a deep sense of self-worth and meaningfulness will be able to better handle a difficult event and not perceive the event as a personal failure. Poor grades may be the result of poor study habits, an undiagnosed learning behavior, or inadequate sleep, and a failed relationship may be the result of a poor match, bad timing, or immaturity.

Physiological Responses to Stress

Stress abounds in life and can be experienced as the result of happy and unhappy events. Regardless of the stressor, each time a stressful event occurs, a series of neurological and hormonal messages are sent throughout the body.

The nervous system serves as a reciprocal network that sends messages between the awareness centers of the brain and the organs and muscles of the body. Part of this system is referred to as the *limbic system*. The limbic system contains centers for

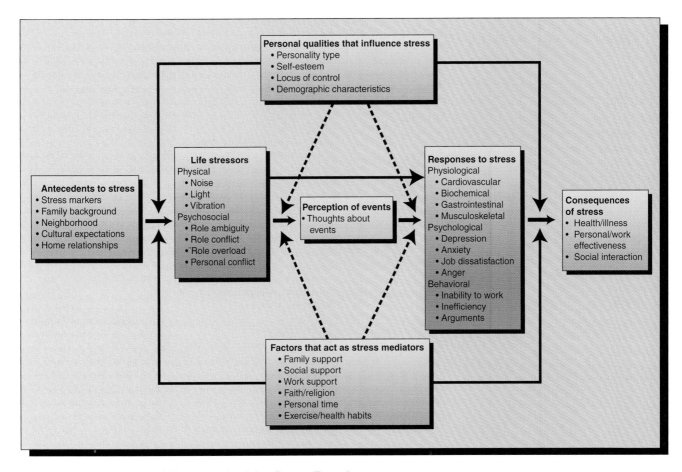

Figure 9-4 Theoretical Framework of the Stress Experience

emotions, memory, learning relay, and hormone production and includes the pituitary gland, thalamus, and hypothalamus.

When a stressor is encountered, the body sends a message to the brain via the nervous system. The brain then synthesizes the message and determines whether it is valid. If a message is not verified by the brain as being threatening, the limbic system overrides the initial response and the body continues to function normally. If the initial response is translated as accurate and a stressor is detected, the body responds with some emotion (fear, joy, terror), and the hypothalamus begins to act.

The hypothalamus sends a hormonal message to the pituitary gland, which then releases a hormone (ACTH) that helps signal other glands in the endocrine system to secrete additional hormones, providing fuel to respond with the fight-or-flight reaction. Systolic blood pressure may rise 15 to 20 mmHg while fluid is retained. The adrenal cortex increases blood pressure to facilitate transportation of food and oxygen to active parts of the body.[7] Blood volume is increased.

The hypothalamus also sends a message to release the hormones epinephrine and norepinephrine, which initiate a variety of physiological changes. These changes include increased heart rate, increased metabolic rate, increased oxygen consumption, and the release of hormones called *endorphins*, which decrease sensations of pain.

The autonomic nervous system is responsible for a second major set of physiological responses. In reaction to a threat, the autonomic nervous system increases heart rate, strength of the skeletal muscles, mental activity, and basal metabolic rate; dilates the coronary arteries, pupils, bronchial tubes, and arterioles; and constricts the abdominal arteries. This system also returns the body to a normal, relaxed state.

Stress and the Immune System

The mind and body act on each other in remarkable ways. Our immune system is a part of the body's defense against illness and disease originating from factors and conditions both outside and inside our bodies.

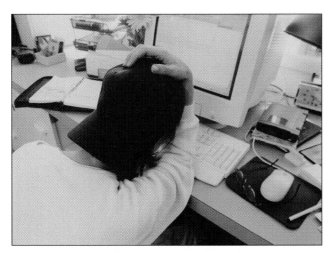

Everyday problems can trigger the stress response. What are your biggest stressors?

The immune system consists of a variety of mechanical and chemical defenses that serve to protect against such outside invaders as microorganisms, allergens, and other substances as well as inside factors such as mutating cells or improperly functioning tissue. The immune system is a functional system rather than an organ system and, as a result, seems to be prone to the effects of stress when fighting off the situations and conditions previously mentioned.[8]

The biological link between emotions and disease and even death is strong. Mortality is three times higher in people with few close relationships than in those with numerous such relationships, and people with strong support groups have additional protection against life stressors. Death rates are higher for cancer patients with pessimistic attitudes. Illness is more common among people who feel locked into strife-ridden marriages. AIDS patients with healthy psyches seem better able to withstand disease.[9]

The immune function seems to be affected by the relationship between the brain and nervous system. This relationship among brain, nervous system, and immune response has been the outgrowth from the field of study called **psychoneuroimmunology (PNI)**. This relatively new medical discipline seeks to explain the connection between the brain, the nervous system, and the body's response to infections and deviated cell division. Several studies have shown that chronic stress suppresses the body's ability to initiate an effective immune response. This suppression is attributed to an increase in corticosteroids, produced during chronic stress. This increase in corticosteroid levels delays and weakens the immune response.[10] O'Leary found that chronic stress suppresses the immune system, particularly when the stress is associated with social disruption (leaving home for the first time), psy-

chological depression (feeling "down" for prolonged periods), or some negative personality attribute (lack of self-confidence).[11] It has also been found that immunosuppression is associated with loneliness and feelings of hopelessness.[12] Stress has also been demonstrated to be associated with infertility.[13,14] No known specific reason exists for this correlation. Whether the stress is the result of infertility problems or another source, stress reduction intervention results in significant improvement in conception rates.

Because stress affects the immune system, the body becomes more susceptible to a multitude of ailments, from colds to cancer. Respiratory conditions, such as asthma, may become worse. The cardiovascular system reacts by constricting the blood vessels while increasing blood volume. The result is a rise in blood pressure throughout a stress-ridden day. Multiple increases in blood pressure can eventually contribute to chronic high blood pressure. More forceful contraction of the heart elevates levels of free fatty acids, enhancing the development of clogged arteries leading to and including the heart. In extreme cases, sudden death can occur, especially for a person who has been experiencing high levels of uncontrolled stress for an extended period.

Headaches, including migraines, have long been associated with stress. Tension headaches are caused by involuntary contractions of the scalp, head, and neck muscles. Typical muscular reaction to stress is contracting or tensing. When chronic stress occurs, the body reacts by being constantly ready to respond, and the muscles become braced, always in a state of tension. More stress magnifies the tension the muscles are already undergoing. Increased muscular tension manifests in headaches, backaches, neckaches, and other pains. The smooth muscles that control internal organs also experience pains. More intense contractions can lead to stomachache, diarrhea, hypertension, heartburn, gastritis, bloating, inflammation of the pancreas, and blockage of the bile ducts.

Stress decreases saliva in the mouth, often making speaking awkward. Swallowing may become difficult, and the increase in stomach acids contributes to ulcer pain. People tend to perspire more, and electrical currents are transmitted more quickly across the skin. Skin conditions such as acne, psoriasis, herpes, hives, and eczema are exacerbated.

Stress also seems to affect the body's nutritional status. Individual nutritional patterns can also influence stress management efforts. For example, eating too much or too little, eating the wrong kinds of food, and overusing products such as caffeine or alcohol upset homeostasis. Diets high in fat, sugar, and processed foods place a heavy burden on various body systems. Ingesting too few calories can lead to the breakdown of lean tissue. To meet the demands of stress, you should

Wellness Across the Generations
Women's Changing Roles

As many families now have two-career households and more women work outside the home, it is natural to wonder if the double demands of household and worksite pose a threat to women's physical and psychological health. A study done at Duke University Medical Center by Linda Luecken and her colleagues, suggests that they do.

The study focused on 109 women with full-time clerical and customer-service jobs. Some had children and some did not. The results indicated that working women with children at home had higher levels of cortisol (a stress hormone thought to reflect high levels of distress), a greater lack of personal control, and more risk for cardiovascular disease than working women with no children. Both groups of women reported similar levels of work strain, but the working mothers reported higher levels of home strain, including greater demands and less control. This increased strain seemed to be caused by the reality that these women performed most of the child-rearing and household duties. Such chores as laundry, cleaning, cooking, chauffeuring, and homework more often fell to the women in the study than to their male partners.

Luecken and her colleagues estimated that working women with children have up to twenty-one hours more work per week than men have. They also found that working mothers have little chance to "unwind," so they have increased sympathetic nervous system arousal both during and after work. Even if male partners help with household duties, they often finish their duties with enough time to relax. The presence of a spouse or significant other did not significantly reduce the physiological and psychological consequences of stress on the working mother. Interestingly, higher income, ethnicity, and the number of children at home did not influence the level of stress.[23]

Here are some ways working mothers might balance the demands of work and household duties:

- Set limits. Schedule and honor your time to relax. Learn to say "no."
- Make lists of your priorities, from most important to least important. Get done what is really important and let the rest go.
- Remember that perfection is the enemy of happiness.
- Team up with other parents to share the load: child care, dinner clubs, or shuttling.
- Pay attention to the moments of joy that parenting and connecting with a partner and friends have to offer.[24]

maintain adequate nutrition through a balanced and varied diet. (Chapter 6 provides guidelines for developing a beneficial nutritional plan.) Table 9-3 provides some insight into the interactive natures of stress, nutritional status, and immunity.

Ultimately, no body system escapes the effects of stress. Long-term presence of certain stress-associated hormones in the brain damages receptors and cells found in the hippocampus. (The hippocampus sends messages when stress is occurring.) Because brain cells do not regenerate, these cells are lost forever. The effects of this loss are unknown, but indications are that eventually affected people become less able to respond to stress appropriately.[15] Assessment Activity 9-3 provides guidelines for identifying stress style and suggests relaxation activities.

Self-Esteem and Stress

How people feel about themselves and others and their perceptions of the stressors in their lives are part of the psychology of stress. Ability to cope with stress often hinges on impressions of how detrimental a stressor is and how adequately resources can deal with the situation. How much stress people feel themselves experiencing is closely associated with their sense of self-esteem. Self-esteem includes beliefs and attitudes about changes, personal talent, skills, and one's ability to deal with the changes and challenges that inevitably occur in life. It is also the basis of self-efficacy and the locus of control (see Chapter 1). The most influential factor in determining response to stress may be people's perceptions of themselves.

Attitude and Stress

The question many researchers have asked is why one person is more susceptible to stress than another. The answer is not altogether clear, but evidence is mounting that one's perception or attitude is a key factor in the stress equation. The realization that our attitude has such a significant impact on our health has led to a new movement in psychology termed "positive psychology." Dr Martin Segilman of the University of

Table 9-3 Stress, Nutritional Status, and Immunity: An Interactive Effect

Although the mechanism is not completely understood, stress significantly affects nutritional status and therefore immunity. Several nutritional factors have implications for how your body responds to stress.

Energy

Stress can increase the body's basic caloric needs by as much as 200%. The stress hormones increase body heat production. When this heat is released, it is not available for cell metabolism. The caloric inefficiency induced by stress accounts for the increased need for energy intake.

Protein

Stress may increase the body's need for protein from 60% to as much as 500%. The integrity of the body's tissues, such as the skin and the tissue lining the mouth, lungs, and nose (called *mucosal tissue*), depends on adequate protein repair and maintenance of secretions of biochemicals that serve as protective agents. The formation of antibodies also requires protein.

Fats

Dietary fatty acids influence the synthesis of a group of fatty acid derivatives called *prostaglandins*. Prostaglandins stimulate or depress other cellular and immune functions in relation to stress.

Vitamins

Vitamin A functions to maintain healthy skin and mucous membranes. Vitamin A—deficient individuals have fewer mucous-secreting cells and those they do have produce less mucous—thus the protection provided by the mucous lining is diminished. Vitamin C has been shown to enhance the engulfing or "eating" actions of the immune cells called *macrophages.* If vitamin C is deficient, macrophages are less mobile and less able to consume disease-causing organisms. Deficiencies of vitamins A, B_{12}, and folate can impair production of the cells that enable antibody responses. Large doses of vitamin E have been associated with suppression of B cells, vital to the immune response. Finally, metabolic requirements for thiamin, riboflavin, and niacin are increased in response to a stressful situation.

Minerals

Deficiencies of zinc impair immune cell reproduction and responsiveness.

Pennsylvania is the founding father of positive psychology. He believes that optimism is a key in maintaining not only our mental health but our physical health as well. Other writers have examined the differences between optimism and pessimism and the impact that these attitudes have on health. What researchers have found is that the fundamental difference between a pessimist and an optimist is the degree of control one feels over the amount of control they have concerning their lives.[16] What is suggested is that we learn feelings of helplessness and this becomes a major factor in depression and stress. Not surprisingly both depression and stress are highly correlated with pessimism. Researchers report that optimists are much better at coping with the anxiety and distress associated with everything from infertility, heart surgery, cancer, to higher grade point averages in law students. Another study by Mayo Clinic researchers compared the health of 839 men and women to scores on a personality test they took thirty years previously. It was found that those who had an optimistic attitude in their younger years were 19 percent more likely to still be alive than their pessimistic counterparts.

To help develop more positive optimistic attitudes:

1. **Teach yourself a lesson.** Find something positive in a sad or stressful situation by what you have learned from the experience. Don't ignore the negatives but do learn from them without dwelling on them.

2. **Interrupt negative thoughts.** Get out of the pessimistic frame of mind. Force yourself to think positive thoughts. Think of pleasant memories. Don't allow the negative to set you off on a "pity party" or a self-flagellation.

3. **Set realistic goals.** Set achievable realistic goals. Positive thinkers have developed the art of meeting goals (see the section on time management).

4. **Be good to yourself.** Treat yourself to the things you love—it is essential to building confidence and creating a sense of control over your life. Keep in mind that the purpose is to take control; don't do something because it is a habit—do it because you want to.

5. **Go digging for silver.** Seek the bright side of things. Make sure you find at least one positive thing that happens each day. Take an appreciation appraisal each day. When irritating or disappointing events occur, ask yourself, "What did I learn from this that will make me a better person?"

6. **Be glad it's not worse.** When you are low, think of someone less fortunate than you. Write down or say "I'm glad that . . . " or "I'm lucky to. . . ." People who can find positives to reflect on report more satisfaction with their lives than those who are always pointing to the negative.

7. **Fake it.** When all else fails, keep on smiling. Project the mood you want to get back. Find something that makes you laugh. It is hard to be down if you are smiling and laughing.

Gender and Stress

Researchers have found interesting differences between men and women in their reactions to stress. Women's blood pressure goes up less than men's in reaction to stress. However women tend to react to a wider range of outside stressors than men. Women feel stress more often because they take a holistic view of everyday life. A man tends to worry if his family is sick; his wife takes on the burdens of the whole neighborhood.[17] For certain, life is more stress filled than 200 years ago. Stress and anxiety have become a core theme in our lives. The challenge we face in our quest for high level wellness is not to master the threats (stressors), but our all-too-human responses to them.

Personality and Stress

Two physicians, Friedman and Roseman,[18] have written extensively about personality, cardiovascular disease, and stress. These researchers have described two stress-related personality types—type A and type B. Most people are neither type exclusively but fall somewhere between the two.

Type A personality is characterized by an urgent sense of time, impatience, competitiveness, aggressiveness, insecurity over status, and inability to relax. People with type A behavior characteristics are likely to be highly stressed. Type B people have a more unhurried approach to their lives. The type B personality does not become as upset at losing or not attaining a goal. Type B people also tend to set more realistic goals.[19] Researchers disagree on whether there is a possible relationship between the stress-prone type A personality and cardiovascular disease.[20]

In general, researchers believe that being a type A personality is not a problem if there is no underlying hostility. However, regardless of whether type A people are more susceptible to heart disease, they do experience more negative effects, such as tiredness and frustration, from short-term stress.

"Stress survivors"—people who handle stress successfully or have successful coping abilities—have several common characteristics. Psychologist Suzanna Kobasa[21] has isolated these attributes and characterized the type of person who exhibits them. A hardy personality tends to remain healthy even under extreme stress. Characteristics of a hardy personality or hardiness are challenge, commitment, and control (see Assessment Activity 9-5).

Challenge is the ability to see change for what it is—that is, not only inevitable but an opportunity for growth and development of unique abilities. *Commitment* is delineated by a strong sense of inner purpose. It is necessary to want to succeed to achieve success.

Wellness Across the Generations

The Time of Our Lives

Although middle age is often dreaded, the changes that inevitably occur as we grow older are not necessarily bad. In fact, more and more elderly adults report that the best time in their lives was not their youth, but rather their midlife years.

One recent study of this question involved more than 3000 people, each of whom answered more than 1100 questions. Researchers found that more than 70 percent of respondents viewed themselves as being in excellent health and felt their lives had purpose and meaning. In fact, nine of ten study participants said they had never experienced the proverbial midlife crisis. Most middle-aged people reported that they had been able to make the adjustment nesessary for life to remain rewarding. Most said that they did not have arthritis, backaches, skin problems, indigestion, constipation, depression, gum disease, high blood pressure, or migraines. And contrary to popular belief, most middle-aged women reported that menopause was a fairly benign experience.

One negative finding of the study is that middle-aged adults are not working hard to maintain a high quality of life. In addition, respondents reported not having enough money and sex—probably two things lacking at any age, not just middle age. However, while sexual satisfaction was low, middle-aged adults seemed to be content overall with their marriages and relationships. Seventy-two percent said that their relationships were very good or excellent, and 90 percent felt that their relationships were unlikely to break up.

Finally, the survey found that by the time adults reached age 65, men felt an average of 12.6 years younger than their actual age and women felt 14.7 years younger than their actual age. As we grow older, our lives can become even more fulfilling, particularly if we can maintain a sense of control over our well-being by practicing healthful lifestyle habits. How can *you* ensure optimal health as you age?

Adapted from Johns Hopkins InteliHealth Online, www.intelihealth.com/IH?ihtIH?d=dm

Commitment is the ability to become involved while maintaining the discernment to know when dedication and desire are harmful. *Control* is the recognition that one has power over one's life and attitudes. People who have a sense of control act in situations rather than react to them.

Dealing with Stress

All events in life precipitate a reaction. How people react or respond to situations differs. **Coping** is the attempt to manage or deal with stress. Coping is independent of outcome—it does not necessarily result in success.

Dealing successfully with stress may require using a variety of techniques (see Real-World Wellness: Guidelines for Dealing with Stress). Because stress-related responses are based primarily on mental perceptions, coping strategies that achieve desirable results may need to originate in a change in attitude or outlook. If specific situations or people are perceived as disruptive, one solution is to avoid them.

Although there are no easy answers, there is always some type of answer or solution. When dealing with a stressor reaches a point where it seems there are no solutions, the tension from the situation becomes increasingly detrimental. It may then become necessary to consider changing attitudes, goals, and values.

Real-World Wellness

Guidelines for Dealing with Stress

Being in school can be so overwhelming. I have many classes, extracurricular activities, and a pile of homework each night. How can I balance it all?

Following are guidelines for effectively dealing with potential harmful stress:

- **Schedule time effectively.** Practice good time-management techniques by using time wisely. This means taking time out for yourself every day and scheduling work when you are usually at your peak ability (see Assessment Activity 9-7).

- **Set priorities.** Know what is important to you. Do not attempt to work on four or five projects simultaneously. Keep your efforts focused on one or two major items.

- **Establish realistic goals.** Goals must be achievable. Do not establish impossible expectations and then become frustrated when they are not accomplished as quickly as you would like. Write down long-range goals and then establish checks for keeping yourself on track and monitoring progress. Short-term goals help you see how you are moving toward your goal and provide rewards as you advance toward success.

- **See yourself as achieving the goals.** Visualize yourself as being successful. Go over in your mind what it will look and feel like to accomplish a goal.

- **Give yourself a break.** Take time every day to exercise and relax.

Seeking the help of a professional counselor is frequently beneficial when attempting to resolve particularly stressful situations. Assessment Activity 9-4 identifies ways to recognize some of the positive and negative behaviors that can be used to deal with stress.

Learning about and using relaxation techniques can help alleviate or even prevent detrimental effects associated with stress. Engaging in positive self-talk and relabeling negative experiences (viewing difficulties as "challenges" rather than as problems, for example) are positive steps in reducing stress-related disorders. Eating well, taking time to enjoy life, laughing, exercising, and living in the present reduce stress. People can handle stress effectively when they work on developing all of their abilities to the fullest, when they develop lifestyles compatible with personal values, and when they develop realistic expectations for themselves. Working toward these goals is the way to establish a wellness lifestyle (see Real-World Wellness: Marta's Day).

Real-World Wellness

Marta's Day

This semester I've been getting up late for class, putting off studying, and eating poorly. I'm feeling very stressed out, and *my grades have begun to suffer. What can I do to get out of this downward spiral?*

Here is an analysis of Marta's day including her stress responses to events in her day and suggestions for other ways to react.

Event	Marta's Stress Response	A Better Approach
Morning: Is late rising for first class; stayed up late studying the night before	Skips first class to study for exam; misses notes from that class and cannot contact friend to see if she can use her notes; skips breakfast	Begin studying for a test a few days before the exam; do not attempt to cram everything into one night; get a good night's rest and get up early to review your notes; eat breakfast and attend first class.
Is late for test	Stays home too long and gets caught in traffic; arrives late for the test; does not have a full hour to complete the test	Leave early to allow for traffic and parking problems; be on time to concentrate on the test and have time to relax a few minutes.
Lunch	Skips lunch—has a soft drink and potato chips	Have a nutritionally balanced meal in a relaxing atmosphere; go with a friend just to chat.
Afternoon: Is late for work because had to return overdue library book	Rushes to library; has to pay fine; has to stand in line at the library for 15 minutes	Write down when books are due and return them on time; use a daily calendar to plan activities and allot time to take care of personal business.
Evening: Watches TV until midnight; neglects to study for test the day after tomorrow	Is too tired and "stressed out" to study so watches TV all evening; has a hamburger and soda for dinner	Take a short nap after work and have a nutritious meal; plan the evening so that some time is spent watching TV and some is spent studying; go to bed early so you can get to school on time and rested.
Next morning: Gets up late for class again	Begins the same cycle of feeling tired and pressured and being late	Analyze current time constraints to determine where more time needs to be allotted and how to develop a more efficient plan (see Assessment Activities 9-6 and 9-7).

Successful coping includes being aware of incidents and situations that you might perceive as being stressful. Recognition of stressors means being aware of how your body responds to stress. Recognition requires continuous monitoring of your body and mind for evidence of excessive stress.

Successful coping takes real effort. One suggestion is to focus on the signals your body is sending when experiencing stress and then to think back to the event or situation that might have triggered those feelings. Another suggestion is to recreate a recent event that has been stressful. After visualizing the episode, write down six ways that the outcome could have been different—three ways it could have been worse and three

ways it could have been better. The latter will increase awareness of how to better handle similar situations in the future. A last suggestion is to try something new. The idea is that you be challenged and meet that challenge successfully. Trying something new and meeting the challenge reinforces your sense of being able to deal with life successfully.[21]

Relaxation Techniques

The ultimate goal in stress coping and management is to reduce the negative effects of stress. Different **relaxation techniques** have proved successful. Brief descriptions of various techniques follow. If you are interested

Real-World Wellness

Progressive Muscle Relaxation

When I'm uptight, my muscles get so tense that I can't relax. What can I do to loosen them again?

There are numerous progressive muscle relaxation activities. The exercises are frequently structured by a facilitator. Some exercises begin with the feet, hands, or face, but because of space constraints, only the relaxing of the face will be described here. You can add the other parts of the body by recording the entire process on audiotape and listening to the tape as often as desired—usually once a day or two to three times a week. Take your time (3 to 4 minutes) for each area of the body.

- Assume a comfortable position and concentrate on the instructions. You may find it beneficial to lie down or sit in a comfortable chair.
- Close your eyes.
- Allow all your muscles to relax and feel loose and heavy. Take several deep breaths.
- Wrinkle your forehead and hold for 6 seconds.
- Notice the feelings.
  - Relax; allow the forehead to become smooth.
  - Notice the feeling of relaxation.
- Frown with your eyes, forehead, and scalp and hold for 6 seconds.
  - Experience the sensation of tension.
  - Relax the muscles.
  - Notice the feelings of relaxation.
- Keeping your eyes closed, clench your jaw and push your teeth together.
  - Hold for 6 seconds.
  - Notice the tension.
  - Relax your jaw and allow your lips to part slightly.
- Now press your tongue against the roof of your mouth and feel the tension.
  - Hold for 6 seconds.
  - Allow your tongue to return to its normal position, experiencing the sensation of relaxation.
- Now press your lips together as tightly as possible.
  - Hold for 6 seconds.
  - Relax and notice the feelings of relaxation over your lips.
- Using the same principles, gradually move through the body from the shoulders to the arms, hands, fingers, back, chest, abdomen, hips, legs, ankles, feet, and toes.

in pursuing the use of these techniques, you can find more information about them in books or on tapes. These books and tapes can be purchased at bookstores or may be found at your library.

Deep Breathing

Deep breathing is the most basic technique used in relaxation and is often the foundation for other methods. The primary benefit of this technique is that it can be done anywhere and anytime. It is beneficial to practice deep breathing several times a day. The methodology consists of completely filling the lungs when breathing so that the abdomen expands outward. Begin by taking a deep breath and then exhaling slowly through the mouth. A hand can be placed on the stomach to ensure that it is fully expanded. If the stomach does not rise, the breath is not deep enough or the abdomen is being held too tightly. Repeat this cycle several times and then rest quietly for 3 to 5 minutes.

Progressive Muscle Relaxation

Progressive muscle relaxation creates awareness of the difference between muscular tension and a relaxed state. This is a three-step process that begins with tens-ing of a muscle group and noticing how the tension feels. Next, make a conscious effort to relax the tension and notice that feeling. The third phase consists of concentrating on the differences between the two sensations. Beginning at either the head working down or at the feet working up, tense and relax all major muscle groups (see Real-World Wellness: Progressive Muscle Relaxation).

Autogenics

Autogenics is the use of self-suggestion to produce a relaxation response. Autogenics begins with a deep breath and a conscious effort to relax. This technique may follow a progression from head to feet or feet to head. Repeat the phrase "My arm feels heavy and warm" several times before moving on to the next muscle group. You can repeat other phrases that carry a calming message such as "I am completely calm and relaxed." End the session by thinking, "I am refreshed and alert." Autogenics takes practice, time, and commitment and should be practiced twice a day for about 10 minutes. Commercial tapes may help guide people wanting to learn autogenics (see Real-World Wellness: Performing Autogenic Training).

Real-World Wellness

Performing Autogenic Training

I'm looking for a practical technique I can use to reduce my stress. I know it's important to relax, but I have a hard time relaxing sometimes. Merely telling myself to relax doesn't work. What can I do to help myself relax?

Autogenic training is a form of hypnosis that helps the practitioner develop images of warmth and relaxation. With practice, autogenic training can increase peripheral blood flow and reduce muscle tension. *Autogenic* means "self-generating." The technique is a type of self-hypnosis that uses deep breathing and conjures images through a series of phrases to evoke the relaxation response. Here are guidelines for practicing autogenics:

- Either sitting or lying down, begin by taking five to six deep breaths and contract any tense muscles.

- Repeat to yourself, "My breathing is slow and even, my breathing is smooth and rhythmic."

- Continue with the deep breathing and imagine you are on a warm, sunny beach with the waves moving in and over your body, generating a warm and relaxed feeling.

- Feel the waves move over your stomach, hips, back, legs, and feet.

- Repeat to yourself, "I am relaxed, I am calm, I am quiet. My breathing is smooth and rhythmic. My heartbeat is calm and regular."

- Starting with your right arm, repeat the following as the breathing continues slowly and regularly: "My right arm and hand are heavy and warm." Continue with your left arm.

- Focus on both arms and repeat the phrase, "My arms and hands are heavy and warm."

- Move the focus to your legs and feet and repeat, "My legs and feet are heavy and warm." Focus on the right side, the left side, and finally both legs at the same time.

- As you proceed through the session, visualize the waves of warmth and relaxation washing over your entire body. Continue to breath slowing and deeply.

- As you prepare to wrap up the session, continue to breath deeply and slowly and begin to get back in touch with where you are. Tell yourself you are warm, safe, secure, and relaxed.

- Count down from 5:
  4. Take a deep breath and visualize the room.
  3. Take a deep breath and begin to stretch.
  2. Take a deep breath and slowly open your eyes.
  1. You are mentally alert and ready to get back to your activity. You are fully awake.

Meditation

Meditation can be approached from a variety of perspectives. As a stress-reduction technique its purpose is to help the practitioner temporarily tune out the world and to invoke relaxation. During a meditation session, the person meditating concentrates or focuses his or her attention on a *mantra*, or particular word or sound, while attempting to eliminate all outside distractions.

Begin by taking a comfortable position on a couch or in a chair. Take several deep breaths, slowly inhaling and exhaling. Shut your eyes or softly focus them on an object so that the details are blurred. Concentrate all your thoughts on a word or phrase that you have selected to use, such as *peace* or *relax*, while continuing to breathe slowly and deeply.[22] The relaxation response can also be initiated by counting breaths backward from 100 or by imagining a white light that slowly travels throughout your body, letting in light and energy while expelling tension and fear. Many commercial meditation tapes are available.

Visualization

Visualization (imagery) is a form of relaxation that uses the imagination. Begin by finding a comfortable position, shut your eyes, and take several deep breaths. Several variations of visualization can then be used. You can imagine a tranquil scene, such as a beach on a sunny day or a valley with a stream or forest, and then place yourself in the scene. Imagine all of the scene's sights, sounds, smells, and feelings. People suffering from a terminal illness frequently imagine scenes in which their immune system attacks or destroys their disease, or they envision themselves as healthy and disease free. People who want to make major life changes, such as losing weight or stopping smoking, can envision themselves slim or not smoking or imagine themselves in trouble situations such as a situation in which you are tempted to overeat or smoke. Then people can envision themselves making wise choices or not engaging in undesirable behaviors. Visualization can also be used to improve athletic performance. Tapes are available that can assist people in learning how to develop this technique.

Biofeedback

Biofeedback, based on scientific principles, is designed to enhance awareness of body functions—it is an educational tool. Sensory equipment demonstrates subtle body changes, such as increases or decreases in skin temperature, muscle contraction, and brain wave variations.

This biofeedback, or feedback on biological processes, enables people to become aware of what is happening in their bodies when stressed and learn how to control tensions through awareness of relaxing sensations. After a few sessions, people should begin to recognize and thereby alter their typical bodily responses to situations that serve as stressors for them.

Massage Therapy

Massage therapy has become an acceptable form of stress reduction and a healing alternative. Some people consider today's American society to be in the midst of a "touch famine." Appropriate touching is lacking even though we recognize the need for physical interaction. Babies who are not handled can die from this type of deprivation. Although adults are not likely to respond so extremely to lack of touch, the need to be touched does not disappear with age. Research findings indicate that massage can promote physical relaxation and well-being. Certified massage therapists are licensed by the American Massage Therapy Association.[26]

Music

The power of music is undisputed. A strong beat and rhythmic music instill in almost all people of any age the desire to respond by moving or dancing. Quiet music soothes by causing people to breathe more deeply, stilling turbulent emotions, reducing metabolic response, and calming the autonomic nervous system.

Humor

Laughter is a powerful stress-reducing agent. A deep laugh temporarily raises pulse rate and blood pressure and tenses the muscles. After a good laugh, however, pulse rate and blood pressure go down and the muscles become more relaxed. Laughter works in two ways. Being able to laugh at a situation reminds you that life is seldom perfect or predictable. Laughing helps keep events in perspective. Laughing also works to reinforce a positive attitude. Laughing or even smiling can improve mood.

Time Management

A major contributor to stress is the pressure associated with time constraints. By effectively using time, you can eliminate a great deal of stress. For the college student, effective use of time is crucial, especially when the student is working and attending school at the same time. Procrastination can add to stress and undermine academic work, personal relationships, and work efforts. Good time management including appropriate prioritizing, scheduling, and the completion of personal responsibilities can contribute to feelings of personal satisfaction.

Certain behaviors or habits can unnecessarily rob you of time:[27]

1. **Workaholism.** *Workaholism* is spending excessive amounts of time working, even though the activity may not be productive. Generally, people who engage in workaholic behavior like to work long hours and do not use time-saving techniques. They also may become overinvolved in unimportant tasks that eat away at their time, requiring them to use extra time to accomplish important tasks.

2. **Time juggling.** Time jugglers constantly overschedule themselves, often making promises to be in more than one place at a time. Because it is frequently impossible to do several things at once or be in two places at the same time, this behavior often results in the neglecting of important activities.

3. **Procrastination.** Procrastinators consistently put off until later things that could just as easily be done now. Some procrastinators choose the simplest of two tasks to do now to avoid the really important ones until the last possible minute, when the pressure is on.

4. **Perfectionism.** Perfectionists go beyond trying to do their best to achieve perfection. Because standards of perfection vary from one person to the next, this behavior rarely results in a sense of accomplishment, and the inability to achieve impossible goals contributes to feelings of dissatisfaction and failure.

5. **Yesism.** *Yesism* is the inability to tell anyone "no." Extremely nice people often suffer from this condition because they don't like to disappoint others or they fear being rejected, even if saying "yes" ends up costing them.

Time Management Suggestions

Effective time management allows us to have a sense of direction and to fulfill the requirements for using time in a productive satisfying fashion. Some suggestions for appropriate use of your time:

1. **Set goals.** Spend time planning your goals. Think of short-term (one year or less) goals and long-term (1–3 years) goals. Ask yourself if the goals established are essential, important, or trivial. A good question is "When does this task have to be completed?" Your goals should cause you to "stretch" but not "break" as you strive to achieve them.

2. **Prioritize.** Use the 80/20 rule, which states that 80 percent of the reward comes from 20 percent of the effort. Prioritize time to concentrate your efforts on those items that will provide the greatest reward for fulfilling your short- and

long-term goals. Once your priorities have been established, start with the most important tasks to be accomplished—don't procrastinate.

3. **Develop a time framework.** To help alleviate stress, establish the amount of time to be spent on each activity. Some tasks cannot be completed in a day's time. Estimate the days or weeks required to complete the task. This is especially important in accomplishing long-term goals. Allotting blocks of time each day of each week helps to alleviate the pressure of completing a difficult task in a short time. For example, if a term paper is due at the end of a semester, you can spend a certain number of hours each week working on the paper. You can establish benchmarks for the completion of the paper and devise rewards for yourself each time you achieve a benchmark.

4. **Use a to-do list.** Several suggestions for using a to-do list are to: (1) Develop a list of activities each day and create priorities for accomplishing the list. (2) Combine your daily list with a calendar or schedule. This allows you to see a running agenda of the important tasks to be accomplished over time. The important thing is to find a method that works for you. Don't be afraid to experiment with a variety of methods to help provide focus on your priorities.

5. **Ask for help.** If responsibilities become overwhelming, ask for help. Say "no" when there are too many tasks to handle. Do not feel guilty about saying "no"; this only adds more stress. For example, if sorority or fraternity demands are too great, either ask others to share the workload or refuse the responsibility.

6. **Be flexible.** Allow time for interruptions and distractions. Time management experts suggest planning for just 50 percent of your time. With 50 percent of your time planned, you will have the flexibility to handle interruptions and the unplanned "emergency." When you expect to be interrupted, schedule routine tasks. Save larger blocks of time for your priorities.

7. **Take a break.** Every day should provide for fun, leisure, time alone, and relaxation. Make the most of every day. Schedule in time every day for yourself.

Assessment Activity 9-6 is a prioritization worksheet to help you organize your tasks. Assessment Activity 9-7 provides you with a log. Use it to record your daily activities for several days to a week. Then review it and see if you are spending your time as effectively as you thought or if you have overscheduled what you can do in twenty-four hours. This can provide you with a basis for devising improved time-management plans.

Exercise

Because the fight-or-flight syndrome stimulates the body into action, exercise is a logical method of responding to that physiological command. Exercise has been found to directly affect brain chemistry. Studies have shown an increase in endorphin levels after an easy or a strenuous run.[28] (Endorphins are natural pain killers that function to help alleviate sensations of pain and stimulate a positive response from the immune system.) Exercise is a positive stressor (eustressor) and, when properly used, seems to offset the adverse effects of distress.[26] Studies have demonstrated that exercise reduces the severity of the stress response, shortens the recovery time from the stressor, and diminishes vulnerability to stress-related disease. The higher the fitness level, the more beneficial the exercise in reducing stress. (The recommended types of exercise programs are discussed in Chapter 3.)

A correctly designed exercise program produces beneficial physiological responses and can induce psychological effects that serve to reduce anxiety, promote feelings of accomplishment, and evoke muscle relaxation.

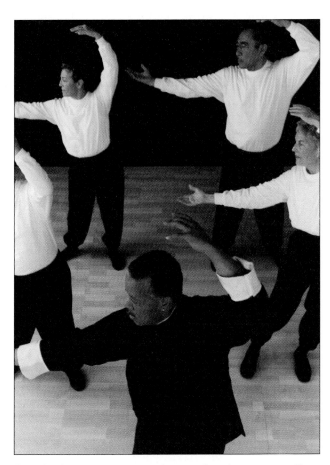

Exercise is a great way to reduce anxiety, increase positive feelings, and relieve stress.

Nurturing Your Spirituality

Enjoying Healthy Pleasures

Certain lifestyle patterns have detrimental effects upon our well-being and quality of life: not exercising, smoking, drinking to excess, not wearing a seat belt, and eating poorly. However, just as important as avoiding lifestyle patterns that can negatively affect quality of life is appreciating the joys, thrills, delights, and happiness that are part of our lives. The idea is to minimize the negative and maximize the positive in our lives. Pleasure has gotten a bad name and we have become almost phobic about enjoying ourselves and having fun. In their book *Healthy Pleasures*, Sobel and Ornstein[25] point out that, even though certain negative habits and addictions are unhealthy, we also must seek to feel good mentally and emotionally. We need to seek enjoyment to enhance our survival. Ornstein and Sobel emphasize that no better way exists to ensure healthy, life-saving behaviors than to make them pleasurable. From eating to reproduction to caring for others, pleasure can guide us to better health. Doing what feels good is often beneficial for health and survival.

A pleasurable experience can be as simple as taking time to enjoy a sunset, smell the air after a rain shower, napping for half an hour in the afternoon, making a kind comment to a stranger or friend, or letting go of anger toward another human being. Seeking out pleasure may involve giving ourselves positive self-talks, looking for humor, and hanging out with happy people. Enjoying our gifts of pleasure is powerful medicine and can be contagious. It is cheap and effective, and its only side effect is a happy life. The following website provides a storehouse of information on the importance of adding pleasure to your life: www/arise.org.

Many people consider stretching a means of invoking feelings of relaxation, and stretching is also associated with reduced tension. Moderate levels of exertion are frequently considered most beneficial for most people. (A moderate-level activity is a walk at the rate of approximately 3 miles an hour.) Excessive or addictive exercise habits can have the reverse effect and contribute to feelings of tension and irritability. When engaging in exercise as a stress-reduction technique, strive to find the level that creates the greatest sense of well-being upon completion.

Selecting a Stress-Reducing Technique

No single stress-reduction technique automatically reduces stress for everyone. People are comfortable with and enjoy different activities, and personal preference is what determines long-term use. When dealing with stress, you must first become aware that a stress response is occurring. People are frequently unaware that the reason they are always tired or irritable or have body aches is they are experiencing stress's negative effects. Second, find the stress-reduction techniques that work best for you. Usually, more than one approach is required, depending on the person and his or her type of stress response. Any technique that helps create a sense of relaxation, provides personal time, and allows you to gain control can lead to a happier, healthier, more enjoyable life. Third, the best form of stress management is the prevention of negative effects before they become unmanageable. Well-thought-out, prudent lifestyle decisions based on knowledge of health behaviors and understanding of your needs and expectations may be the best contribution you can make to your stress-management plan. Finally, it is not the goal of stress reduction strategies to overcome every stressor we face in our lives, but to find effective responses to those stressors for purposes of managing our responses to them.

Summary

- Stress is the nonspecific response of the body to any demands on it.
- Anything that creates stress is a stressor.
- Stressors may generate eustress (good stress) or distress (bad stress).
- The general adaptation syndrome (GAS) explains how the body responds to a stressor. The three stages of GAS are alarm, resistance, and exhaustion.
- The stress response can enhance physical and mental performance. This is referred to as the *inverted-U theory*.

- Whether positive or negative, a stressful event always produces a series of neurological and hormonal messages that are sent through the body.
- The responses to stress can be physiological (cardiovascular, gastrointestinal, musculoskeletal), psychological (causing depression, anxiety, anger), or behavioral (generating an inability to work, arguments).
- The immune system can be compromised as the result of prolonged stress, resulting in increases of susceptibility to comunicable diseases and chronic conditions.

- High stress has been associated with infertility problems.
- People's perceptions of stress are associated with self-esteem, self-efficacy, and locus of control.
- People who deal effectively with stress seem to view stressful situations as opportunities for growth, have a sense of inner purpose, and view themselves as having power over their lives.

- Coping is the effort(s) made to manage or deal with stress.
- Many techinques—including autogenics, deep breathing, visualization, muscle relaxation, meditation, massage, biofeedback, exercise, yoga, music, and humor—can help reduce stress.
- Effective time management can be a key to stress reduction.

Review Questions

1. What is stress? What are stressors?
2. What are the stages the mind and body go through when exposed to a stressor?
3. What are some potential signals that a person is experiencing chronic stress, and what are the possible effects?
4. What factors influence how a person perceives and copes with stress?
5. Define *hardiness* and how it may help a person effectively deal with stress.
6. What are some guidelines for handling stress positively?
7. Discuss various stress-reducing techniques.

References

1. Siegal, B. S. 1988. *Love, Medicine and Miracles.* New York: Perennial Library.
2. Selye, H. 1975. *Stress Without Disease.* New York: New American Library.
3. Hanson, P. G. 1986. *The Joy of Stress.* Kansas City, Kans.: Andrews, McMeel & Parker.
4. Selye, H. 1978. *The Stress of Life* (rev. ed.). New York: McGraw-Hill.
5. Girdano, D., and E. George Jr. 1989. *Controlling Stress and Tension.* Englewood Cliffs, N.J.: Prentice Hall.
6. Folkman, S. 1984. Personal control and stress and coping processes: A theoretical analysis. *Journal of Personal and Social Psychology* 46:839.
7. Seward, B. L. 1994. *Managing Stress.* Boston: Jones and Bartlett.
8. Blonna, R. 1996. *Coping with Stress in a Changing World.* St. Louis: Mosby.
9. Gelman, D., and M. Hager. November 7, 1988. Body and soul. *Newsweek* 88.
10. Glaser, R., et al. 1987. Stress-related immune suppression: Health implications. *Brain Behavior-Immunity* 1(1):7.
11. O'Leary, A. 1990. Stress, emotion, and human immune function. *Psychology Bulletin* 108(3):363.
12. Pellitier, K., and D. Herzing. 1988. Psychoneuroimmunology: Toward a mind-body model: A critical review. *Advances* 5(1):27.
13. Domar, A., and H. Dreher. 1996. *Healing Mind, Healthy Woman: Using the Mind-Body Connection to Manage Stress and Take Control of Your Life.* New York: Henry Holt.
14. Domar A., P. Zuttermeister, and R. Friedman. 1997. *The Relationship Between Distress and Conception in Infertile Women.* Paper presented at the Annual Meeting of the American Society of Reproductive Medicine, Cincinnati, Ohio.
15. Greenberg, J. 1990. *Stress Management.* Dubuque, Iowa: Wm. C. Brown.
16. Newman, J. 2000. C'mon get happy. *Health* 14(6): 130.
17. Adler, J. 1999. How stress attacks you. *Newsweek* 133(24):54.
18. Friedman, M., and R. Roseman. 1984. *Type A Behavior and Your Heart.* New York: Alfred A Knopf.
19. Flannery, R. B. 1987. Toward stress-resistant persons: A stress management approach to the treatment of anxiety. *American Journal of Preventive Medicine* 3(1):25.
20. Fischman, J. 1987. Type A on trial. *Psychology Today* 21(2):42.
21. Kobasa, S. 1984. How much stress can you survive? *American Health* 5(7):64.
22. Benson, H. 1985. *The Relaxation Response.* New York: Berkley.
23. Luecken, L. J., et al. 1997. Stress in employed women: Impact of marital status and children at home on neurohormonal output and home strain. *Psychosomatic Medicine* 59:352.
24. Light, K. C. 1997. Stress in employed women: A women's work is never done if she's a working mom. *Psychosomatic Medicine* 59:360.
25. Sobel, D. S., and R. Ornstein. 1989. *Healthy Pleasures.* Reading, Mass.: Addison Wesley.
26. Lamb, L. E. 1992. Understanding stress. *Health Letter* 39(suppl.):12.
27. Crews, D., and D. Landers. 1987. A meta-analytic review of aerobic fitness and reactivity to psychosocial stressors. *Medicine and Science of Sports Exercise* 19:5114.
28. Appenzeller, D., et al. 1980. Neurology of endurance training versus endorphins. *Neurology* 30:418.

Suggested Readings

Maskach, C., and M. Leiter. 1997. *The Truth About Burnout: How Organizations Cause Personal Stress and What To Do About It*. San Francisco: Jossey-Bass Publishers.

The authors encourage employees and managers to view the problems of burnout as an opportunity to address the major contributing pressures, such as exhaustion, cynicism, and ineffectiveness at work. The book is based on the real-world experiences of the authors working with companies to prevent and deal with burnout.

Schiraldi, G. R. 1997. *Conquer Anxiety, Worry and Nervous Fatigue: A Guide to Greater Peace*. Ellicott City, Md.: Chevron Publishing Corporation.

The purpose of this book is to help readers learn to recognize and understand the symptoms of worry and anxiety. It provides a guide to stress-management strategies, including relaxation, rational thinking, confiding past trauma, solution-focused problem solving, meditation, proper sleep, nutrition, exercise, time management, assertiveness training, building self-esteem, and strengthening spiritual commitment.

Williams, V., and R. Williams. 1998. *Lifeskills*. New York: Times Books.

This review of the research on relationships and health goes on to describe a systematic self-help program to build better relationships to strengthen physical well-being. Eight basic life skills are described.

Name _____ Date _____ Section _____

Assessment Activity 9-1

Life Stressors

The following stress scale was developed by Miller and Rahe. It includes positive and negative events, because both require adaptation. Research has confirmed that stress can have a significant impact on physical and emotional health. The total score on this self-test offers you insight into your risk for illness as a result of recent life events. Stressful changes won't necessarily harm you; the potential for damage rests in how you handle stress.

Directions: To determine the possible impact of various recent changes in your life, circle the "stress points" listed that you experienced during the past year.

Health

An injury or illness that
- kept you in bed a week or more or sent you to the hospital — 74
- did not require long bed rest or hospitalization — 44

Major dental work — 26
Major change in eating habits — 27
Major change in sleeping habits — 26
Major change in your usual type or amount of recreation — 28

Work

Change to a new type of work — 51
Change in your work hours or conditions — 35
Change in your responsibilities at work
- to more responsibilities — 29
- to fewer responsibilities — 21

Home

Major change in living conditions — 26
Change in residence
- within the same town/city — 25
- to a different town/city/state — 47
Change in family get-togethers — 25
Major change in health or behavior of family member — 55
Marriage — 50
Pregnancy — 67
Miscarriage or abortion — 65
Addition of a new family member
- through birth of a child — 66
- through adoption of a child — 65
- through a relative moving in — 59
Spouse beginning or ending work — 46
Changes at work involving
- promotion — 31
- demotion — 42
- transfer — 32

Troubles at work
- with your boss — 29
- with coworkers — 35
- with persons under your supervision — 35
- involving other issues or people — 28
Major business adjustment — 60
Retirement — 52
Loss of job
- due to being laid off from work — 68
- due to being fired from work — 79
Correspondence course to help you in your work — 18

Personal and Social

Change in personal habits — 26
Beginning or ending school or college — 38
Change of school or college — 35
Change in political beliefs — 24
Change in religious beliefs — 29
Change in social activities — 27
Vacation trip — 24
New close personal relationship — 37
Engagement to marry — 45
Girlfriend or boyfriend problems — 39
Sexual difficulties — 44
Child leaving home
- to attend college — 41
- to marry — 41
- for other reasons — 45
Change in the marital status of your parents
- through divorce — 59
- through remarriage — 50
Change in arguments with spouse — 50
In-law problems — 38
Separation from spouse
- due to work — 53
- due to marital problems — 76
Divorce — 96
Birth of grandchild — 43
Death of spouse — 119
Death of
- child — 123
- brother or sister — 102
- parent — 100

Financial

Major change in finances
- through increased income — 38
- through decreased income — 60
- through investment or credit difficulties — 56
Loss or damage of personal property — 43
Moderate purchase — 20

Major purchase	37
"Falling out" of a close personal relationship	47
Accident	48
Minor violation of the law	20
Being held in jail	75
Death of a close friend	70
Major decision about your immediate future	51
Major personal achievement	36
Foreclosure on a mortgage or loan	58

Total score: _____

Interpreting your score: Add up your points. A total score of 250 to 500 is considered a moderate amount of stress. If you score higher than that, you may face an increased risk of illness. If your score is lower than 250, consider yourself fortunate.

From Miller and Rahe. 1997. Life changes scaling for the 1990s. *Journal of Psychosomatic Research* 43.

Name _____ Date _____ Section _____

Assessment Activity 9-2

How Stressed Are You?

Directions: The stress categories and stressors originally listed in figure 9-1 are also listed here. Underneath the stressors in each stress category is a blank. You can use this blank to rank yourself on each category and then to give yourself an overall stress rating. To rate yourself in each category, select a number from 1 to 10. A 1 indicates that you are currently experiencing no stress in that area of your life. A 10 indicates that the amount of stress you are experiencing in that area is overwhelming. This is a subjective rating and should be based on how you feel right now. After completing the assessment, note the areas currently creating difficulty for you and try to plan ways to reduce your overwhelming emotions in the next few days. Recheck your scores over the next few months to see how they change. If you chronically experience overwhelming stress in any area, you might want to seek the advice of a professional, such as a counselor or clergy.

Physical	**Social**	**Intellectual**	**Emotional**	**Spiritual**	**Environmental**
Pathogens	Embarrass-	Mental fatigue	Uncontrolled	Guilt	Noise
Drugs	ment	Overload	anger	Moral conflicts	Overcrowding
Smoking	Teasing	Frustration	Unexpressed	Lack of purpose	Poverty
Lack of sleep	Ridicule	Mental stagnation	anger	Lack of philosophy	Extreme
Injury	Arguments		Inability to love	of life	temperatures
Sedentary	Lack of social		Lack of love		
lifestyle	interaction		Poor self-esteem		
	Rejection				

_____ _____ _____ _____ _____ _____

Overall stress: _____

Questions to consider:
1. Is the stress created from personal pressure or outside factors?
2. What changes could you make to reduce or eliminate the identified stressor(s)?
3. With whom could you discuss your feelings concerning the identified stressor(s)?

Name _____ Date _____ Section _____

Assessment Activity 9-3

Stress Style: Mind, Body, Mixed?

Directions: Imagine yourself in a stressful situation. When you are feeling anxious, what sensations do you typically experience? Check all that apply.

_____ 1. My heart beats faster.

_____ 2. I find it difficult to concentrate because of distracting thoughts.

_____ 3. I worry too much about things that don't really matter.

_____ 4. I feel jittery.

_____ 5. I get diarrhea.

_____ 6. I imagine terrifying scenes.

_____ 7. I cannot keep anxiety-provoking pictures and images out of my mind.

_____ 8. My stomach gets tense.

_____ 9. I pace up and down nervously.

_____ 10. I am bothered by unimportant thoughts running through my mind.

_____ 11. I become immobilized.

_____ 12. I feel I am losing out on things because I cannot make decisions fast enough.

_____ 13. I perspire.

_____ 14. I cannot stop thinking worrisome thoughts.

There are three basic ways of reacting to stress—physically, mentally, or with a combination of the two. Physical stress type people feel tension in the body—jitters, butterflies, the sweats. Mental types experience stress mainly in the mind—worries and preoccupying thoughts. Mixed types react with both responses in about equal measure.

Give yourself a *Mind* point if you answered "yes" to each of the following questions: 2, 3, 6, 7, 10, 12, 14. Give yourself a *Body* point for each of these: 1, 4, 5, 8, 9, 11, 13. If you have more Mind than Body points, consider yourself a mental stress type. If you have more Body than Mind points, your stress style is physical. Do you have about the same number of each? You are a mixed reactor.

Choosing a Relaxer

Mind

If you experience stress as an invasion of worrisome thoughts, the most direct intervention is anything that will engage your mind completely and redirect it—meditation, for example. Some people find the sheer exertion of heavy physical exercise unhooks the mind wonderfully and is fine therapy. Suggestions:

Meditation	Autogenic suggestion
Reading	Crossword puzzles
TV, movies	Games like chess or cards
Any absorbing hobby	Vigorous exercise
Knitting, sewing, carpentry, or other handicrafts	

Body

If stress registers mainly in your body, you will need a remedy that will break up the physical tension pattern. This may be a vigorous body workout, but a slow-paced or even lazy muscle relaxer may be equally effective. Here are some suggestions to get you started:

Aerobics	Progressive relaxation
Swimming	Body scan
Biking	Rowing
Walking	Yoga
Massage	Soaking in a hot bath, sauna

Mind/body

If you are a mixed type, you may want to try a physical activity that also demands mental rigor:

Competitive sports, (racquetball, tennis, squash, volleyball, etc.)	Meditation
	Any combination from the Mind and Body lists

Name _____ **Date** _____ **Section** _____

Assessment Activity 9-4

Identification of Coping Styles

Directions: There are a variety of ways to deal with stress. Following is a list of positive coping behaviors. Indicate how much you currently use them to deal with stress.

	Often	Rarely	Not at All
Listen to music			
Go shopping with a friend			
Watch television/go to a movie			
Read a newspaper, magazine, or book			
Sit alone in the peaceful outdoors			
Write prose or poetry			
Attend an athletic event, play, lecture, symphony, etc.			
Go for a walk or drive			
Exercise (swim, bike, jog)			
Get deeply involved in some other activity			
Play with a pet			
Take a nap			
Get outdoors, enjoy nature			
Write in a journal			
Practice deep breathing, meditation, autogenics, muscle relaxation			
Straighten up your desk or work area			
Take a bath or shower			
Do physical labor (garden, paint)			
Make home repairs, refinish furniture			
Buy something—records, books			
Play a game (chess, backgammon, video games)			
Pray, go to church			
Discuss situations with a spouse or close friend			
Other:			
_____			
_____			
_____			

Directions: Following is a list of negative coping behaviors. Indicate how much you currently use them to deal with stress.

	Often	Rarely	Not at All
Become aggressive			
Use negative self-talk			
Yell at spouse/kids/friends			
Drink a lot of coffee or tea			
Get drunk			
Swear			
Take a tranquilizing drug			
Avoid social contact with others			
Try to anticipate the worst possible outcome			
Think about suicide			
Smoke tobacco			
Chew your fingernails			
Overeat or undereat			
Become irritable or short-tempered			
Cry excessively			
Kick something or throw something			
Drive fast in your car			
Other: _____ _____ _____			

Scoring Instructions Count the number of positive and negative coping techniques you use.

Number of negative techniques: _____

Number of positive techniques: _____

How often do you employ negative coping strategies?

_____

Do you use more positive than negative strategies or the reverse? _____

Do you recognize a need to change some of the techniques you are now using? If so, which ones? _____

_____

What are some ways in which you can maximize your positive coping behaviors? How can you minimize your negative ones? _____

Name _____ Date _____ Section _____

Assessment Activity 9-5

How Hardy Are You?

Directions: Following are twelve items similar to those that appear on a hardiness questionnaire. Evaluating an individual's hardiness requires more than one quick test, but this simple exercise can be a good indication of your hardiness. Write down how much you agree or disagree with the following statements, using this scale.

0 = Strongly disagree
1 = Mildly disagree
2 = Mildly agree
3 = Strongly agree

_____ A. Trying my best at work makes a difference.
_____ B. Trusting to fate is sometimes all I can do in a relationship.
_____ C. I often wake up eager to start on the day's projects.
_____ D. Thinking of myself as a free person leads to great frustration and difficulty.
_____ E. I could sacrifice financial security in my work if something really challenging came along.
_____ F. It bothers me when I have to deviate from the routine or schedule I have set for myself.
_____ G. An average citizen can have an impact on politics.

_____ H. Without the right breaks, it is hard to be successful in my field.
_____ I. I know why I am doing what I'm doing at work.
_____ J. Getting close to people puts me at risk of being obligated to them.
_____ K. Encountering new situations is an important priority in my life.
_____ L. I really don't mind when I have nothing to do.

Scoring These questions measure control, commitment, and challenge. For half of these questions, a high score (agreement) indicates hardiness; for the other half, a low score (disagreement) does.

To get your scores on control, commitment, and challenge, first write in the number of your answer—0, 1, 2, or 3—above the letter of each question on the score sheet. Then add and subtract as shown. (To get your score on control, for example, add your answers to questions A and G; add your answers to B and H; and then subtract the second number from the first.)

Add your scores on control, commitment, and challenge to get a score for total hardiness. A total score of 10–18 = hardy personality; 0–9 = moderate hardiness; below 0 = low hardiness.

(_____ + _____) – (_____ + _____) = _____ = Control score
   (A)   (G)   (B)   (H)

(_____ + _____) – (_____ + _____) = _____ = Commitment score   = _____ = Total hardiness score
   (C)   (I)   (D)   (J)

(_____ + _____) – (_____ + _____) = _____ = Challenge score
   (E)   (K)   (F)   (L)

Paths to Hardiness Three techniques are suggested for becoming happier, healthier, and hardier:

- **Focusing:** Recognize signals from the body that something is wrong. Focusing increases the sense of control over plans and puts people in a psychologically better position to change.
- **Reconstructing stressful situations:** Think about a stress episode and then write down three ways the situation could have turned out better and three ways it could have been worse. Doing this helps you feel better about the way situations turn out and appreciate other coping strategies.
- **Compensating through self-improvement:** It is important to distinguish between what can be controlled and what cannot. A way to regain control is by taking on a new challenge or task to master.

Assessment Activity 9-6

Goals and Priorities

Directions: What follows is an activity designed to help establish your short-term (less than a year, a month, a week) goals and long-term (one year or more) goals. Try to set goals that are specific, realistic, measurable, and achievable. Your goals should require effort on your part but should not cause you to burn out or fail. Your goals should give you a sense of direction. Once your short- and long-term goals have been estab-lished, determine what priorities you need to accomplish. Remember the 80/20 rule (see discussion in this chapter). Use a "to-do" list and establish your priorities for each day of the week. You may wish to prioritize your lists by number, letter, or color. Whatever works best for you. Keep in mind the tips for time management. Be sure to schedule time for yourself regularly. It is vital to your stress management.

Goals
Long-term (one year)

1. _____

2. _____

3. _____

Etc. _____

Short-term (semester/month)

1. _____

2. _____

3. _____

Etc. _____

Priorities for next week

1. _____

2. _____

3. _____

Etc. _____

Day _____ To-Do List

    Must Do

    Important To Do

    Things I Would Like To Get Done

Day _____ To-Do List

    Must Do

    Important To Do

    Things I Would Like To Get Done

Day _____ To-Do List

> Must Do
>
> Important To Do
>
> Things I Would Like To Get Done

Day _____ To-Do List

> Must Do
>
> Important To Do
>
> Things I Would Like To Get Done

Day _____ To-Do List

> Must Do
>
> Important To Do
>
> Things I Would Like To Get Done

Day _____ To-Do List

> Must Do
>
> Important To Do
>
> Things I Would Like To Get Done

Day _____ To-Do List

> Must Do
>
> Important To Do
>
> Things I Would Like To Get Done

Name _____ Date _____ Section _____

Assessment Activity 9-7

Analyzing Your Use of Time

Managing your time effectively can significantly contribute to your feeling of being in control of your life. A by-product of this sense of control is reduced stress and tension; with effective time management you will be able to meet daily demands with less effort. The basis of change is recognizing that there needs to be a change and then determining the areas in your life that require change, so a good way to begin meeting your time management needs is to analyze how you are currently managing your time.

Directions: Make several copies of this log and keep track of your time for a week. Include all your activities—from classes to meals to driving time to conversations with friends. At the end of the day and week, rate each hour as to how important the activities that occurred during that time were. Taking time to relax, talk to friends, and be alone are considered important to total well-being and should not be discounted.

Daily Log

Time	Activities	Where	Essential, important, or trivial
6:00–7:00 AM			
7:00–8:00			
8:00–9:00			
9:00–10:00			
10:00–11:00			
11:00–12:00			
12:00–1:00 PM			
1:00–2:00			
2:00–3:00			
3:00–4:00			
4:00–5:00			
5:00–6:00			
6:00–7:00			
7:00–8:00			
8:00–9:00			
9:00–10:00			
10:00–11:00			
11:00 PM–6:00 AM			

Analyzing Your Log

1. What activities did you find to be the most productive for you? Which were the least productive? _____

_____

2. Where were your most productive activities performed? Your unproductive activities? _____

_____

3. What time of day did you find to be the most productive for you—morning, afternoon, or evening? _____

_____

The analysis should be based on the full week's activities. You are looking for patterns of behavior that provide the best effects for you. You may find that you work best at home or in the dormitory in the after-noons or at the library in the evenings. Using this assessment, try to find the best patterns of achievement for you.

10

Taking Charge of Your Personal Safety

Online Learning Center

Log on to our Online Learning Center (OLC) for access to these additional resources:

- Chapter key term flashcards
- Learning objectives
- Additional goals for behavior change
- Concentration game
- Self-scoring chapter quizzes

- Additional lab activities

The OLC also offers weblinks for study and exploration of wellness topics. Access these links through **www.mhhe.com/anspaugh5e**, click on "Student Center," click on "Chapter 10," and then click on "Web Activities."

Goals for Behavior Change

- Identify and change three risky behaviors you now engage in.
- Make at least two alterations to your home environment to protect yourself and your family.
- Assess your safety precautions when participating in sports and recreational activities.
- Develop a personal safety plan for helping prevent unintentional injury.

Key Terms

acquaintance rape
carbon monoxide
date rape
elderly abuse
homicide

partner abuse
rape trauma syndrome
road rage
unintentional injury

Objectives

After completing this chapter, you will be able to do the following:

- Identify potential dangers associated with unintentional and intentional injuries.
- List protective measures for maintaining a safe home environment.
- Discuss steps necessary to participate safely in recreational activities.
- Describe guidelines for the safe operation of a vehicle.

- Discuss measures for avoiding or dealing with road rage.
- Identify measures to protect against rape.
- Discuss wellness in relationship to homicide, abuse, and hate crimes.
- List measures that help protect against crimes of violence, such as car jacking and ATM robberies.

his chapter follows the stress chapter for good reason. As we rush through our daily lives, one of the consequences of our high-stress, tension-filled lifestyles is accidents. Many of us experience close calls or minor mishaps during the periods when we are experiencing stress. Too often during these periods, we do not pay close attention, are careless in our behavior, or engage in behavior that puts us at greater risk for accidents or personal harm.

Statistics indicate that accidents are the leading cause of death for people between 1 and 45 years. Even if HIV does become the leading killer for certain subgroups within this age range, accidents will still be the number two killer. College students and other young adults tend to give too little thought to their personal safety. As they participate in their daily academic and recreational activities they encounter many potential dangers. No longer can the college campus be considered a safe haven from the violence and crime that are such significant parts of our society. Plenty of evidence indicates that people in a university environment are at significant risk for violence. Because you feel safe does not necessarily mean you are. The chapter explores those areas where the decisions you make can greatly influence your safety.

The first section of this chapter examines **unintentional injury**, which can occur in the home, during recreational activities, or while driving. The second section deals with violence and intentional injury.

Home Safety

We like to think that our homes are places where we can be safe. However, within the confines of the home, dormitory, or apartment many potential hazards exist. By conducting a personal survey and remaining alert to these dangers, you can minimize many risks. Here are some suggestions for safe living in one's home:

- Install smoke detectors and make sure they are in working order.
- If you are going to live above the fifth floor, make sure your fire department has the equipment necessary to reach above that level.
- Properly maintain all electrical and heating equipment.
- Plan and practice escape in case of an emergency.
- Plan alternative methods of escape in case your first-choice plan fails.
- Know how to get emergency help. Most areas of the country have 911 service, but many universities

have special telephone numbers other than 911. Know your number.
- Never smoke in bed or leave lighted cigarettes unattended.
- Inspect living areas for surfaces, objects, or room design that can lead to slipping or tripping.
- Make sure all rugs have skid-proof backing.
- Never overload electrical outlets.
- Do not place extension cords under rugs or where people walk.
- Never use a portable heater in an unvented area or near flammable materials.
- Keep outside doors locked at all times. Install chain locks on all doors.
- Check carefully before allowing anyone to enter.
- Look through the peephole or ask who is there before opening the door.
- Require people who claim to be maintenance workers to show identification before you allow them to enter.
- Place metal poles in the tracks of sliding doors so that they cannot be opened unless you remove the poles.
- Be especially careful in parking garages, laundry rooms, and hallways, and when entering and leaving living quarters.
- Always tell someone where you are going, and whenever possible have a friend accompany you.
- See Just the Facts: Firearms in the Home for firearm safety guidelines.

This list is not all-inclusive, but it includes items for which you need to take responsibility. Discuss the rules for safe living with your housemates to help ensure each person's safety (see Assessment Activity 10-1).

Fire Detection Devices

There are two types of devices that warn of fire: (1) heat detectors, which activate when the temperature reaches a certain point, and (2) smoke detectors, which sense the first traces of smoke and set off an alarm before toxic levels of smoke and gas are reached. Heat detectors are not recommended for the home. Smoke detectors are either photoelectric or ionization chamber detectors. Both types are effective and reliable. Both types come in battery-operated models and models that depend on household electrical current. It is advisable to have a smoke detector for each level of an apartment or home. In placing the detector, be aware that it should (1) be on the ceiling or a sidewall 6 to 12 inches from the ceiling, (2) not be placed in the corner of a room because air does not circulate well in the corners, and (3) be at least 3 feet from registers and air vents so that drafts will not affect proper functioning.[1]

~~ *Just the Facts* ~~

Firearms in the Home

Many homes in the United States have firearms. If you choose to have a rifle, shotgun, or handgun, follow these guidelines for safely maintaining it:

- Keep all firearms unloaded within the home.
- Make sure firearms are locked and secured in a rack or case and have a trigger lock.
- Check to be sure a firearm is not loaded before storing it.
- Keep firearms in good working order.
- Keep your finger off the trigger when handling any firearm.
- Always point the muzzle in a safe direction (never point it at anything you do not intend to shoot).
- Store ammunition in a place separate from firearms.
- Lock the ammunition in a secure place.
- Educate all members of the household about gun safety.
- Enroll in a gun safety course if you are a new owner of a firearm.

It is estimated that between 40 and 55 percent of fire deaths could be prevented by properly installed and well-functioning smoke detectors.

Carbon Monoxide Detection

A relatively new detector alerts you to carbon monoxide dangers. **Carbon monoxide** is a colorless, odorless, tasteless gas that results from incomplete combustion of carbon-containing fuels. Anywhere fuels that contain carbon are burned there is the potential danger of death from carbon monoxide (CO) poisoning. A report by the National Center for Health Statistics (NCHS) illustrates the magnitude of this problem. According to the NCHS, of 900 deaths reported for inhaled poisoning, 75 percent were the result of CO poisoning.[2] Motor vehicle exhausts are the leading cause of CO deaths, but deaths also result from poorly vented cooking stoves, furnaces, and ventilating systems. Death occurs when the oxygen normally found in the red blood cells is replaced by CO. Thus, to prevent CO accidents, several precautions ought to be observed: (1) never operate a motor vehicle in an enclosed area; (2) never use charcoal in an enclosed area, such as an apartment, garage, or bed of a pickup with

Real-World Wellness

Apartment and Dormitory Insurance

I currently live in the dormitory but hope to move into a nonuniversity apartment. Do I need a rental policy? What about remaining in the dorm—do I need insurance there?

While living in the dormitory, your possessions are generally covered under your parents' homeowners coverage. To be absolutely certain, you should check with your family insurance agent to confirm the type and amount of coverage. If you are not a dependent of your parents, you should check with an insurance agent to determine what coverage is available.

If you decide to move to an apartment check with an insurance agent. Each insurance company offers slight variations, but in general good apartment/renters insurance protects your personal property against loss or damage in the dwelling caused by fire and lighting, windstorms and hail, explosion, riot and civil commotion, aircraft, vehicles, smoke, vandalism, theft, falling objects, weight of ice or snow, glass breakage, accidental overflow of water, and accidental electrical damage to appliances. For additional costs, some insurance companies will cover computers, guns, tools, jewelry, cameras/camcorders, or money/coins/gold. Some companies will provide personal liability, which covers claims against bodily injury, sickness, disease, and accidental death of others.

The important thing is to check with an insurance specialist to determine your personal needs when living either in a dorm or when moving into an apartment.

a camper top; and (3) make sure furnaces and all ductwork are inspected annually. Very small amounts of CO are potentially harmful, and anyone renting an apartment or living in a house should be aware of this danger. There are several clues you can look for to detect CO in your home. Consistently stuffy, stale, or smelly air; high humidity; moisture on the windows; no draft in the chimney; soot gathering around the outside of a furnace or fireplace; and the smell of exhaust fumes all point to the presence of CO.

Battery-operated and wired CO detectors are available. Although these detectors are usually more expensive than smoke detectors, it is recommended that all homes and apartments have at least one. Placement should be in approximately the same location as fire detectors. If a second CO detector is used, it should be placed near the heating source.

Ten percent blood level is considered the vital cut off for exposure to carbon monoxide. CO affects children and people with smaller bodies more quickly. A healthy person can withstand a 60 to 80 percent CO blood level. Someone with heart disease may die at CO levels as low as 35 percent.[1]

Recreational and Outdoor Safety

One of the joys of life is participating in recreational or sporting activities. To reduce stress, improve cardiovascular conditioning, and promote personal spirituality, some people find that there is nothing more satisfying than being outdoors. Regardless of the season there are risks if personal alertness is not maintained (see Assessment Activity 10-2). Heat- or cold-related emergencies are always a potential problem. Chapter 3 discusses prevention of these types of emergencies.

In addition to the emergencies created by extreme heat or cold, many other injuries can result from involvement in recreational activities. Some of the more common injuries are blisters, bruises, sprains, muscle cramps, nosebleeds, wounds, and sunburns. Table 10-1 provides information on how to deal with these injuries.

The list of outdoor recreational activities is almost inexhaustible, as is the potential for the unexpected to happen. As you prepare to engage in outdoor or recreational activities, be familiar with the safety rules of your endeavor, have safe and appropriate equipment for the activity, and maintain an attitude of alertness to potentially dangerous situations. Although not all-inclusive, the following rules will help keep you safe in a variety of recreational settings:

- Seek training and instruction from certified or respected instructors.
- Purchase appropriate safety equipment for the activity. Make sure your eyes and head are properly protected.
- Make sure all equipment is in proper operating order.
- Obey the laws related to your recreational pursuit.
- Begin any activity slowly and do not attempt advanced skills or actions until you are experienced enough to meet the necessary skill level.
- Stay aware of weather conditions. Always prepare for the worst possible weather.
- Never use alcohol when engaged in a dangerous recreational endeavor or during extremely hot or cold conditions. Alcohol increases the likelihood of emergency situations.
- Take a first-aid course that will prepare you to deal with a variety of unexpected situations.[3]

 Table 10-1 Recreational Injuries and Conditions

Injury	Signs and Symptoms	Prevention	Treatment
Blisters	Fluid under skin	Wear shoes that fit and gloves on your hands.	Avoid breaking them; if painful, clean area, puncture, squeeze, leave skin, cover with sterile dressing.
Contusions (bruises)	Swelling, pain, discoloration	Wear protective equipment.	Rest; apply cold compression; bandage.
Sprains	Pain, tearing sensation, tenderness, loss of function, swelling	Warm up before activity; strengthen your muscles.	Apply RICE—Rest, Ice, Compression, Elevation.
Muscle cramps	Painful muscle contractions (legs most often affected)	Condition for the activity; warm up before the activity; strengthen your muscles.	Stretch affected muscles.
Nosebleeds	Bleeding from nostrils	Protect your face; moisten your nose linings in dry air or high altitude.	Pinch your nose with your fingers for 5 minutes; apply ice.
Wounds (skin)	Cut, bleeding skin	Wear protective equipment and clothing; inspect equipment before use.	Apply direct pressure, elevate, clean with soap and water, and apply a sterile dressing.
Sunburns	Redness, pain, chills, blisters	Use sunscreen with a protection factor of at least 15; avoid sun exposure during peak hours.	Apply cool compresses; after pain has stopped, use a cream to keep skin moist; don't treat with oil-based products.

Bicycling

The National Safety Council estimates that 57 million Americans ride bikes. Biking can be a highly enjoyable and, with proper precautions and common sense, safe activity. Safe biking begins with the rider. Defensive riding is the key to protecting against injury or even death. The National Safety council reported that, in 1995, 900 bicyclists were killed and more than 600,000 cyclists suffered disabling injuries. To ensure safe biking, taking precautions in traffic and wearing protective equipment are essential. Follow these guidelines for safe riding:[5]

- Always wear a helmet with a stiff outer shell designed to distribute impact and protect against sharp objects. Wear protective gloves. Wear sunglasses to reduce glare.
- Obey traffic rules. Cyclists must follow the same rules as motorists.
- Ride in single file with traffic, not against it. Watch for opening car doors, sewer gratings, soft shoulders, broken glass, and other debris.
- Use hand signals so that drivers will know your intention to make a turn, change lanes, or stop.
- When riding at night, wear reflective clothing. During the day, wear bright, visible clothing.
- Make sure your bicycle has the proper safety equipment: a red rear reflector; a white front reflector; a red or colorless spoke reflector on the rear wheel; an amber or colorless reflector on the front wheel; pedal reflectors; a horn or bell; and a rearview mirror. A bright headlight is recommended for night riding.
- Keep a safe distance from others and never hitch a ride on another vehicle.
- Be especially careful on wet surfaces, because stopping is much more difficult when brake pads and rims are wet. Be careful when applying the front brakes in wet conditions, because it is easy to be thrown over the front handlebars.

Skateboarding

More than 59,964 people require hospital emergency room treatment each year from injuries associated with skateboarding. Common skateboarding injuries range from fractures to death as a result of falls or collision with motor vehicles. Wrist injuries (fractures or sprain) are the primary injuries associated with skateboarding. Irregular surfaces account for more than half of the skateboarding injuries involving falls. To make skateboarding as safe as possible, observe the following guidelines:[6]

- Wear protective equipment, including slip-resistant shoes, a helmet, and specially designed padding. This may not protect from fractures, but it will protect against the number and severity of cuts and scrapes.
- Use a helmet that fits properly and has a chin strap. The helmet should have a hard outer shell with ample padding to help absorb any blows to the head. Because there are no government standards, all equipment should be selected carefully.
- Wear wrist braces, knee and elbow protectors, and skateboarding gloves. You might also consider padded shorts and shirts.
- Learn how to fall. Although it is difficult to do, try to relax your body as you are falling. Attempt to roll rather than absorb the force with your arms.
- Check your skateboard each time before beginning to ride. Check the wheels and the board for cracks, loose screws, and nuts.
- Never ride in the street.
- Obey the city laws. Pay attention to traffic and avoid areas where skating is prohibited.

In-Line Skating

One of the most popular forms of recreational activity is in-line skating. The concept of in-line skating originated with hockey players who wanted to extend their off-season training options. In-line skating is now used by everyone from hockey players to skiers to fitness and recreation enthusiasts. In-line skating burns as many calories as cycling or running. In addition, it is low impact, causing less stress to the lower body joints than caused by other sports. In-line skates protect ankles well because they are heavy, are made of thick plastic, and rise above the ankle.[5] Be sure to follow these safety tips:[7]

- Select good skates. If the plastic of the boot can be squeezed, the material is not strong enough to support your ankle.
- When buying skates, try them on with thick socks to ensure proper fit and comfort.
- Wear safety equipment, including a helmet, knee and elbow pads, and wrist braces.
- Know how to fall. See skateboarding guidelines for recommendations for falling.
- Learn how to skate on a smooth surface while learning how to stop and slow down. Achieve a basic skating proficiency before tackling more challenging surfaces.
- Be conscious of other skaters, joggers, walkers, and bicyclists.
- Watch for changes in skating surfaces and conditions such as potholes, sewer grates, gravel, broken pavement, or obstacles. Do not skate on wet or oily surfaces.
- Check your skates regularly to make sure they are in good condition. Replace worn wheels and brake rubbers.
- Warm up before beginning to skate.

Boating and Using Personal Watercraft

Everyone who plans to operate a boat should take a course on boat or personal watercraft (PWC) safety. Most boating deaths are caused by drowning and are preventable through the use of a personal flotation device (PFD), according to spokespeople for the U.S. Coast Guard. Most major accidents and deaths while boating are caused by "operator error." The four major factors associated with operator error are the following:

1. Inattention: looking away from the direction in which the boat is moving
2. Carelessness: boating in bad weather or rough water conditions
3. Intoxication
4. Speeding[4]

Operator safety awareness is key to saving lives and preventing injury. It is the responsibility of the operator to know and practice Coast Guard safety recommendations and to ensure that every passenger has, and preferably is wearing, a PFD. The National Safety Council, the Coast Guard, and most boat dealers have information about the various types of PFDs.

The number of people using PWCs is also growing. This growth in use has resulted in an increase in injuries and fatalities. From 1987 to 1996 there were 349 fatalities and almost 8500 PWC-related injuries.[8] These small boats (sometimes referred to as *jet skis* or *wave riders*) range in size from one-person to three-person machines. They tend to be quick and maneuverable. The key to the safe operation of PWCs is understanding their nature and practicing safe operation through proper adherence to the safety rules. The Underwriters Laboratories and the National Safety Council make the following recommendations to PWC operators:[9]

- Remember that a PWC is jet propelled. This means that, when the throttle is released, the ability to steer the craft is lost. Operators must know the characteristics of their boats and the space and time needed to safely slow their boats.
- Never get on a PWC without first putting on a vest-type PFD. This vest should be worn even when launching the PWC from a trailer.
- Take a safe boating class.
- Use extra precautions when operating a PWC. Know the state laws regarding age limits for operation, other regulations, and PFD requirements.
- Never loan your PWC to an inexperienced operator.
- Never rent a PWC without learning and practicing, with supervision, the operation of the craft.
- Don't jump the wakes of other boats. Maintain a safe distance from other boats and PWCs.
- Don't operate a PWC after drinking alcoholic beverages or while intoxicated.

Snowmobiling

A highly enjoyable cold weather recreational activity is snowmobiling. The Snowmobile Safety and Certification Committee (SSCC) is a nonprofit organization sponsored by the manufacturers of various types of snowmobiles. Through the efforts of this group, standards have been developed for brakes, controls, seats, lights, shields, guards, handgrips, fuel systems, and sound levels. Anyone considering buying or renting a snowmobile should look for Certification 1 of the SSCC on the right side of the machine.

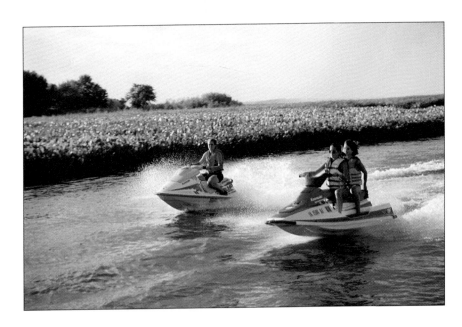

Outdoor recreation is safer when you use proper safety equipment, observe appropriate safety rules, and learn as much as you can about each activity you engage in.

The SSCC also promotes safe operation. Here are some of their guidelines for safe operation of a snowmobile:[10]

- Always perform an inspection of the machine before attempting to start it (check the brakes, throttle, steering controls, loose fittings, screws, and nuts).
- Make sure no one is standing in front of the machine when you turn on the ignition.
- Before operating a snowmobile, receive basic instruction in how to start it, steer it, turn it, and stop it and in how to shift your weight when on the machine.
- Ride only on easy trails at first. Don't attempt difficult trails or off-trail riding until your experience level permits it.
- Ride with an experienced operator until you are accomplished at riding safely.
- Wear protective clothing that provides protection from the cold and also wear safety equipment, such as a helmet with a full-face shield. A full-face shield helps provide warmth as well as protection from branches or other debris.
- Never drink alcohol and operate a snowmobile at the same time. A study in Wisconsin found that more than 60 percent of those fatally injured in snowmobile accidents had elevated blood alcohol concentrations.[11]

Vehicle Safety

Human error accounts for nearly 85 percent of vehicle accidents.[9] Experts use the term improper driving for speeding, failure to yield right-of-way, driving left of center, incorrect passing, and following too closely. Figure 10-1 provides information on the types of accidents and ages of victims.

~ *Just the Facts* ~

A Word Concerning Air Pollution

Many of the activities discussed occur outdoors. One of the factors seldom discussed in relationship to the safety of these activities is the quality of air breathed while participating. There are two types of pollutants: primary and secondary. The primary pollutants include carbon monoxide (CO), carbon dioxide (CO_2), sulfur dioxide (SO_2), nitrogen oxide (NO), and materials called particulates. Secondary air pollutants are formed by the chemical actions of the primary pollutants and the natural chemicals found in the atmosphere. Secondary pollutants include ozone (O_3), sulfuric acid (H_2SO_4), nitric acid (HNO_3), and a host of other compounds.

Harvard researchers found that people living in the most polluted areas of six cities in the United States had death rates from cancer and cardiovascular disease 26 percent higher than in areas with less pollution. Mortality was most strongly associated with the fine particulates such as soot, acid condensates, and sulfate and nitrate particles breathed deeply into the lungs.[12] Another pollutant is ozone. Ozone is produced by the photochemical reactions of sunlight, hydrocarbons, and nitrogen dioxide from automobile exhaust. Symptoms are caused by the irritation to pulmonary membranes and include headache, chest tightness, coughing, throat irritation, burning of the eyes, and nausea. The long-term effects of ozone exposure are unknown. When engaged in outdoor activities, caution should be taken to avoid heavily polluted areas, especially on days of high pollution levels.

Type of accident	Collision with railroad train	Collision with pedalcycle	Pedestrian accidents	Collision between motor vehicles	All motor-vehicle accidents
Death total	400	700	5700	21,300	43,200
Change from 1996	0%	0%	-2%	+9%	.05%
Death rate	0.1	0.3	2.1	8.0	16.1

Figure 10-1 Accident Types, 1997

SOURCE: From National Safety Council, *Accident Facts, 1998.*

One major cause of accidents is speed. In 13.6 percent of fatal motor vehicle accidents, speed is the major factor. Another persistent hazard is the use of alcohol and other drugs. Estimates are that two of five Americans will be involved in an alcohol-related crash at some point in their lives. In 1999, alcohol was involved in 38 percent of fatal crashes.[13] The role that other drugs play in accidents is not clear, but a study by the National Highway Traffic Safety Administration reported that drugs other than alcohol were found in the blood samples of 18 percent of people killed in vehicle accidents.[14] In most cases these other drugs were used in combination with alcohol.

Alcohol and high speeds are not the only factors that affect driving. Drowsiness is another important factor. See Real-World Wellness: Driving Drowsy for ways to minimize your risk of injury while driving your vehicle. The type of vehicle you or others drive is another factor in accidents. See Real-World Wellness: Kings of the Road for a discussion of sport utility vehicle safety.

One of the most important factors in vehicle safety is the use of restraint systems (seat belts and air bags). The National Highway Traffic Safety Administration now requires all 1998 passenger cars and all 1999 multipurpose vehicles (jeeps, SUVs) to have dual airbags. It is estimated that at least 5000 deaths and 70,000 critical injuries could be prevented if people would wear their seat belts.[1]

However, for restraint systems to improve safety, they must be used properly. Children and infants should be placed in the back seat in car seats designed for their age and size. Deaths of young children have been caused by deployed air bags. Some companies have reduced the force of air bags' deployment and/or have provided drivers with the ability to disengage the passenger side air bag. Many states have passed laws requiring that all children riding in cars be in a restraint system. All drivers transporting children should become familiar with the related state laws and be sure to use the type of car seat and restraint system recommended, according to age and size, for their child passengers. The use of restraint systems is not a luxury for adults, either. Proper restraint use is imperative to significantly improve the chances of surviving an automobile accident.

In the last few years, two other factors in vehicle safety have received a great deal of public attention. The first is the use of car phones while driving. While car phones are convenient and can add a measure of safety for people traveling on highways and in areas of high risk, too often car phones are a distraction that can cause accidents. The National Safety Council recommends that drivers who do use cellular phones when

Real-World Wellness

Driving Drowsy

Sometimes when I'm driving, I seem to get really tired. What can I do to help myself remain awake and alert when driving?

A number of conditions lead to driver drowsiness. First, today's cars and trucks have interiors with comfortable seats, are quiet and carpeted, and have temperature-regulated environments. Many vehicles also have cruise control, which can allow a driver's concentration to drift. Second, highways are constructed to eliminate sharp curves, hills, and bumps, which contributes to drowsiness while driving. Third, the repetitive patterns of oncoming light and of white and yellow lines during night driving can cause a trancelike state known as *highway hypnosis*. To prevent drowsiness and falling asleep behind the wheel of a vehicle, the National Safety Council offers the following tips:[17]

- Before starting a trip, get enough sleep—at least seven to eight hours—the night before.

- Don't start a trip late in the day. Driving long distances is hard work and you need to be fresh and alert.

- If possible, don't drive alone. Passengers can take turns driving and help keep each driver awake. Never allow all passengers to sleep in the vehicle at the same time.

- Avoid long drives at night because night driving increases the risk of "highway hypnosis."

- Make sure the vehicle environment is cool in both the summer and winter. Turn the radio volume up and switch stations frequently; avoid soft, sleep-inducing music.

- Stay involved in the driving process—don't use cruise control. Don't allow yourself to become too comfortable. Drive with your shoulders back, your buttocks against the seat back, and your legs flexed at about a 45-degree angle.

- Never use alcohol when driving.

- Take frequent breaks—stop for light meals, stop at a gas station, walk in a safe area for a few minutes.

- If you feel yourself drifting off and no one else can share the driving, stop at a safe place such as a truck stop, well-lit gas station or rest area and sleep for a short time; even twenty minutes will help. Always keep the doors locked.

- If you feel yourself getting drowsy, getting off the road may determine not only whether you stay awake but also whether you stay alive!

Real-World Wellness

Kings of the Road

I'm considering buying a new vehicle. Should I buy a sports utility vehicle because I've heard they are safer than other types of vehicles?

The answer to the question is "yes and no." When involved in an accident you are probably safer in a sports utility vehicle, or SUV, particularly if the accident involves a collision with a regular automobile. Here are some thoughts to ponder about cars and SUVs:[18,19,20]

- When a car is involved in a head-on collision with an SUV, the occupants of the car are four times more likely to be killed than are the occupants of the SUV.

- If there is a side crash, occupants of a car are nearly three times more likely to be killed than are the occupants of the SUV.

- In general, occupants of small cars are nearly fifty times more likely to be killed than are occupants of SUVs.

- Large SUVs can weigh more than 5000 pounds, more than 2.5 times the weight of some automobiles.

- A Chevy Metro is 12 feet 8 inches long, 5 feet 2 inches wide, and 4 feet 7 inches tall. Compare this size to that of a Ford Expedition, 17 feet long, 6 feet 6 inches wide, and 6 feet 2 inches tall. Designed for off-road use, the Expedition weighs 5497 pounds and still meets all government safety requirements.

- Because of an SUV's height, its bumpers tend to be much higher than those of a normal car. An SUV bumper may be at windshield height on some cars.

- Because of their higher centers of gravity, SUVs have a greater tendency to tip over than do cars.

Here are some ways our society might reduce the high risks involved in collisions between SUVs and other types of automobiles:

- Base the SUV on a car frame rather than a truck frame. This would make the SUV smaller, cheaper, and more fuel efficient. SUVs would, however, be less safe for their occupants.

- Raise insurance premiums of drivers of SUVs to discourage people from buying them.

- Give cars and SUVs equal chances in accidents: Make SUVs lighter and closer to the ground. Mercedes did this with its SUV (M-class) by making it with crumple zones and lower bumpers. However, this has made the SUV less safe.

- Improve the safety of automobiles to more closely resemble that of SUVs.

driving should be sure to use a phone that allows the driver to keep both hands on the steering wheel, a phone that features a microphone that can be installed on the sun visor, out of the driver's line of vision. Here are some guidelines for car phone users:

- Safe driving should be the priority, not talking on the phone.
- Do not attempt to use the phone in heavy traffic conditions that require complete concentration.
- Program frequently called telephone numbers into speed dial to minimize the loss of concentration on driving required by dialing a bunch of numbers.
- Do not attempt to dial a number when the vehicle is moving. Wait for a stoplight or pull into a safe area.
- Do not attempt to take written notes while the vehicle is moving. If you need to write something down, pull off the road to a safe location.
- When using the phone, drive in the slow traffic lane in case you have to pull over.

The second factor of concern is overaggressive driving. The United States seems to have become a nation of rude, unthinking, aggressive drivers, manifested in what has become known as **road rage** (see Assessment Activity 10-3). According to one report, in ten years, aggressive driving killed an average of 1500 people each year; injured another 800,000; and cost the country roughly $24 billion in medical costs, property damage, and lost time from work.[15] This study, conducted by the National Highway Traffic Safety Administration, used information from 400 police departments nationwide at which some 500,000 accidents were analyzed from 1988 through 1997. The investigators believe the actual numbers were underreported because many aggressive driving crashes do not cause injuries, and in many such crashes there is not enough evidence to justify a citation. Also, aggressive driving does not always result in an accident.[15]

Men have typically been considered more aggressive drivers than have women. The profile of an aggressive driver is of a poorly educated man, with some record of criminal activity or a history of violence and substance abuse. Such a profile makes many people feel better about themselves, but there are hundreds of examples of successful men and women of all ages and with no violent histories committing acts of belligerence, hostility, and physical violence against fellow drivers.[15] Women are now viewed as being as aggressive as their male counterparts and are increasingly displaying the aggressive driving characteristics once associated primarily with men. As a nation of road ragers, we have come to use our cars as weapons, along with tire irons, golf clubs, guns, pepper spray, and even crossbows.[15]

What we must remember, in our overaggressive commutes to our daily destinations, is to give our fellow drivers a break. It is not our responsibility to teach others how to drive. To respond with less anger to our fellow drivers, we may have to leave a few minutes early to reach our destinations; listen to quiet, relaxing music while driving; and even pretend that the person in the next car (the one possibly driving dangerously or carelessly or too slowly or stupidly) is a loved one. Each of us must assume the personal responsibility to drive in a courteous manner. Be willing to give up the right-of-way and don't take another's foolish, inconsiderate behavior personally. Some guidelines that may help to prevent road rage are provided in Just the Facts: Preventing Road Rage.

Motorcycle Safety

Motorcycles and mopeds offer several advantages over other modes of transportation. Their cost of operation is low, they consume less fuel, they take up less room on already overcrowded roads, and they provide their drivers with an often exhilarating feeling of freedom. Unfortunately, they are also two of the most dangerous transportation modes. The only protection most riders have is

a helmet, and some states do not require that riders wear one. Each year 2000 motorcyclists are killed and more than 50,000 are injured. Of fatal motorcycle crashes, 60 percent involve collisions with other vehicles. It has been reported that 65 percent of motorcycle-vehicle collisions are caused by the actions of vehicle operators and not motorcyclists.[21] The weather, malfunctioning equipment, and the surface of the road play a role in 10 percent of accidents. In addition, most cyclists do not receive formal training in safe riding. This becomes evident in analysis of the evasive actions of motorcycle riders. When avoidance actions are taken, 77 percent of those actions are improper.[21] Skidding from overbraking is the most common problem, and failure to use both brakes when attempting to avoid a collision is the second. A constant problem is the use of alcohol. Approximately 55 percent of motorcycle accidents involve use of alcohol by the cyclist.[11] Finally, motorcycles present a visibility problem: Even with their headlights on, many cyclists are not seen or are overlooked by vehicle drivers.

~ Just the Facts ~

Preventing Road Rage

Here are some guidelines for reducing the incidence of road rage:[16]

- Give the other person a break.
- Do not tailgate.
- Do not let the car phone distract you.
- Do not switch lanes without signaling.
- If you are moving more slowly than most of the traffic, use the right lane.
- Do not drive in the passing lane when not attempting to pass another vehicle.
- Do not park in handicap parking if you are not disabled.
- Do not let your doors hit another person's car in a parking lot.
- Do not make obscene gestures to another motorist.
- Do not make faces at other drivers.
- Do not roll down the window and scream at other drivers.
- When confronted with an aggressive driver, slow down and back off.

Wellness On the Web
Behavior Change Activities

Home Sweet (Safe) Home

We like to believe our home is a safe haven—but to a large degree, safety is something we must create for ourselves. Whether you live in a dormitory or an off-campus apartment, your personal safety depends on being alert to potential hazards and knowing what you can do to prevent or minimize them. Go to your textbook website at **www.mhhe.com/anspaugh5e**, click on "Student Center," "Chapter 10," "Wellness on the Web," and then "Activity 1" to learn more about the dangers related to living on or near campus and what you can do to lower your risk. Select areas where you may be most vulnerable and write down things you can do now that will reduce your risk.

What's Your Domestic Violence "IQ"?

Domestic violence shouldn't happen to anybody, ever. But it does—and when it does, help is available. Maybe you've lived with abuse, maybe experienced it just once; maybe you work or live next to someone who is being abused. Today, family patterns are much more complex than years ago. Sociologists indicate that families, and the individuals in those families, are under more stress than ever. To test your knowledge of this problem, go to the website listed previously; click on "Activity 2," and select "True or False." Answer the questions related to domestic violence. How much did you know?

Here are some "rules of the road" that make motorcycle and moped riding safer:

- Always wear a helmet. Even though some states do not require you to, you significantly improve your chances of surviving an accident on a motorcycle or moped if you wear an approved helmet.
- Helmets should meet the federal safety standards set by the Department of Transportation, indicated by the word *DOT* appearing on the helmet. Some helmets will read, "Approved by the Snell Memorial Foundation," which means they have passed tests even more stringent than the federal standards.
- Wear gloves, boots, and heavy clothing to protect your body if you slide on the pavement, sidewalk, or gravel.
- Seek proper training in how to ride your vehicle; take a course in safe riding.
- Do not ride after drinking alcohol or taking medications that can diminish alertness or performance.
- Ride defensively. Motorcycles are harder to see and some motorists take advantage of their superior vehicle size and weight.
- Avoid riding in the rain or other wet conditions.

Pedestrian Safety

In their haste to get from one class to another, college students are notorious jaywalkers. The majority of the time nothing of consequence happens. However, nearly 60 percent of pedestrian accidents involve attempts to cross a street at either an intersection or between intersections. Usually, such accidents are the pedestrians' fault. Pedestrians make poor choices on when and where to cross streets, or they do not adequately observe traffic before attempting to cross. The student who darts suddenly from between two parked cars puts the motorist at a distinct disadvantage for seeing him or her and for stopping the vehicle. An invention of modern society, the stereo headset, causes users to be unaware of traffic noise and other sounds that would alert them to possible hazards or dangers.

The implication of statistics about accidents involving pedestrians is to be extremely careful when crossing a street. Remaining alert at all times, not wearing stereo headsets, crossing only at designated crosswalks, and not entering the street from between parked vehicles are important safety precautions. When walking or jogging at night, wear light-colored clothing. Even better, wear a jacket or other apparel with reflective strips to make you visible to oncoming motorists. Statistics indicate that alcohol was a factor in 36 percent of fatal pedestrian accidents involving adults. These adults had blood alcohol content (BAC) levels at or above 0.10 (the legal level of intoxication in most states).[22]

Violence and Intentional Injury

As we go about our daily activities, we are constantly conscious of violence. Acts of violence include assault, homicide (murder), sexual assault, domestic violence, suicide, and various forms of abuse (see Just the Facts: Crime Facts). Each year in the United States, intentional violence accounts for 50,000 deaths and more than 2 million nonfatal injuries.[1] Violence has the potential to touch the lives of the college student regardless of school, gender, or ethnicity (see Assessment Activity 10-4). This section deals with one aspect of violence—assault.

Safety at the Automated Teller Machine

Many people use automated teller machines (ATMs) to carry out various banking transactions. These machines provide a convenient way to make deposits or withdrawals in a variety of locations and at almost anytime, when banks are closed, during holidays, evenings, and weekends. Over the last few years many violent crimes have been committed at ATM sites. If you must make an ATM transaction, keep the following rules in mind at all times:

- Use the ATM during daylight hours if possible. If you must use an ATM at night, take someone with you and only use a machine in a well-lighted area.
- Before using the machine, check to make sure no one is acting suspiciously or hanging around the

Crime Facts

What follows are data[23] that represent the annual ratio of crime to fixed time intervals in the United States.

- One violent crime occurs every 22 seconds.
- One property crime occurs every 3 seconds.
- One burglary occurs every 11 seconds.
- One motor vehicle theft occurs every 20 seconds.
- One murder occurs every 22 minutes.
- One forcible rape occurs every 5 minutes.
- One robbery occurs every 47 seconds.
- One aggravated assault occurs every 28 seconds.

(Federal Bureau of Investigation: Uniform Crime Reports, 1996)

~~ *Just the Facts* ~~

Safe Exercising

Unfortunately even when we exercise, precautions must be taken to protect ourselves from harrassment, mugging, or rape. Previously discussed was the detrimental effects of pollutants and dangers from vehicles. Also of concern is the potential of physical dangers. Particularly when in an unknown city or area, we must be aware of the potential of physical danger. Some guidelines to help protect against an unwanted incidence are:

1. Exercise with a partner. There is safety in numbers.
2. Avoid exercising during rush-hour traffic. Locate a relatively quiet place. Ask at the hotel/motel if an area is safe for exercise.
3. Exercise only during the daylight.
4. Carry either an alarm or spray device—know how to use it. These devices can protect against both human and animal pests.
5. Carry a whistle and/or cell phone.
6. Always survey the situation, regardless of time of day. Always be on the safe side.

area. Trust your instincts if you feel uneasy. Seek a machine in another area if you sense something is not right where you are.

- Make sure no one attempts to crowd you while you are using the ATM. Take all receipts with you—do not discard your receipt nearby.
- Do not write down your personal identification number (PIN) or carry it in your billfold or purse.
- If you drive to an ATM, park in a highly visible location and under a light at night. Always lock your car and hold your keys in your hand.
- Do not assume that a drive-up ATM is free of assault potential. Always be alert to your surroundings.

Car Jacking

One of the crimes of the 1990s that seems to be becoming more prevalent is car jacking, a crime in which someone attempts to steal a car while the driver or owner is present. Of car jackings, 45 percent occur on the street and another 30 percent occur in parking lots or garages. A gun is used in 70 percent of car jackings, which makes this crime potentially violent.[9] To protect yourself against such crime and to help reduce the risk of potential assault, do the following:

- Keep the doors of your car locked at all times, even when you are in it.
- Always park in a well-lighted, busy area. Avoid parking in underground or enclosed parking because the security may be poor.

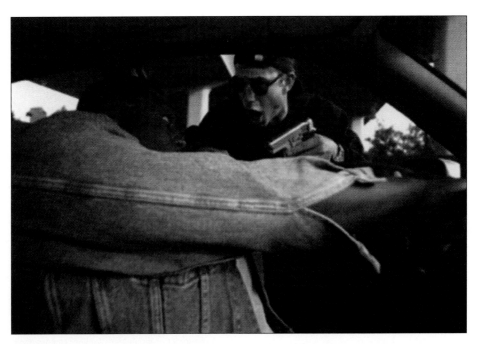

Car jacking is an increasingly frequent crime.

- Always check the backseat before entering your car.
- When walking to your car at night, have a friend or a security guard accompany you. Take your friend to his or her car.
- If you become lost, go to a police station or well-lighted service station for directions. Do not ask bystanders or other motorists for directions.
- If you break down on the road, raise the hood, put a white cloth on the antenna, turn on your flashers, and stay in the car. If approached, lower the window slightly and ask the person to call the police. Do not get out of the car or accept a ride.
- If you are bumped from behind and the circumstances seem to be suspicious, stay in the car and drive to a police station or well-lighted service station and ask for help.
- Never pick up a hitchhiker.

Acquaintance or Date Rape

The terms *acquaintance* and *date rape* have been brought to the national consciousness over the last fifteen years. **Acquaintance rape** is forced sexual intercourse between people who know one another well. **Date rape** is a form of acquaintance rape that involves forced sexual intercourse between people in a dating situation. Statistics indicate that 50 percent of rapes are committed by people the victims know or are dating.[24,25] Researchers reported that 24 percent of college women claimed to be victims of attempted rape, and 17 percent claimed to have been forced to have sex against their will.[26]

In the college setting, poor communication is associated with behavior that results in attempts at seduction. One survey of 600 college men and women found there was substantial agreement among both genders that aggression and coercion usually occurred when one partner felt "led on" and the other did not make it clear how far she or he was willing to go.[27] One solution is for couples to learn that "no" really means "no" regardless of the tone or hesitancy with which it is stated. See Just the Facts: Guidelines for Avoiding Acquaintance and Date Rape.

Researchers also point to a special problem on some college campuses on which there are strong fraternity or sorority organizations. Just because some athletic and other campus groups have condoned inappropriate actions on the part of their group members does not mean that all student social organizations are suspect. However, given the drinking, potential for intimacy, sexual teasing, and competitiveness characteristic of the house party, such gatherings sponsored by social organizations may provide social settings that encourage aggressive sexual behavior.[4] Many sorority and fraternity organizations have classes that educate

Just the Facts

Guidelines for Avoiding Acquaintance and Date Rape

Men should observe these guidelines:

- *Know your sexual desires and limits.* Be aware of the effects of social pressure. It's okay not to "score."
- *Being turned down when you ask for sex is not a rejection of you personally.* If someone says "no" to sex with you it does not mean you are being rejected personally; what is being expressed is the desire not to engage in a single sex act. Personal actions are within your control.
- *Accept the woman's decision.* Don't read other meanings into the situation; "no" means exactly that!
- *Don't assume that the way a woman dresses or flirts indicates she wants to have sexual intercourse.*
- *Don't assume that previous permission for sexual contact applies to the current situation.*
- *Avoid excessive use of alcohol and drugs.* Alcohol and drugs interfere with clear thinking, perception, and effective communication.

Women should observe these guidelines:

- *Know your sexual desires and limits.* Believe in your right to set limits.
- *Communicate your limits clearly.* If you are offended, say so in a firm manner and do so immediately. Say "no" when you mean no.
- *Be assertive.* Men sometimes interpret passivity as permission. Be direct and firm with anyone pressuring you sexually.
- *Be aware that your nonverbal actions send a message.* If you dress in a sexy manner and flirt, men sometimes assume you want to have sex. You should be able to dress as you please and flirt without it meaning anything. However, be aware of the possibility for someone to misunderstand and misinterpret your actions.
- *Pay attention to your surroundings.* Do not put yourself in vulnerable situations.
- *Trust your intuitions.* If you feel you are being pressured, you are!
- *Avoid excessive use of alcohol and drugs.* Alcohol and drugs interfere with clear thinking, perception, and effective communication.

members in an effort to improve mutual understanding and avoid date coercion or rape.

An important strategy in avoiding date and acquaintance rape is to not use alcohol or drugs. Statistics indicate that 75 percent of male students and 55 percent of female students involved in rape had been drinking or using drugs when rape occurred.[18] For a discussion of Rohypnol, the so-called date-rape drug, see Just the Facts: Rohypnol—Setup for Rape.

When a traumatic, often violent experience occurs, such as acquaintance or date rape, the victim usually experiences a great amount of enduring and substantial psychological damage. Date rape victims are particularly vulnerable because they are the victims of misplaced trust. Once the trust in a relationship is broken because of forced sex, developing new relationships becomes much more difficult for the victim.[6]

Regardless of how psychologically strong they are, most rape victims are likely to experience shock, anxiety, depression, shame, and a host of other psychosomatic symptoms. The psychological reactions following a rape are referred to as **rape trauma syndrome.** The syndrome is characterized by fear, nightmares, fatigue, crying spells, and digestive upset. Sexual function and desire may be impaired. The victim of violent sex may want her partner to be warm, tender, affectionate, and understanding, but she may not desire sexual intercourse for a long time after the rape. Sometimes lengthy counseling is necessary to help the rape victim reestablish a trusting attitude toward her relationships and sexuality.[24]

Another common psychological effect of rape is self-blame (the victim blames herself for what occurred). The victim tends to review every single aspect of the attack to understand what she could have done differently to have prevented the rape. Although victims are blameless, self-accusation is common.[28] Self-blame is particularly prevalent in the cases of acquaintance or date rape because victims believe such rapes occurred because they created situations that permitted sexual coercion. Victims also tend to view their friends as being successful in the dating situation; it is common for victims to believe they are the only ones who have "failed." Rape victims tend to perceive themselves as having permitted a social occasion to turn into a painful event. Victims need the understanding of friends, family, significant others, and possibly professional counselors to help them work through these feelings.[29] Just the Facts: What to Do If You Are Raped describes the steps a rape victim should follow or be encouraged to follow as soon as possible after the assault.

The best protection against date or acquaintance rape is preparation and remaining aware that the potential always exists for unwanted sexual advances and

Just the Facts

Rohypnol—Setup for Rape

The drug Rohypnol is a type of sleeping pill (flunitrazepam), which is illegal in the United States and Canada. Here is some key information about the drug:[30]

- It is produced legally in Mexico by Hoffmann-LaRoche.
- It is the most widely prescribed sedative or hypnotic in Europe.
- Manufactured illegal versions are available—the branded product seems to be preferred by illicit users.
- In the United States, it appears to be most frequently used in conjunction with alcohol, creating an enhancing (synergistic) effect.
- It is odorless and tasteless when mixed with alcohol.
- The drug seems to produce amnesia and a loss of inhibition.
- Several arrests have been made in conjunction with alleged date rape involving the use of Rohypnol. Allegations are that the drug was added to women's drinks without their knowledge.
- Adverse effects can include loss of memory, impaired judgment, dizziness, and prolonged periods of blackout. Although a sedative, Rohypnol can produce aggressive behavior.
- Use appears to be spreading among high school and college groups.
- Street names include *rophies, roofies, ruffies, R2, roofenol, Roche, roachies, larocha, rope,* and *rib.*

potentially traumatic sexual experiences. Planning what to do if faced with unwanted advances and acting assertively may prevent or terminate many potentially devastating situations.

Homicide

Murder, or **homicide,** is a crime that has been on the decline for the last several years. FBI statistics indicate that the number of murders in 2000 was estimated at 15,517. This number is virtually unchanged from 1999.[31] Although the latest statistics are encouraging, two trends seem to emerge from the data. First, young African-American males (ages 14–25) are still at high risk for being murdered—they face a one in twenty-one lifetime chance of becoming murder victims.[31] Second,

∿ *Just the Facts* ∿

What to Do If You Are Raped

If you are raped, you should do the following:

- Call the police and tell them you were raped. Provide your location.

- Don't wash or douche before the medical exam. Take a change of clothes, but do not change until you have been examined.

- At the medical facility you will have a complete examination. Point out any bruises, cuts, scratches, and so on.

- Tell the authorities exactly what happened. Be honest and thorough.

- Be sure you are checked for pregnancy and STDs.

- Contact the campus agency that can help with rape counseling or contact the nearest Rape Crisis Center for counseling.

a great many murders involve illegal drug activity. Some research has indicated 25 to 50 percent of homicides are drug related—these murders often result from disputed drug transactions. Many of the buyers involved in these transactions are college-age people. Even if making a one-time buy for fun or experimentation, a person engaging in a drug transaction is at high risk for losing his or her life. The message is to stay out of harm's way.

Domestic Violence

Today's families take many shapes, including single parents, blended families, and two-career families. More and more children are being left unattended while parents are either working or commuting home. Parents frequently feel overworked and children may feel neglected. The mix of related and unrelated people living in the same home can create new problems.

What can emerge from such situations and many others in our volatile society are various forms of domestic violence, including partner abuse, child abuse, or abuse of an elderly family member. (It is beyond the scope of this text to comprehensively discuss the particulars of these three areas of abuse.)

It is estimated that more than 2.5 million women are the victims of some form of violence each year.[14] **Partner abuse** cuts across all social and economic groups, but reported cases tend most often to involve young, unmarried, African-American and Hispanic women living in large cities and lacking economic power.[32] Authorities estimate that only about half of crimes of violence against a partner are reported. It is easy to be critical of people who do not report these crimes, but there are compelling reasons for their silence: Many women do not report abuse for fear of being killed or further injured and concern for the lives of any children that are part of the household. Many abused women may have little or no financial support other than the abuser, so they feel trapped. See Nurturing Your Spirituality: Learning to Communicate for some insight into the basis for some domestic violence.

Perhaps no form of abuse is more discussed than child abuse. The most frequent form of child abuse is neglect, followed by physical abuse, and then sexual abuse.[32] Any form of child abuse has both short- and long-term, and frequently devastating, consequences. Research has shown that abused children are more likely than other children to become abusers, perform poorly in school, and become involved in adult crime and violence.[32]

More than 1.5 million elderly are estimated to be abused in the United States. Most often the abuser is the adult child of the victim. **Elderly abuse** can take the form of denial of food and medical care or of hitting, kicking, or robbing the victim. Suggested causes for such abuse range from the stress involved in caring for the victim to the abuser's having also been abused. For some elderly abusers, chemical dependence may be involved.

Regardless of the causes for any of the three types of abuse mentioned, there is no reason any person should have to suffer the indignity of abuse. Every person has the right to the highest quality life possible and no one has a right to inflict physical or psychological pain on anyone else. Anyone aware of an abusive situation has the moral and ethical responsibility to report the suspected abuse to authorities so that action can be taken to protect the innocent victim and to help ensure either the punishment or rehabilitation of the abuser.

Hate Crimes

Hate crimes are crimes directed at people or groups because of perpetrators' hatred of their race, nationality, ethnicity, religion, or sexual orientation. In 2000, 8063 hate-motivated criminal incidents were reported to the FBI. Of these offenses, 53.8 percent were motivated by racial bias; 18.3 percent by religious bias; 16.1 percent by sexual-orientation bias; 11.3 percent by ethnicity or national origin bias; and 6 by multiple biases.[33] In 1996 the majority of hate crime incidents

Nurturing Your Spirituality

Learning to Communicate

Much of what occurs in relationships can be traced to how couples learn to communicate. As couples fall in love, it is important that, as they experience the wonderful, sometimes overwhelming emotions of being in love with another person, they become aware of how their communication patterns are developing. Each person brings to a relationship a different history and different perceptions and expectations. Dating couples who find that their methods of communication (or lack thereof) lead to periods of intense angry or physical confrontation, such as pushing or hitting one another, should seek to find more effective ways to communicate or, perhaps better yet, end the relationship.

Growing relationships should involve a maturing of love, care, trust, and concern. Such growth can occur only if people learn to communicate effectively and in a nonthreatening manner. Although everyone wants to avoid physically and emotionally abusive situations, learning how to understand and communicate with a person whom you care deeply about is not just something that happens. Couples must work at developing communication. The starting point is how each person views the other: No one "belongs" to someone else, no one is anybody else's property. People make choices to be with and share their lives with others and actively attempt to do so by behaving with kindness and thoughtfulness and by exhibiting a desire to grow with their partners along the journey of life. For continued personal growth, we must find ways to communicate effectively with our partners.

The starting point for good communication is mutual *trust* between partners. Honest communication requires some vulnerability. An untrustworthy partner may misuse personal, private information by mocking it, revealing it to others, or using it to justify behavior. When both partners respect and treasure verbal intimacy, trust is created.

Partners should agree on the ground rules for approaching conversations in which there is potential for disagreement. Each partner should listen carefully to what the other is saying—not to try to win the conversation, but to understand. Each person should be allowed to speak about his or her perceptions and feelings without interruption or fear of verbal or physical abuse. Each person should ask clarifying questions and attempt to repeat what the other expressed. Anger does not lead to effective communication, and people should know when to take a time out and move away from each other for a few minutes to allow their anger to subside.

When communicating, it is important to use *I* messages whenever possible. *I* messages convey what the speaker is feeling, not what the speaker thinks his or her partner is feeling or doing. For example, "You make me feel angry" is not an *I* message, but "I feel angry when you mention my family" is an *I* message. Through *I* messages, the speaker takes responsibility for his or her feelings and does not attribute them to a partner.

When communicating, it is also important to demonstrate an interest in listening and understanding. This entails maintaining eye contact and nodding or saying yes.

Finding ways to resolve conflict can improve the quality and extend the longevity of relationships. Remaining silent only serves to foster anger and indifference. Failing to discuss issues in a relationship merely builds walls, one brick at a time. The feelings of frustration and anger may eventually manifest in extreme verbal or physical abuse or they may lead to indifference and loss of love.

(31 percent) occurred in or on residential properties. Twenty-one percent of incidents were perpetrated on highways, on roads, in alleys, and on streets. Nine percent of hate crimes occurred at schools or colleges.[34] Perhaps the 9 percent occurring at schools or colleges is one of the most alarming statistics, because colleges are institutions in our society that we might expect to celebrate diversity. Hate crimes can occur anywhere, but educated college students and faculty should understand the importance of tolerance and acceptance of individual differences. No person should have to suffer a diminished quality of life because of another's hatred of his or her race, religion, sexual orientation, ethnic background, nationality, or political beliefs.

Just the Facts

Being Safe in Our New World

Since the September 11, 2001 terrorism attacks on the World Trade Center in New York City and the Pentagon in Washington, D.C., many of our thoughts concerning personal safety have changed drastically. For the first time, we realize that there are dangers here in the United States; we are not immune to foreign invasion; and, extremist groups can create havoc on our society psychologically, emotionally, and physically. The way we knew life prior to September 11th has probably changed forever.

The question many of us are asking is, "What are we in danger of next?" Certainly, the possibility of further attacks such as those on the World Trade Center exist. We know that the threat of bioterrorism is ever present in forms of anthrax (cutaneous, intestinal, and inhalation). Other potential threats include smallpox, the plague, botulism, and viral hemorrhagic fevers such as the Ebola virus, and chemical weapons such as sarin, mustard gas, chlorine, phosgene, and hydrogen cyanide.

What can we do? One certainty is that fear is contagious. As a nation we must not panic, but instead use common sense, be alert to suspicious activity, and report it to authorities. Further, we need to be alert to suspicious packages and letters. They may have characteristics such as excessive postage, incorrect titles, discoloration, odors, no return address, or excessive tape or string. If a suspicious letter or package is encountered, place it on a stable surface, leave and secure the area, wash your hands, and seek instructions from law enforcement. If you come in contact with any type of gas or chemical weapon, cover your mouth and nose and leave the area immediately. Use water to quickly rinse your eyes and skin exposed to the agent, then remove any contaminated clothing. Whatever the situation—don't panic! Certainly, we need to live our lives as normally as possible, but we must stay alert to questionable or suspicious situations and maintain a heightened sense of awareness to potential dangers.

There are several useful websites that can provide continually updated information. Some examples are The Center for Disease Control and Prevention available at **www.bt.cdc.gov/**, the Federal Emergency Management Agency at **www.fema.gov/library/terrorf.htm**, the FAA Fly Smart Guide at **www.faa.gov/apa/traveler.htm**, and the National Transportation Safety Board at **www.ntsb.gov/aviation/aviation.htm**.

Summary

- Accidents are the leading cause of death for people 1 to 25 years of age.
- Awareness of potentially hazardous situations is imperative for accident prevention.
- A personal survey should be conducted to determine potential hazards, dangers, and risks in the home.
- Heat detectors and smoke detectors are the two types of devices for warning of fire. Heat detectors are *not* recommended for the home.
- Carbon monoxide is a colorless, odorless, tasteless gas that results from incomplete combustion of carbon-containing fuels. It can be potentially deadly in very small amounts.
- Knowing and obeying the rules for safe participation in recreational activities is the first step to fully enjoying a wide variety of activities.
- Common recreational injuries include blisters, bruises, sprains, muscles cramps, nosebleeds, wounds, and sunburns. A first-aid course that teaches how to manage emergencies is most helpful for safe participation in recreational activities.
- Over 57 million Americans ride bikes. Defensive riding is the key to protecting against injury and death.
- More than 80,000 people require hospital emergency room treatment each year for skateboarding accidents. Protective gear is essential. Wrist fractures and sprains are the number-one injury to skateboarders.
- In-line skating is a popular recreational activity. Protective gear and knowing how to fall are imperative.
- Anyone planning to operate a powerboat or personal watercraft (PWC) should be familiar with safe boating practices and the rules of boating.
- Being familiar with how to operate watercraft and wearing a personal flotation device (PFD) are essential to boating safety. Alcohol should be avoided when operating watercraft.
- Snowmobiling is an enjoyable activity in cold climates. Knowing how to safely operate the machines and wearing proper protective clothing are essential. Alcohol and operation of a snowmobile should not be mixed.
- All firearms in a household should be stored in a locked area and have trigger locks. Ammunition should be stored in a separate location from firearms.
- Trampolines are not good equipment to have for backyard recreation.
- Most vehicle accidents are caused by human error.
- Alcohol is involved in 39 percent of fatal crashes.
- All occupants of a vehicle must use a restraint system (seat belts).
- Car phones can contribute to inattention and accidents during driving.
- Aggressive driving contributes to many accidents and other verbal and physical assaults.

- The United States is a nation of road ragers who commit acts of belligerence, hostility, and physical violence.
- Helmets are essential for riders of motorcycles and mopeds.
- Sixty percent of fatal motorcycle crashes are caused by collisions with other vehicles.
- Fifty-five percent of motorcycle accidents involve the use of alcohol.
- Nearly 60 percent of pedestrian accidents involve jaywalking.
- A pedestrian should always remain alert, never wear stereo headsets, and cross only at designated crosswalks.
- Acts of violence can occur anywhere and anytime. Acts of violence include assault, homicide, sexual assault, domestic violence, suicide, and various forms of abuse.
- Try limiting use of ATM machines to daylight hours. Never use an ATM machine at night alone.
- To help protect against car jacking, always lock the doors, park in a well-lighted area, and check the backseat before entering the vehicle.

- Acquaintance rape is forced sexual intercourse between people who know one another well. Date rape is a form of acquaintance rape.
- Most rape victims suffer psychological effects, such as shock, anxiety, depression, and shame.
- Rape trauma syndrome is characterized by fear, nightmares, fatigue, crying spells, and digestive disturbances.
- Rohypnol is a drug associated with rape. It induces loss of inhibition and amnesia.
- Homicide has been declining for the last several years.
- Domestic violence can take the form of partner abuse, child abuse (physical and sexual), and elderly abuse.
- Hate crimes are crimes directed at people or groups solely because of the perpetrators' hatred of victims' sexual orientation, race, ethnicity, nationality, or religion. Nine percent of hate crimes occur at schools or on college campuses.

Review Questions

1. What is the difference between intentional and unintentional injury?
2. Discuss some of the guidelines to follow to maintain a safe home environment.
3. What precautions should be taken to prevent fires and to protect oneself if one occurs?
4. What are the guidelines for safely participating in any recreational activity?
5. How should a firearm in a household be stored?
6. What does the term *improper driving* connote and what are some guidelines for safer driving?
7. What guidelines should men and women consider following to prevent rape?
8. How can rape trauma syndrome affect a victim?
9. Why does alcohol seem to be associated with intentional and unintentional injury and violence?
10. What needs to be done to prevent crimes such as abuse, murder, car jacking, and robbery?
11. What steps need to be taken to prevent hate crimes on college campuses?

References

1. Bever, D. L. 1996. *Safety: A Personal Focus* (4th ed.). St. Louis: Mosby.
2. The National Safety Council. 1994. *Accident Facts: 1998 Edition.* Chicago: The National Safety Council.
3. Payne, W. A., and D. B. Hahn. 1996. *Understanding Your Health* (4th ed.). St. Louis: Mosby.
4. Consumer Reports. 1998. Consumer reports on health—special report on health guide to medication. *Consumer Reports* 10(4):1.
5. The National Safety Council. 1998. *Safe Bicycling Fact Sheet.* Itasca, Ill.: The National Safety Council.
6. The National Safety Council. 1998. *Skateboarding Fact Sheet.* Itasca, Ill.: The National Safety Council.
7. The National Safety Council. 1998. *In-Line Skating Fact Sheet.* Itasca, Ill.: The National Safety Council.
8. Acerrano, A. 1997. Danger afloat. *Sports Afield* 49.
9. The National Safety Council. 1998. *PWC Popularity Continues—Underwriters Laboratories Inc. and the National Safety Council Offer Recommendations for Riders.* Itasca, Ill.: The National Safety Council.
10. International Snowmobile Industry Association. 1982. *Snowmobile Fact Book.* Annandale, Va.: ISIA. Available online at **www.snowmobile.org/ t_safety.htm**.
11. Peter, R., and F. Wenzel. 1986. A ten-year survey of snowmobile injuries and fatalities in Wisconsin. *The Physician and Sports Medicine* 14(1):140.
12. Dockery, D. W., et al. 1993. An association between air pollution and mortality in six U.S. cities. *New England Journal of Medicine* 329:1753–1759.
13. The National Safety Council. 1998. *Accident Facts: 1998 Edition.* Itasca, Ill.: The National Safety Council.
14. The National Highway Traffic Safety Administration. 1994. *Traffic Safety Facts 1993: State Alcohol Estimates.* Washington, D.C.: NHTSA.
15. Bowles, S., and P. Overberg. November 23, 1998. Aggressive driving: A road well-traveled. *USA Today* 17A.
16. AAA Foundation. 1997. *Road Rage on the Rise.* Available online at **www.webfirst.com/aaa**.
17. The National Safety Council. 1998. *Driver Fatigue Fact Sheet.* Itasca, Ill.: The National Safety Council.
18. Fix, J. I. February 10, 1998. Cars lose in crashes with sport-utilities—weight, height of impact lethal study shows. *Detroit Free Press.*
19. **www.auto.com/autonews**

20. King of the Road, **www.hypatia. wright.edu/dept/eng/kings.htm**.

21. National Highway Traffic Safety Administration. 2001. *Traffic Safety Facts 1993: Motorcycles*. Washington, D.C.: NHTSA.

22. National Highway Traffic Safety Administration. 1994. *Traffic Safety Facts 1993: Pedestrians*. Washington, D.C.: NHTSA.

23. FBI. 1996. *Uniform Crime Reports, 1996*.

24. Bureau of Justice Statistics. 1989. *Injuries from Crime: Special Report*. Washington, D.C.: U.S. Department of Justice, U.S. Government Printing Office.

25. Rynd, N. 1988. Incidence of psychometric symptoms in rape victims. *The Journal of Sex Research* 24:155.

26. Ledserman, D. 1995. College report rise in violent crime. *The Chronicle of Higher Education* A32, vol. 45.

27. Copenhaver, S., and E. Grauerhola. 1991. Sexual victimization among sorority women: Exploring the link between sexual violence and institutional practices. *Sex Roles* 24:3142.

28. Muelhlenhard, C. L., and M. A. Linton. 1987. Date rape and sexual aggression in dating situations: Incidence and risk patterns. *Journal of Counseling Psychology* 34(2):186.

29. Hass, K., and A. Hass. 1993. *Understanding Sexuality*. St. Louis: Mosby.

30. National Institute of Drug Abuse. 1995. *Epidemiologic Trends in Drug Abuse—Advanced Report by the Community Epidemiology Work Group*. NIDA. Washington, D.C.

31. U.S. Department of Justice. 2000. *Federal Bureau of Investigation Crime Statistics for 1997*. Uniform Crime Reporting Program Press Release. Available online at **www.fbi.gov/ucr/ urr97prs.htn**. Washington, D.C.

32. Department of Justice. 1992. *Drugs, Crime, and the Justice System: A National Report*. Washington, D.C.: U.S. Department of Justice, U.S. Government Printing Office.

33. Bachman, R. 2000. *Violence Against Women: A National Crime Victimization Survey Report*. Washington, D.C.: U.S. Department of Justice. U.S. Government Printing Office.

34. Federal Bureau of Investigation. 1997. *Uniform Crime Reports—Hate Crimes Statistics, 1996*. U.S. Department of Justice, U.S. Government Printing Office.

Suggested Readings

Dreissman, B. and Kreissman. 1997. *The Complete Winter Sports Safety Manual: Staying Safe and Warm Snowshoeing, Skiing, Snowboarding, Snowmobiling and Camping*. Helena, Mt.: Falcon Publishing Company.

This book provides the information needed to stay safe while participating in winter sports, including information about emergency equipment and emergency field procedures.

Gillis, J., A. B. Cheng, K. Fierst, and A. B. Curran. 1998. *The Car Book 1998: The Definitive Buyer's Guide to Car Safety, Fuel Economy, Maintenance, and Much More*. New York: Harper-Perennial Library.

Easy-to-read ratings concerning crash tests, fuel economy, preventive maintenance, insurance costs, and consumer satisfaction are provided for all vehicles.

Gutman, B. 1996. *Be Aware of Danger (Focus on Safety)*. Breckenridge, Colo.: TwentyFirst Century Books.

This book focuses on helping children deal safely with strangers and dangerous situations in school and on the streets. It is an excellent resource for parents who have children ages 9 through 12.

Marques, L., L. Carter, and M. Nelson. 1998. *Child Safety Made Easy*. Concord, Calif.: Screamin' Mimi Publications.

This humorous, easy-to-read publication explores poignant issues about safety for children and families. Excellent safety tips for people caring for newborns and children up to 5 years of age.

Tilton, B. 1995. *Camping Healthy Hygiene for the Outdoors*. Merrillville, Ind.: Ics Books.

This publication provides tips on how to camp safely and protect yourself from disease and illness at the campsite.

Name _____ **Date** _____ **Section** _____

Assessment Activity 10-1

How Safe Is Your Home?

Directions: This activity is designed to help you assess the safety of your living environment—apartment, dormitory, or house. Indicate whether each statement is or is not true for you or if you are unsure about it. A scale is provided at the end of the assessment.

General Concerns	Yes	No	Not Sure
I have homeowners or renters insurance.			
I have personal liability insurance.			
There is at least one smoke detector per floor (including the basement).			
There is a carbon monoxide detector on each floor.			
All detectors are in working order.			
There is at least one fire extinguisher in the house.			
I know (and my housemates know) the location and operation of the fire extinguisher.			
Electrical outlets are never overloaded.			
There is a rehearsed plan of escape from the house.			
Everyone in the household knows how to protect herself/himself in a fire emergency.			
Emergency phone numbers are posted near every phone.			
All guns are safely stored with trigger locks engaged.			

Entryways and windows
	Yes	No	Not Sure
Doors and windows are locked at all times.			
There are deadbolts on all the doors.			
I use the peephole before allowing anyone to enter.			
Strangers are not allowed to enter without first showing identification.			
There are safety bar locks on all the sliding doors.			

Surfaces, Hallways and Stairs	Yes	No	Not Sure
There are slip-proof floor coverings on all floors.			
There is sufficient lighting in halls, stairs, and entryways.			
Electrical outlets are childproofed.			
Halls, stairs, and entryways are clear of obstacles.			

Kitchen
	Yes	No	Not Sure
Surfaces are clean and free of dangerous objects and substances.			
Sharp objects are properly stored.			
There are slip-proof floors and throw rugs.			
I position panhandles safely while cooking.			
All food preparation surfaces are clean.			
Household cleaning agents and other dangerous products are kept in a safe location.			

Bathroom
	Yes	No	Not Sure
Electrical appliances are not near sinks or tubs.			
There is a bath mat or nonskid strips in each tub.			
Toilets are clean, free of mildew, and bacteria.			
Drugs and other dangerous products are kept out of reach of children			
Drugs and other products are stored in their original containers.			

Living room and den
	Yes	No	Not Sure
Electrical cords are placed in safe locations and do not trail across the floor.			
Unused outlets are covered.			
Rugs are secured with slip-proof backing.			

Bedroom and nursery

Smoke and carbon monoxide
detectors are installed and
working.   _____ _____ _____
There are night-lights in the
room or adjoining hallway.   _____ _____ _____
There is no high threshold to
trip over.   _____ _____ _____
Unused electrical outlets are
covered.   _____ _____ _____

Scoring Although this assessment is designed only to
be a thought-provoking activity, the following scale
may help increase awareness of the potential dangers
within your house. Give yourself one point for each
"yes" answer. Give yourself zero points for each "no"
or "not sure" answer:

39–34:   Good score, but stay alert
33–28:   Check carefully for potential hazards
27 and below: Significant risks; changes are necessary

Name _____ Date _____ Section _____

Assessment Activity 10-2

Recreational Safety—How Safe Are You?

Directions: This activity is designed to assess your susceptibility to accidents and events when participating in recreational activities. Indicate whether each statement is always, sometimes, or never true for you. Skip over the activities in which you never participate.

General Considerations	Always	Sometimes	Never
I seek proper instruction before participating in a recreational activity.	_____	_____	_____
I take a safety class for each new recreational activity.	_____	_____	_____
I use appropriate safety equipment.	_____	_____	_____
All my equipment is in excellent working order.	_____	_____	_____
I do not use alcohol or drugs when engaging in a recreational activity.	_____	_____	_____
I can swim well enough to save myself in a given situation.	_____	_____	_____
I know the basic first aid and CPR for a given situation.	_____	_____	_____
I can effectively deal with heat and cold emergencies.	_____	_____	_____
I use sunscreen when in the sunlight.	_____	_____	_____
I obey rules, laws, and regulations related to my activity.	_____	_____	_____
I am aware of weather conditions when engaging in my activity.	_____	_____	_____

Bicycling

	Always	Sometimes	Never
I obey traffic rules and follow the same rules as motorists.	_____	_____	_____
I use hand signals to inform others of my intentions.	_____	_____	_____
I wear a helmet.	_____	_____	_____

General Considerations	Always	Sometimes	Never
I wear a helmet with the following features:			
—a stiff outer shell designed to distribute impact and protect against sharp objects	_____	_____	_____
—an energy-absorbing liner 1/2-inch thick	_____	_____	_____
—a chin strap and fastener	_____	_____	_____
—lightweight, cool, and comfortable clothing	_____	_____	_____
At night I wear brightly colored, reflective clothing.	_____	_____	_____
I ride in single file with traffic, not against it.	_____	_____	_____
I remain alert to holes, sewer gratings, soft shoulders, broken glass and other debris, and people opening car doors.	_____	_____	_____

Motorcycling

	Always	Sometimes	Never
I wear a helmet (regardless of state laws).	_____	_____	_____
I wear boots, gloves, and heavy clothing to protect my skin when riding.	_____	_____	_____
I keep abreast of safety techniques and regulations through proper training.	_____	_____	_____
I avoid riding in wet or icy weather.	_____	_____	_____
I do not take drugs or drink alcohol when riding.	_____	_____	_____
I ride defensively, giving up the right-of-way.	_____	_____	_____

Boating & personal watercraft (PWC)

	Always	Sometimes	Never
I know the latest rules of operation for a power boat.	_____	_____	_____
I do not operate a boat while drinking alcohol or intoxicated; I do not ride in a boat operated by someone who is or has been drinking alcohol.	_____	_____	_____

General Considerations	Always	Sometimes	Never
I wear a personal flotation device (PFD) when in a boat.	___	___	___
I make sure I have an observer when water skiing or operating a watercraft pulling a skier.	___	___	___
I am alert to changing weather conditions.	___	___	___
I do not ride or operate a PWC without wearing a securely fastened PFD.	___	___	___
I do not drink alcohol when operating a PWC.	___	___	___
I look in all directions when operating a PWC.	___	___	___
I do not jump the wakes of boats.	___	___	___
I remember that, when I release the throttle, the PWC cannot be steered or controlled.	___	___	___
I cruise an area to check for hazards before skiing, operating a PWC, or operating a boat at increased speed.	___	___	___

In-line skating

	Always	Sometimes	Never
I wear protective equipment (helmet, elbow and knee pads, light gloves, wrist guards).	___	___	___
I practice stopping, turning, and making general movements on the skates before skating on streets.	___	___	___
I am skilled at skating backwards.	___	___	___
I can safely stop by using the heel stop, T-stop, or power stop.	___	___	___
My skates fit me properly.	___	___	___
I obey all traffic laws.	___	___	___
I am watchful of pedestrians, cyclists, and autos when skating.	___	___	___
I do not pass other skaters or pedestrians without alerting them.	___	___	___
I inspect my equipment before skating.	___	___	___

Skateboarding

	Always	Sometimes	Never
I wear protective equipment (helmet, elbow and knee pads, light gloves, wrist guards).	___	___	___

General Considerations	Always	Sometimes	Never
I wear slip resistant shoes.	___	___	___
My skateboard has a slip resistant surface.	___	___	___
I inspect my board prior to riding.	___	___	___
I do not ride in the street.	___	___	___
I do not skate in crowds of nonskateboarders.	___	___	___
I obey the laws about where and where not to skate.	___	___	___
I know and practice how to fall.	___	___	___
I do not hitch a ride from a car, bicycle, or other vehicle.	___	___	___

Firearms

	Always	Sometimes	Never
Gun safety is a high priority.	___	___	___
I obey the gun possession laws in my state.	___	___	___
My guns are in proper operating condition.	___	___	___
I consider every gun to be loaded.	___	___	___
I keep the safety on until ready to shoot.	___	___	___
I keep the gun barrel pointed down.	___	___	___
When stored, my gun has a trigger lock on it.	___	___	___
I do not store a loaded gun.	___	___	___
I do not handle a firearm when drinking or intoxicated.	___	___	___
I target practice only at approved ranges.	___	___	___

Assessment

This activity is designed to help you assess your behavior when participating in a variety of activities. Evaluate your participation in any of your activities. Any check in the "never" or "sometimes" column means that precautions should be taken to correct the situation. Safe participation in any activity requires careful planning—not doing so can place you at serious personal risk. Here are some questions to consider:

1. What needs to be done to correct each of the "sometimes" or "never" items?
2. What are the potential consequences of not taking corrective action(s)?
3. Are you endangering others through your present actions?

Assessment Activity 10-3

Road Rage and You

Directions: The best way to avoid problems and conflicts when driving is to prohibit yourself from becoming an aggressive driver. Following is a series of questions designed to help you determine how prone you are to provoking rage in other drivers. Indicate how often you adhere to each driving safety guideline.

	Never	Rarely/ Sometimes	Often	Always
I give the other driver the benefit of the doubt when there is confusion about who has the right-of-way	_____	_____	_____	_____
I practice driving courteously.	_____	_____	_____	_____
I try to leave early so I don't feel pressure to drive aggressively.	_____	_____	_____	_____
I do not block the passing lane.	_____	_____	_____	_____
I use my horn sparingly.	_____	_____	_____	_____
I do not make or return obscene gestures.	_____	_____	_____	_____
I use my signal when switching lanes.	_____	_____	_____	_____
I do not tailgate or talk on my car phone when driving.	_____	_____	_____	_____
If I am moving slowly, I pull over to allow traffic to pass.	_____	_____	_____	_____
I do not stop in my car to talk to another driver or pedestrian.	_____	_____	_____	_____
I do not allow my door to hit another parked car when I'm exiting or entering my car.	_____	_____	_____	_____
I avoid using my high beams in the city or when there is oncoming traffic.	_____	_____	_____	_____

Points to Ponder

Consider the following questions:

1. As you reflect on the items in the list, what are the driving situations that anger you the most?
2. How do you handle these situations? What could you do to better handle them?
3. How many of the statements in the list reflect your driving habits? What might you do to improve your current patterns of behavior?
4. In your opinion, what should be done about aggressive driving?

Name _____ Date _____ Section _____

Assessment Activity 10-4

Encounters of the Dangerous Kind

Unfortunately, our everyday lives seem to be associated with many aspects of violence. This activity is designed to help you determine how at risk you are for such violence as car jacking, ATM robbery, gang violence, domestic violence, rape, and even homicide. This survey will ask you to think about some issues and situations that can have dangerous, life-threatening consequences.

Directions: Indicate whether each statement is always, sometimes, or never true for you.

General Safety Considerations	Always	Sometimes	Never
I am aware of my surroundings.	_____	_____	_____
I tell someone where I am going when leaving my home.	_____	_____	_____
I am careful about providing personal information and daily schedule information to people I do not know.	_____	_____	_____
I vary my daily routine and walking patterns.	_____	_____	_____
If I walk at night, I walk with others.	_____	_____	_____

Car jacking

	Always	Sometimes	Never
I look in the backseat before entering my car.	_____	_____	_____
I survey the location before parking, stopping, or getting into or out of my car.	_____	_____	_____
I keep my car doors locked.	_____	_____	_____
I have a plan of action if my car should break down.	_____	_____	_____
I check my mirrors and scan ahead for potential dangers.	_____	_____	_____
I avoid driving alone at night.	_____	_____	_____

General Considerations	Always	Sometimes	Never
I avoid dangerous areas that have a reputation for being high-risk areas.	_____	_____	_____
If hit from behind, I travel to the nearest police station, motioning to the person who hit me to follow.	_____	_____	_____
If I notice anyone loitering near my car, I do not go near it but go to a safe place and call the police.	_____	_____	_____

ATM safety

	Always	Sometimes	Never
I avoid using an ATM at night.	_____	_____	_____
I attempt to take someone with me when going to use an ATM.	_____	_____	_____
I look for suspicious people or activity before entering an ATM area.	_____	_____	_____
If I drive to an ATM, I park under a light in a highly visible area.	_____	_____	_____
I remember my PIN number.	_____	_____	_____
I take all receipts with me.	_____	_____	_____
Even if using a drive-up ATM, I survey the area carefully.	_____	_____	_____

Violence, rape, and homicide

	Always	Sometimes	Never
I avoid dangerous areas of my city or campus.	_____	_____	_____
I watch my alcohol intake carefully when at parties.	_____	_____	_____
I do not drink alcohol on a first date.	_____	_____	_____
I avoid arguments or potentially violent situations after drinking alcohol.	_____	_____	_____
I refuse to be with anyone who seems to be violent.	_____	_____	_____

I do not strike or allow myself to be struck by another person.

————   ————   ————

I do not allow myself to be around anyone who has a gun and is drinking alcohol or using other drugs.

————   ————   ————

I break off a verbally or physically abusive relationship.

————   ————   ————

Scoring   In each section of the survey give yourself 3 points for each time you checked the "always" column and 2 points for each check in the "sometimes" column. Give yourself 0 points for any checks in the "never" column. Although not scientific, the following point scheme may help you assess your total risks. Even though your score may reflect a high level of safety, make sure to examine each section for too many "sometimes" or "never" answers, which could indicate you are at serious risk.

87–81:   You are probably safe if you continue to observe current precautions.

80–70:   You may have some areas to reexamine and change.

69 and below: You may engage in some behaviors that require significant change.

11

Taking Responsibility for Drug Use

Online Learning Center

Log on to our Online Learning Center (OLC) for access to these additional resources:

- Chapter key term flashcards
- Learning objectives
- Additional goals for behavior change
- Concentration game
- Self-scoring chapter quizzes

- Additional lab activities

The OLC also offers weblinks for study and exploration of wellness topics. Access these links through **www.mhhe.com/ anspaugh5e**, click on "Student Center," click on "Chapter 11," and then click on "Web Activities."

Goals for Behavior Change

- Make more informed decisions about alcohol, tobacco products, and other drugs.
- Assess your personal attitudes about drugs and drug use behavior.
- Discontinue any risky behaviors related to drug use.
- Develop a personal plan for your use of alcohol.

Key Terms

addictive behavior
alcohol
binge drinking
caffeine
cocaine
depressants
designer drugs
drug
inhalants
mainstream smoke

marijuana
narcotics
nicotine
passive smoking
psychoactives
reward deficiency
 syndrome
sidestream smoke
stimulants

Objectives

After completing this chapter, you should be able to do the following:

- Identify reasons people use drugs.
- Define specific terms associated with drugs and drug use.

- Explain how drugs are classified.
- Describe the dangers associated with the use of various drugs.

uality of life is a frequently used term that refers to the "how" of life—how well you live, how healthy you are, how much you are able to accomplish your goals, and how happy you are. The primary determinants of quality of life are the decisions you make that affect your life either positively or negatively. As suggested by this book, a high quality of life balances the physical, mental, emotional, social, and spiritual needs of a person for optimal health, satisfaction, and enjoyment. Achieving this goal means making intelligent choices—ones that contribute to your well-being—both for the moment and for your future. To make informed choices, you must have accurate information and you must understand that your actions have consequences. The decisions you make are cumulative. As time goes on and as you age, the consequences of previous decisions, actions, habits, and modes of behavior increasingly affect the way your body and your mind function. The emphasis of much of this book is on personal behaviors, such as exercise, weight maintenance, proper nutrition, and the prevention of disease through lifestyle. Other factors and decisions also influence your quality of life.

This chapter deals with drugs. Drug use or nonuse can strongly affect your health and quality of life. Drugs used for treatment, cure, prevention, or relief of pain or disease are categorized as medicines. Many people are alive because of the therapeutic effect of drugs used to prevent or manage disease and maintain health. However, not all drugs are used as medicines. When usage involves reasons other than medicinal, even if usage is considered recreational, the potential exists for tragic consequences. Understanding potential problems can help you make wiser decisions about drug use.

Reasons for Drug Use

A **drug** is any substance that kills organisms (such as bacteria and fungi) in the body or that affects body function or structure.[1] (Other terms that may be important for understanding drugs are listed in Just the Facts: Understanding Drug Terminology.) People use drugs for many reasons. Some need drugs for health reasons—to maintain a normal life or to alleviate symptoms or complications of diseases or other conditions. Others indulge in drugs to alter their moods. Researchers have identified several reasons people use drugs:[1]

- *Medicinal purposes:* Medicines are used for a wide range of purposes—from reducing symptoms of the cold and flu or treating headaches to lowering blood pressure or cholesterol to extend life and maintain quality of life. People who suffer from chemical imbalances such as with bipolar disorder or depression would be unable to live normal lives without the availability of certain drugs. Methylphenidate (Ritalin), commonly used illegally as a stimulant, is also used to treat adults and children who have attention-deficit disorder. When used in this capacity, Ritalin frequently helps such people focus on and complete tasks—something difficult for these people to do without medical intervention. Medicines, although dangerous even under a physician's supervision if misused or prescribed incorrectly, are invaluable to many for maintenance of an active, positive lifestyle.

- *Recreational/social facilitation:* People frequently use drugs with the belief that they will lessen the tension associated with social encounters. Marijuana and alcohol are particularly popular in social situations. Potential dangers of using drugs for this purpose include mental dependency on the drug and an inability to cope with social events without using the drug.

- *Sensation seeking:* Some people enjoy taking risks. For them, drugs fulfill the need for excitement and adventure. Others turn to drugs out of boredom or a feeling of inadequacy in their lives. Unfortunately, when they become tolerant to the drug or they do not find the type of "high" they were looking for, users frequently turn to increasingly dangerous drugs or to increased doses to provide equivalent or more exciting thrills.

- *Religious or spiritual factors:* Throughout history people have used drugs to enhance their spirituality or to achieve spiritual states or awarenesses. Too often in these situations, the drug becomes the object of worship. Though many people have tried, the spiritual realm has not been achieved through use of mind-altering drugs.

- *Altered states:* Drugs are sometimes used to increase the intensity of a mood or create a state of euphoria. Some people attempt to enhance physical performance or stimulate artistic creativity. Evidence indicates that perceptions of improved abilities induced by drugs are false.

- *Rebellion and alienation:* The use of drugs can be a deliberate act of rebellion against social values, especially the values of parents or society. Many people who experience extreme pressures and have difficulty coping turn to drugs as an escape. These people include college-age students facing academic pressure and increased personal freedom.

- *Peer pressure and group entry:* People who have a great desire to feel accepted socially often use drugs to demonstrate their sameness with other members of their group. People claim to use drugs to feel accepted, to imitate people they admire, and to attempt

Just the Facts

Understanding Drug Terminology

Here are possibly unfamiliar terms that are useful for understanding the effects of substances:

- **Addiction:** Compulsive, uncontrollable, chronic dependence on a drug or drugs to the degree that severe emotional, mental, or physiological reactions occur; a desire to use drug(s) contrary to legal and/or social prohibitions.

- **Antagonistic:** Opposing or counteracting.

- **Binge drinking:** Consuming five or more drinks in a row for males and four in a row for women.

- **Designer drugs:** Illegally manufactured psychoactive drugs similar to controlled drugs on the FDA's schedule.

- **Drug abuse:** The excessive and pathological use of a drug that has dangerous side effects.

- **Drug misuse:** The use of a drug for purposes other than intended.

- **Effective dose:** The amount that produces the desired effect.

- **Habit:** As pertains to drug use, a patterned, regular, and possibly involuntary involvement with a particular drug.

- **Lethal dose:** The amount capable of causing death.

- **Medicines:** Drugs used to prevent illness or to treat symptoms of an illness.

- **Over-the-counter (OTC) drugs:** Nonprescription drugs.

- **Physical dependence:** A physiological need for a drug.

- **Polyabuse:** The use of multiple drugs.

- **Potentiating:** Describes an exaggerated drug response obtained when two drugs are taken together; a much greater effect is obtained than when either drug is taken separately.

- **Prescription drugs:** Drugs obtained only by order of a physician or dentist.

- **Psychoactive:** Affecting mood and/or behavior.

- **Psychological dependence:** An emotional or mental need to use a drug.

- **Synergistic:** Describes a combined effect greater than the sum of the individual effects when two or more drugs are used at the same time; the combination produces an exaggerated effect or a prolonged drug action.

- **Therapeutic index:** The difference between the minimum amount of a drug needed for a therapeutic effect and the minimum amount that has a toxic concentration or effect.

- **Toxic dose:** The amount that produces a poisonous effect.

---

to create an identity or project a specific image. Self-esteem seems to be a vital component. People with high self-esteem see themselves as competent, successful, self-sufficient, accepting, outgoing, and well rounded. People with low self-esteem tend to feel isolated and unloved and have a reduced capacity for joy or self-fulfillment. To overcome these sensations and perceptions, many people turn to drugs.

Curiosity: Many people first experiment with drugs out of curiosity—the desire to see what using the drug feels like or what the attraction is for chronic users. Although curiosity is normal and healthy in many circumstances, the primary problem associated with experimentation with drugs out of curiosity is the inability to know how a drug will affect any one person. Whereas one person may consider the effects of a drug pleasurable, someone else may have a different, occasionally fatal, reaction. Most people try alcohol during their lives. For most people this creates no problem; they can choose to use it or not use it. For some people, however, one act of curiosity of alcohol can result in the disease of alcoholism.

The reasons any person uses drugs are usually not easily categorized. (List yours in Assessment Activity 11-2.) Most drug-use situations depend on personality, experience, perceptions of the environment, and expectations (see Just the Facts: What's the Cause of Addiction?).

Drug Classification

Drugs can be classified in a number of ways. For example, they can be classified according to legality (legal or illegal), whether their effects are primarily physiological or psychological, or whether their use has more medicinal benefits or a greater potential for abuse. This latter system is based on the Controlled Substance Act of 1970, which classifies narcotics and other dangerous drugs. The system contains five classifications called *schedules*. Schedule I drugs have no medical use and a high potential for abuse (such as heroin and LSD); schedule II through V drugs have approved medicinal uses with varying potentials for abuse and significant psychological and physical dependence. Excluded from this classification system are two of the most deadly drugs found in modern society: alcohol and tobacco products.

∼ *Just the Facts* ∼

What's the Cause of Addiction?

Addiction has been defined as "a condition characterized by the compulsive abuse of a drug or drugs."[1] In other words, addiction is a pathological relationship with a substance that has life-damaging potential. Here are some theories about addiction:

- The spectrum of addictions ranges from alcohol and tobacco to behavior such as eating and working.
- The causes of addiction are complex and interrelated. A number of interacting variables may contribute to the development of addiction.
- Variables that may contribute to addiction include genetics, family influences, friends, life events, social and cultural values, availability, and personality.
- Studies indicate that some inherited traits may lead to alcoholism.[8,9] For instance, alcoholics may have an inherited inability to determine their levels of intoxication when drinking alcoholic beverages.
- Studies have found that addictive, impulsive, and compulsive disorders may have a common genetic origin.[10] These disorders may result from the failure of cells to signal molecules in the brain's reward system, so that the brain is unaware of certain sensations of pleasure or success. This failure is viewed as a type of sensory deprivation of the brain's pleasure mechanisms. The manifestation of this disorder is referred to as **reward deficiency syndrome**.
- Personality type, temperament, and attitudes may also contribute to drug use and addiction. **Addictive behavior** is any behavior that is excessive, compulsive, and psychologically or physically destructive.
- Personality traits associated with drug abuse include rebelliousness, resistance to authority, independence, and low self-esteem. In addition, people who abuse drugs seem to have a high tolerance for deviance in others, place a low value on education and religion, display low levels of competence in task performance, have low degrees of obedience, and have an underdeveloped sense of diligence.[11]
- Because innumerable circumstances, factors, and conditions influence personality and predisposition to addiction, it has not yet been determined whether predetermination of addiction is chemical, genetic, or psychological.

Drugs are also classified according to the physiological effect they have. Categories include stimulants, depressants, hallucinogens, narcotics, and inhalants. Two other types are also important. Designer drugs are manufactured to mimic the effects of drugs found in the previously mentioned categories, and marijuana, or cannabis, is difficult to classify but is usually included as a hallucinogen. Depending on the dose, marijuana can mimic a variety of substances found in other categories. The following is a list of drug categories and the effects they have on the body:

- *Stimulants:* **Stimulants** speed up the central nervous system, producing an increase in alertness and excitability. Examples are amphetamines, cocaine, crack cocaine, methamphetamines, and drugs such as Ritalin and phentermine (Ionamin).
- *Depressants:* Also known as *sedatives* and *tranquilizers,* **depressants** slow down the central nervous system, causing a feeling of relaxation. Examples of the depressant drugs are barbiturates; methaqualone (Quaaludes or "quad"); and tranquilizers such as diazepam (Valium), chlordiazepoxide HCI (Librium), and meprobamate (Miltown).
- *Psychoactives:* **Psychoactives** can alter feelings, moods, and/or perceptions. Marijuana is classified as a psychoactive drug but can exhibit effects similar to those of stimulants, depressants, and narcotics. Some examples of psychoactive drugs are lysergic acid diethylamide (LSD), mescaline, peyote, phencyclidine (PCP), and psilocybin.
- *Narcotics:* **Narcotics** are powerful painkillers. They also produce pleasurable feelings and induce sleep. The narcotic drugs include codeine, heroin, methadone, morphine, opium, and substances such as oxycodone (Percodan), propoxyphene (Darvon), pentazocine (Talwin), and difenoxin (Lomotil).
- *Inhalants:* **Inhalants** are volatile nondrugs that cause druglike effects if inhaled. Examples are glue and gasoline. Some, such as nitrous oxide and amyl nitrate, have medical uses.
- *Designer drugs:* **Designer drugs** are drug analogs of amphetamines, methamphetamines, narcotics, and hallucinogens manufactured in illegal laboratories to mimic controlled substances. They are often more powerful and less predictable than the drugs they imitate. The number and variations of designer drugs available are increasing rapidly.

Currently, three main types of illegal synthetic analog drugs are available: (1) analogs of phencyclidine (PCP); (2) analogs of synthetic narcotic analgesics, such as Demerol; and (3) analogs of amphetamines and methamphetamines. Perhaps one of the best known analogs in the third category is MDMA, known as *ecstasy* or *Adam*. It is widely used in the college setting as a euphoriant.[3]

Commonly Abused Substances

This section briefly examines some of the most well-known and frequently used drugs—caffeine, alcohol, tobacco products, designer drugs, club drugs, cocaine, and marijuana. This section is not intended to be all-inclusive. There is a wide range of other substances that are potentially dangerous if misused or abused. Because these drugs are so frequently used, it is important for you to understand their positive and negative effects so that you may make decisions based on information rather than myth.

Caffeine

Caffeine is probably the most commonly used drug in American society. Each day millions of Americans drink, chew, or ingest approximately 4 mg of caffeine for every 2.2 pounds of body weight. Approximately 3 percent of the population consumes 600 mg or more of caffeine daily.[3] Caffeine is a stimulant that speeds heart rate, temporarily increases blood pressure, and disrupts sleep. It also relieves drowsiness, helps in the performance of repetitive tasks, and improves work ability.[4] Negative effects include insomnia, anxiety, heart dysrhythmias, gastrointestinal complaints, dizziness, and headaches.

The active ingredient in caffeine belongs to a group of drugs with similar structures known as *xanthines.* Xanthines include a substance found in cocoa beans, which are used to make chocolate, and in tea leaves. In the past, caffeine consumption was thought to cause birth defects, breast-feeding problems, cardiovascular disease, cancer, and fibrocystic breast disease. Current research has found no substantial association with these conditions.[5,6] However, pregnant and nursing women should consume no more than two cups of coffee a day and should consume tea and caffeinated soft drinks only in moderation (fewer than 300 mg per day).[6] Furthermore, women who suffer from premenstrual tension (PMS) should eliminate caffeine. Research has indicated that women who drink one-half to four cups (25 to 200 mg) of caffeinated tea a day are twice as likely to suffer PMS symptoms as are women who drink none at all.[6]

The majority of adults can consume relatively low doses of caffeine (the equivalent of two to three cups of coffee per day) safely. Approximately 10 percent of the adult population experiences *caffeinism,* a condition in which frequent high-dose use causes psychological and physical problems. Doses as low as 250 mg per day can produce restlessness, nervousness, excitement, insomnia, flushed face, diuresis, muscle twitching, rambling thoughts and speech, and stomach complaints. Doses greater than 1 gram per day can cause muscle twitch-

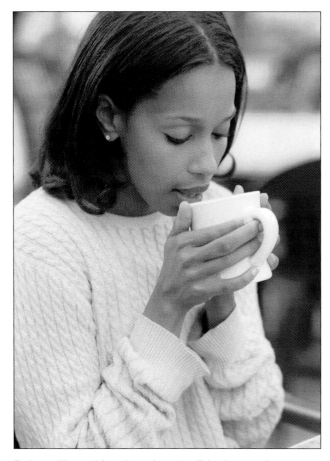

Today, millions of Americans ingest caffeine in some form.

ing, rambling thoughts and speech, heart dysrhythmias, and motor agitation. Higher doses can cause ringing in the ears and flashes of light.[3]

It is easy to consume a great deal of caffeine. By becoming familiar with the amount of caffeine in a product and restricting your consumption to fewer than 400 mg of caffeine per day, you can benefit from the effects of the drug without suffering any negative effects.[4]

Alcohol

Alcohol use is pervasive. **Alcohol** is a drug generally deemed socially acceptable. Nevertheless, no other drug causes so much physical, social, and emotional damage to people and their families. People drink alcoholic beverages in many situations and for many reasons. They drink when they are among friends and when they are upset or depressed. People drink to spark romantic feelings, to put themselves at ease in social situations, and to celebrate special occasions. In addition, people drink because their role models drink and because the advertising industry has convinced them that alcohol contributes to self-enhancement. Unfortunately, the devastation associated with alcohol is

Table 11-1   Effects of Alcohol Use

Short-Term or Immediate			Long-Term	
Number of Drinks*	Blood Alcohol Concentration (BAC)	Effect(s)	System/Organ	Health Risks
1–2	0.00–0.05	Usually relaxation and euphoria; decrease in alertness	Breast	50% higher risk for cancer in women who drink any alcohol; 100% increase for women having three or more drinks per day
2–3	0.05–0.10	Exaggerated feelings and behavior, emotional instability, increased reaction time and diminished motor coordination, impaired driving; a legally drunk designation in most states	Cardiovascular	High blood pressure; irregular heartbeat; chest pain/angina; myocardial infarctions; damage to coronary arteries
4–5	0.10–0.15	Loss of peripheral vision; highly impaired driving ability; unsteady walking/standing	General gastrointestinal	Risk of mouth, tongue, throat, esophageal, stomach, and liver cancer; pancreatitis; malnutrition; digestive impairment
5–10	0.15–0.30	Significant impairment of sensory perceptions; slurred speech; decreased sensitivity to pain; difficult and staggering walk	Immune system	Lower resistance to infectious diseases
			Liver	Hepatitis; cirrhosis
			Pancreas	Interference with insulin production
10+	>0.30	Stupor or unconsciousness; anesthetization; possible death at levels greater than 0.35	Small intestine	Interference with or prevention of absorption of proteins, iron, calcium, thiamine, and vitamin B_{12}
			Stomach	Bleeding from irritation, ulcers
			Muscular system	Destruction of muscle fibers
			Nervous system	Destruction of brain cells; interference with neurotransmitters; slowing of reaction time
			Reproductive system	Impotence; decreased testosterone production; fetal alcohol syndrome; miscarriage

*1 drink = 12 oz. beer, 6 oz. wine, 1 oz. hard liquor

often not mentioned. Table 11-1 summarizes the short- and long-term effects of the drug. Because society has labeled alcohol appropriate and even necessary for some occasions, abstinence may seem unrealistic for many people.

As with many drugs, there are times and places where medicinal and health reasons are cited for alcohol use. Current research suggests that moderate amounts of alcohol may help reduce the risk of heart disease. The possible benefits and pleasures of the use of alcoholic beverages do not eradicate the dangers that result from misuse or abuse, however (see Assessment Activity 11-1). Nearly half of annual traffic deaths are caused by accidents involving alcohol consumption.

This figure does not include permanent physical injuries and emotional damages caused by alcohol-induced traffic accidents and deaths nor does it include the increased number of violent acts associated with alcohol intoxication. Drinking of alcohol, if it occurs, ought to be approached responsibly, with recognition of the potential for harm to self and others. Real-World Wellness: Responsible Drinking provides suggestions for responsible drinking.

Although there are several types of alcohol, the intoxicating agent in all alcohol drinks is ethyl alcohol, a colorless liquid with a sharp, burning taste (see Just the Facts: How Much Alcohol Is in Beer, Wine, and Other Drinks?). The percentage of alcohol in a beverage is

Real-World Wellness

Responsible Drinking

I enjoy an occasional drink, and I often invite friends to my home to celebrate holidays and special events. How can I make sure I'm drinking and hosting parties responsibly?

Following are suggestions to help each person be a responsible drinker and host:

• Drink slowly; never consume more than one drink per hour.

• Eat while drinking, but do not eat salty food.

• When mixing drinks, measure the amount of alcohol; never just pour.

• Serve and choose nonalcoholic drinks as an alternative.

• As host, always serve the guests or hire a bartender. Do not have an open bar or serve someone who is intoxicated.

• Stop using or serving alcohol one hour before a party is over.

• Don't drink and drive. Have a nondrinker drive or call a cab.

How Much Alcohol Is in Beer, Wine, and Other Drinks?

Did you know that all of the following contain the same amount of alcohol? Each contains the equivalent of 3 ounces of pure alcohol. A 160-pound person who consumed these amounts within a two-hour period would be considered legally intoxicated in most states:

• Six 12-oz. glasses of beer

• 15 ounces of fortified wine (about 2 glasses)

• 24 ounces of table wine (about 4 glasses)

• Six servings of liquor (1.3 oz. of 80 proof)

• One measure of vermouth

• One jigger (1 1/2 oz.) of whiskey

Jason Alan Bitter was killed on November 19, 1994, by a drunk driver who crossed the center line. The offender's BAC was .36, more than three times the legal limit in Missouri. Dina Khoury-Hager was also killed in the crash. Both were 17 years old and would have graduated from college in 1999.

measured by its proof, twice the percentage of alcohol. A beverage that is 40 percent alcohol has a proof of 80. The blood alcohol concentration (BAC) is the percentage of alcohol content in the blood. This percentage determines the alcohol's effect on a person (table 11-1). The more quickly the alcohol is absorbed, the quicker the BAC increases.

Alcohol enters the bloodstream quickly from the stomach and even more quickly from the small intestine. In the stomach, food inhibits absorption of alcohol. Food does not affect absorption in the small intestine.[7]

Here are some other factors that affect the rate of absorption and effect of alcohol:

• *Rate of consumption:* How quickly is the beverage consumed? Large amounts of alcohol quickly consumed expose the brain to higher peak concentrations, altering perceptions and response times.

• *Type of beverage:* Beer and wine contain substances that slow the rate of absorption; thus, the effects are experienced more slowly than are the effects of drinking distilled spirits, even when the same amount of alcohol is consumed. Carbonated beverages added to liquor speed absorption, but diluting them with water slows the process.

• *Body weights:* Body weight and body composition do not influence the rate of absorption, but they do influence the effects of alcohol. More weight and/or more muscle mass (muscle with more fluid volume than fat) results in a greater distribution of the alcohol, lowering its concentration in the body and weakening its effects.

Tolerance to alcohol: Some people seem to remain sober while others react quickly to the same amount of alcohol. One drink for a novice may have the same effect as three drinks for a more experienced drinker. This indicates that the experienced drinker's body has adapted to the alcohol at the cellular level and is encouraging increased consumption. Tolerance consists of an increase in the rate of alcohol absorption metabolism as well as a reduced response to the drug. It is the reduced response that is frequently associated with physical and psychological dependence. Increased tolerance to alcohol can also result in a decreased response to other drugs, specifically other central nervous system depressants.

Alcoholism is a disease in which a person loses control over drinking. According to a definition approved by the National Council on Alcoholism and Drug Dependence and the American Society of Addiction Medicine, alcoholism is a "primary, chronic disease with genetic, psychosocial, and environmental factors influencing its development and manifestations. The disease is often progressive and fatal."[8] An alcoholic is a person who suffers from the disease of alcoholism. For alcoholics, alcohol increasingly becomes the focus of life, and family, social, work, or school responsibilities become less important and are eventually disrupted by the desire and need for alcohol. Some alcoholics make this transition rapidly, whereas others maintain the appearance of being social drinkers for many years. Unfortunately, predetermining who will have trouble with alcohol is impossible. Alcoholism crosses all social and economic barriers and can affect everyone from clergy, medical doctors, high school students, and college students, to professors.

Women who are alcoholics face certain unique problems, and women who use alcohol or tobacco during pregnancy put their children at risk of developing certain health problems. The rate of alcoholism is increasing among younger women (see Wellness Across the Generations: Alcohol and Tobacco Use Among Young Women).

There is no single accepted reason why any person becomes an alcoholic. Most researchers think that a variety of events, genetic tendencies, and situations working together result in alcoholism for some people. The medical model of alcoholism includes biological or genetic explanations of abuse. It views alcohol abuse as uncontrollable because of physiological differences between alcoholics and nonalcoholics. Each year, more research seems to link alcoholism to an inherited susceptibility or predisposition for the disease:[6] Children

HealthQuest Activities

- The alcohol self-assessment activity in the Alcohol Module, will help you understand your current drinking behavior and determine how that behavior may affect your health. You can assess your beliefs about alcohol and take a critical look at your ideas about whether alcohol use harms various aspects of your life, such as your friendships, family relationships, and appearance. *HealthQuest* will help you estimate your risk of becoming a problem drinker or alcoholic. After completing the assessment activity, briefly record your answers to the following questions: Do your beliefs about alcohol reflect your drinking behavior? What factors might cause a person's beliefs and behaviors to be incompatible? What life experiences or influences, such as family, religion, and advertising, have helped form your beliefs about alcohol? Do you think your beliefs and behavior patterns are fixed, or will they change over time?

- The *Alcohol Decision Maze*, found in the Alcohol Module, simulates an evening out with a friend. The activity prompts you to make a variety of choices throughout the evening that may influence whether or how much you drink. First you will choose among several companions for the evening. Then you must decide where to go. At each location, such as a restaurant or sporting event, you can choose from a list of activities in which to participate. The choice to buy or drink alcohol surfaces often. *HealthQuest* will then provide feedback on the outcome of the evening and estimate your blood alcohol content. Complete this activity several times, making different decisions each time. Does the outcome of the evening reflect the drinking behavior resulting from your decisions?

of alcoholic parents are four times more likely to become alcoholics even when raised by nonalcoholics.

Treatment for alcoholism is often long-term. The course of treatment usually occurs in three stages: (1) detoxification (eliminating the alcohol from the body), (2) medical care (attending to any health-related problems), and (3) changing long-term behavior (helping the recovering alcoholic overcome long-established drinking patterns and destructive behaviors). Several sources provide long-term medical and psychological support to people with drug or alcohol problems.

Alcoholics remain alcoholics for life, regardless of whether they drink. Recovering alcoholics must therefore be careful about any products they consume, including

Wellness Across the Generations

Alcohol and Tobacco Use Among Young Women

At one time it was thought that alcohol-related problems occurred more often in men than women. Now mounting evidence indicates that women—especially young women—are drinking more. This fact is reflected in the increased number of admissions of younger women to treatment centers.[15] Women who are alcoholics often drink for reasons different from those that prompt men to abuse alcohol, and some of the consequences of drinking are different between the genders. Smoking, too, poses special risks for women, especially those who are pregnant. Here are some of these gender differences:

- More women than men who abuse alcohol can identify a specific triggering event that prompted them to start drinking, such as a death, a divorce, a job change, or the departure of a child from home.

- Women tend to begin abusing alcohol later in life than men do and to progress more quickly in their abuse pattern.

- Women are prescribed more mood-altering drugs than men are and are thus at greater risk for drug interactions and cross-tolerance.

- Alcoholic women are less likely than men are to have a family support system to aid them in their recovery attempts.

- Women alcoholics tend not to receive as much social support as men do during their treatment for and recovery from alcoholism.

- Women tend to have more financial problems than men do, which makes entry into a treatment program more difficult.[16]

Here are some alcohol- and tobacco-related effects of concern to parents and couples considering pregnancy:

- The children of pregnant women who drink are at a high risk for fetal alcohol syndrome (FAS), which causes a variety of birth defects ranging in severity from abnormal eye alignment to nose and jaw irregularities, cleft palate, joint defects, heart defects, and inadequate brain development. FAS has been reported in children of women who drank as little as 30 milliliters of alcohol per day (about two mixed drinks, three bottles of beer, or two glasses of wine). Thus it is recommended that women abstain from drinking any alcohol during pregnancy.

- Babies born to mothers who smoke have a lower average birth weight and length and have a smaller head circumference.[17]

- Infants born to mothers who smoke are more likely than children born to nonsmokers to die from sudden infant death syndrome (SIDS).[17]

- Smoking during pregnancy may cause hyperactivity in children.

Finally, men and women who smoke should know the following:

- Smoking by both men and women is associated with premature facial wrinkling.

- Osteoporosis (loss of calcium from the bone) is associated with smoking.

medicines and mouthwashes, which sometimes contain alcohol. Currently, an estimated 10 million adults and 3 million adolescents under the age of 18 are alcoholics.[8]

Alcohol use has been demonstrated to have a strong association with crime and violence. Data clearly indicate that homicide is more likely to occur in a situation in which drinking has occurred.[12] In this same study all incidents of spousal and child abuse were correlated with drinking. A Canadian study found that at least 42 percent of violent crimes involved alcohol.[2] In addition, 75 percent of suicide attempts involved alcohol use.[1]

As explained in the safety chapter, alcohol and driving can be a lethal combination. Alcohol is linked to at least half of all highway fatalities, and this figure in-cludes only crashes involving drivers classified as legally intoxicated. Finally, in single-vehicle fatal wrecks occurring on weekend nights, the driver is legally intoxicated almost 70 percent of the time.

Binge drinking among college students

Binge drinking is defined as consuming five or more drinks in a single session for men and four or more for women at least once within the previous two weeks. According to a national survey conducted by the Harvard School of Public Health, nearly half of college students surveyed drank four or five drinks in the previous two weeks prior to the survey.[28] Another study reported that 39 percent of college women binge drank within a two-week period prior to the survey.[29] In a multicampus survey, white non-Hispanic students reported the highest percentage of binge drinking in a two-week period (43.8 percent), followed by Native American (40.6 percent) Hispanic (31.3 percent), Asian (22.7 percent), and black non-Hispanic (22.5 percent) students.[13]

(For a discussion of how much alcohol is contained in various types of alcoholic drinks, see Just the Facts: How Much Alcohol Is in Beer, Wine, and Other Drinks? on p. 343.) This information is alarming in light of the number of deaths in the last few years caused by binge drinking during fraternity or campus rituals. Problems associated with student binge drinking include residence hall damage, fights, sexual assault, and drunk driving. The greater a student's alcohol use, the poorer his or her academic performance.[14] The most distressing fact is that binge drinking too often causes unnecessary deaths of drinkers, their friends, and other innocent victims.

Many colleges and universities have begun programs that emphasize responsible, rather than total, abstinence. Guidelines published for reducing the risk associated with heavy or binge drinking are:

1. *Pace your drinking*—Allow time between drinks and sip the drink.
2. *Do not drink every day*—Tolerance is developed and a person must increase the amount of alcohol consumed before effects are noticed. BAC is still rising even though effects are unnoticed.
3. *You decide when to drink*—Do not allow others or situations to determine your drinking. Drink on your terms.
4. *Consider alternating nonalcoholic drinks with those containing alcohol*—Drink a soft drink without alcohol every other drink or drink plain orange juice every other drink.
5. *Don't drink on an empty stomach*—Food with fats and/or protein slow the absorption of the alcohol.
6. *Measure the alcohol*—Pay attention to the size of containers. Do not provide kegs of beer or use larger sized wine, beer, or shot glasses. No "chugging" contests or other drinking games.
7. *Don't drink for more than one hour*—Decide what nonalcoholic drink you are going to drink after the hour.
8. *Learn how to calculate your BAC*—Know how many drinks are allowed within your hour period.
9. *If you are a female, drink less*—Women become more intoxicated than men after drinking the same amount of alcohol even when differences in body weight are take into account. Women have proportionately less water in their bodies than

men, thus they become more highly concentrated in BAC.

10. *Avoid taking over-the-counter (OTC) or prescription medications*—More than 100 medications interact with alcohol. If you are taking any OTC or prescription drugs, ask your doctor or pharmacist whether you can safely drink alcoholic beverages.

Fortunately, most college students moderate their drinking after their college years. However, about 12 percent are unable to control their drinking and continue to abuse alcohol. You should weigh carefully the potential harmful consequences of alcohol use and abuse before partaking in binge or heavy drinking. Is it worth the price?

Tobacco Products

All tobacco products, including cigarettes, cigars, pipes, and smokeless tobacco (snuff and chewing tobacco), contain the drug **nicotine**. Nicotine is an addictive substance and an alkaloid poison. It affects the body by increasing heart and respiratory rates, elevating blood pressure, increasing cardiac output and oxygen consumption, and constricting the bronchi (the two main branches of the trachea that lead to the lungs). A person inhales nicotine when smoking a tobacco product. Nicotine in smokeless tobacco is absorbed through membranes of the mouth and cheek.

Smoking is directly or indirectly responsible for the conditions and diseases listed in Just the Facts: Risks of Smoking. Some components of cigarette smoke are known as *carcinogens* (substances that cause cancer or foster the growth of cancer cells). Nicotine, tars, and carbon monoxide are found in cigarette smoke. The tar in tobacco is a black, sticky, dark fluid composed of thousands of chemicals. Many of the chemicals found in tar are cancer causing. Carbon monoxide is a deadly gas emitted in the exhaust of cars and in burning tobacco. The carbon monoxide level in cigarette smoke is 400 times greater than what is considered safe in industrial settings. Carbon monoxide binds to hemoglobin more readily than oxygen, interfering with the ability of blood to transport oxygen to the body. Carbon monoxide impairs the nervous system and increases the risk of heart attacks and strokes.

The addictive nature of nicotine has come under substantial public scrutiny. Some experts consider nicotine to be as addictive as cocaine and other drugs. Tobacco is considered the leading preventable contributor to disease and early death in the United States (from heart disease and cancer specifically) and is listed as a primary risk factor for heart disease by the American Heart Association. Cigarettes are responsible for 435,000 deaths annually.[18] Because of the health risks and because of what is seen by many as an

Just the Facts

Risks of Smoking

Here is some information about the risks of smoking:

Conditions and Diseases That Can Be Caused by Smoking and Tobacco Products

Risks	Results
Coronary heart disease	An estimated 430,700 die each year of smoking-related illnesses. Largest portion of these deaths is related to cardiovascular disease (AHA).
Peripheral arterial disease	Smokers are 2 to 3 times more likely to suffer from abdominal aortic aneurysm than are nonsmokers. Smokers have more atherosclerotic occlusions.
Lung cancer	Smoking cigarettes is the major cause of lung cancers in men and women. Rates are currently increasing faster among women than men.
Cancer of the larynx	Laryngeal cancer is 2.0 to 27.4 times more likely in smokers than in nonsmokers.
Oral cancers	Use of smokeless tobacco and snuff is associated with an increased risk of oral cancer. Pipes and cigars are also major risk factors. Use of alcohol seems to enhance the possibility of developing oral cancer.
Cancer of the esophagus	Smoking cigarettes, pipes, and cigars increases by as much as 9 times the risk of dying from esophageal cancer. Alcohol use in combination with smoking adds to that risk.
Bladder cancer	The percentage of bladder cancer attributed to smoking is estimated at 40 to 60 percent in men and 25 to 35 percent in women.
Cancer of the pancreas	Smokers have twice the risk of nonsmokers for cancer of the pancreas.
Chronic obstructive pulmonary (lung) disease (COPD)	Between 80 and 90 percent of more than 60,000 deaths per year from COPD are caused by smoking.
Peptic ulcers	Cigarette smokers develop peptic ulcers much more frequently than do nonsmokers. Ulcers are also more difficult to cure in smokers.
Complications in pregnancy, illnesses in children	Smoking mothers have more stillbirths and babies with low birth weight. The hospital admission rate for pneumonia and bronchitis is 28 percent higher for children of smoking mothers than for children of nonsmoking mothers. Asthma is more common among children of smoking mothers. Parental smoking is a risk factor associated with persistent middle-ear effusion in young children.

Source: American Cancer Society, 2000. Surveillance Research

effort on the part of tobacco companies to intentionally increase nicotine addiction to increase sales of cigarettes, some people suggest that tobacco should be made an illegal drug.

Secondhand and sidestream smoke

Passive smoking is the inhalation of what is known as *secondhand cigarette smoke* from the environment by a nonsmoker. Smokers inhale what is known as **mainstream smoke;** passive smokers most frequently inhale **sidestream smoke,** which results from burning tobacco products (the end of the lighted tip of a cigarette, cigar, or pipe).[19] Because it is not filtered by either a cigarette filter or the smoker's lungs, sidestream smoke contains higher concentrations of carbon dioxide and carbon monoxide. For each pack of cigarettes smoked indoors by a smoker, a nonsmoker in the vicinity passively smokes the equivalent of three to five cigarettes.[1] Research shows that nonsmokers living with smokers have a 20 percent higher mortality rate than do the nonsmoking partners of nonsmokers. Nonsmoking wives of smokers have been found to be at greater risk of lung cancer than the wives of nonsmoking husbands. Other studies have reported that nonsmokers living with smokers have a greater risk of developing respiratory problems and that nonsmoking women living with smokers have a greater risk of cervical cancer.[20] The bottom line about passive smoking is that there is no safe level of exposure to tobacco smoke.

Wellness On the Web
Behavior Change Activities

When "Social Drinking" Becomes Antisocial

Despite the proven health risks, the ruined lives, and the rising toll of fatal drunk-driving accidents, alcohol use continues to be pervasive in our society. Alcohol is a drug that many people deem socially acceptable. Slick TV and magazine advertisements glamorize drinking and portray it as the pastime of attractive, healthy, affluent people. The grim reality is that no other drug causes so much physical, social, and emotional damage to both individuals and families. People drink alcoholic beverages in many situations and for many reasons, and many people don't know why they drink. To test your knowledge of alcohol use, go to www.mhhe.com/anspaugh5e, click on "Student Center," "Chapter 11," "Wellness on the Web," and then "Activity 1," and complete the alcohol quiz. How much did you know about alcohol and our society?

Kicking the Habit

If you've ever tried to quit smoking, you know how hard it can be. That's because nicotine is a highly addictive drug. For some people, it can be as addictive as heroin or cocaine. Within seconds of your taking a puff of smoke, nicotine travels to your brain. It tells your brain to release chemicals that make you want to smoke more. Although quitting is difficult, the health benefits you gain far outweigh the temporary discomfort of withdrawal. Most people make two to three tries, or more, before finally being able to quit. Studies show that each time you try to quit, you'll become more determined and learn more about what helps and what hurts. Regardless of age, health, or lifestyle, anyone can quit smoking. The decision to quit and your chances of success are strongly influenced by how much you want to stop smoking. Go to the website listed previously and click on "Activity 2" to learn about the steps the CDC recommends to help you quit—and win.

Cigars and pipes

In the hope of avoiding the dangers associated with cigarette smoking, some smokers have turned from cigarettes to cigars or pipes. Since pipe and cigar smokers don't inhale, they do seem less likely to develop lung and heart disease. However, pipe and cigar smokers have a much higher risk of developing mouth, larynx, and esophageal cancers because they hold the nicotine and tars from their tobacco products in their mouths instead of inhaling them. Furthermore, when a cigarette smoker switches to cigars or a pipe, he or she tends to continue to inhale and, thus, to remain at the same risk for lung and heart disease while the risk of other cancers increases.[30]

Smokeless tobacco products

Smokeless tobacco products consist of snuff and chewing tobacco. Snuff is a finely shredded or powdered tobacco sniffed by the user, allowing nicotine to be absorbed through the mucous membranes of the nose and mouth. Chewing tobacco consists of loose-leaf tobacco mixed with molasses or other flavors and pressed into what are called *plugs* or twisted into rope-like strands. This material is then placed between the gums and cheek or lower lip, where the nicotine is absorbed. In 1994 it was estimated that more than 6 million men and 730,000 women used smokeless tobacco products.

Smokeless tobacco is not a safe alternative to cigarettes. It contributes to the development of periodontal (gum) disease, which can result in bleeding gums, loss of teeth, staining of teeth, and tooth decay. Periodontal disease is less significant than the oral cancers that may be caused by frequent contact of the cells of the gums and cheek with the carcinogenic agents in the tobacco. Two early danger signs of such cancers are the formation of leukoplakia (white spots) or erythroplakia (red spots), which indicate precancerous conditions and should be evaluated by a physician immediately. If treatment is delayed, cancer can quickly spread to the jaw, neck, brain, and digestive and urinary systems.[1]

Clove cigarettes

Some people smoke clove cigarettes as an alternative to regular cigarettes. Clove cigarettes usually consist of 60 percent tobacco and 40 percent clove buds. Clove cigarettes generate even more nicotine, tar, and carbon monoxide than do regular cigarettes, so the dangers are even greater. Some users have developed serious lung and respiratory illnesses.[21]

Advantages of quitting

Smoking is an extremely strong addiction. To quit completely, many people require the help of trained professionals (see Real-World Wellness: Charting a Plan to Quit Smoking or Stop Using Tobacco Products and Real-World Wellness: Choosing a Smoking Cessation Aid). Although quitting is difficult, the health benefits gained far outweigh the problems. When people stop smoking, their risk of developing heart disease and some kinds of cancer (if not already present in the body) eventually decreases to that of nonsmokers; in other words, some of the effects of smoking are reversible (see figure 11-1).

Real-World Wellness

Charting a Plan to Quit Smoking or Stop Using Tobacco Products

I've tried several times to quit smoking, but I'm still lighting up. This time I want to be prepared. Is there a plan I can follow that will help me quit for good?

The *Mayo Clinic Health Letter* offers the following suggestions:[13]

- *Set a date:* Make the date reasonably soon. Make a list of reasons you want to quit.

- *Start stopping before you reach the date:* Taper off the number of cigarettes you are currently smoking. Choose a milder brand.

- *Make your plans known:* Tell a friend, your family, and colleagues of your plans. Ask for their support.

- *Take it one day at a time:* Get up every morning and decide not to smoke that day. Focus your attention on that day only.

- *Change your routine:* Avoid or change situations in which you have previously smoked.

- *Alter your surroundings:* Start new activities, such as exercising or needlepoint.

- *Time the urge:* Identify when your urge to smoke is the strongest. Being prepared will help you resist.

- *Use substitutes:* Substitutes can include gum, celery, carrots, and pickles.

- *Prepare a daydream:* Have a pleasant daydream ready to help fight off the desire to smoke. This can be an image of yourself without a cigarette in a situation you find highly desirable.

- *Use relaxation techniques:* Deep breathing or progressive muscle relaxation can help.

- *Stay busy:* Find ways to keep yourself and your mind occupied so you do not miss smoking or having a cigarette in your hand.

- *Practice positive thinking:* Tell yourself, "I can make it." Remember that you *can* do it.

Your first year as a nonsmoker

Immediately
- The air around you is no longer dangerous to children and adults.

20 minutes
- Your blood pressure improves.
- Your pulse rate decreases.
- The temperature of your hands and feet increases to more normal levels.

12 hours
- Your body's carbon monoxide level starts to decrease.

1 year
- Your risk of early heart disease falls by 50%.

1 to 9 months
- You have fewer coughs, colds, and flu episodes.
- Fatigue and shortness of breath decrease.
- Your lungs increase their ability to remove impurities and reduce infection.

Your future years
- Within 10 to 15 years your life expectancy is comparable to that of people who never smoked.

24 hours
- Your chance of heart attack decreases.

36 hours
- The carbon monoxide in your blood decreases to healthier levels.
- The oxygen in your blood increases to healthier levels.

2 to 12 weeks
- Your circulation improves.
- Your lung function improves.

48 hours
- Nerve endings start to regrow.
- Exercise gets easier.
- Your senses of smell and taste improve.

Figure 11-1 Health Benefits of Quitting Smoking

Quitting smoking results in benefits that begin immediately and become more significant the longer a person stays smoke-free.

Real-World Wellness

Choosing a Smoking Cessation Aid

I've been smoking since my freshman year in high school, and I'm about to graduate from college and enter the workforce. I'd like to quit, but I'm confused about all the smoking cessation products available. How do I choose the one that's best for me?

Several tools are available to help smokers wean themselves off cigarettes. These smoking cessation aids can be purchased over the counter (OTC) or with a doctor's prescription. The dosages for both versions can vary widely. For this reason, it is probably better to seek a prescription version, which will more specifically be targeted to your needs. Read the following information about three commonly used methods, and then talk to your doctor to choose the one best suited to your needs.

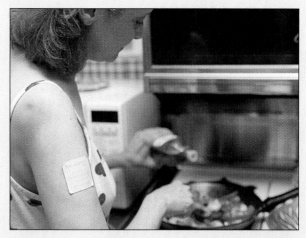

Many people have used nicotine patches to help them quit smoking. If you're a smoker, have you considered trying the patch?

- *Nicotine-containing gum:* Nicotine gum requires immediate smoking cessation. The dosage is 2 to 4 mg of nicotine per piece of gum. When used under a physician's guidance, the success rate is about 40 percent. Chewing the gum may cause mouth ulcers and nausea in some people, and the product should not be used by pregnant or nursing women. Initial doses of the chewing gum cost about $50, with weekly refills costing about $30.

- *Transdermal patches:* The patch is designed to aid smoking cessation by relieving nicotine withdrawal cravings. Two types are available: a step-down version and a single-dose version. The single-dose version provides the same milligrams of nicotine in each dose (15 mg). The step-down version provides different levels of nicotine for various periods after cessation, theoretically reducing the amount of nicotine available as the person is weaned away from the drug. The step-down method is designed to ease withdrawal by making the symptoms less severe and withdrawal more gradual. The patches contain 15 to 21 mg of nicotine a day for the first weeks. After four to twelve weeks, the dosage is reduced

to 10 to 14 mg a day. A final set of patches used for two to four weeks contains 5 to 7 mg of nicotine. Single-dose patches eliminate the step-down effect. Used alone, both versions of the patch seem to be less than 25 percent effective. When used with the prescription medication mecamylamine, however, the effectiveness rate rises to 40 percent. The patch can cause skin irritation, redness, and irregular heart rate in some users. The cost is about the same as for nicotine-containing gum.

- *Nicotrol™ inhaler.* A federal advisory panel to the FDA recently endorsed a prescription inhalation device that is an alternative to chewing gum and transdermal patches. The Nicotrol inhaler is meant to simulate cigarette smoking. The device has a mouthpiece with a nicotine plug attached to it. Seventy to eighty puffs on the inhaler provide the amount of nicotine in ten puffs on a regular cigarette. Having the inhaler to handle may help smokers who miss having something to do with their hands while simultaneously providing a low level of nicotine to ease cravings.

HealthQuest Activities

- The Tobacco Module of HealthQuest allows you to assess your risk of disease caused by exposure to tobacco smoke. If you're a smoker, you can evaluate the reasons you may be ready to quit or cut back. If you have loved ones or friends who smoke, you will also benefit from this exercise—the feedback you'll receive in the personal risk section will take into account both direct and indirect exposure to tobacco smoke. Feedback about reasons for quitting is based on the relative importance of each reason to the smoker. For

example, you might want to quit for health reasons, while a friend of yours might want to quit because smoking is inconvenient at work.

- The *Tobacco Ads and You* activity in the Tobacco Module introduces you to the messages that tobacco advertisements send to consumers and the ways in which young people are manipulated to become smokers. This exploration activity helps you examine your beliefs and feelings about cigarette advertising by rating how each ad appeals to you. You can also participate in a survey about the messages the ads are trying to convey and your use of tobacco products and promotional items.

Illegal Drugs

Designer Drugs

Designer drugs resemble those controlled by the Federal Drug Administration (FDA); that is, they act like known drugs but have a different chemical composition. Probably the two best-known designer drugs currently being used are *China white*, an analog of heroin, and *ecstasy*. Ecstasy is an analog of the amphetamines and hallucinogens under FDA control since 1985. Designer drugs appear so rapidly that it is difficult or impossible to restrict sales. Poor quality control and combinations with other, often poisonous, substances can result in neurological damage or death. Brain damage is often caused by a single dose.

Club Drugs

Club drugs are among a group of drugs used by teens and young adults who are part of a bar, rave, or trance scene. Raves and trances are generally night-long dances, often held in warehouses. Not everyone attending these events uses drugs, but those who do are attracted to the low cost, the seemingly increased stamina, and the intoxicating highs said to increase the rave or trance experience.[26]

The drugs of concern are MDMA (Ecstasy), Rohypnol, GHB, and Ketamine. Researchers are finding that critical parts of the brain are showing changes from use of these drugs. When used in higher doses, most of these drugs can cause a sharp increase in body temperature, which leads to muscle breakdown, cardiovascular incidents, and kidney failure.[26]

MDMA (Ecstasy)

MDMA is a chemical substance that combines methamphetamines with hallucinogenic (LSD-like) properties. Ecstasy is the street name for MDMA. Other names include Adam, X-TC, Hug, Beans, Love bug, Clarity, and Lover's Speed. Ecstasy is a combination of several illicit drugs. Because so many different recipes are used to make Ecstasy, the risk of death and permanent brain damage is heightened. The drug works primarily by affecting nerve cells that produce serotonin, one of several chemicals transmitting signals from one nerve to the next. Ecstasy causes nerve cells to release all the stored serotonin at once and then keeps it from being reabsorbed, further increasing the concentration in the synapse. The result can lead to long-term or permanent damage to those areas of the brain critical to thought, memory, and pleasure. The aftermath of use can include a depressive hangover, sometimes called "Terrible Tuesday." Other psychological effects are confusion; sleep problems; severe anxiety; paranoid thinking; enhanced

mental and emotional clarity; sensations of floating; and violent, irrational behavior. Some reported physical effects of the drug include muscle tension, involuntary teeth clenching, blurred vision, hypertension, loss of control over voluntary body movements, tremors, kidney failure, heart attack, stroke, seizures, and malignant hyperthermia (increased body temperature).[27]

Rohypnol

Rohypnol, a trade name for flunitrazepam, has been a serious concern for several years because of its abuse in date rape (see Chapter 10). When mixed with alcohol, Rohypnol incapacitates its victims and prevents them from resisting sexual assault. Slang names for the drug include "rophies," "roofies," "roach," and "rope." The drugs (alcohol and Rohypnol) produce a form of "amnesia" in which individuals may not remember events they experienced while under the effects of the drugs. Further, Rohypnol may be lethal when mixed with alcohol or other depressants.

GHB

GHB (gammahydroxbutrate) has been abused in the United States for euphoric, sedative, and anabolic (body-building) effects. It is a central nervous system depressant widely available over the counter in health food stores during the 1980s and until 1992. It was purchased mostly by body builders to aid in muscle building and fat reduction. Street names include Liquid Ecstasy, Soap, Easy Lay, and Georgia Home Boy. GHB is difficult to distinguish from water. Coma and seizures can occur with abuse and, when combined with methamphetamines, there appears to be an increased risk of seizure, nausea, and difficulty breathing. Withdrawal effects include insomnia, anxiety, tremors, and sweating. The drug is sold over the internet and is available in some workout gyms, rave night clubs, gay male parties, college campuses, and on the street. The duration of the drug is short, but may cause unconsciousness when mixed with alcohol.

Ketamine

Ketamine is an anesthetic approved for both human and animal use in medical settings. Over 90 percent of the drugs sold legally is used for practice of veterinary medicine. Ketamine can be injected or snorted. On the street, it is known as "Special K" or "vitamin K." At high doses, Ketamine can cause delirium, amnesia impaired motor function, high blood pressure, depression, and potentially fatal respiratory problems. Certain doses can cause dreamlike states and hallucinations. Because of the latter characteristics, it has become common in club and rave scenes and has been used as a date rape drug.

Cocaine

At one time **cocaine** was considered the drug of upper-class America. Unfortunately, the use of cocaine and its derivative, crack, is now epidemic. It is estimated that 25 to 30 million people have experimented with cocaine in the United States. Approximately 5 million people use the drug regularly. Among young adults, 6.7 percent have tried crack and 40 percent have tried cocaine.[22] From 1987 to 1991, cocaine use reportedly decreased. However, since 1991, the use of cocaine appears to have rebounded, especially among young people.[23]

A powerful stimulant, cocaine is derived from the leaves of the South American coca shrub and ground into a crystalline powder. The most common methods of using the drug are either snorting it, liquefying it and then injecting it, or freebasing (smoking). When snorted, the white powder is sniffed up through the nose. The most potent and expensive method of cocaine use is freebasing. The drug is usually smoked in a water pipe because this provides faster absorption into the bloodstream.

Crack is relatively easy to make and fairly inexpensive to buy. At $10 to $15 a dose, crack is the form of cocaine most prevalent on the streets. When snorted, crack reaches the brain in about 5 minutes. When injected or smoked, it takes only a few seconds for the drug to take effect.

Use of cocaine produces feelings of well-being, euphoria, and extreme exhilaration. Mental alertness seems to increase. Blood vessels constrict, causing heart rate and blood pressure to rise. Cocaine is rapidly metabolized by the liver. Snorting cocaine results in a 5- to 15-minute "high," and the effects of crack last 20 to 30 minutes. Psychological and physical dependency on crack develop rapidly because of the brief period of stimulation. The feelings of exhilaration experienced while under the influence of the drug are quickly followed by depression.

The physical consequences of cocaine use are extreme and highly dangerous. Cocaine use can cause headaches, exhaustion, shaking, blurred vision, nausea, impaired judgment, hyperactivity, loss of appetite, loss of sexual desire, and paranoia that can lead to violence. Snorting cocaine can destroy the septum in the nose. Freebasing may damage the liver and the lungs; fluid buildup in the lungs caused by freebasing has resulted in death. Cocaine can initiate strokes, bleeding in the brain, heart attacks, irregular heartbeat, and sudden death.[22]

Cocaine addiction is extremely difficult to overcome. Addiction researchers currently believe a broad-based treatment program, including medical, psychiatric, pharmacological, and psychosocial elements, is the most successful.

Marijuana

Approximately twenty-five years ago, **marijuana** became a cultural phenomenon, the symbol of one generation's disregard for or anger with another. The marijuana found on the streets at that time, however, lacked the potency of current crops. Crossbreeding of more potent varieties, improved cultivation, and use of different parts of the plant all contribute to increased levels of delta-9-tetrahydrocannabinol (THC), the major psychoactive drug found in marijuana. Some marijuana currently grown in the United States rivals the previously stronger varieties of Mexico, Jamaica, and other areas. The THC percentage of *Cannabis sativa* (the Indian hemp plant from which marijuana is derived) in plants grown in the United States can range from 2 percent to as high as 7 percent. A variety of marijuana know as *sinsemilla,* made from the buds of flowering tops of female plants, can have a potency as high as 24 percent.[3] The higher the percentage of THC, the more potent the drug. Marijuana is composed of the dried leaves and flowering tops of the cannabis plant. Hashish, which has stronger effects, is processed from the resin of the plant. The resin is either dried and pressed into cakes or sold in liquid form called *hash oil.* Marijuana is used more extensively than hashish in the United States.

More than 400 known chemicals constitute marijuana. More than sixty of these are *cannabinoids,* chemicals found only in cannabis. THC is the cannabinoid that appears most responsible for the sensations experienced by marijuana users. Cannabinoids are different from other drugs in that they are fat soluble rather than water soluble; they have a decided affinity for binding to fat in the human body. Although other drugs enter and then leave the body within relatively short periods, marijuana tends to attach to fatty organs, such as the gonads and brain, and remain.[24] A single ingestion of THC may require up to thirty days to be eliminated from the body.

Marijuana can be eaten in baked goods, such as brownies, but the effects tend to be less predictable. Because it better controls amount ingested, smoking is generally a more efficient and powerful technique for achieving the desired effect. When inhaled, THC reaches the brain in as few as fourteen seconds. Hashish is so concentrated that a single drop can equal the effects of an entire marijuana joint (cigarette). Cannabis products are difficult to classify but are considered hallucinogens.

Small doses or short-term use of marijuana creates sensations of euphoria and relaxation often accompanied by hunger or sleepiness. Time seems to slow, and the senses appear heightened. Memory of recent events, physical coordination, and perceptions may be impaired. Students, for example, may have difficulty remembering events that occurred when they were high. Even with small amounts of marijuana, driving ability can be affected. Physiologically, heart rate speeds up and certain blood vessels become dilated, which may create problems for people with any types of heart problems. Some users experience anxiety, panic, and paranoia. In rare cases or with stronger doses, people may suffer from a sense of depersonalization, image distortion, and hallucinations. Chronic use seems to lead to behavioral changes in some people that may be permanent. Lack of motivation or interest in activities unrelated to drug use is one result. Use by teenagers leads to impaired thinking, poor reading comprehension, and reduced verbal and mathematical skills.

All the long-term effects of marijuana use have not been determined. This is partly because of the lesser potency of marijuana used previously. In addition, people vary greatly in their responses to the drug. Chronic users may experience psychological dependence and need increased doses as tolerance develops. Very heavy users experience withdrawal symptoms of restlessness, irritability, tremors, nausea, vomiting, diarrhea, and sleep disturbances.[24]

Physically, marijuana appears to be more carcinogenic than tobacco. Known carcinogens occur in larger amounts in marijuana, and when marijuana is smoked, the smoke is held in the lungs. Cannabis smoke contains more tars than does tobacco smoke. Marijuana use quickly affects pulmonary function adversely, and long-term use causes cellular changes in the lungs. People who have angina pectoris (chest pains associated with heart disease) may be significantly at risk because more oxygen is required during marijuana use. Marijuana binds readily to hemoglobin, reducing the amount of oxygen carried to the heart and other tissues.

Many people consider cannabis an aphrodisiac. Over time it has the opposite effect, depressing the sex drive and causing impotence. Regular male users show a decrease in sperm count and reduced motility of sperm. Proportionately, more sperm appear abnormally shaped, a phenomenon associated with lessened fertility. In women, THC blocks ovulation. Pregnant women who smoke marijuana frequently use other drugs, all of which have a detrimental effect on the fetus. Marijuana also depresses the immune system.[24]

Therapeutic use is still being explored. At this time the most promising application seems to be as an anti-nausea drug for chemotherapy patients. Glaucoma patients may have access to and may use marijuana to reduce intraocular pressure (pressure within the eye).

Marijuana is an illegal drug. Many people who use marijuana eventually experiment with or use other harder drugs. Some researchers consider marijuana thus to be a *gateway drug*. As with alcohol and all other drugs, the way a person reacts to marijuana or is most adversely affected by it cannot be predicted. People do not begin use with the intention of having a drug become the focus of their lives, but some ultimately allow the drug to control them. Marijuana is a drug that has that potential.

Other Drugs of Concern

Drugs discussed in the following sections have been abused for many years. Unfortunately, some that had become less popular seem to be reappearing, along with a dangerous new generation of illicit drugs. All illegal drugs have quality control problems: Because there is no federal regulation of these drugs and because people involved in the transportation and distribution of illegal drugs are not always concerned about purity or quality, dangerous and even poisonous substances may be added to drugs. Also, it is frequently impossible to determine the potency of a drug. A very pure form of a drug can easily be lethal for a person who has been using a less potent form.

Heroin

Heroin is a narcotic synthesized from morphine. This drug induces a strong sensation of euphoria but quickly leads to physical and psychological dependency. The physical tolerance for heroin develops rapidly. Because heroin is usually injected, addicts often share needles, which increases the risk of contracting diseases, such as AIDS and hepatitis. Experts fear the younger generation may become addicted to heroin through a substance called *moonrock*—a mixture of heroin and cocaine that can be injected, smoked, or snorted. Heroin is used in this way to reduce the paranoia and depression that follow a cocaine high. Heroin use is considered to be on the rise.

In recent years heroin use has increased significantly, especially among well-educated people, often women, employed in white-collar and other professional jobs.[25] Heroin use has also reportedly increased among junior high and high school age groups. One reason for this trend may be the availability of more potent forms of heroin, which allow the user to experience a more pronounced effect by snorting it instead of injecting it, which people may be reluctant to do in part because of fear of HIV transmission. In addition, many users believe that smoking or snorting heroin, unlike injecting it, is nonaddicting.[25] Heroin may appeal to children because it is cheap and can be purchased fairly easily on the street. Users may not realize they are becoming addicted because they may function normally for some time after starting to use the drug before their behavior changes significantly enough for friends and family to become aware of their use. Heroin is undeniably rearing its ugly head again in the form of increased use, and it has reached the country's youth regardless of educational attainment, social class, or ethnic and racial background.

Methamphetamine (Crank)

Methamphetamine is a potent stimulant that can cause uncontrollable manic behavior or paranoid thinking. The most current use of this drug is as crystal methamphetamine, or *ice*. Although crystal methamphetamine has been touted as a safe alternative to cocaine, evidence indicates otherwise. Recent headlines told about a father who, under the influence of methamphetamine, decapitated his son. Overdoses are often fatal, and the drug is extremely addictive. In many areas of the United States, use of ice is a widespread problem.

Lysergic Acid Diethylamide (LSD)

LSD is a hallucinogenic drug that has become more popular, especially among the upper class. The substance induces altered perceptions of shapes, images, time, self, and sound. Tolerance to the drug develops quickly with daily use.[12] Flashbacks can occur in some people.

Phencyclidine (PCP)

PCP was originally intended for use as a surgical anesthetic for humans. However, the drug was determined unsuitable for this purpose because of its unusual and undesirable effects on patients.[9] Also called *angel dust*, PCP provokes a variety of unpredictable responses in users. These reactions include feelings of unreality, depersonalization, confusion, depression, anxiety, aggressive and violent behavior, acute or permanent psychosis, and coma. Users often fail to experience sensations of pain and report feeling uncoordinated in their movements. Classified as a hallucinogen, PCP has been used as an additive to cocaine, a combination that multiplies the toxic effects of both drugs.

Over-the-Counter Drugs

An area of drug use that is sometimes overlooked and assumed to be safe is the use of over-the-counter drugs (OTCs). The power of OTCs is often underestimated. As with all drugs, the ultimate responsibility for correct use of OTC drugs rests with each person. Because OTCs are readily available, abuse is a real possibility. OTCs may potentiate the effects of prescription drugs, herbs, vitamins, alcohol, or other OTCs, especially when not taken according to directions. OTCs can cause physiological damage to various body structures, with symptoms ranging from disorientation to kidney or liver damage. Here are some guidelines for safe use of OTCs:[3]

- Always know what you are taking and the product's active ingredients.
- Know the drug's effects (including its undesired ones) and possible side effects. Be sure you understand how the drug is supposed to work.
- Read and heed warnings and cautions concerning use of the product.
- Don't use any OTC product continuously for more than two weeks. If the problem for which you took the drug persists, consult your physician.
- Be particularly cautious if you are also taking any prescription drugs, because serious interactions can occur.
- If you have any questions about an OTC product, consult a pharmacist.
- If you don't need a drug, don't use it.

A Final Thought

To develop a high level of wellness, you must address the issue of drug use. Drugs prescribed as medicine can promote quality of life, but unwise use severely diminishes quality of life. Alcohol continues to be the most abused drug among college students. Perhaps as people become more aware of the dangers associated with alcohol and drug use, a smaller percentage of college students will use them (see Nurturing Your Spirituality: Finding Alternatives to Drug Use).

Nurturing Your Spirituality

Finding Alternatives to Drug Use

The best treatment for any alcohol or drug abuse problem is to prevent it. Adolescents and college-age students need attractive alternatives to drugs, such as participation in organizations or groups that fulfill in safe, constructive ways their need for camaraderie, acceptance, and group involvement. These organizations or groups can be developed around athletics, recreational activities, career development, or service opportunities. Involvement in enjoyable and meaningful activities tends to discourage drug use by providing a strong reinforcement system that helps people feel good about themselves and their abilities. All people, young and older, need a positive group atmosphere that fosters self-esteem, develops participants' ability to help others, and provides role models who pursue selfless, achievement-oriented goals.

At the college and university level, students aged 25 and younger may be faced with an autonomy never before experienced when they leave home to go to school. They are faced with the fact that no one is standing over them to ensure their attendance at and productivity in school, at work, or in other areas. Their decision-making power is increased as well as is the pressure to conform to peer standards, many of which they are encountering for the first time. This newfound freedom sometimes requires a continuation of prevention education and activities that direct them toward positive activities and behaviors. University administrators should seek to make such programs highly visible within the institutions they serve. It

is helpful for everyone connected with a college or university to demonstrate positive behaviors concerning the prevention of drug and alcohol abuse on campus. This may require that the president not serve alcoholic beverages at receptions and that faculty actively discourage binge drinking and other dangerous forms of drinking and be willing to engage in activities outside the classroom that involve positive alternatives to alcohol and other drug use. Another important component of any alternative program is a strong peer education network, in which student leaders promote a healthy campus life by discouraging alcohol and drug abuse and related problems, such as property destruction, violence, and sexual assault.

Other prevention-oriented programs are recreational activities, such as hiking, camping, and canoeing, and leadership challenge courses, such as rope courses and outward-bound experiences. The programs should offer diverse opportunities that appeal to a wide variety of student interests. Art exhibits; musical events; movie or book clubs; and community service programs, such as Humanity for Mankind, can all offer further opportunities for students to engage in personally and socially beneficial activities. Having mentors assigned to incoming first-year students and holding group discussions of various problems associated with collegiate life, perhaps with mandatory attendance by first-year students, may also be helpful. In addition, the college or university should emphasize to students that the purpose of higher education is to gain the experience and expertise to better serve one's family, community, and country. To truly accept responsibility for their lives, all people need to understand and accept responsibility for their behavior and recognize that alcohol and drug use never offers a long-term solution to personal, emotional, or spiritual difficulties.

Summary

- People use drugs for a variety of reasons, including for recreational or social enjoyment, to seek novel sensations, to enhance religious or spiritual experiences, to alter consciousness, to rebel or alienate oneself from society, and to submit to peer pressure.
- Drugs are commonly classified in a variety of ways, including according to their physiological effects.
- Caffeine is probably the most commonly used drug in the United States. It is a stimulant that speeds heart rate, increases blood pressure, and can cause insomnia.
- Alcohol is a socially acceptable drug that is a major source of physical and emotional damage and death.
- The blood alcohol concentration (BAC) of ethyl alcohol is affected by the rate of consumption, the type of alcoholic beverage being consumed, and the drinker's body weight and tolerance to alcohol.

- Binge drinking often occurs on college campuses and can lead to property destruction, sexual assault, and even death.
- Alcoholism is a disease in which a person loses control over drinking.
- Determining who will become an alcoholic is impossible because alcoholism crosses all social, economic, gender, educational, and racial lines.
- Nicotine is an addictive drug contained in tobacco. The tars found in tobacco are carcinogenic agents.
- No tobacco product is safe. Cigarettes, cigars, pipes, and smokeless products all pose threats to health.
- Carbon monoxide, formed when tobacco is smoked, interferes with the body's ability to transport oxygen and increases the risk of heart attack and stroke.
- Sidestream smoke has a higher concentration of tar and nicotine than the smoke inhaled by the smoker.

- Clove cigarettes contain even more nicotine and carbon monoxide than do regular cigarettes.
- Cocaine use has become epidemic in the United States. Cocaine can be snorted, injected, or freebased (smoked).
- The primary psychoactive ingredient in marijuana is delta-9-tetrahydrocannabinol.
- Carcinogens can be found in more potent levels in marijuana than in tobacco.
- Hashish is more potent than regular marijuana. Sinsemilla is a form of marijuana that can have a potency as high as 24 percent.
- Short-term effects of marijuana use include euphoria and perceptual impairment. Some people experience anxiety, a sense of depersonalization, and hallucinations.

- Some drugs, such as heroin, methamphetamine (crank), and LSD, have been abused in our society for many years.
- The newest form of methamphetamine is ice, which is smokable and more addictive, potent, and destructive than crack cocaine.
- Heroin use has been increasing among college and high school students.
- Designer drugs are analogs of controlled substances and are more powerful and less pure and have less predictable effects than do controlled substances.
- OTC drugs must be used carefully to avoid psychological and physiological problems.

Review Questions

1. What are some reasons people choose to use drugs?
2. Discuss the ways in which drugs can be classified.
3. What are the positive and negative effects of caffeine use?
4. What factors affect a drinker's blood alcohol concentration (BAC)?
5. How can a person practice responsible drinking?
6. What are some potential effects of long-term alcohol use?

7. Discuss the risks of using any tobacco product.
8. Discuss the specific benefits of quitting smoking.
9. Why is heroin use increasing among high school and college students?
10. What makes cocaine such a dangerous drug?
11. What factors should you consider before using any OTC product?

References

1. Pinger, R., W. Payne, D. Hahn, and E. Hahn. 1998. *Drugs: Issues for Today.* Dubuque, Iowa: WCB/McGraw-Hill.
2. Schlaadt, R. G., and P. T. Shannon. 1994. *Drugs: Use, Misuse, and Abuse.* Needham Heights, Mass.: Allyn and Bacon.
3. Hanson, G., and P. J. Venturelli. 1998. *Drugs and Society.* Boston: Jones and Bartlett.
4. Consumer Reports. September 1997. What caffeine can do for you—and to you. *Consumer Reports on Health.* 97–101. Vol 9:9.
5. Mayo Clinic. February 1992. Second opinion. *Mayo Clinic Health Letter.* 8. Vol 10:2.
6. Tufts University. February 1990. Grounds for breaking the coffee habit. *Tufts University Diet & Nutrition Letter* 3–6. Vol 7:2.
7. Carroll, C. R. 1993. *Drugs in Modern Society* (3d ed.). Dubuque, Iowa: Wm. C. Brown.
8. Morse, R. M., and D. K. Flavin. 1992. The definition of alcoholism. *JAMA* 268:1012–1014.
9. National Institute on Drug Abuse. 2001. Genetic factors in drug abuse and dependence. In *The Biobehavioral*

Etiology of Drug Abuse, eds. H. W. Gordon and M. D. Glantz. Research Monograph. 159.
10. Blum, K., G. Cull, E. Braverman, and D. Comings. 1996. Reward deficiency syndrome. *American Scientist* 84: 132–145.
11. Hawkins, J. D., D. M. Lishner, and R. F. Catalano. 1985. Childhood predictors and the prevention of adolescent substance abuse. *National Institute on Drug Abuse Research Monograph 56:* 87–1335.
12. National Clearinghouse for Alcohol and Drug Information. 2001. *Mind Over Matter—The Brain's Response to Hallucinogenic.* Rockville, Md.: Government Printing Office.
13. U.S. Department of Health and Human Services. 1996. *National Household Survey on Drug Abuse: Population Estimates.* Washington D.C.: U.S. Government Printing Office.
14. American Academy of Pediatrics. 1998. *AAP Releases New Findings on Teen and Underage Drinking.* Washington, D.C.: AAP.
15. U.S. Department of Health and Human Services. 1995. *Alcohol and Health: Seventh Special Report to the*

U.S. Congress. Washington, D.C.: U.S. Government Printing Office.
16. Kinney, J., and G. Leaton. 1999. *Loosening the Grip: A Handbook of Alcohol Information* (6th ed.). Dubuque, Iowa: WCB/McGraw-Hill.
17. Bartecchi, C. E., T. D. MacKenzie, and R. W. Shrier. 1995. The global tobacco epidemic. *Scientific American* 49.
18. Aldrich, L. 1995. Tobacco tax increase would reduce smoking. In *Smoking,* ed. K. L. Swisher. San Diego, Ca.: Greenhaven Press, 28–29.
19. Ray, O., and C. Ksir. 1999. *Drugs, Society, and Human Behavior* (8th ed.) Dubuque, Iowa: WCB/McGraw-Hill.
20. Environmental Protection Agency. 1993. *Respiratory Health Effects of Passive Smoking.* Fact sheet. Washington, D.C.: EPA.
21. Clark, G. C. 1990. Comparison of the inhalation toxicity of kretek (clove cigarette) smoke with that of American cigarette smoke. *Archives of Toxicology* 64(7):515–521.
22. Editors. November 1988. Hour by hour crack. *Newsweek,* 64–75.
23. Johnson, L. 1996. *University of Michigan Annual National Surveys of Secondary Students.* Lansing, Mich.:

University of Michigan. Available from author at 412 Maynard, Ann Arbor, MI.

24. Nahas, G. G. 1994. *Marijuana in Science and Medicine.* New York: Raven Press.

25. Fields, R. 1998. *Drugs in Perspective* (3rd ed.). Dubuque, Iowa: WCB/McGraw-Hill.

26. National Institute on Drug Abuse. 2000. *NIDA infofax—club drugs.* Available online at **www.nida.nih.gov/infofax/clubdrugs.html**.

27. National Institute on Drug Abuse. 2000. *Community drug alert bulletin on club drugs.* Available online at **www.clubdrugs.org**

28. Wechsler, H., et al. 1998. Changes in binge drinking and related problems among American college students between 1995 and 1997. *Journal of American College Health* 47:57–68.

29. Lyall, K. 1999. Binge drinking in college: A definitive study in binge drink-ing on American college campuses: A new look at an old problem. Report supported by the Robert Wood Johnson Foundation. Princeton, N.J.: The Foundation.

30. American Heart Association. 2001. *Biostatistical fact sheet—risk factors cigarette and tobacco smoke.* Available online at **www.americanheart.org/statistics/biostat/bioci.htm**.

Suggested Readings

Nakken, C. 1996. *The Addictive Personality: Understanding the Addictive Process and Compulsive Behavior.* Center City, Minn.: Hazelden.

This book examines genetic factors tied to addiction, cultural influences on addic-tive behavior, the progressive nature of the disease, and the steps necessary for a successful recovery.

Whelan, E. M. 1997. *Cigarettes: What the Warning Label Doesn't Tell You: The First Comprehensive Guide to the Health Consequences of Smoking* Amherst, N.Y.: Prometheus Books.

Noted experts detail all the known health risks of smoking, explaining clearly how cigarette smoking, can damage the body.

Assessment Activity 11-1

Do You Have a Drinking Problem?

Many self-tests have been published for people to use to determine whether they are alcoholics or have drinking problems. None can provide a definite diagnosis; deciding whether someone should seek help is usually a complex, subjective matter. One of the most popular printed self-tests appeared in a "Dear Abby" advice column, and it is offered here as a guide. If these questions seem to indicate that you or a friend needs to seek help, you should visit a counselor, psychologist, or physician experienced in the assessment of chemical dependency.

Directions: Check all that apply.

_____ 1. Have you ever decided to stop drinking for a week or so but only lasted for a couple of days?

_____ 2. Do you wish people would stop nagging you about your drinking?

_____ 3. Have you ever switched from one kind of drink to another in the hope that this would keep you from getting drunk?

_____ 4. Have you had a drink in the morning in the past year?

_____ 5. Do you envy people who can drink without getting into trouble?

_____ 6. Have you had problems connected with drinking during the past year?

_____ 7. Has your drinking caused problems at home?

_____ 8. Do you ever try to get "extra" drinks at a party because you did not get enough to drink?

_____ 9. Do you tell yourself you can stop drinking anytime you want, even though you keep getting drunk when you don't mean to?

_____ 10. Have you missed days at work (or school) because of drinking?

_____ 11. Do you have blackouts?

_____ 12. Have you ever felt that your life would be better if you did not drink?

If you checked four or more of these items, you should seek the guidance of a specialist in chemical dependency or seek help directly through Alcoholics Anonymous (AA) or a similar organization. It is acceptable to go to an open AA meeting, listen to what is being said, and decide for yourself if their program would be useful to you.

Name _____ Date _____ Section _____

Assessment Activity 11-2

What Are Your Reasons for Drug Use?

Directions: In the following table are listed various drugs and products that can affect your life either positively or negatively. Think about how you view each product and what the long-term and short-term conse- quences of use might be. You might wish to consult other sources to help you determine possible effects. In the last column, explain briefly why you choose to use or to refrain from using the drug or product.

Drug	Possible Negative Effects	Possible Positive Effects	Reasons for Using or Not Using
Caffeinated drinks (tea, coffee, cola)			
Alcohol			
Cigarettes			
Pipe or cigar			
Cocaine (any form)			
Marijuana (any form)			
Designer drugs (any form)			
Heroin			
Over-the-counter medications			

Points to Ponder
1. Which drugs do you view positively?
2. Are you unsure of your feelings about any sub- stance? If so, why?
3. What potential is there for abuse or misuse of any of the drugs (even those you have positive feelings about)? If so, what is the potential source of problems?

12
Preventing Sexually Transmitted Diseases

Online Learning Center

Log on to our Online Learning Center (OLC) for access to these additional resources:

- Chapter key term flashcards
- Learning objectives
- Additional goals for behavior change
- Concentration game
- Self-scoring chapter quizzes

- Additional lab activities

The OLC also offers weblinks for study and exploration of wellness topics. Access these links through **www.mhhe.com/anspaugh5e**, click on "Student Center," click on "Chapter 12," and then click on "Web Activities."

Goals for Behavior Change

- Make choices regarding your personal sexual behavior.
- Practice safer sex if you have chosen to be sexually active.
- Take responsibility for the potential consequences of your sexual behavior.
- Learn how to talk with your partner about your sexual history.

Key Terms

acquired immunodeficiency syndrome (AIDS)
chlamydia
cunnilingus
fellatio
genital warts
gonorrhea
hepatitis B
herpes

human immunodeficiency virus (HIV)
nucleoside analogs
protease inhibitor
safer sex
sexually transmitted diseases (STDs)
syphilis
viral hepatitis

Objectives

After completing this chapter, you will be able to do the following:

- Discuss the difference between being HIV positive and having AIDS.
- Identify the signs and symptoms of various STDs.
- Evaluate the risks of having multiple sex partners.
- Discuss the meaning of having a monogamous relationship.
- Identify safer sex practices.

exuality is a lifelong part of a person's life, affecting and being affected by relationships, anatomy, behaviors, thoughts, and values. Sexual behavior is only one aspect of sexuality.

Decisions concerning sexual behavior have many far-reaching consequences. These choices can enhance or severely diminish feelings of well-being. Sex can be wonderful and fulfilling but may also cause serious problems. This chapter examines some of the **sexually transmitted diseases (STDs)** that can result when people engage in behavior that puts them at risk. The chapter also identifies how to avoid contracting and spreading STDs. The chapter examines viral, bacterial, and other common STDs and infections.

Safer Sex

This book discusses the various components of optimal wellness. Sexual behavior can have a strong positive or negative impact on physical and emotional health (see Assessment Activity 12-2). Making decisions concerning sexual behavior is not easy (see Nurturing Your Spirituality: Making Decisions About Sex). If people (whether heterosexual or homosexual) choose to have multiple sexual partners, they must realize that each time a sexual act occurs, the potential sexual histories of two people are brought together. Even though it may be the first experience for one, the other partner may have had sex with three other people. In this case, the person for whom it is the first experience is essentially exposed to the sexual histories of four others. The diseases or infections of any of those four people may be brought to the present relationship (see Assessment Activity 12-1).

Unfortunately, people are not always honest about their past relationships. For many reasons, they may not tell the truth about the number of past partners or about the frequency of condom use. The potential for dishonesty in others makes prevention of STDs a personal responsibility for everyone.

Some people choose abstinence. Abstinence means voluntarily refraining from all sexual acts—which includes practicing sexual activities that involve vaginal, anal, or oral stimulation or penetration. People choose abstinence for a number of reasons, most frequently moral or religious.

A second frequent choice is to have sexual contact within a monogamous (involving only one long-term partner) relationship. Monogamy obviously is dependent upon both partners' willingness to maintain a monogamous relationship. Monogamy may be a choice for two people who have never had sexual intercourse with anyone else or for two people who have had sex partners in the past but have decided to limit their future sexual practices to those they share with each other. Having sex with only one uninfected and faithful partner is as equally effective in preventing STDs (not pregnancy) as abstinence—if it is practiced consistently by both partners. However, even with monogamy, precautions are necessary to prevent unwanted pregnancies.

People embarking on a monogamous relationship who have had partners in the past need to discuss their sexual histories as well as their commitment to the present relationship. This commitment may involve a willingness to be tested for possible STDs (see Real-World Wellness: Communicating with Your Partner About STDs). Some STDs take time to manifest and so testing for them may have to be done several times over a period of years. Assuming that the people involved are committed to monogamy and are honest about their sexual histories, monogamy can serve to protect against the spread of STDs.

In modern society, many relationships are not of long duration, and the practice of *serial monogamy* is common. *Serial monogamy* is monogamy for as long as a relationship is intact; for the duration of their relationship, two partners only have sex with each other. Because relationships may be of relatively brief duration (ranging from weeks to years) and each partner may then seek new partners, the risk with serial monogamy for contracting and spreading an STD is significant.

A third choice is to have sex with more than one partner but to practice **safer sex.** There is no such thing as *safe* sex with multiple partners, but steps can be taken to help ensure *safer* sex. Regardless if you are heterosexual or homosexual, or male or female, you can follow certain practices to limit your exposure to STDs. The starting point for safer sex is using some of the guidelines outlined in Real-World Wellness: Communicating with Your Partner About STDs. Anyone who is sexually active with multiple partners should be checked every three to six months for possible STDs. It is often the case that people, especially women, who are not disease free are asymptomatic (have no symptoms);[1] no persons should let their lack of symptoms lull them into assuming they are disease-free.

Here are some practices for people who are straight or gay that represent safer sex:

Safer practices

- Hugging
- Kissing (not deep or French kissing)
- Petting
- Watching erotic videos, reading erotic books, and so on
- Masturbation (solo or mutual unless there are sores, lesions, and/or abrasions on the genitalia or hands)

Nurturing Your Spirituality

Making Decisions About Sex

Everyone must decide at some point whether to engage in sexual activity. For some people the decision is ongoing. Even after having a sexual experience, a person must decide whether to have sex with the first partner again, to have sex with another person, or not to have sex. Having sex *is* always a choice, unless rape or abuse is involved.

People sometimes change their minds about wanting to have sex. A person may have sex with someone once or many times and then decide to refrain from having sex with that person again. Some people decide to wait to have sex until they are married or until their financial, social, or emotional circumstances change. Some decide to change their sexual behavior to be more closely aligned with moral, ethical, or religious beliefs.

Why do people change their minds about sex? The decision to refrain from further sexual intercourse is sometimes referred to as *secondary virginity*. Couples choosing to engage in sex must make sure that their choice fits with their value systems and understand that they are emotionally, socially, and financially responsible for the results of their decisions. Before initiating sexual intercourse, couples should discuss the following:

- Their thoughts and feelings about sexual activity
- Whether sexual intercourse fits their moral and ethical codes
- Willingness to practice safer sex to protect themselves as well as to deal with the potential pregnancy created as the result of their decision

What considerations are important when deciding whether to have sex? Reasons for having or not having sex are varied. Some couples may believe their feelings are strong enough for one another that sex would seal their commitment to the relationship. Others may decide that if two people love one another it is okay to have sex. Some

people engage in sexual activity because they see it as a way to be popular or as evidence that they are attractive. Some people have sex because they think everyone else is and that not to have sex would make them outsiders. (Not everyone is having sex! Many people, young and old, choose to abstain until marriage or some other long-term commitment.)

Some people choose to refrain from having sex until marriage because they view sex outside marriage as morally wrong. Another reason for abstinence may be a desire to get to know one's partner well (which takes time) before sex. Having sex may alter expectations and the nature of a relationship; some people do not have sex because they don't want their relationship to change. If the physical component of a relationship is emphasized over other aspects, partners may find it difficult to get to know each other well. Many people choose to abstain because they do not want to risk unwanted pregnancy; STDs; or the financial, emotional, and social responsibility of having sex. Some say that not having sex allows them to know themselves better and to figure out what they are looking for in a potential mate. Still others say that not having sex reduces the stress in their lives, freeing them from worries about problem pregnancies or STDs.

How do you decide whether to have sex? It is vitally important to know what your values are and to do only what furthers your total wellness. If you are choosing to have sex because of peer pressure or fear of being alone, then you are not acting out of a wellness perspective. If you are having sex for what you consider to be valid reasons and you are truly comfortable with your decision, then having sex may be an overall positive experience for you. Young adults often fail to realize that, during the next few years, they will be going through many changes as they move from home and from school out into the work world. These changes will alter their self-perceptions and their values. Making the wrong decision now may put that future in jeopardy. Taking time to consider behaviors carefully is crucial, because the regret of an unwanted pregnancy or a lifelong STD can be life altering or even fatal.

What factors will affect your decision to have or not have sex?

Possibly safer practices:

- Deep, French kissing, unless there are sores in the mouth
- Vaginal intercourse with a latex condom with nonoxynol-9
- **Fellatio** with a latex or polyurethane condom
- **Cunnilingus** with a latex dental dam, unless a female partner is menstruating or has a vaginal infection
- Anal intercourse with a latex condom with nonoxynol-9, but there is a great amount of dis-

agreement concerning the safety of this practice even with a condom—this is the most risky sexual behavior

Unsafe practices:

- Vaginal or anal intercourse without a latex condom with nonoxynol-9
- Fellatio or cunnilingus without a condom or latex dental dam
- Oral-anal contact
- Contact with blood, including menstrual blood

Real-World Wellness

Communicating with Your Partner About STDs

My partner and I have been very close to having sex on several occasions. I am very worried about contracting an STD. I really don't know much about my partner's past sexual history. How do I open the discussion or ask the questions concerning safe sex practices? How do I find out if there is anything I should be aware of in this person's past?

The decision about whether to have sex is extremely important. Considerations include the possibility of contracting an STD, the potential for an unwanted pregnancy, and the psychological and emotional ramifications of intimate contact should the relationship end. Sex represents a psychological, physical, emotional, and financial commitment to another person. Don't be reluctant to bring up the topic of safer sex. The ability to discuss important issues is a sign of personal and social maturity. Here are some suggestions on ways to introduce the topic. What others can you suggest?

- "I feel that we both are thinking about sex, but before I make a final decision, I have some concerns I'd like to discuss with you."
- "I've always practiced safer sex in the past and, if we're going to have sex, I think it's important for us to use condoms."
- "What type of protection do *you* have if we decide to have sex? This is the type of protection *I* have."
- "I know if you really care about me you'll be willing to use a condom."
- "Before this relationship goes any farther, I want to ask you about your past sexual history and our plans for practicing safer sex."
- "I really like you and I hope we can have a more intimate relationship at some point. But I think there are some important things we should talk about first."
- You're so sexy sometimes I just get carried away when I'm close to you. Why don't we have a quiet dinner together to discuss our sexual past and what we want from this relationship?"

You can probably think of even better ways to approach a conversation concerning sex. What is important to remember is that sex can be a wonderful emotional and physical experience, but it's not worth dying for.

Just the Facts

Effective Condom Use

Condoms can be effective in protecting against STDs if used properly. Here are some guidelines for proper use:

- Use one every time you have sexual intercourse or oral sex involving a penis.
- Use only latex or polyurethane condoms.
- When having vaginal or anal intercourse, make sure the condom has nonoxynol–9.
- Put the condom on before any contact with the vagina.
- When the condom is on the penis, there should be about a half-inch of space left at the condom tip to hold the ejaculate.
- Withdraw the penis soon after ejaculation. Hold the base of the condom firmly against the penis as it is withdrawn so the condom does not come off.
- Use foam, spermicide, or a female condom in combination with a condom.
- Check for possible breaks immediately after use of any condom.
- Always use a water-based lubricant such as K-Y jelly. Vaseline or other oil-based lubricants can cause the condom to break down and become ineffective.
- Never reuse a condom.

- Taking semen in the mouth
- Sharing a vibrator or other sex toys without washing them between uses

See Just the Facts: Effective Condom Use.

Sexually Transmitted Diseases (STDs)

Each year in the United States it is estimated that more than 12 million people contract an STD.[2,3] Approximately 25 percent of new cases occur among teenagers. Two-thirds of STD cases occur in people under the age of 25.[4] Another particularly disturbing fact is that young women under 24 years of age may be at more risk of STDs than are older women because the cells of the cervix in young women are immature and more easily infected.[5] An important component of these statistics is that a large number of STD cases go unreported because many are asymptomatic (particularly in women) or because they are treated by a private physician and never reported. Consequently, the estimated

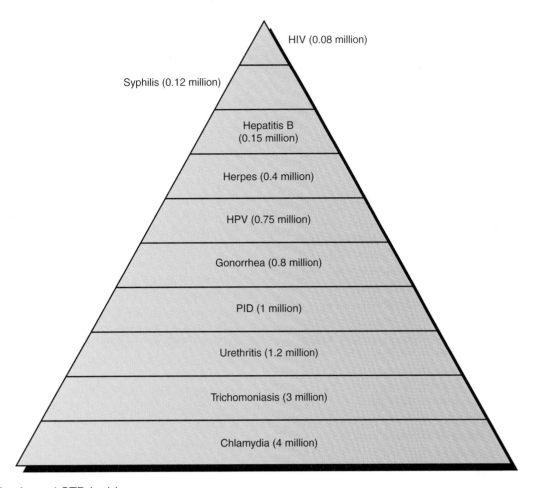

HIV (0.08 million)

Syphilis (0.12 million)

Hepatitis B
(0.15 million)

Herpes (0.4 million)

HPV (0.75 million)

Gonorrhea (0.8 million)

PID (1 million)

Urethritis (1.2 million)

Trichomoniasis (3 million)

Chlamydia (4 million)

Figure 12-1 Annual STD Incidence

12 million may reflect a vast underreporting of the number of cases. The estimates for annual STD incidence are shown in figure 12-1.[5]

Viral Diseases

Human Immunodeficiency Virus and Acquired Immunodeficiency Syndrome

Damage to the immune system as a result of infection with **human immunodeficiency virus (HIV)** leads to a complex of rare diseases called **acquired immunodeficiency syndrome (AIDS).** The Centers for Disease Control (CDC) lists two conditions to be used in diagnosing AIDS. These are an HIV seroconversion and a T-cell count below 200 cells per millimeter regardless of other specific symptoms that may or may not be present.[6] A normal range of T-cells is 800 to 1000. In the presence of these two conditions, some other conditions may be used to diagnose AIDS. These conditions

fall into several categories and are presented in Just the Facts: Conditions Used to Diagnose AIDS.

People infected with HIV may experience a variety of symptoms or may appear to be quite healthy. A small percentage of HIV-positive people seem to have been able to suppress and survive HIV infection for more than twenty years without ever developing AIDS. The reason for this is not understood by experts. It has been suggested that suppressor compounds formed by the immune system cells may be responsible. However, even people with no obvious symptoms can transmit HIV to others. The indicators of possible HIV infection include persistent diarrhea, dry cough, and shortness of breath; fatigue; skin rash; swollen lymph nodes (neck, armpits, groin); candidiasis; unexplained fever or chills; night sweats (over several weeks); and unexplained weight loss of 10 pounds or 10 percent of body weight in fewer than two months. Women may experience these symptoms as well as abnormal Pap smears, persistent vaginal candidiasis, and abdominal cramping as a result of pelvic inflammatory disease (PID). These infections are a result of HIV infection and are caused by

~ *Just the Facts* ~

Conditions Used to Diagnose AIDS

Here are some conditions besides HIV seroconversion and low T-cell counts used to diagnose AIDS:

Opportunistic infections (infections that take advantage of a weakened immune system)

- Pneumocystis carinii pneumonia (PCP)—a type of lung disease caused by a protozoan or fungus, usually not harmful to humans

- Tuberculosis—either *Mycobacterium avium-intracellulare* (MAI) or *Mycobacterium tuberculosis* (TB), with MAI being most common among AIDS patients

- Bacterial pneumonia—caused by several common bacteria

- Toxoplasmosis—a disease of the brain and central nervous system

Cancers

- Kaposi's sarcoma, a cancer that causes red or purple blotches on the skin

- Lymphomas, cancers of the lymphatic system

- Invasive cervical cancer—more common in women who are HIV positive

Other conditions

- Wasting syndrome, which involves persistent diarrhea, severe weight loss, and weakness

- AIDS dementia, impairment of mental function, mood changes, and impaired movement as a result of HIV infection of the brain

Other infections

- Candidiasis (also called *thrush*), a fungal infection that affects the vagina, mouth, throat, and lungs

- Herpes, a common viral STD described later in this chapter

- Cytomegalovirus, a virus that, in AIDS patients, can lead to brain infection, infection of the retina, pneumonia, or hepatitis

immunodeficiency, but they are not AIDS (see Wellness Across the Generations: HIV and AIDS Pose Special Risks to Women and Their Children).

The reason some people develop AIDS rapidly and others do not is not known. Factors that may contribute to the advancement of the condition are weakening of the immune system through other infections, alcohol or drug abuse, poor nutrition, and stress.[2] The

Wellness on the Web
Behavior Change Activities

What Do You Know About STDs?
More than twenty sexually transmitted diseases (STDs) have been identified, and all are preventable. But STDs are thriving, and it's largely because of ignorance and inaction. People who have multiple sex partners are at the highest risk of contracting STDs. The only sure ways of preventing STDs are to abstain from sex, or for two uninfected people to participate in a mutually monogamous relationship. Another effective but not foolproof way to reduce the risk of infection is the proper use of condoms.

Education about STDs is another form of prevention. How much do you know about STDs? To learn about STDs, including their symptoms and common treatment practices, visit www.mhhe.com/anspaugh5e, Student Center, Chapter 12, Wellness on the Web, Activity 1.

Breaking the Silence: Talking About Sex
Safer sex sounds like a great idea, but it can be difficult to achieve because few people want to discuss it. In this case, silence definitely is *not* golden. Having sex should be viewed as a major decision that may have lifelong consequences. The choice to engage in safer sexual behavior rests with each individual. One of the best ways to protect yourself is to know as much as possible. To find the answers to a number of questions about sex frequently asked by adults go to www.mhhe.com/anspaugh5e, Student Center, Chapter 12, Wellness on the Web, Activity 2, and select from the categories of questions listed. You are sure to find some questions whose answers you will find helpful.

longer the virus is in the system, the greater the chances of developing AIDS. In one study spanning six years, 30 percent of the participants with the virus developed AIDS, 49 percent displayed symptomatic HIV infections, and 21 percent remained free of symptoms. All these people could continue to spread the disease.[7] Another problem is the rapid development and emergence of new drug-resistant strains of HIV.[11]

Two types of HIV have been identified.[8] Almost all cases of HIV in the United States are a virus known as HIV-1. Another type of virus, HIV-2, is found mainly in West Africa and appears to take longer than HIV-1 to damage the immune system. The virus replicates inside human cells and is transmitted by blood, blood products, semen, vaginal secretions, and breast milk. HIV is an extremely fragile virus in that it does not survive in air and can be destroyed readily by soap and water, household bleach, and chlorine used in swimming pools. Just the Facts: How HIV Is and Is Not Transmitted explores transmission in greater detail.

In 2000 women represented 16 percent of all AIDS cases reported.[7] Also in 2000, 64,373 women died from AIDS-related deaths.[7] Most women are infected through use of injected drugs or through sex with infected partners. Activities that put women at high risk include being a partner of an injected-drug user or of a gay or bisexual man or having multiple sex partners. Although lesbians with HIV are in a small minority, they can and do contract HIV in the same ways as heterosexual women. Lesbians who share sex toys without first washing and cleaning them are at greater risk for HIV than are those who practice safer sex.

Heterosexual women are at greater risk for contracting HIV from an infected man than are non-HIV-positive men from HIV-positive women. Women are more susceptible to HIV infection because they have more surface area of contact in the vagina and the tissue there is softer and more easily scratched or torn. Further, semen is often ejaculated directly into the uterine and cervical canal. Semen normally contains 10 to 100 times more migratory lymphocytes than does cervical mucus, thus placing more virus in the area for potential infection.[8]

Wellness Across the Generations

HIV and AIDS Pose Special Risks to Women and Their Children

Women tend to be diagnosed at a later stage in the HIV process than are men and they have almost a 30 percent greater chance than men do of dying before they have an AIDS-defining condition.[1] Further, women tend to be excluded from many clinical trials. Because female physiology is different from male physiology, women need to participate in clinical trials to ensure that new experimental drugs and therapies work for them as effectively as they do for men.

A pregnant woman has about a 25 to 35 percent chance of passing the virus to her newborn. The Centers for Disease Control and Prevention has recommended HIV testing for all pregnant women. HIV transmission from mother to infant can be reduced from almost 26 percent to slightly more than 8 percent when both the HIV-positive mother (predelivery) and infant (postdelivery) are given doses of a drug called *AZT*. An HIV-positive mother can infect her newborn by breast-feeding. The exact risk for this form of transmission is not known, but the risk can be completely avoided through the use of formula as opposed to breast milk.

Just the Facts

How HIV Is and Is Not Transmitted

Here are possible means of transmission of HIV and some activities that, contrary to misinformed opinion, do not transmit HIV:

How HIV is transmitted

Sexual activity

- Homosexual, between men
- Heterosexual, from men to women and women to men

Blood

- Through needle sharing among intravenous drug users
- Through transfusion of blood and blood products
- To health care workers through a needle stick, an open wound, or mucous membrane exposure
- Through injection with an unsterilized needle (including needles used in acupuncture, medical injections, ear piercing, and tattooing)

Childbirth

- Intrauterine (within the uterus)
- Peripartum (during labor and delivery)

How HIV is not transmitted

- Through food and water
- Through sharing of eating and drinking utensils
- Through shaking or holding hands
- Through use of the telephone
- Via a toilet seat
- Via insects
- In whirlpools or saunas
- Through coughing or sneezing
- Via domestic pets
- Through an exchange of clothing
- From swimming in a pool
- Through bed linens

The HIV virus attacks the helper T-lymphocytes, specifically the T-4 cells, possibly the most critical element in the body's immune system. HIV attaches to the part of the T-cell that recognizes viral infections and blocks its ability to react to them. Over time, HIV may even multiply and destroy T-cells, leaving the body more defenseless against invasion by opportunistic organisms that can lead to illness and eventually death.[9] Among adults ages 25 to 44, AIDS is the leading cause of death for men and it is the fourth for women.[7,12]

In the United States, whether through homosexual or heterosexual contact, anal intercourse is still the most prevalent means of spreading HIV infection. This may be because this activity increases the likelihood of making small tears that facilitate the spread of the virus from semen to blood. Vaginal and oral sex are also considered highly dangerous.[10] Sharing of needles among drug users and having sex with an IV drug user are high-risk activities. Sex with a prostitute is a significant risk factor. Anyone who has had multiple sexual partners during the last five to ten years is at risk because there is no way of knowing the sexual histories of all the sex partners of one's multiple sex partners. People who are not sexually active are not at risk. People in monogamous relationships in which neither partner has an STD or has used IV drugs are considered safe. It is estimated that HIV infections among non–drug-using heterosexuals in the United States doubled during the 1990s.[16]

AIDS is a preventable disease, and education is still the best defense. People who have sex outside a monogamous relationship and those who share needles from intravenous drugs are still at extremely high risk for infection.

HIV is spread through intimate sexual contact; through transfusion of blood from an infected individual; and from an infected mother to her fetus during the prenatal period, the birth process, or breast-feeding (see Just the Facts: Preventing the Spread of AIDS). In no case has HIV been spread through casual contact—this includes close contact between family members or friends and infected adults or children. Very few health care professionals working with AIDS patients have contracted the disease, and their infection was caused by rare mishandling of blood. The AIDS virus is not transmitted from toilet seats, foods, beverages or social kissing. The virus is found in small amounts in tears and saliva, although transmission through these mediums is undocumented.

Of great concern in the AIDS epidemic is the loss of life's most productive years; because 25- to 44-year-olds made up more than half the work force in 1992, loss of life in that age group has been disruptive to society. It was projected that more than 80,000 American children lost their mothers to AIDS by the year 2000.[13]

Just the Facts

Preventing the Spread of AIDS[7]

The spread of AIDS can be stopped by preventing the transmission of the AIDS virus from one person to another. This means eliminating direct sexual contact with infected people and not using contaminated needles. Recommendations to reduce the possibility of becoming infected include the following:

- Practice abstinence or mutual monogamy.

- Always use protection (that is, latex condoms and spermicide, such as nonoxynol-9) if having sex with multiple partners or with people who have multiple partners.

- Do not have unprotected sex with people with AIDS, those who engage in high-risk behavior, or those who have had a positive test for the AIDS virus.

- Avoid sexual activities that might cut or tear the rectum, vagina, or penis.

- Do not have sex with prostitutes.

- Do not use IV drugs or share needles. Refrain from having sex with IV drug users.

Probably no other infectious disease has taken or is taking such a devastating toll on Americans. By the end of December 2000, more than 774,467 Americans had been diagnosed with AIDS and more than 448,060 people had died since the disease was first reported in 1991.[14] It is estimated that the average costs of treating one AIDS patient is $20,000–$24,000 per year.[15]

Testing for HIV

Two tests are currently being used to detect HIV. The ELISA is the antibody test initially used. If the ELISA result indicates that the patient has HIV, another test—the Western blot technique—is administered for confirmation. A person may not have abnormal results on the ELISA if the virus has not been present long enough for antibodies to develop. Antibodies may develop within two months or may take up to thirty-six months to develop.[11] Usually, Western blot results are clearly either HIV positive or negative. If there is an inconclusive Western blot test, the person should be retested in six months. A third test, the single-use diagnostic system (SUDS), is currently being readied for determining if HIV infection has occurred. A home test is now available for over-the-counter use. However any positive HIV home test should be followed up with one of the aforementioned tests for HIV. Remember: Anyone who tests positive is infected with HIV and can transmit the infection.

Treatment for HIV and AIDS

At present no cure exists for HIV and AIDS, which results in a multitude of infections leading to death. The type of treatment that seems most effective in the treatment of AIDS is the use of a triple-drug therapy, consisting of a **protease inhibitor,** which blocks an enzyme (protease) that helps the virus develop at a later stage in the viral life cycle, and two drugs from another group of antiviral drugs called **nucleoside analogs** (AZT, ddI, and ZVD), which work by blocking reverse transcriptase, the enzyme used by HIV to copy itself in a host cell.

Early, aggressive treatment with a combination of a protease inhibitor and two nucleoside analogs (AZT and ddI), sometimes called a *cocktail,* has cut the death rate by 70 percent and inhibited opportunistic infections by 73 percent.[16] However, dangerous side effects seem to accompany this type of therapy, including diabetes, abnormally high cholesterol and triglyceride levels, shrinking limbs, and the bizarre appearance of disfiguring deposits of fat on parts of the body.[16]

Even with this dramatic improvement, the AIDS crisis is far from over. Although some patients appear virus free, no one knows that the virus is not "hiding" in other locations of the body or if the HIV virus will find a way to mutate so that the current cocktail is no longer useful. Further, no one knows, if the current therapy is discontinued, whether HIV will return. The cost for this type of treatment is high, and only a few people can access the treatment. Even with all the advancements, the best protection for those choosing to be sexually active is education and the practice of safer sex.

AIDS is the most deadly of all STDs, but it is preventable. With education, wisdom, and reduction in high-risk behaviors, AIDS can be prevented (see Just the Facts: Preventing the Spread of AIDS). Information on AIDS can be obtained through various sources (see Just the Facts: AIDS and HIV Sources of Information).

Herpes

Herpes is caused by the herpes simplex virus (HSV). Five different strains of the herpes virus infect human beings. The most common strains are herpes simplex-1 (HSV-1) and herpes simplex-2 (HSV-2). Type 1 is usually confined to congenital areas in the form of cold sores or fever blisters. It is a common form of herpes but is not categorized as an STD. Type 2 generally causes lesions on and around the genital areas and is an STD. However, through either direct or indirect contact, type 1 can affect the genital area and type 2

AIDS and HIV Sources of Information

Contact the following organizations for information about HIV and AIDS:

CDC National AIDS Hotline
(800) 342-2437
Free information on HIV and AIDS available in several languages

CDC National AIDS Clearinghouse
(800) 458-5231
www.cdcnac.org
Information on services and education services; copies of Public Health Service publications available

Linea Nacional de SIDA
(800) 344-7432
Twenty-four–hour hotline that provides in Spanish information and referrals for HIV and AIDS

HIV Insite Gateway to AIDS Knowledge
www.hivinsite.vcs8.edu
Information concerning prevention, education, treatment, and clinical trials

Local health departments also offer valuable information concerning HIV and AIDS.

A severe herpes infection.

can produce sores in the mouth. The common sites for type 1 and type 2 can thus be reversed. Estimates indicate that 30 million people in the United States are infected with genital herpes.[17]

Type 2 herpes usually appears as a single blister or a series of painful blisters on the penis or inside the vagina or cervix. The blisters may also be present on the buttocks and thighs and in the groin area. Following a short prodromal (time interval between the earliest symptoms and appearance of actual disease) of tingling, discomfort, or itching, small red lesions appear. This phase is followed by the formation of a small blister filled with clear fluid. This fluid is highly contagious. The infection usually lasts one to three weeks and then abates, but it does not leave the body. The virus retreats to the nerve endings where it remains dormant. Herpes can become active again without any warning; that is, the disease may be recurrent. Menstruation, stress, trauma to the skin (such as too much sunlight), lack of sleep, and poor nutrition seem to trigger recurrences. Recurrences are generally less severe and of shorter duration than the initial episode.[18]

Genital herpes is acquired by sexual contact. It was once believed that herpes could be transmitted only when the virus was active and causing symptoms, such as the presence of blisters or sores. It is now known that the virus can be spread even when there are no symptoms.[23] Research does indicate that the risk of transmission is greatest among couples during the first three months of a sexual relationship. Estimates are that half of couples transmit within this period, indicating the possibility that partners develop a natural immunity to the virus over time.[23]

Men do not seem to experience any major long-term complications from herpes. Women, however, may be faced with the possibility of cancer of the cervix and infection of their newborns during the birth process. Any woman with a history of herpes should have an annual Pap smear test. Physicians attending the pregnancy of a woman with a history of herpes should be informed so that the course of the pregnancy can be monitored. If herpes becomes active or the physician feels the baby would be at risk through a vaginal birth, caesarean section delivery (surgical removal of the fetus through the abdominal wall) is often used. Additional hazards of herpes infection are herpes encephalitis, in which the virus invades the brain, and herpes keratitis, or eye infection. These two conditions are rare and can be effectively treated with antiviral drugs.

Three antiviral prescription drugs are now available for treating herpes. Acyclovir (brand name Zovirax, now available as a generic) promotes healing and helps suppress future outbreaks. Two newer drugs, valacyclovir and famciclovir, are similar to Zovirax but are designed to make higher levels of the drug's active ingredient available to the body. Some physicians prescribe a course of suppressive therapy with one of these drugs, which keeps herpes from recurring in up to 90 percent of patients. Patients must start taking the drugs at the first hint of symptoms. This therapy works only as long as the drug is taken, and if the drug is stopped there may be recurrences.[17] Warm compresses, sitz baths, and aspirin may help relieve discomfort.

Hepatitis B

Hepatitis is an inflammation of the liver caused by one or more viruses. There are five distinct types of **viral hepatitis** known: Hepatitis A (formerly *infectious hepatitis*), hepatitis B (formerly *serum hepatitis*), hepatitis C (non-A, non-B hepatitis), hepatitis E (another form of non-A, non-B), and hepatitis D, or *delta hepatitis.*

Hepatitis B is considered the most serious of the five types of hepatitis. It has an incubation period of between 45 and 160 days. The symptoms of hepatitis B include vomiting, abdominal pain, loss of appetite, and jaundice (an excess of a bile pigment in the blood that causes the skin to look yellow). Some infected people do not develop the worst symptoms of the disease but experience mild flulike illness without jaundice. However, the CDC estimates that approximately 25 percent of carriers suffer chronic symptoms, and these people are at the greatest risk for one of the most serious consequences of infection, cirrhosis of the liver. Cirrhosis is a degenerative disease in which liver cells are damaged and scarred with the eventual outcome of death or the necessity of liver transplantation. All carriers of hepatitis B are at greater risk of developing primary liver cancer than are noncarriers. At one time, hepatitis B was spread primarily through tattoo needles, the sharing of needles by drug users, and transfusions of contaminated blood. Today, it is more commonly spread through body secretions, including sweat, breast milk, and semen. A vaccine has been developed to immunize against the disease.

Symptoms of all forms of viral hepatitis are similar. They include fatigue, loss of appetite, mild fever, nausea, vomiting, diarrhea, aching muscles and joints, and tenderness in the upper right abdomen. A few people may have jaundiced (yellowed) skin and eyes, itching skin, darkened urine, and light-colored feces. Still others may exhibit no symptoms except those usually associated with the flu. This group does not usually seek treatment but still can transmit the infection to others.

Viral hepatitis is a type of liver injury. Most patients with hepatitis recover without serious problems. However, serious scarring of the liver or even death may occur. In some cases of hepatitis B the person with the disease becomes a chronic carrier or can develop chronic progressive hepatitis that eventually leads to liver failure.

Genital Warts

Warts on the genitalia, around the anus, in the vagina, and on the cervix are called **genital warts,** or *condyloma.* These warts are caused by the human papilloma virus (HPV). There are more than fifty forms of HPV. Experts postulate that this condition is the third most prevalent STD after chlamydia and gonorrhea. It is also

Genital warts are the result of human papilloma virus.

estimated that 1.2 million people are infected annually. Approximately one in ten Americans may be carrying the virus.[18] Genital warts most commonly involve people between the ages of 15 and 24.

Genital warts are cauliflowerlike. In moist areas, they are soft and either pink or red. On dry skin, they are usually yellow-gray and hard. The warts are transmitted sexually and generally appear one to six months after exposure. There are fifty-six distinct varieties of HPV, some of which have been specifically linked to cervical cancer and cancers of the rectum, vulva, skin, and penis. The warts appear most often on the shaft of the penis, the vulva, the vaginal wall, the cervix, and the perineum. They may also be found in the anal area of both sexes and are associated with anal intercourse with an infected partner. Cryosurgery (freezing) is the treatment of choice, although electrocautery (burning) and use of the topical agent podophyllin also are successful methods of treatment. Podophyllin should not be used during pregnancy or on warts in the cervical area. If the infected person has had a variety of partners, the genitalia of all partners should be examined so that treatment can be initiated if appropriate.

Bacterial Diseases

Chlamydia

Chlamydia is thought to be the most common STD in the United States, with an estimated 3 million new cases each year.[19] The causative agent is the bacterium *Chlamydia trachomatis*. Chlamydia is frequently found with other STDs, such as gonorrhea, herpes, and syphilis, and it may be contracted through oral, anal, and vaginal intercourse. Approximately 75 percent of women and 50 percent of men have no symptoms. Most people infected with chlamydia are not aware of their infections and therefore do not seek medical help.

In men the infection is usually manifested by inflammation of the urethra (urethritis). Infected men generally experience a burning sensation during urination and possibly a mild discharge.

Symptoms in women include vaginal discharge, intermittent vaginal bleeding, and ill-defined discomfort or pain on urination. Infected mothers may pass the infection to their babies during the birth process. This may result in conjunctivitis in the baby or a more serious condition known as *chlamydial pneumonia*. As many as one in ten adolescent girls tested for chlamydia was infected.[19]

When left untreated, chlamydia can lead to arthritis and can damage the heart valves, blood vessels, and heart muscle. In men the condition can also lead to sterility. In women the disease can infect the uterus, fallopian tubes, and upper reproductive areas, producing the chronic condition pelvic inflammatory disease, or PID. This scarring of the fallopian tubes by PID causes sterility and an increased risk of ectopic pregnancy (a condition in which the embryo is implanted outside the uterus). Women infected with chlamydia have a three to five fold increased risk of acquiring HIV, if exposed.

Tetracycline, erythromycin, and doxycycline are the drugs used for treatment. They are taken orally for one to three weeks. Taking the full course of medication is extremely important because relapse can occur. All sexual partners should be treated or the disease can be passed among them.[21]

Gonorrhea

Nearly 2 million cases of **gonorrhea** are reported each year, making it the second most prevalent STD. Gonorrhea is caused by the bacterium *Neisseria gonorrhoeae*, which attacks the mucous membranes of the penis, vagina, rectum, throat, and eyes. The disease is spread by vaginal, oral, and rectal contact.

Gonorrhea produces symptoms in 80 percent of men. The symptoms appear two to ten days (an average three to five days) after contact with the bacteria and include a thick, milky discharge from the penis and a painful, burning sensation on urination. These signs should cause men to seek medical treatment immediately. Untreated gonorrhea can result in sterility.

The symptoms in women are discharge and burning on urination, but they may be so mild that they are unnoticed. The bacteria can survive in the vagina and other areas of the female reproductive system for years. During this time, women can infect any sex partners and their fetuses if they become pregnant. Contact by the baby with the bacteria during childbirth can lead to an eye infection resulting in blindness. Untreated gonorrhea can lead to PID, the leading cause of sterility in women. In both men and women, rectal and oral gonorrhea may go unnoticed. The disease can develop into a serious infection, resulting in arthritis; meningitis; skin lesions; and liver, heart, brain, and spinal cord problems.

Gonorrhea is either diagnosed by obtaining a smear from the penis or cervix or through a urine test. Physicians commonly treat for chlamydia as well when gonorrhea has been diagnosed. This dual therapy can be most cost-effective because the cost of treatment is less than the cost of testing. Most gonococci in the United States can be cured with doxycycline and dzithromycin, therefore cotreatment might hinder the development of antibiotic-resistant strains of gonorrhea.[21] Gonorrhea can be completely cured, although there is no immunity to the disease. If a person has multiple sexual partners, medical help and advice must be sought regularly.

Syphilis

Syphilis is caused by a corkscrew-shaped bacterial spirochete called *Treponema pallidum*. Kissing, oral-genital contact, and intercourse are the most common forms of transmission. The spirochete dies quickly when exposed to air, so primary entry to the body is through a break in the skin. Once in the bloodstream, it exists in a variety of organs and mimics the symptoms of many major chronic diseases. Because of this ability to mimic other diseases, it is referred to as *the great imitator.*

One interesting fact concerning syphilis is that some HIV infections seem to be exacerbated by it. The lesions caused by syphilis seem to help the HIV virus seep into or out of the body. Not everyone who has sex with a person who is HIV positive becomes infected, but if either partner also has primary or secondary syphilis, the risk of transmission increases sixfold.[20] There are four stages of syphilis.

Primary syphilis

The initial sign of primary syphilis is a lesion called a *chancre* located at the site of entry of the pathogen. The incubation period can range from ten to ninety days (an average of twenty-one days) before symptoms appear. The chancre can vary from the size of a pinhead to the size of a dime. Even though the chancre may look painful, it is not and may go unnoticed. If the lesion occurs on the labia, vagina, or rectum, it can easily remain undetected. The chancre disappears within three to six weeks. In 90 percent of women and 50 percent of men the chancre is difficult to identify.

Secondary syphilis

From four to twelve weeks after the chancre disappears, the symptoms of secondary syphilis may appear. Symptoms include headaches, swollen glands, low-grade fevers, skin rash, white patches on the mucous membranes of the mouth and throat, hair loss, arthritis pain, and large sores around the mouth and genitals. These sores contain the bacteria responsible for syphilis, and contact with them can spread the disease. Symptoms may be mild or severe, and in rare instances no symptoms appear. If left untreated, symptoms usually run their course, lasting anywhere from a few days to several weeks. The pathogen remains active in the body even with the absence of symptoms and will reappear later—perhaps as long as twenty years after the initial infection.

Latent syphilis

During latent syphilis there are few or no clinical signs that the disease exists, although the spirochetes are invading the various organs and systems of the body, including the brain, heart, and central nervous system. The spirochetes multiply relentlessly and begin to destroy the tissues, bones, and organs. At this stage a person is not contagious.

Late syphilis

From fifteen to twenty years after the onset of latent syphilis, the disease progresses to its most devastating stage. Late syphilis can cause heart damage, central nervous system damage, blindness, deafness, paralysis, and psychosis. Death from the effects of this stage of syphilis is probable.

Penicillin is the preferred drug for treating syphilis. People who are penicillin sensitive are placed on other antibiotics, such as tetracycline or erythromycin. For an individual who has syphilis less than a year, a single dose will cure the disease. Larger doses are needed for those who have had the disease longer than a year.[22] Antibiotics can kill the pathogen at any stage, but any damage incurred cannot be reversed. People with syphilis commonly have other STDs, such as gonorrhea and chlamydia, thereby requiring greater doses of antibiotics.

Other Common STDs

In addition to the STDs mentioned, there are several others that have potential for harm. Table 12-1 lists several other common STDs.

Table 12-1 Other Common STDs

STD	Causative agent	Symptoms	Treatment
Candidiasis (yeast infection)	A fungus (*Candida albicans*) that can be transmitted through sexual coitus or an imbalance of the acidity of the vagina	White "cheesy" discharge, irritation of vaginal and vulva tissue	Vaginal cream or suppositories, such as miconazole (Monistat)
Chancroid	A bacteria (*Haemophilus ducreyi*) that can be contracted through a lesion or its discharge	Cluster of small bumps or blisters on the genitals or around the anus that rupture and ulcerate	Antibiotics, such as erythromycin
Granuloma inguinale	A bacteria (*Calymmatobacterium granulomatis*) that can be contracted through contact with a lesion or its discharge	Painless red bumps or sores in the groin that ulcerate and spread	Antibiotics, such as tetracycline or doxycycline
Nongonococcal urethritis (NGU)	A bacteria (mostly *Chlamydia trachomatis*) that can be transmitted during coitus	Inflammation of the urethra; for men, discharge and irritation during urination; for women, possible mild discharge of pus from the vagina or no symptoms	Antibiotics, such as tetracycline, doxycycline, or erythromycin
Pediculosis (Crabs)	*Phthirus pubis* (pubic lice)	Intense itching in the genital area	Shampoos, such as those with lindane solution (Kwell)
Pelvic inflammatory disease (women only)	Caused by untreated chlamydia or gonorrhea; may lead to infertility or arthritis	Low abdominal pain, bleeding between menstrual periods, persistent low fever	Penicillin or other antibiotics
Trichomoniasis (trich)	Protozoan parasite (*Trichomonas vaginalis*) contracted through sexual intercourse; can be spread by towels, toilet seats, or bathtubs used by an infected person	White to yellow discharge with a most unpleasant odor	Anti-infectives, such as metronidazole (Flagyl)

Summary

- The only way to completely avoid acquiring an STD is to abstain from sex or to have sex in a purely monogamous relationship.
- Practicing safer sex helps reduce the possibility of contracting an STD. The use of condoms is associated with decreased risk.
- The human immunodeficiency virus (HIV) attacking the immune system causes a complex of rare diseases called *acquired immunodeficiency syndrome* (AIDS).
- Although no cure exists for AIDS, some of the latest combinations of drugs seem to be prolonging life and reducing the HIV content in the body.
- Genital herpes is a viral disease characterized by lesions around the genital area. The disease can recur at any time and represents a serious threat to women by increasing their risk of cancer of the cervix. Three drugs are used to treat the disease (acyclovir, valacyclovir, and famciclovir).

- Viral hepatitis is an injury to the liver. There are several types of hepatitis. Hepatitis B is perhaps the most serious.
- Genital warts, or condyloma, are caused by the human papilloma virus (HPV) and have been linked to some cancers.
- Chlamydia is a bacterium that produces the most common STD in the United States. Untreated, it can cause arthritis, sterility, damage to the heart and blood vessels, and ectopic pregnancies.
- Gonorrhea is probably the second leading STD. It can lead to sterility in both men and women. The symptoms are often unnoticed by women.
- Syphilis is a bacterial disease that has four stages. The stages are primary, secondary, latent, and late.
- Several other STDs that have damaging potential are candidiasis, chancroid, granuloma inguinale, nongonococcal urethritis (NGU), pediculosis, pelvic inflammatory disease (PID), and trichomoniasis.

Review Questions

1. How can people accept responsibility for their sexual behavior?
2. What makes HIV an extremely dangerous infection?
3. What precautions can you take to protect against the spread of AIDS?
4. What are the various kinds of viral hepatitis and how are they spread?
5. Discuss why HPV is more dangerous for women than for men.
6. Why does chlamydia represent a serious problem?
7. Why is gonorrhea a more serious problem today than it was just a few years ago?
8. List and explain the four stages of syphilis.
9. Discuss some other common STDs.
10. If one STD is present, why may it be necessary to get treatment for more than one?

References

1. Strong, B., C. DeVault, and S. B. Werner. 1999. *Human Sexuality—Diversity in Contemporary America* (3d ed.). Mountain View, Calif.: Mayfield Publishing Co.
2. Center for Disease Control and Prevention. 1997. *1996 Report* available online at www.wonder.cdc.gov/wonder/STDSTDD007.PCW.html.
3. National Women's Health Resource Center. 2001. *Women and Sexually Transmitted Diseases (STDs).* Available online at www.healthywomen.org.
4. U.S. Department of Health and Human Services. 1996. *HIV/AIDS Surveillance Report* 8(20):18.
5. American Social Health Association. Jan. 1999. STD statistics available online at www.ashastd.org/std/stats/html.
6. Center for Disease Control and Prevention. 1997. *HIV/AIDS Surveillance Report* 9(2):1.
7. Cox, F. D. 1999. *The AIDS Booklet* (5th ed.). Boston: WCB/McGraw-Hill.
8. Stine, G. J. 1993. *Acquired Immune Deficiency Syndrome—Biological, Medical, Social, and Legal Issues.* Englewood Cliffs, N.J.: Prentice-Hall.
9. Nevid, J. S. 1995. *Choices: Sex in the Age of STDs.* Boston: Allyn and Bacon.
10. Notes from the Twelfth World AIDS Conference, Geneva, Switzerland. June 26–July 12, 1998. Available online at www.mhhe.com/hper/health/personal health/aidsnotes.mhtml.
11. Nowak, M. A., and A. J. McMichael. 1995. How HIV defeats the immune system. *Scientific American* 273(2):58.
12. Center for Disease Control and Prevention. 1996. *HIV Surveillance Report* 7(2):10.
13. Editors. 1994. Heterosexual AIDS is no myth. *Newsweek* 52(3):70.
14. Center for Disease Control. 2001. HIV/AIDS—United States 1981–2000. *Morbidity and Mortality Weekly Reports* 50(21): 430.
15. Hellinger, F., and J. Fleishman. 2000. Estimating the national costs of treating people with HIV disease. *Journal of Acquired Immunodeficiency Syndrome* (24):2, 182–188.
16. Palella, F. L., et al. 1998. HIV outpatient study investigators. Declining morbidity and mortality among patients with advanced human immunodeficiency virus infections. *New England Journal of Medicine* 338(13):853.
17. University of California at Berkeley. 1999. Herpes: new strategies. *University of California, Berkeley, Wellness Letter* 15(4):4.
18. Nuovo, G. J., et. al. 1990. Human papillomavirus types and recurrent cervical warts. *Journal of the American Medical Association* 263:1223.
19. Center for Disease Control and Prevention. 2001. Chlamydia in the United States. Available online www.cdc.gov/nchstp/dstd/fact_sheet/chlamydia_facts.htm.
20. Editors. December 22, 1998. Syphilis eradication: So near, so elusive. *USA Today* 6D.
21. Center for Disease Control and Prevention. 2001. Guidelines for treatment of sexually transmitted diseases. Available online at www.cdc.gov/wonder/STD/STD98TG.
22. Center for Disease Control and Prevention. 2001. Syphilis fact sheet. Available online at www.cdc.gov/nchstp/dstd/fact_sheets.
23. National Women's Health Resource Center. 2001. Health Topics—Genital Herpes. *Available online at* www.healthywomen.org.

Suggested Readings

Center for Disease Control and Prevention. 1998. *1998 Guidelines for Treatment of Sexually Transmitted Diseases.* New York: International Medical Publications.
This replaces the *1993 Guidelines for Treatment.* It was developed by CDC staff members after consultation with a group of experts on the treatment of STDs.

Nevsid, J. S., and F. Gotfried. 1993. *201 Things You Should Know About AIDS and Other Sexually Transmitted Diseases.* Boston: Allyn and Bacon.
This book provides information on all the common STDs, offers guidelines for prevention, and lists available treatments.

Shilts, R. 1987. *And the Band Played On: Politics, People, and the AIDS Epidemic.* New York: St. Martin's Press.
This classic book written by a gay man with AIDS expresses his views about the political aspects of AIDS and the difficulties in receiving treatment.

Name _____ **Date** _____ **Section** _____

Assessment Activity 12-1

Are You at Risk for a Sexually Transmitted Disease?

Directions: Review each of the following sexual behaviors listed. If you engage in any of the listed activities, assess your personal risk for contracting a sexually transmitted disease through that activity by checking the appropriate line.

There is no risk for activity 1. The risk is low for activity 2. The risk is high for activities 3, 4, 5, and 6.

After reviewing the different categories of activities, are there areas of concern for you?

Activity	Risk	Precautions
1. _____ No sex	No risk: There is virtually no chance of getting an STD.	No precautions are necessary.
2. _____ Sex with only one partner	Low risk: If both partners have no other sexual partners and no disease, there is almost no risk of getting an STD.	Remain monogamous.
3. _____ Sex with a variety of partners	High risk: Each time there is another partner, the risk increases.	Choose partners carefully, use condoms and spermicides, wash after sex, do not douche, and urinate after sex.
4. _____ Sex with a partner who has sex with a variety of partners	High risk: The more partners, the greater the risk an STD will be transmitted.	Be aware of symptoms.
5. _____ Sex with someone who is or has been an IV drug user	High risk: If needles are shared, the risk is great, particularly of getting AIDS and hepatitis B.	Know the social and sexual history of your partner.
6. _____ Oral sex	High risk.	Know your partner; do not engage in oral sex if you do not know the history of your partner.

Assessment Activity 12-2

Making a Decision

The decision to have sexual intercourse is a major one. Many factors affect this decision, and many factors will be affected by it. People engage in sexual activity for a variety of reasons that are often unrelated to love and often without regard to the consequences of that behavior.

Directions: Listed here are factors that may influence your decision to engage in sexual activity. Rank each of these factors as to how they affect your behavior now and when you are in a situation in which you have to make a decision. Answer as truthfully as possible—you do not need to submit this activity to your instructor.

Factor	Not Important	Slightly Important	Important	Very Important	Extremely Important
Risk of AIDS					
Risk of other STD					
Risk of pregnancy					
Sexual history of partner					
History of partner with regard to IV drug use					
Biological gratification (physical sensations)					
Need for money					
Desire to be accepted by partner or social or cultural group					
Chance to reduce stress or to get mind off other problems					
Intense need to feel loved or cared for					
Desire to show commitment to a relationship					
Desire to express love for partner					
Monogamous nature of relationship					
Desire for a variety of partners					
Chance to feel desirable					
Chance to prove sexual prowess					

Consider asking your potential partner to also take this assessment as a basis for discussion. As you assess your responses, note the factors that are important to you in making this decision.

What are the most important factors? _____

_____

_____

Does the person you are considering having sex with have any history, behaviors, or other qualities that you consider to be negative in terms of your decision to have sex? What are they? _____

_____

_____

How important are these histories, behaviors, and other qualities to you? _____

_____

_____

How severe are the potential consequences of your or your partner's ideas and/or actions? _____

_____

_____

13

Reducing Your Risk of Cancer

Online Learning Center

Log on to our Online Learning Center (OLC) for access to these additional resources:

- Chapter key term flashcards
- Learning objectives
- Additional goals for behavior change
- Concentration game
- Self-scoring chapter quizzes

- Additional lab activities

The OLC also offers weblinks for study and exploration of wellness topics. Access these links through **www.mhhe.com/ anspaugh5e**, click on "Student Center," click on "Chapter 13," and then click on "Web Activities."

Goals for Behavior Change

- Identify and change two behaviors that put you at risk for cancer.
- Begin an exercise program for preventing cancer as well as promoting overall wellness.
- Regularly perform the self-examinations for cancer described in this chapter.
- Consult your physician to arrange any appropriate medical screening tests, such as a mammogram or a PSA test.

Key Terms

basal cell carcinoma	lymphoma
benign	metastasis
cancer	oncogene
carcinogens	sarcoma
carcinoma	squamous cell carcinoma
leukemia	

Objectives

After completing this chapter, you will be able to do the following:

- Define *cancer*.
- Identify the various types of cancer.
- List the signs and symptoms of the various types of cancer.

- Identify ways of protecting against various cancers.
- Discuss treatments for cancer.

ith the possible exception of AIDS, there is probably no disease that strikes more fear in people than cancer. The term **cancer** refers to a group of diseases characterized by uncontrolled disorderly cell growth. It is the second leading cause of death, accounting for 25 percent of deaths.[1] It is the leading cause of death among adults ages 25 through 64.[2]

Between 1991 and 1995, the national cancer death rate fell 2.6 percent. Most of the decline was attributed to decreased mortality from cancers of the lung, colon-rectum, and prostate in men and breast, colon-rectum, and gynecologic sites in women.[1] In 2000 almost 552,200 Americans were expected to die of cancer, almost 1500 people a day.[1] (Heart disease deaths, the number-one cause of deaths, fell 50 percent during the same period.)

Death rates for many major cancers have leveled off or declined over the past fifty years. Still, one of four Americans will eventually develop one or more of the 100 different forms of cancer; 40 percent of people who get cancer will be alive five years after diagnosis and considered cured. Others, however, who survive for five years may still show evidence of cancer.[3] *Cured* means that a patient has no evidence of disease and has the same life expectancy of a person who never had cancer. Although it strikes more frequently with advancing age, cancer causes the deaths of more children than any other disease (see Wellness Across the Generations: Children and Cancer). The chances of developing cancer can be reduced by assuming control of your daily behaviors and activities (see Just the Facts: Tips for Cancer Prevention; see Assessment Activity 13-2: Are You Practicing Cancer Prevention?).

Wellness Across the Generations
Children and Cancer

Despite its rarity, cancer is the chief cause of death by disease in children under the age of 15. Cancer is a devastating event, particularly when the diagnosis occurs in children. The overwhelming emotional and psychological trauma associated with cancer affects not only the child but also brothers, sisters, parents, and other relatives. If there is any good news to report, it is that mortality rates have declined 57 percent since the 1970s. St. Jude Children's Research Hospital, the only cancer research center in the world devoted solely to children, reports that, since 1962, the survival rates for various childhood cancers have risen significantly. For example, children with acute lymphocytic leukemia (cancer of the blood) now have a survival rate of 80 percent compared with the 1962 rate of 4 percent. Children now have the following survival rates (see list):

Even though the survival rates are significantly better today than they were in 1962, the families of children diagnosed with cancer still need support. St. Jude provides not only medical treatment for the child, but also social support, psychological counseling, and education about the cancer for all the members of the family. Its mission is to serve as an advocate for the family as well as for the child affected, regardless of the prognosis.

As researchers move slowly toward providing cures and increasing life expectancy of children affected by cancer, we can all hope that, one day, we will only know of children dying from cancer through reading about them in textbooks. For more information about childhood cancers, visit the following website: **www.stjude.org**.

	Now	*1962*
• Hodgkin's lymphoma (cancer of the lymph nodes):	90%	50%
• Non-Hodgkin's lymphoma (malignant tumor):	80%	7%
• Retinoblastoma (cancer affecting the eyes):	90%	75%
• Neuroblastoma (cancer of the nervous system):	56%	10%
• Wilms' tumor (cancer of the kidney):	90%	50%
• Osteosarcoma (bone cancer):	70%	20%
• Rhabdomyosarcoma (cancer affecting the muscles):	75%	30%

Cell growth is controlled by deoxyribonucleic acid (DNA) and ribonucleic acid (RNA) in the nucleus of each cell in the body. If the nuclei lose the ability to regulate and control this growth, cellular metabolism and reproduction are disrupted and a mutant cell is produced that varies in form, quality, and function from the original. When a mass of these cells develops, it is considered a neoplasm, or tumor. It may be malignant (cancerous) or **benign** (noncancerous). A benign tumor will not spread throughout the body. It is enclosed by a membrane that prevents it from invading other tissues. A benign tumor is not life threatening unless it is in an area that interferes with normal functioning. A malignant tumor is the most dangerous tumor because it has a tendency to spread from its original location to other parts of the body, which can make it life threatening. Cancer cells can crowd out normal cells, invade surrounding tissue, and move through the lymphatic or circulatory system to infiltrate other areas of the body. (The lymphatic system is a network of nodes and vessels that serves to drain fluid from tissues and return it to the bloodstream. It is also part of the body's immune system.) The process by which cancerous cells spread from their original site (primary site) to another location (secondary site) is called **metastasis**. The ability of cancerous cells to metastasize makes early detection critical. Table 13-1 describes the types of cancer (**carcinoma, sarcoma, lymphoma,** and **leukemia**) and where they are most often found.

Just the Facts

Tips for Cancer Prevention

More than 200 studies demonstrate a strong association between diets high in vegetables and fruits (5–9 servings a day).[5] Observe the following guidelines to improve your chances of avoiding cancer:

What to Do

- Eat more broccoli, cauliflower, and brussels sprouts. Eat more cabbage-type vegetables, such as cabbages and kale. These vegetables protect against cancers of the colon, rectum, stomach, and lung.

- Add more high-fiber foods to your diet. Eat more peaches, strawberries, potatoes, spinach, tomatoes, wheat and bran cereals, rice, popcorn, and whole-wheat bread. Fiber protects against cancer of the colon.

- Choose foods containing vitamin A. Eat more carrots, peaches, apricots, squash, and broccoli. Fresh foods are the best sources and are far better than vitamin pills. Vitamin A protects against cancers of the esophagus, larynx, and lung.

- Choose foods containing vitamin C. Eat more grapefruit, cantaloupe, oranges, strawberries, red peppers, green peppers, broccoli, and tomatoes. These help fight cancers of the esophagus and stomach.

- Practice weight control. Exercise and eat foods low in calories. A good exercise for most people is walking. Obese people have a high chance of getting cancers of the uterus, gallbladder, breast, and colon. Check with your doctor before you start an exercise program or a special diet.

- If female, perform monthly breast exams, and get annual mammograms after age 40. Males should get annual digital and PSA exams after age 50 (40, if African American or with a family history). Males over age 16 should perform monthly testicle exams. Males and females over age 50 should get annual colon cancer checks.[6]

What to Avoid

- Avoid fat. Eat lean meat, fish, and low-fat dairy products. Cut extra fat off meats and skin poultry before cooking. Avoid pastries and candies. A high-fat diet increases the chance of getting cancer of the breast, colon, and prostate. Calories loaded with fat cause weight gain.

- Avoid salty foods. Stay away from nitrite-cured and smoked foods. Bacon, ham, hot dogs, and salt-cured fish are examples. People who eat these foods have a greater chance of cancer of the esophagus and stomach.

- Avoid smoking. Smoking is the main cause of lung cancer. Pregnant women who smoke harm their babies. Parents who smoke at home cause breathing and allergy problems for their children. Chewing tobacco can cause cancers of the mouth and throat. Pick a day to quit and call the American Cancer Society for help.

- Avoid alcohol in excess. If you drink a great deal, you may get cancer of the liver. It is worse to smoke and drink. This increases the chances of getting cancers of the mouth, throat, larynx, and esophagus.

- Avoid too much sun. The sun causes skin cancer and other damage to skin. Use a sunscreen. Wear long sleeves and a hat between 11 A.M. and 3 P.M. Do not use indoor sunlamps, visit tanning parlors, or take tanning pills. Be alert for changes in a mole or sore that does not heal. If changes occur, go to a doctor.

Table 13-1   Types of Cancer and Most Common Sites

Type	Most Common Site	Method of Spread
Carcinoma	Tissues covering body surfaces and lining the body cavities are the most common locations. Sites include the breast, lungs, intestines, skin, stomach, uterus, and testes.	Lymphatic and circulatory system
Sarcoma	The connective system is most commonly affected. Sites include bones, muscle, and other connective tissue.	Circulatory system
Lymphoma	The condition develops in the lymphatic system, infectious regions of the neck, armpits, groin, and chest. Hodgkin's disease is an example.	Lymphatic system
Leukemia	The blood-forming tissues, bone marrow, and spleen are particularly affected.	Circulatory system

Table 13-2   Factors That Can Cause Cancer[1]

Carcinogen	Site of Cancer	Comments
Alcohol	Liver, larynx, pharynx, breast, esophagus	Heavy drinking increases the risk of cancer, especially when accompanied by cigarette smoking or use of chewing tobacco.
Smoking	Lungs, mouth, pharynx, larynx, bladder, esophagus	Smoking accounts for about 30 percent of cancer deaths. It is considered the number-one carcinogen in the United States and the most preventable cause of death. It is responsible for 87 percent of lung cancer deaths.
Ultraviolet radiation	Skin	Almost all skin cancers are sun related.
Ionizing radiation	Blood-forming tissues, lungs	Excessive exposure to radiation increases cancer risk. Excessive radon exposure increases the risk of lung cancer.
Smokeless tobacco	Mouth, larynx, pharynx, esophagus	Oral cancer increases with the use of chewing tobacco and snuff.
Estrogen	Endometrium (uterus), liver, breast	Oral contraceptives increase the risk of liver cancer. Estrogen treatment to control menopausal symptoms increases the risk of cancer. The risk is reduced with simultaneous progesterone treatment.
Industrial agents		Industrial chemicals and agents, such as nickel, chromate, asbestos, and vinyl chloride, increase the risk of various cancers.
Dietary fat		High consumption of dietary fat is related to cancers of the colon, prostate, and pancreas; replacing fat with complex carbohydrates provides protection against several cancers (see Chapter 6).

Causes and Prevention

Cancer is caused by both external (chemicals, diet, radiation, viruses, pollutants, etc.) and internal (hormones, immune conditioning, and inherited mutations) factors. Any combination of these factors may initiate or promote carcinogenesis—the development of cancer cells. Ten or more years often pass between exposures or mutations and the detection of cancer.[3]

Although the causes of cancer are not clearly understood, correlations have been found between cancer and everything from genetic factors to exposure to the sun's radiation. Many **carcinogens** (cancer-causing agents) trigger the development of cancer. (Table 13-2 contains a list of substances known to be carcinogenic.)

An inherited tendency for cancer has been theorized for years. Everyone seems to have genes that may cause cancer, but not everyone gets cancer. In most cases environmental factors activate the cancer. A good example of the interplay between genetic and environmental factors is found in cigarette smoking. Approximately

Wellness On the Web Behavior Change Activities

Cancer: An Ounce of Detection Is Worth a Pound of Cure

Time after time, we hear the same tragic story from cancer patients: "I knew I had a lump, but I was afraid it would be cancer, so I didn't go to the doctor," or "By the time I realized something was wrong, the cancer had metastasized." The very word "cancer" strikes fear into the hearts of the bravest—yet reliable studies show that the earlier cancer is diagnosed, the better the chances of survival. Both health care providers and the public look to the American Cancer Society (ACS) for guidelines to help detect cancer at the earliest possible stage. The ACS publicizes its recommendations (and most doctors follow them) about Pap smears and mammograms for women, prostate examinations for men, and colorectal examinations for anyone over age 50. These procedures offer hope of detecting cancer early, when it's most treatable. Go to **www.mhhe.com.anspaugh5e**, "Student Center," and "Wellness on the Web." Then select "Activity 1" and read through the list of recommended early detection tests.

What Causes Cancer?

What is cancer, and how does it originate? Thanks to sophisticated research, medical science is coming closer than ever to solving these riddles and opening the door to possible cures. In the meantime, we're learning a great deal about the risk factors that increase a person's chance of developing cancer. Different cancers have different risk factors. According to the American Cancer Society, existing scientific evidence suggests that about one-third of the cancer deaths that occur in the United States each year are caused by cigarette smoking, and another third are the result of dietary factors. This means that for the majority of Americans who don't use tobacco, dietary choices and physical activity become the most important modifiable determinants of cancer risk. To learn more about individual risk factors, go to the website listed previously, select "Activity 2," and read through the list of risks for different types of cancers. Were you surprised by anything you learned?

HealthQuest Activities

- The self-assessment activity *Cancer: What's Your Risk?* found in the Cancer Module allows you to examine how your family history, personal health history, occupation, environment, and behavior affect your risk of developing cancer. *HealthQuest* will estimate whether you are at decreased, average, or above average risk of developing several kinds of cancer. Complete the self-assessment and then gather more information about the cancers for which you are at increased risk. Use the Cancer Info feature in the Connections section to help you.

- Like other chronic diseases that occur more frequently as people age, cancer may appear to young adults to be an unlikely possibility. Review the *Cancer Info* feature to learn how cancer affects quality of life. Then read the "Connections" article on social support for people with cancer. Finally, increase your awareness of skin cancer prevention by using the *Skin Cancer Exploration*. List the factors that put a person at highest and at lowest risk for skin cancer. Then determine which factors are modifiable and which are not.

87 percent of lung cancers occur in cigarette smokers,[3] but only 15 percent of smokers develop lung cancer. Why not the other 85 percent? The 15 percent who develop cancer are thought to be susceptible to the disease on the basis of their genes. If they had not activated the cancer genes by smoking, they probably would not have contracted the disease.

A gene that causes cancer is called an **oncogene.** Within a tiny segment of DNA is an area that can be activated to form an oncogene. All cells have normal regulatory genes called *proto-oncogenes.* A variety of genetic mutations, viral infections, or other carcinogens cause these normal genes to somehow lose their ability to replicate themselves in a normal genetic fashion. If the gene that is miscopied is one that controls specialization, replication, repair, or tumor suppression, the result is a cancer-producing gene. Unless it is activated, however, it will never cause cancer. If an oncogene is formed, it acts with other oncogenes to produce abnormal cells that can replicate and spread.

Suppressor genes also play a role in cancer. Suppressor genes, which exist in normal cells, control cell growth. If suppressor genes mutate, cells are permitted to grow unrestrained.

Another explanation of cancer is an error in cell duplication on the basis of chance alone. Several trillion new cells are formed each year, and perfect duplication does not occur with each new cell formation. When an abnormal cell develops, the immune system recognizes it as a rogue cell and attacks it. Every cancer cell needs to be killed because almost all cancers arise from a single cancer cell. Cancer develops as a result of the immune system's failure to clear the body of cancer cells. This is one reason the immune system is receiving considerable attention from cancer researchers.

The development of cancer is a process that generally takes years. By stopping this process at any step, the deadly potential of cancer is ended. After the cancer process is initiated, due to environmental or genetic causes, several things must happen. The cancer cells have to grow and reproduce; the immune system must fail to recognize the cancer and leave it alone; and the new tumor must eventually find a way to "feed" itself by forming new blood vessels to supply itself with blood (a process called angiogenesis).[1]

Much research appears to link psychological states with the prevalence of disease in certain people. People with positive, involved attitudes who view life's challenges as opportunities for personal growth seem to have fewer diseases and recover from them more often. People who feel lonely and depressed and lack appropriate social support are more cancer prone than are their mentally healthy counterparts.[1]

Emotional factors, such as stress, lack of social support, and the inability to express and cope with the range of emotions brought on by a frightening diagnosis of cancer, have been linked to the progression of cancer. Several studies have reported that patients who participate in support groups while receiving standard medical care live significantly longer than do those receiving medical care alone. Conversely, cancer patients who are socially isolated have poorer survival rates than do those with more social connections.[8] This doesn't suggest that stress and social isolation cause cancer. It does suggest a significant correlation between emotion and the progression of cancer once the disease is established. Many experts believe that a person's emotional state may somehow bolster the body's natural cancer-fighting power.

Although some of these concepts are controversial, it is generally accepted that substances such as tobacco, tobacco smoke, alcohol, asbestos, herbicides and pesticides are carcinogens. Scientists believe that more than 80 percent of cancers are associated with lifestyle factors that are easily controlled—diet, smoking, and exposure to the sun.[6] Almost two-thirds of cancer deaths are attributed to diet and tobacco (figure 13-1).

Figure 13-1 Percent of Cancer Deaths Caused by Preventable Factors[5]

According to a twenty-year study of 115,195 healthy women ages 30 to 55, one-third of cancer deaths are caused by excessive weight.[7] (Chapter 6 provides guidelines for cancer prevention as related to diet; Chapter 8 provides guidelines for weight maintenance.)

One of the major carcinogens may be sun radiation—more specifically, excessive exposure to the ultraviolet (UV) rays of the sun. People who spend hours in the sun without protection have an increased risk for skin cancers. UV light peaks from 10 A.M. to 2 P.M. (11 A.M. to 3 P.M. during daylight savings time). Avoiding sun exposure during these hours can cut UV-light exposure by up to 60 percent. Most major newspapers now include the UV index as a routine part of the weather report. Using tanning beds also increases the risk for skin cancer.

Finally, the herpes viruses have been connected with cancer of the cervix. Viruses may be involved in the development of some forms of leukemia, Hodgkin's disease, and Burkett's lymphoma. The exact role of

viruses in causing cancer is not known, but they may provide an opportunistic environment for cancer development. Other researchers have suggested that it is a combination of factors, in which the virus may play a part, rather than the virus itself that causes cancer.

Cancer Site

The American Cancer Society reports each year on the incidence and number of deaths from cancer for a variety of sites (figure 13-2). Skin cancer is the most common cancer. More than 1 million people are diagnosed annually with basal and squamous cell skin cancer. Almost all of these are considered sun-related cases.[3] Fortunately, the majority of skin cancers are highly curable. For both genders the cancer that kills most often is lung cancer. Excluding basal cell and squamous cell carcinomas, the breasts are the most prevalent cancer site for women, and the prostate is the leading cancer site for men. Almost 60 percent of cancer deaths

Cancer cases by site and sex

Male	Female
Prostate 184,500	Breast 178,700
Lung 91,400	Lung 80,100
Colon & rectum 64,600	Colon & rectum 67,000
Urinary bladder 39,500	Endometrium (uterus) 36,100
Non-Hodgkin's lymphoma 31,100	Ovary 25,400
Melanoma of the skin 24,300	Non-Hodgkin's lymphoma 24,300
Oral cavity 20,600	Melanoma of the skin 17,300
Kidney 17,600	Urinary bladder 14,900
Leukemia 16,100	Pancreas 14,900
Stomach 14,300	Cervix (uterus) 13,700
All Sites 627,900	All Sites 600,700

Cancer deaths by site and sex

Male	Female
Lung 93,100	Lung 67,000
Prostate 39,200	Breast 43,500
Colon & rectum 27,900	Colon & rectum 28,600
Pancreas 14,000	Pancreas 14,900
Non-Hodgkin's lymphoma 13,000	Ovary 14,500
Leukemia 12,000	Non-Hodgkin's lymphoma 11,900
Esophagus 9,100	Leukemia 9,600
Urinary bladder 8,400	Endometrium (uterus) 6,300
Stomach 8,100	Brain 6,000
Liver 7,900	Stomach 5,600
All Sites 294,200	All Sites 270,600

Figure 13-2 Cancer Incidence and Death by Site and Sex—1995 Estimates*

*Excluding basal and squamous cell skin cancer and in situ carcinomas except urinary bladder.

Source: American Cancer Society, Surveillance Research, 1998.

among males are from four primary sites—lung, prostate, colon, and pancreas. Sixty percent of female cancer deaths occur from five sites—lung, breast, colon, ovary, and pancreas.[12] For any cancer, early detection is imperative (see Assessment Activity 13-1). If cancer is diagnosed while it is still localized, the cure or survival rate may be 90 percent or higher for some cancers such as skin, colon, and rectum cancers.[2]

Exercise and Cancer Prevention

Researchers are continuing to investigate the role of exercise in the prevention of some types of cancer, including of the colon, breast, and reproductive system. In 1996 regular physical activity was added to the list of cancer-prevention measures developed by the American Cancer Society. Mounting research indicates that lack of exercise is a contributing factor to the development of cancer. A panel of cancer experts concluded that as many as 30 to 40 percent of cancers worldwide could be prevented if people exercised, maintained proper weight, and followed a proper diet.[7] Another study found that, over an eight-year period, physically unfit men had four times the overall cancer death rate of the most fit men. For women, an even greater difference exists in the death rate between the fit and unfit.[7] Many researchers have followed various groups for long periods to determine whether those who exercise seem to have some measure of protection against cancer.[9] The most impressive results have shown exercise providing protection against colon, breast, and prostate cancers.

Exercise and Colon Cancer

In a review of many studies, it was found that people who tend to sit the majority of the workday or remain inactive in their leisure time have a 30 to 100 percent greater chance of contracting colon cancer.[10] One study of 17,607 college graduates, ages 30 to 79 years, confirmed a lower risk of colon and lung cancer among physically active men.[20] A study done at Harvard University reported that, among 48,000 men, colon cancer risk decreased 50 percent in the most physically active group. This protective effect seemed to occur when the men exercised on average about one to two hours a day.[20] Another study of nearly 90,000 nurses also confirmed the protective effect of physical activity for women against colon cancer.

There are several possible explanations of why exercise is beneficial in protecting against colon cancer. One theory is that exercise increases peristalsis of the large intestine, thus decreasing transit time and the time during which potential carcinogens can be in contact with the cell lining of the colon. Another theory is

that exercisers tend to be of more normal weight and are less likely to be obese than nonexercisers. Both obesity and lack of exercise increase levels of insulin, which in turn increase the growth rate of cells lining the colon, thereby increasing the likelihood of developing cancer.[18] Another interesting aspect of the Harvard study was the discovery that exercisers ate an average of 29 grams of fiber daily, whereas nonexercisers ate only 12 grams. The increased fiber serves to increase peristalsis.

Exercise and Breast Cancer

In a study of 545 premenopausal women, it was found that women exercising 3.7 hours per week reduced their risk for breast cancer by more than 50 percent.[11] A study of Norwegian women who engaged in regular exercise demonstrated a 37 percent reduction in breast cancer risk.[11] If the women were both lean and exercisers, their risk was reduced by 72 percent.

Some researchers feel that exercise helps reduce the amount of body fat and protects against obesity. As mentioned in the case of colon cancer, obesity is associated with higher blood insulin levels, which promote the growth of breast cancer cells. Thus, exercising women may be protected from breast cancer because of the indirect effects of exercising on exposure to their own hormones.[11]

Exercise and Prostate Cancer

In a study on over 17,000 college alumni, prostate cancer was found to be reduced by 47 percent in highly active men compared to sedentary men 70 years old and older.[13] At the Cooper Clinic in Dallas it was found that men in the highest fitness group had a 74 percent smaller risk than those in the lowest fitness group of developing prostate cancer.[14] This same study found that men expending more than 1000 calories a week in exercise had less than half the risk of prostate cancer of their sedentary counterparts.

The protective nature of exercise against the development of prostate cancer seems to be the result of repeated bouts of exercise that lower blood levels of testosterone. Men who exercise a great deal tend to expose their prostate to less testosterone, thus reducing their risk for cancer.[15]

Cancers of Concern to Everyone

Lung Cancer

Although breast cancer and prostate cancer (see the next sections) receive the majority of attention in the United States, lung cancer is the leading cause of cancer death in the United States[4] and throughout the world.[21] This is largely because lung cancer is more difficult to detect and thereby more deadly than other, even more frequently occurring types of cancer. Lung cancer is one of the most preventable forms of cancer, because the vast majority of cases are directly associated with lifestyle—smoking cigarettes. All cancers caused by cigarette smoking are 100 percent preventable.

The incidence of lung cancer is highest among people who started smoking cigarettes at an early age and who smoke the most cigarettes daily. The single best prevention of lung cancer is never to smoke. Passive, or involuntary, smoke also contributes significantly to lung cancer. A person who lives or works with smokers significantly increases his or her risk of developing lung cancer even if choosing to not smoke. Symptoms of lung cancer typically include a persistent cough, blood in the sputum, chest pain, recurring pneumonia, or bronchitis.

The good news about lung cancer (and nearly all cancer deaths) is that, for the first time, all cancer deaths declined between 1990 and 1995 (by 3 percent).[3] Part of this decrease is due to the reduction in the total number of smokers. The bad news about lung cancer is that early diagnosis tends to be rare. Regular X rays of the lungs and checking for blood in the sputum seem to be ineffective means of early detection, perhaps because of the altered appearance and function of lung cells from smoking. By the time most lung cancers are detected, the cancer is either not treatable because of widespread metastasis or the treatment is limited to ensuring a short-term extension of life. Five-year survival rates following diagnosis of lung cancer are between 7 and 12 percent, which is low.

The colorless, odorless gas radon has been somewhat inconsistently associated with increased risk of lung cancer.[3] People living in areas designated high in radon should have their homes measured. Asbestos inhalation has also been associated with lung cancer.

Although the absolute best ways to prevent lung cancer are to not smoke, not living with a smoker, not working in a smoking environment, ensuring that radon levels in the home are safe, and avoiding asbestos, substantial evidence exists for the role of diet in lung cancer prevention.[4,16,17] A diet high in whole fruits and vegetables seems to protect against lung cancer. Smokers who regularly consume much produce (fruits and vegetables) seem to have reduced incidence. While regular consumption of whole fruits and vegetables does not ensure that a smoker (or anyone else) will not get cancer, especially lung cancer, there is convincing evidence that a healthy diet provides some protection.

Colorectal Cancer

Colon cancer and cancer of the rectum rank as the second leading causes of cancer deaths in the United States (they are the third leading causes for women, behind lung and breast cancers, and the third leading causes for men, behind lung and prostate cancers).[19] When detected early, 90 percent of localized colorectal cancers can be cured. Once the cancer has spread, however, this chance drops to only 10 percent.[19]

A family history of colon cancer doubles the risk, but family history only accounts for 10 to 15 percent of colon cancers.[16] People with a family history need to be extra vigilant, participating in regular screenings, but so do people with family histories of benign polyps in the colon. Frequent constipation has been implicated as a risk factor; experiencing constipation even once a month may double one's risk.[20] Any change or increases in constipation or chronic constipation suggest the need for follow-up screening for abnormal growths. Consuming large numbers of calories may increase colon cancer risk.[3] Symptoms of colorectal cancer include a change in bowel habits, chronic abdominal discomfort, sudden weight loss, lack of appetite, or rectal bleeding. Long-term survival rates are much higher when potential cancers are detected before symptoms develop. Detection of colorectal cancer can frequently be accomplished via screenings, although many people avoid the screenings because they find them somewhat distasteful.

Identification of polyps (growths) is a primary screening method. The occurrence of polyps in the colon and rectum does not mean a person will develop cancer. In cases in which the polyps do become cancerous, the length of time from initiation to cancer may be five to ten years.[19] The type of screening test used depends on the age of the person as well as family and personal history. Anyone over age 50, even without a family history of the disease, should be tested.

Anyone can undertake prevention of colorectal cancer. Diet is believed to be the primary cause for its development. The National Cancer Institute, the American Cancer Society, and the American Institute for Cancer Research recommend a diet high in vegetables (especially cruciferous vegetables) and fiber and low in fat.[4,16,18] Regular physical activity and maintaining recommended body weight are also probably preventive. Long-term (fifteen years or more) ingestion of the B-vitamin folate may reduce the risk of colon cancer.[21] Recent studies suggest that 81 mg of aspirin (the lowest observable amount that produced desirable results) may also have a protective effect against colon cancer.[4,22] Although aspirin is a drug with side effects, some potentially life threatening, it may also be beneficial for people at elevated risk who can tolerate it. However, aspirin as a preventive should never be taken without prior consultation with a physician.

Stomach, Liver, and Pancreatic Cancer

Stomach cancer

Stomach cancer except for cancer of the upper part of the stomach (which may be associated with obesity) has steadily declined in the United States and other developed countries. This decrease seems to be strongly linked to the availability of refrigeration, eliminating the need for salt as a preservative. Refrigeration also provides year-round availability of fresh fruits and vegetables, linked to decreased risk. The popular interest in green tea consumption may prove beneficial in reducing the risk for stomach cancer. Diets high in salt probably increase the risk for stomach cancer. The major nonlifestyle cause of stomach cancer is infection with the *Helicobacter pylori* bacteria.[16]

Most types of stomach cancer can be prevented by diet. Although the numbers of cases are declining, stomach cancer still ranks among the top ten cancer killers in the United States. Symptoms are nonspecific and diagnosis at early stages is not usual.

Liver cancer

Liver cancer is relatively uncommon in the United States and other developed countries. No effective treatment exists for it; the five-year survival rate is only 6 percent. Many liver cancers are lifestyle-related. The primary risk factor for liver cancer is infection with hepatitis B or hepatitis C viruses. The major method of transmission for these viruses is the sharing of needles or sexual contact.[21] Recent findings suggest that hepatitis B can also be transmitted by sharing a rolled paper used for snorting cocaine or other drugs.[23] Regular, heavy (more than moderate) consumption of alcohol, leading to cirrhosis and a condition known as *alcoholic hepatitis,* is closely associated with the development of liver cancer.[21] Ingestion of aflatoxins (a type of food mold) from contaminated food has been demonstrated to produce liver cancer, particularly among people in developing countries,[29] but tends to be rare in the United States.

Pancreatic cancer

Pancreatic cancer, lesser known than the cancers mentioned previously, ranks among the leading five causes of cancer death in the United States. Pancreatic cancer does not seem to get the publicity of many other types of cancer, yet it is extremely deadly and almost impossible to diagnose. In 1998, 29,000 new cases were diagnosed, and 28,900 people died from it.[1] At the time of publication, no effective method existed to screen or diagnose this cancer. Occasionally, depending upon where the tumor originates, jaundice may occur while the tumor is in an early stage. Even so, the five-year survival rate is only 4 percent. Little is known about pancreatic cancer except that smoking increases the risk. Because the pancreas is related to digestion and absorption, speculation is that diet affects the development and course of this cancer, but no specifics are known at this time.

Leukemia and Lymphoma

Leukemia and lymphoma (Hodgkin's disease and non–Hodgkin's lymphoma) are two of the most frequent childhood cancers, but they strike more adults than children every year. **Leukemia** occurs in adults nearly 12 times more often than in children. The causes of leukemia are largely unidentified, although people with genetic abnormalities, such as Down's syndrome, experience it more frequently. Excessive exposure to certain chemicals, such as benzene, or infection with the retrovirus HTLV-I also place people at elevated risk. Symptoms resemble those of many other conditions, so they are frequently overlooked initially. They include fatigue, paleness, weight loss, repeated infections, easy bruising, and nosebleeds or other hemorrhages. Children usually experience the onset of these symptoms abruptly, but adults with chronic leukemia will progress slowly and exhibit few symptoms.

Early, appropriate diagnosis is the key to long-term survival for leukemia. Depending on the type of leukemia and stage of diagnosis, five-year survival rates may be as high as 57 percent for adults and 80 percent for children.[1]

Lymphoma is a condition in which a tumor composed of lymphoid tissue occurs. The two most general categories of lymphoma are Hodgkin's disease and non–Hodgkin's lymphoma, which includes all types of lymphoma other than Hodgkin's. Hodgkin's disease rates have declined, especially in the elderly, but cases of non–Hodgkin's lymphoma have nearly doubled since the 1970s. Studies suggest that eating large amounts of red meat (beef, pork, or lamb) increase the risk.[38] Other causes involve reduced immune function and exposure to infectious agents via organ transplants or viruses like HIV (human immunodeficiency virus) or Epstein-Barr. Herbicides and other chemicals may influence the development of the disease.

Symptoms include enlarged lymph nodes, itching, fever, night sweats, anemia, and weight loss. The fever may come and go over periods of weeks or months. Survival rates vary greatly, according to the type of disease and stage at diagnosis but can be as high as 51 to 81 percent after five years.[3]

Skin Cancer

The most frequently occurring types of cancer are skin cancers. Skin cancers fall into three main categories: basal cell carcinoma, squamous cell carcinoma, and melanoma. Of the three categories, melanoma is by far the most deadly.

Basal cell carcinoma

Basal cell carcinoma is the most common skin cancer and, along with squamous cell, is responsible for approximately 1.3 million cases of skin cancer a year.[1] Basal cell carcinoma occurs in the outermost skin layers and tends to spread by widening rather than by growing deeper into the skin. The cancer develops into a central sore that crusts over and bleeds but does not go away.[24] Basal cell carcinoma grows slowly and rarely spreads to other parts of the body.

Squamous cell carcinoma

The second most common type of skin cancer is squamous cell. **Squamous cell carcinoma** grows faster than basal cell cancer but still grows fairly slowly and can metastasize to other parts of the body. Typically, a squamous cell skin lesion is a firm, red, painless nodule.[24] Both basal cell and squamous cell carcinomas are usually the result of overexposure to sunlight. They occur on a part of the body that has been exposed to the sun.

Malignant melanoma

Although it is the least common type of skin cancer, about 75 percent of skin cancer deaths are due to malignant melanoma. All skin cancers, but especially malignant melanoma, have increased in number in recent years so that the current lifetime risk of developing malignant melanoma is about one in eighty-two. Although the use of sunscreens with an SPF of 15 or higher seems to reduce the number of basal and squamous cell skin cancers, it does not appear to decrease the risk for melanoma. Genetics is a strong factor in getting malignant melanoma, but it does not explain the explosive increase in the disease that has occurred in the last few decades. Melanoma often grows on parts of the body that are rarely exposed to the sun (such as the buttocks or feet) and does not increase in incidence among people whose occupations require them to spend long hours in the sun (such as farmers).[25] Melanoma appears to be more highly associated with intermittent sun exposure and blistering sunburns occurring early in life (before age 15).

All adults are susceptible, but particularly those with the following risk factors:

- A family history of melanoma
- A personal history of one or more severe sunburns as a child
- Fair skin and many freckles, blonde or red hair, and light eyes
- Occupational exposure to industrial radiation or certain chemicals
- Consumption of medications that increase sensitivity to ultraviolet light

People with these factors should check their entire bodies regularly for any change in the size or color of a mole or other spot; any scaling, oozing, or bleeding from a bump or nodule; pigmentation spreading beyond its border; and a change in sensation, itchiness, tenderness, or pain. Any skin growth that bleeds or crusts should be seen by a physician (figure 13-3).[26]

Knowing the ABCDs of skin cancer can help people identify melanoma during the early stages when it is still highly treatable (with a 95 percent five-year survival rate):

- *Asymmetry:* If you drew an imaginary line through the center of the mole or pigmented area, the two halves would be shaped differently.
- *Border:* Most normal moles are regularly shaped and their outside borders are regularly shaped. If a border appears to have scalloped edges or to be poorly defined in areas or uneven, it is not normal.
- *Color:* A mole should be one color. Variation in color—differing shades of black or brown or tan or red or some combination of colors—or an intensely black color indicates a problem and need for further investigation.
- *Diameter:* A mole or pigmented area greater than 6 mm (the size of a pencil eraser) should be looked at by a specialist.

(a) (b)

Figure 13-3 Comparison of Nonmalignant and Malignant Skin Growths

(a) normal mole. Note its symmetrical shape, regular borders, even color, and relatively small size (about a half centimeter). (b) malignant melanoma. Note its asymmetrical shape, irregular borders, uneven color, and relatively large size (about 2 centimeters).

As with all cancers, the first line of defense is prevention. Because most skin cancers are directly related to overexposure to the sun's ultraviolet rays, take caution to limit this exposure. Although the use of sunscreen (with an SPF of 15 or higher) may not prevent malignant melanoma, it does decrease the incidence of basal and squamous cell skin cancers. Newer sunscreens block a wider range of ultraviolet rays and may prove to reduce even melanoma over time. Children particularly should always wear sunscreen when playing outside to prevent the blistering sunburn associated with melanoma later in life. The sun's rays are the strongest between 10 A.M. and 2 P.M. (even on cloudy days) and direct exposure at that time should be avoided, even with a sunscreen. Protective clothing such as hats, long-sleeve shirts, long pants, and ultraviolet-protecting sunglasses (too much sun can lead to cataracts or melanoma in the eyes) should be worn. Avoid tanning booths and sunlamps (see Real-World Wellness: Are

Tanning Devices Hazardous to Your Health?). No matter how dark a person's skin is, he or she becomes darker when exposed to the sun. Although the risk is greatly reduced for darker-skinned people, anyone can get skin cancer.

Oral Cancer

Oral cancers are cancers of any part of the oral cavity, including the lip, tongue, mouth, and throat. Oral cancer occurs more than twice as often in males than in females. This is because the risk factors of cigar and pipe smoking and the use of smokeless tobacco are practiced much more frequently by men than by women. Cigarette smoking and excessive consumption of alcohol (both on the rise among women) are also considered risk factors. Wiser lifestyle choices (choosing not to use tobacco products and reducing the consumption of alcohol) could practically eliminate oral cancers.

Real-World **Wellness**

Are Tanning Devices Hazardous to Your Health?

I want to be tan this summer and thought I would get a head start by using a tanning bed. Is it safe for me to do so?

Sunlight produces two types of ultraviolet radiation: ultraviolet A (UVA) and ultraviolet B (UVB). UVB is 1000 times more likely to cause burns than is UVA. Because it penetrates the skin more deeply, UVA radiation causes the skin to tan or burn more slowly. A small amount of UVB radiation, however, can cause skin damage.

Most tanning devices (for example, sunlamps) give off either mostly UVA or UVB radiation. Newer UVA sunlamps give off as much as 10 times more UVA than is received from the sun or given by older UVB sunlamps. Although exposure to UVA sunlamps is less likely to cause burns of the skin and eyes, UVA radiation in high doses may increase the risks of skin cancer and premature skin aging. Studies also suggest that skin cancer is exacerbated when people combine tanning in the sun with tanning by sunlamps. Here are some facts concerning tans and tanning devices:

- *Skin cancer* risks increase each time the skin is exposed to UV radiation.
- *Burns* of the skin and eyes may occur.
- *Photosensitivity* means being extra sensitive to UV radiation as a result of using or consuming various substances that may cause allergic reactions, severe skin burns, itchy and scaly skin, and rash. Examples of

photosensitizing products are soaps, shampoos, makeup, birth control pills, antibiotics, antihistamines, diuretics, and tranquilizers.

- *Cataracts,* an eye condition in which the lens becomes cloudy, may develop as a result of unprotected exposure to UVA and UVB radiation. For this reason, it is required that tanning devices have labels warning users to wear protective eyewear.
- *Premature skin aging,* in which the skin becomes dry, wrinkled, and leathery, is one of the most noticeable signs of repeated UV exposure.
- *Blood vessel damage and reduced immunity* may result from exposure to UV radiation.
- People who have red or blond hair and blue eyes, are fair-skinned, have freckles, and sunburn easily are at highest risk for skin damage. If you burn and do not tan in sunlight, you will probably burn and will not tan using sunlamps.
- A UVA tan offers some protection against further UV damage—about the same as an SPF of 2 or 3. Even with a dark tan, UV damage continues to accumulate.
- Sunscreens are not recommended for tanning indoors except to protect parts of your body you do not want to tan (for example, the lips). Sunscreens do not prevent UVA allergic-type reactions of photosensitive people.
- Always wear special goggles that block UV radiation, avoid using photosensitizing products, avoid tanning if your skin never tans, and follow the manufacturer's recommended time of exposure for your skin type.

Cancers That Can Affect Women

Breast cancer

Some women are at increased risk for breast cancer. Breast cancer is often fatal (in approximately 25 percent of cases). On the brighter side, advances in breast cancer research have escalated (see Just the Facts: Drugs and Breast Cancer Treatment). Women's groups have done a good job of getting the word out about early detection and have supported efforts for improved treatment. These efforts have led to a decline in cancer deaths, but the surgeries and other treatments associated with breast cancer can still be devastating. Although breast cancer is relatively rare in men about 1600 men were diagnosed with it in 1998.

One in nine women who live to age 85 will develop breast cancer. Being over the age of 60 automatically places a woman in a high-risk category. Having an inherited mutation in the genes known as *BRCA1* and *BRCA2* accounts for about 10 percent of cancers. This means 90 percent of cases are due to causes other than recognized inherited genetic factors. A woman with a mother or sister who has had breast cancer has double the risk of getting breast cancer. This risk is particularly high if the cancer occurred in the relative before menopause or involved both breasts or if it affected more than one first-degree relative (for example, a mother and sister or two sisters) or other close relatives in several generations.

Still, most cases of breast cancer cannot be explained because most women have at least one risk fac-tor. Other risk factors include early menarche (before age 12), late menopause (after age 55), recent use of oral contraceptives or postmenopausal estrogens; never having had children or having given birth to a first child late in life.[3,27] Understanding the role of lifestyle factors remains somewhat nebulous. Although breast cancer is worldwide, a strong cultural relationship exists between diet, especially high fat intake, and cancer. The reasons for this relationship have not been established.[3] Other factors that appear related to the incidence of breast cancer but that are unexplained at this time are alcohol intake (perhaps as few as three to five drinks a week); weight gain, particularly following menopause; and physical inactivity.[28]

Early detection is the best means of reducing mortality (see Just the Facts: Cancer-Related Checkup Guidelines). The five-year survival rate for localized cancers is 96 percent. Localized spread of the cancer lowers that survival rate to 76 percent, and distant metastasis yields only a 21 percent five-year survival rate.[3] Eighty percent of breast cancers are found by the affected women

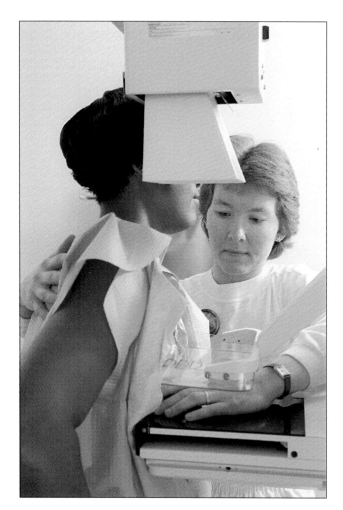

Mammography is important in the early detection of breast cancer.

Just the Facts

Drugs and Breast Cancer Treatment

The drug tamoxifen has received a great deal of coverage in the press about its use as an anticancer drug. As with all drugs, tamoxifen has side effects. These particular side effects can be deadly, and use of the drug should be carefully considered. Tamoxifen has also been used as a cancer preventive among women at high risk (which can include any woman over 60 years of age as well as younger women with several factors, including breast cancer in first-degree relatives). Other drugs that seem to reduce the rate of invasive breast cancer are raloxifene (a drug used to prevent bone loss); taxol, as a treatment in even late-stage cancer; and herceptin, which seems to delay progression of late-stage cancer.[29,30] Good news emerges almost daily about treatment for breast cancer. Early detection can result in a complete recovery.

Just the Facts

Cancer-Related Checkup Guidelines

Listed here are checkup guidelines to help healthy people with early cancer detection. These are guidelines and not rules. They apply only if none of the following seven warning signs is present:

C	hange in bowel or bladder habits
A	sore that does not heal
U	nusual bleeding or discharge
T	hickening or lump in breast or elsewhere
I	ndigestion or difficulty swallowing
O	bvious change in wart or moles
N	agging cough or hoarseness

Summary of American Cancer Society Recommendations for the Early Detection of Cancer in Asymptomatic People

Site	Recommendation
Cancer-related checkup	A cancer-related checkup is recommended every three years for people ages 20 to 40 and every year for people age 40 and older. This exam should include health counseling and, depending on a person's age, possibly examinations for cancers of the thyroid, oral cavity, skin, lymph nodes, testes, and ovaries as well as for some nonmalignant diseases.
Breast	Women 40 and older should have an annual mammogram and annual clinical breast exam (CBE) performed by a health care professional and should perform monthly breast self-examinations. The CBE should be conducted close to the scheduled mammogram. Women ages 20 to 39 should have a clinical breast exam performed by a health care professional every three years and should perform monthly breast self-examinations.
Colon and rectum	Men and women 50 or older should follow *one* of the following examination schedules: • A fecal occult blood test every year and a flexible sigmoidoscopy every five years • A colonoscopy every ten years • A double-contrast barium enema every five to ten years • A digital rectal exam at the same time as the sigmoidoscopy, colonoscopy, or double-contrast barium enema (people at moderate or high risk for colorectal cancer should talk with a doctor about a different testing schedule)
Prostate	The ACS recommends that both the prostate-specific antigen (PSA) blood test and the digital rectal examination be offered annually, beginning at age 50, to men who have a life expectancy of at least ten years and to younger men who are at high risk. Men in high-risk groups, such as those with strong familial predispositions (i.e., two or more affected first-degree relatives) or African Americans, may begin at a younger age (i.e., 45 years).
Uterus	**Cervix:** All women who are or have been sexually active or who are 18 and older should have an annual Pap test and pelvic examination. After three or more consecutive satisfactory examinations with normal findings, the Pap test may be performed less frequently. Discuss the matter with your physician. **Endometrium:** Women at high risk for cancer of the uterus should have a sample of endometrial tissue examined when menopause begins.

Source: ©1998, American Cancer Society, Inc.

through self-examination. Monthly self-examination remains the primary way to find small, localized cancers, especially in young women (see Just the Facts: Breast Self-Examination). Mammograms are useful tools but are more useful for detection in older women whose breast tissue is less dense. Even the best mammogram misses 10 percent of tumors, because breast tissue extends beyond the area X-rayed in a mammogram. Examinations by qualified physicians are helpful in detecting breast cancer, but most examinations occur only on an annual or biannual basis. The time lapse between such exams provides aggressive, fast-growing tumors with time to spread to surrounding tissue or lymph nodes.

Symptoms include a tumor that may feel like a piece of gravel or hard nodule. The tumor will not enlarge and shrink in size from month to month. Other symptoms include thickening, swelling, dimpling, scaling, pain, and tenderness of the nipple or discharge from the nipple. Breast cancer can occur at any age, even in very young women. Anyone (male or female) detecting these symptoms should consult a physician without delay.

Uterine cancer

Uterine cancers can occur either in the cervix (cervical cancer or cancer in the neck of the uterus) or in the endometrium (endometrial cancer or cancer of the lining of the uterus). Cervical cancer is closely linked to sexual behavior, especially through transmission of the human papillomavirus. Because of its close association with sexual activity (sex at an early age, multiple partners, a partner who has had multiple partners, multiple pregnancies, and a history of sexually transmitted diseases such as herpes and genital warts), many experts considered it a sexually transmitted disease. However, this is not the only reason people develop this cancer. As women have participated more frequently in annual Pap smears and preventive reproductive health, the number of deaths from cervical cancer has declined significantly (70 percent decrease).[3] Smoking seems to increase the risk of the disease. Prevention involves following safer sex practices (see Chapter 12), not smoking, and having regular Pap smears.

Symptoms include abnormal vaginal bleeding or spotting or discharge. Late symptoms include pain. When diagnosed early, invasive cervical cancer is one of the most treatable cancers, with a five-year survival rate of 91 percent. Regular Pap smears after either age 18 or after sexual activity if initiated (no matter how young) can detect early, abnormal cells or localized cancers. Women should have regular Pap smears for the rest of their lives.

The lining of the uterus is the endometrium. Endometrial cancers occur in the upper, more broad por-

tion of the uterus, as opposed to in the more narrow opening (the cervix). Endometrial cancer is more common among women over the age of 50, following menopause. Increasing evidence points to high levels of the hormone estrogen as contributing to the course of the disease. This is because estrogen causes the lining of the uterus to grow, which can lead to a premalignant condition that can lead to invasive cancer.

Risk factors include being overweight (extreme obesity), diabetes, high blood pressure, early menarche (before age 12), late menopause (after age 52), never giving birth, and receiving unopposed estrogen replacement therapy. The Pap smear detects endometrial cancer less than half the time. Those with risk factors should check with their gynecologists.[31]

Ovarian cancer

Ovarian cancer is difficult to diagnose, having few symptoms until reaching an advanced stage. Five to 10 percent of ovarian cancers are inherited, meaning that family history and mutations in the same genes that are related to breast cancer (*BRCA1* and *BRCA2*) serve as potential markers. Symptoms are frequently vague and may include cramping, discomfort, distention of the abdomen resulting from fluid buildup, diarrhea or constipation, gas, or a feeling of incomplete emptying of the bladder. Full-term pregnancies and breast-feeding as well as the use of oral contraceptives seem to reduce the risk. A high-fat diet seems to increase the risk. Fertility drugs that stimulate ovulation may be associated with increased risk.

Although considered a relatively rare cancer, late diagnosis can be deadly. If found in stage I, the cure rate is about 90 percent. The average age of women diagnosed with ovarian cancer is 61.[3,32]

Cancers That Can Affect Men

Testicular cancer

About 5000 men and boys, usually ages 15 to 34, are diagnosed with testicle cancer per year. These are usually treatable. Testicular cancer is painless and asymptomatic, but it is detectable by self-examination. Every boy old enough to be in high school and every man should do a monthly self-exam until reaching the age of 40 (see Just the Facts: Testicular Self-Examination). Signs of possible testicular cancer include any lump, enlargement, or hardening of either testis. Any changes should be followed up with an examination by a physician. Undetected, the disease can spread to the lymph nodes and beyond. Early detection results in a high cure rate.[33,36]

Breast Self-Examination

(a)

(b)

(c)

(d)

(e)

(f)

continued

Just the Facts

continued

Here are the proper techniques for examining the breasts.

1. Lying in bed, place a pillow under one shoulder to elevate and flatten the breast. Examine each breast using the opposite hand, first with your arm under your head and again with your arm at your side (a).
2. Make small circular motions with the flat pads (not the tips) of your fingers (b).
3. Examine your breasts in concentric circles from the rims inward toward the nipples. Feel for knots, lumps, thickenings, indentations, and swellings. Be sure to include the armpit (b).
4. Wet, soapy skin makes it easier to feel lumps. Keep one hand overhead and examine each breast with the opposite hand while you are in the shower (c).
5. In front of a large mirror, stand with your arms relaxed at your sides. Examine your breasts for swelling, dimpling, bulges, retractions, irritations, and sores or changes in mole or nipple color, texture, or orientation. Repeat with the arms extended and again with your arms clasped behind your head (d).
6. Repeat the inspection in step 5 while contracting your chest muscles: first clasp your hands in front of your forehead, squeezing your palms together, then place your palms flat on the sides of your hips, pressing downward. This highlights the bulges and indentations, which may signal the growth of tumors (e).
7. Bend forward from the hips, resting your hands on your knees or two chair backs. Use a mirror to examine your breasts for normal irregularities and abnormal variances; both are pronounced in this position.
8. Squeeze your nipples to inspect for secretions and discharge (f).
9. Report any suspicious findings to your doctor without delay.
10. Supplement your self-examination with a breast examination by your doctor as part of a regular physical examination and cancer checkup.

Just the Facts

Testicular Self-Examination

Cancer of the testes (the male reproductive glands) is one of the most common cancers in men 15 to 34 years of age. It accounts for 12 percent of cancer deaths in this group. The best hope for early detection of testicular cancer is a simple, 3-minute monthly self-examination. The best time is after a warm bath or shower when the scrotal skin is most relaxed.

Roll each testicle gently between the thumb and fingers of both hands. If you find any hard lumps or nodules, see your doctor promptly. The lumps or nodules may not be malignant, but only a doctor can make the diagnosis.

After a thorough physical examination, your doctor may perform X-ray studies for the most accurate diagnosis.

Prostate cancer

Most men who live long enough will have some evidence of prostate cancer. The second leading cause of cancer death among men, prostate cancer has a 100 percent cure rate when diagnosed while localized (58 percent of prostate cancers). Improvement in diagnosis has resulted from a blood test for prostate-specific antigen (PSA test). The PSA test, in combination with a digital (manual) rectal exam (DRE), has made prostate cancer much easier to detect at earlier stages.

Men at elevated risk include African Americans (who have incidence and death rates twice as high as those of white men), increasing age (PSAs and DREs should be annual events in men over age 50; prostate cancer is rare in young men), and men with family histories of prostate cancer. Dietary fat intake may also be a factor. African-American men and those with family histories should begin annual checkups at age 40.

Symptoms for prostate cancer tend to be nonspecific and similar to those of a condition known as *benign prostate hypertrophy.* They include weak or interrupted urine flow; inability to urinate; difficulty starting or stopping urine flow; a frequent need to urinate, especially at night; pain or burning on urination; and continuing pain in the lower back, pelvis, or upper thighs.

Treatment

The best treatment for cancer is prevention by leading a wellness lifestyle. Even with a family history, it is impossible to determine at this time who will get cancer. Taking appropriate lifestyle measures may make the difference. Eating a healthy diet high in fruit, vegetable, and grain products; exercising regularly; avoiding tobacco products and excessive alcohol consumption; performing self-exams accurately and regularly; and getting screenings as recommended can save lives. Screenings that result in accurate diagnoses are vital. When detected while still local, prostate and thyroid cancers are considered 100 percent "curable" (the patient is still living with no signs of cancer at five years). The cure rate for melanoma and ovarian cancer, when diagnosed early is 95 percent; breast cancer is 96 percent; and testicular cancer is 99 percent.[38]

Traditional cancer treatment has involved the use of surgery, radiation, chemotherapy, or some combination of these three. Today, these more traditional approaches are being combined with new, experimental approaches, such as gleevec. At the same time, traditional methods are being continuously refined, and every year, more experimental methods are being used. New treatments for cancer are being tested every day. The recent breakthrough of the drug gleevec has some people using the term "cure" for all cancers. Gleevec has performed miraculously thus far, but this drug was approved by the FDA in record time and five-year studies have not been achieved. While the new drugs are promising, cancer remains not one disease, but many diseases, and only time will tell the long-term effects of this and other cancer drugs.

Surgery

Cancers are often treated surgically. A surgeon removes the malignant tissue and some additional normal tissue. Current surgical techniques focus on removing less surrounding normal tissue than before and combining surgery with chemotherapy and/or radiotherapy. Surgery is used most often with breast, skin, gastrointestinal tract, female reproductive organ, prostate, and testicular cancers.

Chemotherapy

Chemotherapy is the use of drugs and hormones to treat cancers. Eight years ago, 124 drugs were being tested as potential anticancer agents. Today there are 402 or more.[8] Some of the most important advances in the treatment of cancer have been in the area of chemotherapy. Most chemotherapeutic agents work by destroying the cancer cells' ability to carry out cell division and replication. Unfortunately, chemotherapy influences all cell division, even in healthy cells that need to divide to function normally. As a result, people having chemotherapy often have side effects, some of which can be dangerous. These side effects include suppression of the immune system, diarrhea, and hair loss.

Newer drug therapies take a different approach. New types of drugs include antigrowth drugs that block the body's signals that promote cancer cell growth (called antigrowth drugs—gleevec falls into this category); drugs that cause the cancer cells to self-destruct; antiangiogenesis drugs that cut off the cancer cell's blood supply; and drugs that "coordinate" radiation dosages with monoclonal antibodies (molecules specifically engineered to fit into the receptacles on certain cells) that target specific cancer cells. These drugs have much fewer and less severe side effects than traditional chemotherapies.[8]

Radiotherapy

Radiotherapy is the use of radiation to destroy cancer cells or their reproductive mechanisms so that they cannot replicate. As a result of radiation, side effects such as diarrhea, itching, and difficulty swallowing can occur. However, as the ability to more carefully plan the preciseness of focus, length of exposure, and time of treatment has improved, the damage to noncancerous cells and the potential side effects have decreased.

Immunotherapy

Immunotherapy is the use of a variety of substances to trigger a person's immune response, which then attacks malignant cells or keeps them from becoming active. The substances being used in this therapy are manufactured through genetic engineering. Among these technologies are interferon, interleukin-2 (proteins produced by the body to protect against viral invasions of healthy cells), tumor necrosis factor (TNF), and bone marrow growth regulators. Interferon is used for treatment of a rare blood cancer called *hairy cell leukemia.* Interleukin-2 is under study in the treatment of kidney cancer and melanoma. Vaccines against several types of cancer are also being developed.

Complementary Therapies

New technologies enhance the diagnosis and treatment of cancer. Magnetic resonance imaging (MRI) and computerized tomography (CT scanning) help to detect and map hidden tumors. Bone marrow transplantation is now a treatment option for select patients with leukemia and lymphoma.

Other approaches that have been used or are under investigation as alternatives to conventional treatment or as methods to use in conjunction with traditional therapies are acupressure, acupuncture, herbs, vitamins (for prevention and free radical removal), biofeedback (monitoring body functions to control bodily functions), homeopathy (use of extremely small doses of toxic substances), reflexology (massaging of certain areas of the feet), therapeutic touch (redirecting the "life forces" of the body), and visualization (envisioning a cure happening) (see Just the Facts: How 1 + 1 = 3: The Power of Synergy). Some of these alternative methods have been proven to help in the treatment process. Others are still being investigated (see Nurturing Your Spirituality: Living Well with Cancer). Some may become part of more traditional treatments.

Today, more than ever, there is hope for anyone with cancer. Cancer trials are ongoing and new drugs are constantly being developed. Even the most deadly cancers have new treatments being tested. As more is learned about cancer, more will be done to stop its deadly attack on the human body.

How 1 + 1 = 3: The Power of Synergy

Although research shows that people who eat diets high in vegetables and fruits have lower risks of developing certain cancers than people who eat less healthy, high fat/high meat diets, these results have not been replicated when people take supplements. The beta carotene in a pill is not the same as the beta carotene in a carrot because the results are not equivalent. One theory uses the word "synergy" to explain the difference. When beta carotene or vitamin A or vitamin C are ingested in food sources, such as fruits and vegetables, more than the vitamin is affecting the body. The phytochemicals and vitamins interact in such a way that their effect is "synergized" or magnified so that greater results are achieved. Taking a pill is never a substitute for healthy food. Vitamins do not have the same ingredients in the same combinations as food, nor do they have the fiber! Don't try to take pills to make you more healthy. Eat healthy. It's as simple as five to nine fruits and vegetables every day![39]

Nurturing Your Spirituality

Living Well with Cancer

Chemotherapy and other drug treatments offer potentially life-saving solutions for cancer patients. But does the cure lie solely in the doctor's office? Perhaps not. Research indicates that spiritual practices may increase a cancer patient's chance of survival and enhance his or her quality of life.

Scientists have recently begun studying how the mind affects the neurological and immune systems.[35] This new discipline, known as *psychoneuroimmunology*, is of great interest to cancer researchers. For example, participation in support groups has been shown to increase the life expectancy of people with cancer. The results of a study reported by Johns Hopkins University are striking: "Women with breast cancer who took part in a support group lived an average of eighteen months longer (a doubling of the survival time following diagnosis) than those who did not participate. In addition, all the long-term survivors belonged to the therapy group."[34]

Although support groups do not improve physical health, they seem to provide a camaraderie that contributes to overall wellness. Belonging to groups such as prayer circles also plays a beneficial role in recovery. Support groups offer patients a sense of connectedness that promotes wellness. Conversely, social isolation—lack of a support network of friends and family—seems to increase the likelihood of death.[37] Although the extent of its influence is unknown, the nurturing of cancer patients' spiritual side as well as care for their physical health seems to help in the effort to maintain wellness.

Summary

- *Cancer* refers to a group of disorders characterized by uncontrolled disorderly cell growth.
- Cancer is the second leading cause of death, and one in four Americans will eventually develop one or more of the 100 different forms.
- There are two types of tumors or neoplasms. A malignant (cancerous) tumor can spread or metastasize (move from one location to another), while the second type of tumor, called *benign*, cannot.
- Cancer is caused by either external (chemicals, diet, radiation, viruses, pollutants), or internal (hormones, immune, inherited) factors.
- A carcinogen is anything that triggers the development of cancer.
- A gene that enables cancer to develop is called an *oncogene*.
- Exercise has been found to help prevent colon, breast, and prostate cancers.
- Lung cancer is the leading cause of cancer death in the United States and throughout the world.
- Lung cancer is almost 100 percent preventable if people never smoke.
- Passive smoke (smoke from other people's tobacco products) is dangerous to the nonsmoker by increasing risk of developing cancer.
- Colon and rectum cancer, when detected early, are very curable. Colon cancer is associated with family history, constipation, and high calorie consumption. Diet is believed to be the primary cause.
- Stomach cancer is relatively uncommon in the United States, although it is still ranked among the top ten cancer killers. It is best prevented by a healthy diet.
- Liver and pancreatic cancers are relatively uncommon. Both are difficult to treat. The five-year survival rate for pancreatic cancer is only 4 percent.
- Leukemia is cancer of the blood-forming mechanisms, involving the white blood cells. It strikes both children and adults.
- Lymphoma is cancer of the lymphoid tissue. The two types of lymphoma are Hodgkin's disease and non–Hodgkin's lymphoma. Non–Hodgkin's includes all lymphomas except Hodgkin's.
- The three types of skin cancer are basal cell, squamous cell, and melanoma. Basal and squamous cell cancers are most treatable. Melanoma, although most deadly, is treatable if detected early. Exposure to the sun's ultraviolet light is most responsible for causing the three types of skin cancer.

- The ABCDs of skin cancer are helpful in identifying melanoma: A = Asymmetry; B = Borders uneven; C = Color (different shades of brown or black); D = Diameter greater than 6 mm.
- Oral cancer affects the lip, tongue, mouth, and throat. Risk factors are cigar and pipe smoking and the use of smokeless tobacco.
- Statistics show that one in nine women who live to age 85 will develop breast cancer.
- A woman with a mother or sister with breast cancer has double the risk for breast cancer. Early detection is the best means of reducing mortality.
- Breast self-examination and mammograms are useful tools for preventing breast cancer.
- Uterine cancers can occur either in the cervix or in the endometrium. Cervical cancer is closely associated with sexual behavior, especially through transmission of the human papillomavirus. Smoking seems to increase the risk.
- Risk factors for uterine cancers include obesity, diabetes, high blood pressure, early menarche, late menopause, never giving birth, and unopposed estrogen replacement therapy.
- Ovarian cancer is difficult to detect. Its symptoms are frequently vague and may include cramping, discomfort, distention of the abdomen, diarrhea or constipation, gas, and the feeling of incomplete emptying of the bladder.
- Testicular cancer is painless and asymptomatic but is detectable by self-examination. Early detection results in a high cure rate.
- Prostate cancer is the second leading cause of cancer death among men. The PSA and a digital rectal exam have made prostate cancer much easier to detect at earlier stages. These should be done annually after age 50. Symptoms include weak urine flow, inability to urinate, frequent need to urinate, painful or burning urination, and continuing pain in the lower back or upper thighs.
- Cancer is treated through the use of surgery, chemotherapy, radiotherapy, and immunotherapy.
- Bone marrow transplantation is now a treatment option for select patients with leukemia and lymphoma.
- Several complementary therapies are under investigation as treatment alternatives to conventional approaches or to be used in conjunction with conventional approaches. These include acupressure, acupuncture, vitamins, biofeedback, homeopathy, reflexology, therapeutic touch, and visualization.

Review Questions

1. Describe the process by which cancer cells develop.
2. What characteristics differentiate cancer cells from other cells?
3. Discuss lifestyle factors that may contribute to the development of cancer.
4. What factors other than lifestyle factors contribute to the development of cancer?

5. Explain the concept of oncogenes.
6. What role does exercise play in the prevention of colon, breast, and prostate cancers? What mechanisms seem to be aiding in the prevention of these cancers?
7. Differentiate between the three types of skin cancer.

8. What are the leading sites of cancer in females? males?
9. Describe the conventional methods of treating cancer.

10. What are some unconventional approaches to cancer treatment and adjunct therapies?

References

1. American Cancer Society. *Statistics 2000*. Available online at wysiwg:// 25/http://www3.cancer.org/can.
2. Fravenkneckt, M. 1995. Cancer prevalence and prevention: Demonstrating the role of personal responsibility. *Journal of Health Education* 26:240.
3. Margolis, S., and J. M. Samet. 1998. *The Johns Hopkins White Papers: Early Detection and Prevention of Cancer*. Baltimore, Md.: The Johns Hopkins Medical Institutions.
4. Hellmich, N. October 1, 1997. Fighting cancer: Diet and exercise. *USA Today* D-1,2.
5. American Institute for Cancer Research. 2001. JAMA findings on diet and breast cancer misunderstood, experts say. *AICR Science News* 20:1–2.
6. American Cancer Society. 2001. Leaflet. *Jesse Harris Cancer Answer Week leaflet*.
7. Lee, I., and R. Paffenbarger. 1994. Physical activity and its relation to cancer risk: A prospective study of college alumni. *Medicine and Science in Sport and Exercise* 26:831.
8. *Atlas of Cancer Mortality*. 2001. Available online at www.dceg.cancer. gov/atlas/text2/full]txt.html.
9. Nieman, D. 1999. *Exercise Testing and Prescription—a Health-Related Approach* (4th ed.). Mountain View, Calif.: Mayfield Publishing Co.
10. Bernstein, L., et al. 1994. Physical activity and the risk of breast cancer in young women. *Journal of the National Cancer Institute* 86: 11403.
11. Thune, I., T. Brenn, E. Lund, and M. Gaard. 1997. Physical activity and the risk of breast cancer. *New England Journal of Medicine* 336: 1269.
12. American Institute for Cancer Research. 2001. Red meat and non–Hodgkin's lymphoma. *Newsletter* (Winter) 80:5.
13. Lee, I., R. Paffenbarger, and C. Hsieh. 1992. Physical activity and risk of prostatic cancer among college alumni. *Journal of Epidemiology* 135:169.
14. Oliveria, S., H. Kohl, D. Trichopoulos, and S. Blair. 1996. The association between cardiorespiratory fitness and prostate cancer. *Medicine and Science in Sports and Exercise* 28:97.
15. Hackney, A. 1996. The male reproductive system and endurance exercise. *Medicine and Science in Sports and Exercise* 28:180.
16. World Cancer Research Fund/ American Institute for Cancer Research. 1997. *Food, Nutrition and the Prevention of Cancer: A Global Perspective*. Washington, D.C.: American Institute for Cancer Research.
17. Consumer Reports on Health. 1998. Fruits and vegetables: Nature's best protection. *Consumer Reports* 10(6):1.
18. Potter, J. D. 1998. Diet and cancer: The big picture. *Nutrition Action Health Letter* 25:10.
19. University of California at Berkeley. 1998. Six tests for colon cancer. *University of California at Berkeley Wellness Letter* 15(2):2.
20. Editors. July 25, 1998. Risks for colon cancer. *Health News* 7.
21. Leibman, B. 1998. Vitamins and colon cancer. *Nutrition Action Health Letter* 25(10):8.
22. Mayo Clinic. 1995. Update—aspirin's effect on colon cancer boosts image as wonder drug. *Mayo Clinic Health Letter* 13(12):4.
23. Editors. November 10, 1998. Hidden cases of hepatitis C damaging livers in millions. *USA Today* A-1.
24. Anderson, K. N., and L. E. Anderson. 1990. *Mosby's Pocket Dictionary of Medicine, Nursing, and Allied Health*. St. Louis: Mosby.
25. University of California at Berkeley. 1998. Casting a shadow on sunscreens. *University of California at Berkeley Wellness Letter* 14(9):2.
26. Editors. 1997. Health news: Evaluating melanoma risk. *The New England Journal of Medicine* 3(8):1–2.
27. Harvard University. 1997. Advances in breast cancer research. *Harvard Women's Health Watch* 5(11):2–3.
28. University of California at Berkeley. 1997. The best advice about breast cancer and exercise. *University of California at Berkeley Wellness Letter* 13(11):1.
29. Harvard University. 1998. Tamoxifen and beyond. *Harvard Women's Health Watch* 5(10):1.
30. Harvard University. 1998. Advances in breast cancer research. *Harvard Women's Health Watch* 5(11):1.
31. Mayo Clinic. 1985. When found and treated early, this form of uterus cancer usually can be cured. *Mayo Clinic Health Letter* 3(11):1.
32. Harvard University. 1998. Ovarian cancer. *Harvard Women's Health Watch* 6(2):4–5.
33. Mayo Clinic. 1985. This painless self-exam can help reveal testis cancer early, when treatment is most effective. *Mayo Clinic Health Letter* 3(11):8.
34. Johns Hopkins University. 1999. *Overview of NIH Office of Alternative Medicine Fields of Practice: Mind/Body Control*. Available online at www.intelihealth.com.
35. Mayo Health Clinic. 1999. *Mind Over Malignancy? Attitude and Cancer Survival*. Available online at www.mayohealth.org/mayo9703/ htm/mindover.htm.
36. Pitre, H. *Prostate Cancer Update: An Interview with Dr. Alan Koletsk*. Patient Resource Center. Available online at www.salick.com/ resource/features/prostate_ update. html.
37. National Cancer Institute. *Cancer 2000 Facts and Figures Graphical Data*. Available online at www. cancer.org/statistics/cff2000/ data/survivalByStage.html.
38. Lemonick, M., and Park, A. 2001. New hope for cancer. *Time* 28:62–69.
39. American Institute for Cancer Research. 2001. The anti-cancer power of synergy. *Newsletter* (Summer) 72:1–3.

Suggested Readings

Anderson, G. 1990. *The Cancer Conqueror: An Incredible Journey to Wellness*. Kansas City, Mo.: Andrews & McMeel.

This book, which describes how a positive attitude affects cancer and may even help contribute to its cure, provides an encouraging message for people with cancer and their families.

Anderson, G. 1993. *50 Essential Things to Do When the Doctor Says It's Cancer*. Bergenfield, N.J.: Plume.

A cancer survivor offers readers fifty proactive steps to take when faced with a diagnosis of cancer.

Sinclair, G. 1997. *All Things Work for Good: A Book of Encouragement for People with Cancer, Their Family and Friends*. Sharon, Mass.: The Positive Press.

A survivor writes about the many spiritual, mental, and physical questions a diagnosis of cancer can elicit. The author writes candidly, humorously, and with clarity about his personal struggle.

Name _____ **Date** _____ **Section** _____

Assessment Activity 13-1

Cancer Early Detection Inventory

This inventory was developed to help in the early detection and treatment of cancer. It presents common symptoms for various cancer sites. If you have symptoms, check with your physician. The chances are that you will not have cancer, but any symptoms suggest a potential problem with your health—it is wise to be safe and consult your physician.

Directions: For each cancer site, check any of the symptoms you experience.

Bladder
1. Blood in urine? _____
2. Unusual change in bladder habits? _____
3. Discomfort during urination? _____
4. Change in flow during urination? _____
5. Urge to urinate more frequently? _____

Bone
1. Pain in the bone or joint? _____
2. Swelling in the bone or joint? _____
3. Unusual warmth in the bone or joint? _____
4. Protruding veins along the bone or joint? _____

Breast
1. Thickening or lump in the breast? _____
2. Lump under the arm? _____
3. Thickening or reddening of the skin of the breast? _____
4. Puckering or dimpling of the skin of the breast? _____
5. Nipple discharge? _____
6. Inverted nipple, if nipple was previously erect? _____
7. Persistent pain and tenderness of the breast? _____
8. Unusual changes in the nipple and surrounding skin? _____
9. Benign breast lumps? _____

Colon and Rectum
1. Continuous constipation or diarrhea? _____
2. Rectal bleeding? _____
3. Change in bowel habits? _____
4. Increase in intestinal gas? _____
5. Abdominal discomfort? _____

Lung
1. Unusual cough? _____
2. Shortness of breath? _____
3. Sputum streaked with blood? _____
4. Chest pain? _____
5. Recurring attacks of pneumonia or bronchitis? _____

Lymphatic System
1. Painless enlargement of a lymph node or cluster of lymph nodes? _____
2. Profuse sweating and fever? _____
3. Weight loss? _____
4. Unexplained weakness? _____
5. Unusual itching? _____

Oral
1. Sore in the mouth that does not heal? _____
2. Lump or thickening that bleeds easily? _____
3. Difficulty in chewing or swallowing food? _____
4. Sensation of something in the throat? _____
5. Restricted movement of the tongue or jaw? _____
6. Poor oral hygiene? _____

Prostate
1. Weak or interrupted flow of urine? _____
2. Inability to urinate or difficulty in starting urination? _____
3. Need to urinate frequently, especially at night?

4. Blood in urine?   _____

5. Urine flow that is not easily stopped?   _____

6. Painful or burning urination?   _____

7. Continuing pain in lower back, pelvis, or upper thighs?   _____

Skin

1. Obvious change in wart or mole?   _____

2. Unusual skin condition?   _____

3. Chronic swelling, redness, or warmth of the skin?   _____

4. Unexplained itching?   _____

5. Overexposure to the ultraviolet rays of the sun?   _____

Testes

1. Enlargement and change in the consistency of the testes?   _____

2. Dull ache in the lower abdomen and groin?   _____

3. Sensation of dragging and heaviness?   _____

4. Difficulty with ejaculation?   _____

Thyroid

1. Lump or mass in the neck?   _____

2. Persistent hoarseness?   _____

3. Difficulty in swallowing?   _____

4. Overexposure to head and neck X-ray treatments?   _____

Uterus and Cervix

1. Irregular bleeding?   _____

2. Unusual vaginal discharge?   _____

3. Positive Pap smear, class 2 to 5, some signs of abnormality?   _____

4. Recurring herpes simplex virus?   _____

5. Fibroid tumors of the uterus?   _____

Application: Carefully evaluate any statement you have checked. If the symptom appears severe (such as blood in the stool), see a physician immediately. However, nonsevere symptoms (such as pain in a joint) may be observed for a short period to see if there is improvement. Never wait longer than two weeks to see a physician if the symptom persists.

1. How many symptoms have you checked? _____

2. How serious do these symptoms seem? _____

_____

3. Should you see a physician now or wait? _____

_____

Name _____ Date _____ Section _____

Assessment Activity 13-2

Are You Practicing Cancer Prevention?

Listed here are several common cancers and the significant risk factors for each. As you look at each risk factor, determine whether you should increase or decrease that factor. If the factor does not apply to you or your lifestyle, leave the I/D column blank.

Cancer	Smoking		Fruits and Vegetable Consumption		Exercise		High Fat Percentage		Smokeless Tobacco Use		Meat Consumption		Obesity		High Alcohol Consumption	
	RF	I/D	RF	I/D	RF	I/D	RF	I/D	RF	I/D	RF	I/D	RF	I/D	RF	I/D
Lung	+		+													
Colon and rectum			+		✓		✓				?		?			
Breast			?		✓		?						✓		✓	
Prostate			?								?		✓			
Stomach	✓		✓													
Kidney	+												✓			
Esophagus	+		✓						+						✓	
Oral	+		✓						+						✓	
Larynx	+		✓						+						✓	

RF = Risk factor

I/D = Increase or decrease?

+ = Solid body of evidence suggests a link between this lifestyle factor and cancer.

✓ = Many studies suggest a plausible link between this lifestyle factor and cancer.

? = Some research suggests a connection; the jury is still out.

Follow-up Questions
1. Are you following a more positive lifestyle for the prevention of cancer?
2. How many lifestyle factors do you need to increase? decrease?
3. What would you say are your main strengths in the effort to prevent cancer?
4. What are your greatest risk factors for cancer?

14

Managing Common Conditions

Online Learning Center

Log on to our Online Learning Center (OLC) for access to these additional resources:

- Chapter key term flashcards
- Learning objectives
- Additional goals for behavior change
- Concentration game
- Self-scoring chapter quizzes

- Additional lab activities

The OLC also offers weblinks for study and exploration of wellness topics. Access these links through **www.mhhe.com/anspaugh5e**, click on "Student Center," click on "Chapter 14," and then click on "Web Activities."

Goals for Behavior Change

- Identify your personal risk factors for the conditions discussed in this chapter.
- Select strategies for prevention of these conditions.
- Initiate a prevention plan for any of the conditions identified as a potential personal risk.

Key Terms

allergens
arthritis
asthma
Crohn's disease
diabetes mellitus
headaches
inflammatory bowel
  disease (IBD)

influenza
osteoarthritis
osteoporosis
rheumatoid arthritis
ulcerative colitis

Objectives

After completing this chapter, you will be able to do the following:

- Differentiate between type 1 and type 2 diabetes mellitus.
- Identify the common forms of arthritis.
- Describe the effects of calcium hormone therapy and exercise on osteoporosis.
- Discuss preventive measures and treatments that help reduce the severity and length of asthma attacks.

- Differentiate between the common cold and influenza.
- Distinguish between the different types of headache.
- Identify environmental factors that may trigger headaches.

his chapter focuses on conditions that are detrimentally affected by lifestyle. If precautions are taken against the onset of these diseases, their impact on the body may be lessened or even avoided. Although every condition affected by lifestyle cannot be described, those that frequently occur and those on which lifestyle has the greatest impact are discussed, including diabetes, arthritis, osteoporosis, asthma, influenza, headaches, and the common cold.

Diabetes Mellitus

Diabetes mellitus is a group of diseases resulting from one of the following situations: The body does not make insulin, the body doesn't make enough insulin, or the body doesn't use insulin properly.[1] Diabetes is a metabolic disorder involving the pancreas. People with diabetes experience an abnormality in the way their bodies use glucose (blood sugar); this results from the deficient production of insulin by the pancreas or from resistance of the body's tissues to the action of insulin.[2] The blood may contain ample glucose (blood sugar), but without enough insulin available for use, the glucose cannot move from the bloodstream into the cells, where it is needed for fuel. As a result, people with diabetes cannot use the energy they consume, and high glucose levels build up in the blood and urine, leading to a condition known as *hyperglycemia* (high blood sugar). Large amounts of sugar in urine require additional water so that the sugar can be diluted for elimination. The increased need by the body for water leads to a depletion of the body's water stores, causing excessive thirst and frequent urination. When the body becomes unable to completely break down glucose as a source of energy, fat must be used. Fat is metabolized differently than glucose, and its breakdown is incomplete when glucose is not available. Incomplete metabolism causes an excess amount of chemicals called *ketone bodies* to build up in the body. The buildup of ketones is used to perform the functions that glucose would perform under normal conditions (supplying energy), but the excess amounts of ketone bodies disrupt the body's chemical balance, altering the blood's chemistry and making it more acidic. Acidic conditions in the body are extremely hazardous.

Diabetes can be a serious disorder. Symptoms include excessive thirst; increased urination; hunger; a tendency to tire easily; wounds that heal slowly; blurred vision; and frequent skin, vaginal, and urinary tract infections. Dehydration and buildup of ketones can cause ketoacidosis (the accumulation of ketones)

and nausea, vomiting, abdominal pain, lethargy, and drowsiness. Ketoacidosis often leads to severe sickness, coma, and even death. Of equal significance is that prolonged periods of elevated glucose levels disrupt normal enzyme and membrane functions. Chronic complications that may result are eye disease, kidney disorders, painful nerve and muscle symptoms, and decreased circulation. Diabetes is a leading cause of foot and leg amputations. Diabetes can also produce impotence in men and increased risk of heart disease and heart attacks in both genders. Of the 16 million people with diabetes in the United States, nearly one-half are unaware they have it (see Assessment Activity 14-1). By the time people realize they have this condition, they may have already suffered severe consequences.[1]

Type 1 Diabetes

Diabetes consists of two diagnostic categories. *Type 1 diabetes* occurs most commonly in children and young adults, although it may develop at any age. Type 1 is an autoimmune disease in which the body produces antibodies that attack and damage its own cells, in this case the insulin-producing cells of the pancreas.[2] Symptoms may be sudden and sometimes progress rapidly, requiring quick intervention to prevent death. People with type 1 diabetes produce little or no insulin and require insulin injections to function. Before insulin was discovered, the average life span for a person with type 1 diabetes was two years after diagnosis. Properly treated, these people now live almost as long as the general population.

Type 2 Diabetes

Type 2 diabetes is the most common type and is found primarily in people over the age of 40 (see Just the Facts: Type 2 Diabetes in Youth). Scientists believe that it is strongly linked to genetic factors. If an identical twin develops type 2 diabetes, the other most likely will as well. People with type 2 either develop a resistance to insulin activity or experience insufficient insulin action. Their bodies are usually capable of producing adequate amounts of insulin—something a person with type 1 diabetes cannot do. The difficulty in type 2 diabetes is that body cells become resistant to insulin at the receptor sites (the place where insulin attaches to the cell). Type 2 is linked strongly to obesity. Almost 80 percent of diabetics with type 2 are overweight at the time of diagnosis.[2] Often the only treatment necessary for type 2 is weight loss, although some people still require medication or injections of insulin to help control the condition.

Type 2 Diabetes in Youth

A growing number of children and adolescents are developing type 2 diabetes. Typically, type 2 diabetes occurs in youngsters who are overweight, older than ten years of age, in middle to late puberty, and have a family history of type 2 diabetes. Researchers expect that as the American population becomes even more overweight, the frequency of type 2 diabetes will increase in younger, prepubescent children. Since the development of type 2 diabetes in children and adolescents is relatively new, accurate statistics regarding the number of type 2 cases have not been reported, but it is estimated that between 8 and 45 percent of children with newly diagnosed cases of diabetes will have type 2 diabetes.[24]

Causes

Type 1 diabetes is an autoimmune disease. This means the body's immune system attacks a part of the body that is well. In type 1 diabetes, the body produces antibodies that attack and damage the area of the pancreas that produces insulin. Initially, the ability to produce insulin is impaired, but eventually, usually in less than a year, little or no insulin is produced. The onset is usually before age 35 and often in childhood. Type 1 diabetes is sometimes associated with a viral infection within the insulin-producing cells, resulting in the inability to produce insulin.[1]

Heredity plays a role in type 2 diabetes. In a study of 218 people with type 2 diabetes, 66 percent reported at least one relative with diabetes, and 46 percent reported at least two relatives with diabetes. Patients whose mothers had diabetes were twice as likely to develop the disease than were those whose fathers had diabetes.[1]

Obesity also is an important factor (see Just the Facts: Preventing and Controlling the Effects of Diabetes). Not all people who are obese develop diabetes, but 90 percent of people with diabetes are overweight. Tumors of certain endocrine organs such as the pituitary gland, adrenal glands, and pancreas can all interfere with or destroy insulin production. Taking corticosteroids, used to treat asthma or arthritis, may result in latent diabetes.[1]

Treatment

Although there is no cure for diabetes, the disease can be controlled by diet, exercise, and/or insulin. People with type 1 have to have insulin injections, usually several a day, and they must manipulate dosage levels according to dietary and activity levels (see Just the Facts: American Diabetes Association Guidelines for Diabetes Screening). Self-administered blood glucose tests help them monitor blood sugar levels and determine the appropriate insulin dose. Good blood sugar control reduces the risk of the complications associated with type 1 diabetes.

People with type 2 diabetes can often control the disease through weight loss, exercise, and adequate nutrition. Losing weight helps to lower insulin resistance, enabling the body to make more efficient use of the insulin available. New nutrition guidelines developed by the American Diabetes Association (ADA) dispel the notion of a diabetic diet that is good for everyone with the disease. For example, the previous emphasis on sugar consumption has given way to an emphasis on carbohydrate consumption.[3] The total amount of carbohydrate, regardless of its source, is what affects blood sugar levels.[4] Another example is that diabetics are now encouraged to consume monounsaturated fats. Type 2 studies at four different medical centers showed better control of blood glucose levels when 45 percent of the calories came from fat, with highly monounsaturated olive oil as the predominant fat, and 40 percent from carbohydrate than when 55 percent came from carbohydrate and 30 percent came from fat.[5]

Evidence that links exercise to a decreased incidence of type 2 diabetes is increasing. A study of 5990 men showed that incidence rates declined as energy expenditure increased. For each 500-calorie increment in physical activity, the risk of type 2 diabetes decreased by 6 percent. Men who increased their energy expenditure

Preventing and Controlling the Effects of Diabetes

Several lifestyle behaviors can significantly reduce the likelihood of developing type 2 diabetes:

- Maintaining normal weight
- Exercising regularly
- Not smoking
- Maintaining blood pressure levels or treating high blood pressure
- Maintaining normal blood lipid levels
- Eating a low-fat, high-fiber diet

Just the Facts

American Diabetes Association Guidelines for Diabetes Screening

Here are the cutoff points for diagnosis. They are based on fasting glucose levels:

- Blood glucose levels of 126 mg/dl or higher, in at least two tests done on separate days, indicate diabetes.

- Blood glucose levels between 110 mg/dl and 125 mg/dl indicate impaired fasting glucose.

- Normal blood glucose levels should be less than 110 mg/dl.

The ADA offers the following guidelines for testing frequency:

- People 45 years and older should be tested every three years if their results fall within the normal range.

- More frequent testing, beginning at a younger age, should be considered for people with the following factors:

    Obesity

    First-degree relative with diabetes

    Membership in a high-risk ethnic group, including African Americans, Hispanics, and Native Americans

    Having delivered a baby weighing more than 9 pounds or having developed diabetes when pregnant (gestational diabetes)

    Hypertension

    Low level of HDL cholesterol (35 mg/dl or lower) or triglyceride level more than 250 mg/dl

    Impaired glucose tolerance detected by a previous test

- Testing should be done immediately if the classic symptoms of diabetes are observed: abnormal thirst, frequent urination, and unexplained weight loss.

Wellness Across the Generations

Are Illness and Chronic Disease Inevitable as We Age?

As the population of the United States continues to age, chronic conditions are becoming increasingly common. The largest group of maturing adults, known as *baby boomers,* were born after World War II between 1946 and 1964. Are they doomed to develop age-related conditions? Will you or someone close to you inevitably have to face a chronic condition or disease associated with aging?

The answer for all age groups is a resounding "NO." We may have genetic predispositions of which we should be aware; however, we can embrace the concepts of wellness, including maintaining an active lifestyle, eating properly, not smoking, and controlling stress. By doing so, we may be able to delay the onset of many chronic conditions, diminish their severity, or prevent the factors that cause them. The earlier we begin to practice positive behaviors, the greater the likelihood of healthy outcomes.

All people can make health-related choices that enhance their well-being and that of their families and communities. It is imperative that we accept responsibility for improving our lives. Regardless of age, we are empowered through our attitudes and actions to create a high quality of life. Wellness is a journey, not a destination, filled with opportunities for joy, happiness, learning, and making the most of each day.

---

by 2000 calories decreased their risk by 24 percent.[4,6] In a study of more than 21,000 male physicians, men who exercised just once a week had 23 percent less chance of developing type 2 diabetes than did men who did not exercise.

Exercise lowers blood sugar levels by reducing the body's resistance to insulin. Cells become more sensitive to insulin and more capable of absorbing glucose. The effect is lower levels of circulating blood sugar. This benefit of exercise, however, lasts for only twenty-four hours, which means exercise must be done every

day. Regular activity doesn't seem to have the same dramatic effect on type 1 diabetes, but it does lower the amount of insulin needed and the risk of cardiovascular disease.[1]

Many of the complications associated with diabetes are preventable or treatable, but diagnosis and proper treatment are necessary (see Wellness Across the Generations: Are Illness and Chronic Disease Inevitable as We Age?). Neglect of diabetes and its complications may result in early death (see Just the Facts: Major Complications of Diabetes).

Just the Facts

Major Complications of Diabetes

Several serious complications can result from diabetes. Most of the following complications are caused by blood vessel damage:

- *Coronary heart disease (CHD):* People with diabetes have two to four times more risk of dying from CHD than do people without diabetes.
- *Nerve damage:* Between 60 and 70 percent of people with diabetes have some form of nerve damage.
- *Foot problems:* Because of peripheral nerve damage, foot problems can go unnoticed. Proper treatment for conditions such as athlete's foot, blisters, and calluses is extremely important. Any sign of infection should be treated immediately to avert the need for amputation.
- *Kidney damage:* Thirty to 40 percent of people with type 1 diabetes and 20 percent of those with type 2

diabetes eventually develop kidney disease, which can lead to kidney failure.

- *Peripheral vascular disease (PVD):* Diabetes and smoking can double or triple the risk of PVD (atherosclerosis) in the arteries of the legs, which increases the risk of foot and leg problems, including the possibility of amputation.
- *Skin problems:* People with diabetes are at increased risk for skin infections.
- *Stroke:* People with diabetes have a two to four times greater risk of stroke.
- *Vision loss:* Diabetic retinopathy (retina disease) is the leading cause of blindness. People with diabetes are also at increased risk for glaucoma and cataracts.

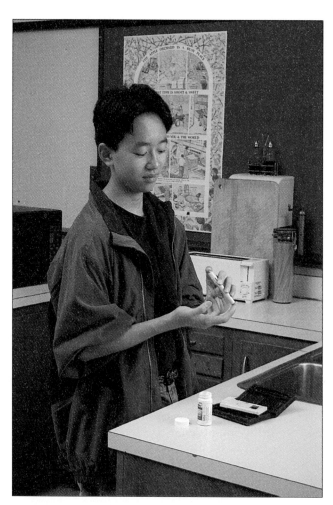

To successfully manage their condition, people with type 1 diabetes must periodically test their blood glucose level.

Arthritis

Arthritis is an inflammatory disease of the joints. The more than 100 varieties of arthritis include gout, ankylosing spondylitis, systemic lupus erythematosis, osteoarthritis, and rheumatoid arthritis. Osteoarthritis and rheumatoid arthritis are found most often. Both result in pain and deformed joints.

Osteoarthritis, also known as *degenerative joint disease,* is the most common form of arthritis, affecting more than 20 million Americans. By age 40, about 90 percent of people have X-ray evidence of osteoarthritis in the weight-bearing joints, such as the hips and knees, although symptoms generally do not appear until later in life.[7] Men typically develop symptoms before age 45, whereas women usually have them after age 55. Men more often have osteoarthritis in the hips, knees, and spine, and women are more likely to have it in the hands and knees.[7] It is the most limiting chronic condition affecting women in the United States.[7]

Osteoarthritis is characterized by the gradual breakdown of cartilage, which comes with age. The first signs are microscopic pits and fissures on the cartilage surface that cause the cartilage to crack and lose its resilience.[8] Tiny pieces of cartilage may break off into the joint cavity. The result is a change in the contours of the articular surfaces. Finally, patches of exposed bone appear, causing mechanical-type friction and irritation. The bone responds by trying to repair itself, but the repair is disorderly. As a result, joint surfaces thicken and bone spurs (osteophytes) form.

The deterioration associated with osteoarthritis seems related to the wear and tear of daily living, age,

Wellness On the Web Behavior Change Activities

Breathing Easier: Getting the Facts on Asthma

If you're an asthma sufferer or have ever been with someone who's had an asthma attack, you know how hard it is to catch your breath and fill your lungs when your airway is closing. Asthma is a chronic respiratory condition characterized by attacks of wheezing and difficulty in breathing. The cause of asthma attacks is partial obstruction of bronchi and bronchioles resulting from the contraction or spasm of the muscles in the bronchial walls. Attacks may be mild or severe and may last anywhere from a few minutes to a few days. Asthma is a condition surrounded by myths, such as that it's psychosomatic or that it affects children with certain personality traits. See how your knowledge stacks up against the facts. Go to www.mhhe.com/anspaugh5e, "Student Center," "Chapter 14," "Wellness on the Web," "Activity 1," and answer each statement true or false. How many statements were you able to answer correctly?

and injury. Other factors may include heredity, diet, abnormal use of joints (for example, throwing a curve ball every day year after year), excessive weight, stress, and impaired blood supply to affected joints.

Treatment for osteoarthritis includes aspirin and cortisone drugs to relieve pain. Mild exercise, heat, cold, or a combination of heat and cold application accompanied by massage can be used. Exercise is used for therapeutic purposes to help maintain range of motion and to strengthen the muscles that can help alleviate joint problems. Exercise is usually prescribed by a physical therapist. Occasionally, surgery is performed to replace joints or repair tendons and ligaments.

Should a person with osteoarthritis exercise to avoid deconditioning, or will the exercise cause further damage to the arthritic joints? The answer seems to be "yes" and "no" to both questions, depending on the person. An eight-week walking study[9] involving patients with osteoarthritis of the knee (one of the most common arthritic problems) provides a reason for optimism regarding exercise. Patients who walked thirty minutes three times a week reported a 27 percent decrease in pain and an improved ability to walk longer distances compared with a nonwalking control group. The researchers concluded that supervised walking can be helpful for people with significant arthritis of the knee. Stretching exercises also help to relieve arthritis pain by lengthening tendons, which reduces muscle spasms, the source of much of the pain in osteoarthritis. However, the results of other studies have shown

that exercise may not contribute to relief of pain. In addition, exercise of an arthritic joint may cause pain that can be relieved only by rest.

Rheumatoid arthritis is one of the most crippling forms of arthritis. It affects about 1 percent of the adult population worldwide. More than 2.5 million Americans have this condition, and more than 60 percent of those affected are women.[10] Onset of rheumatoid arthritis is usually between the ages of 20 and 45. Although the exact causes are unknown, this form of arthritis may be an autoimmune disease. The most obvious damage occurs in joints, but the disease affects the whole body. Symptoms of rheumatoid arthritis include joint swelling, redness, stiffness, pain, muscle atrophy, joint deformity, and limited mobility. The condition is unpredictable because it can suddenly flare up and just as suddenly go into remission. Emotional stress is often associated with an attack. The disease frequently results in disability.

Treatment includes a mixture of rest periods, gentle exercise, physical therapy, and medication. Emphasis is on relieving pain, reducing inflammation, maintaining function of the joints, and preventing deformities (see Nurturing your Spirituality: Living Well with a Chronic Condition).

Osteoporosis

Osteoporosis is a chronic disease in which the mineral content of the bones progressively decreases so that the bones become brittle and are easily broken. It is linked to more than 1 million fractures of the hip, spine, and other bones each year. Vertebral bones in the spine shrink and fracture, causing a deformed spine. Bones in the wrist are also common fracture sites. Some 25 million Americans, 80 percent of whom are postmenopausal women,[11] are affected by osteoporosis. Although postmenopausal white and Asian women are at highest risk, men and women of all ages and ethnicities can be affected.[12]

Though bones may seem hard, they are made of living cells that require calcium and vitamin D (necessary for optimum absorption of calcium) to grow and stay strong. Almost all of the body's calcium stores are located in bone.[12] During growth and development, bones typically receive more calcium than they give up. By age 25, when bone density peaks, calcium absorption levels off; at age 30, the bone-building process is over. This is when bone-mass maintenance and calcium are especially important.[13] If blood levels of calcium drop, the body withdraws what it needs from its bones. With adequate dietary intake of calcium, bones are spared the effects of calcium depletion that may accelerate osteoporosis.

Calcium is not the only factor associated with bone loss. Estrogen depletion during menopause triggers

Nurturing Your Spirituality

Living Well with a Chronic Condition

Many people have potentially debilitating or even life-threatening conditions, such as asthma, diabetes, and high blood pressure. Proper management of these conditions makes it possible for these people to live long lives. A person with a chronic condition may even have a quality of life as high as that of someone who does not have a chronic condition. If you have a chronic disease, you can learn to manage it effectively.

First, you need to know as much as you can about your condition. Knowledge is power. The more you know, the better you will be able to understand the condition and its treatment. More important, great strides are being made every day in the treatment of many diseases, and a cure may be possible in your lifetime. A trusted physician who takes the time to listen to you and to explain your options can be helpful. You should explore your alternatives and participate in making decisions. Taking an active role helps

physically, because no one knows your body like you do, and it empowers you to avoid feeling like a victim.

Second, having a support system, such as your family or a group of people who have the same condition you do, can foster your emotional well-being in many ways. Having someone to whom you can express your frustrations or fears and from whom you can receive unconditional support provides security. Knowing others who share your feelings can make you feel less alone. Often, those who have the same condition as you can offer solutions you hadn't considered. You can also find ways to laugh together about those moments of utter distress when you feel different from everyone else. The bonds people create when they share their problems can be lifelong, making the difficult times easier to bear.

Life lessons can be learned in many situations. Everyone has his or her share of problems. Sometimes having a chronic condition may seem unfair, but we are all less lucky than some and better off than others. All people struggle to find ways to be grateful for life every day and to jump life's hurdles. Take care of yourself, make friends, find inner peace, and share with others. Then your life will be full no matter what challenges life hands you.

---

bone loss of up to 1 percent a year. By the time a woman is 80, she may have lost 30 to 40 percent of her bone mass. When bone-mass loss becomes excessive, a fall may not be needed to fracture bones. Bending over and lifting 25 pounds—a heavy bag of groceries—could cause injury. During menopause, hormone-replacement therapy in the form of estrogen supplementation is recommended for many women as protection against osteoporosis.[11]

Because nicotine is thought to decrease blood levels of estrogen, smoking also contributes to bone loss. Smokers go through menopause on average at least two years earlier than nonsmokers.[12] Genetics may also play a role in osteoporosis. Researchers have identified an osteoporosis gene that determines how well vitamin D facilitates the absorption of calcium. People who have the gene are more resistant to absorbing available calcium. Caffeine and alcohol have also been implicated in bone loss. A recent study found that women who drank two or more cups of caffeinated coffee a day and drank no milk experienced significant loss of bone density after menopause. The effects of caffeine can be negated with consumption of milk. In the same study, coffee drinkers who drank at least one glass of milk per day had 6.5 percent higher bone density than the coffee-only group.[12]

The National Osteoporosis Foundation recommends several steps to reduce the risk of contracting this disease. First, consume adequate amounts of calcium, preferably from food. If this doesn't work, cal-

cium supplements are recommended. The Foundation suggests 1500 mg, almost double the amount given in the RDA.[14] Second, consume enough vitamin D (400 IU) to permit absorption of the calcium. Third, consider hormone-replacement therapy (estrogen) and discuss its use with your medical doctor, especially if you have a family history of osteoporosis. And fourth, participate in weight-bearing activities, such as walking, running, and weight training, to prevent bone loss. In one study, women who participated in a year-long exercise program and received daily doses of estrogen experienced a 7 percent increase in bone density and fared better than women on estrogen alone.[11] Physical exercise forces bones to adapt to the stresses imposed on them, and they hypertrophy in response. Bones atrophy when they are unstressed.

People with osteoporosis can and should exercise, but the type of physical activity and the intensity of exercise must be carefully selected. Forceful contractions of muscles and high-impact activities should be avoided because they may stress the bones beyond their breaking point. Swimming, water aerobics, stationary cycling, walking, and light weight training are good starting activities for those with osteoporosis.

Asthma

Asthma is a chronic respiratory condition characterized by attacks of wheezing and difficulty in breathing. The cause of asthma attacks is partial obstruction of bronchi and bronchioles resulting from the contraction or spasm of the muscles in the bronchial walls. Attacks may be mild or severe and may last anywhere from a few minutes to a few days. Asthma may develop at any age, although many children with asthma outgrow the condition as they get older and the bronchial passages widen. Asthma may be hereditary.

The two major types of asthma are extrinsic and intrinsic. Extrinsic asthma is the most common type and is typically triggered by a hypersensitivity to irritants or **allergens,** such as dust, pollen, feathers, animal dander, molds, smoke, extremely cold or dry air, and air pollutants. (Allergens are substances that cause allergic reactions, such as asthma, in some people.) For some asthmatics, drugs, food allergies, and exercise may induce an attack.

Intrinsic asthma is caused by factors such as stress or frequent respiratory tract infections. This form of asthma is less common than extrinsic asthma, but its symptoms are similar.

There is no cure for asthma, but there are preventive measures and treatments that help reduce the severity and length of an attack. One form of prevention is immunotherapy in which the asthmatic is desensitized through injections of weakened allergens. Medications, such as corticosteroid drugs, reduce in-

flammation and serve as a primary intervention for many asthmatics.

Bronchodilator drugs (medicines that open the bronchioles) are used routinely by asthmatics when an asthma attack occurs. These drugs are breathed in through an inhaler and usually restore normal breathing in several minutes.

One way to anticipate an impending attack or to determine the severity of an actual attack is to use a peak-flow meter, a small hand-held device (available at drugstores) that measures airflow. Peak airflow will go down hours and sometimes even a day or two before an attack, so the meter can serve as an early warning system. During an attack, it provides an objective way to determine how much the air passages in the lungs narrow.

Exercise-induced asthma is common among asthmatics. Symptoms include a coughing attack and tightness in the chest during or shortly after exercise. It appears to be most common when the asthmatic exercises in cold, dry air. Still, physical activity remains an integral part of wellness for people with exercise-induced asthma. Improvements in fitness and health status occur in asthmatics who exercise. An added benefit is that for many asthmatics exercise is accompanied by a decrease in the frequency and severity of exercise-induced attacks (figure 14-1). See Assessment Activity 14-2, Managing Your Asthma.

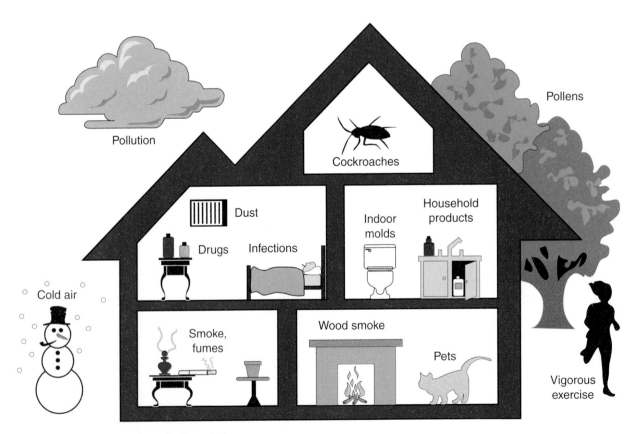

Figure 14-1 Common Asthma Triggers

If you have asthma, do you know which triggers are troublesome for you?

The Common Cold

More than 200 viruses, known as *rhinoviruses*, can cause the common cold.[15] A person may develop a temporary immunity to one or two viruses and still be infected by another. Any time people are together, viruses that cause the common cold are present. Adults average two to three colds each year, and children experience six to ten. Colds can be spread by shaking hands, sneezing, and breathing. Evidence indicates that hand-to-hand contact is the most common way a cold is spread. When infected people blow or touch their noses, the virus is transferred to their hands. When an uninfected person touches the infected person's hands, the virus is again transferred. Touching the face with hands that carry the virus leads directly to developing a cold. Frequent hand washing may prevent the spread of the virus.

The signs and symptoms of a cold are easily recognized. They include a feeling of listlessness, general aches and pains, watery eyes, and runny nasal passages. As the cold progresses, the nasal membranes swell, resulting in a stuffy nose. Infections affecting the throat can lead to sore throats and coughing. These symptoms tend to last seven to ten days. As an old axiom points out, if a cold is treated, it will go away in seven days and if left alone, it will last a week. A cold may occasionally persist for several weeks, but complications are infrequent in adults and older children. When they do occur, they most often are middle ear or sinus infections.

Antibiotics do not cure the common cold because they fight only bacterial infections. Over-the-counter decongestants—in spray or pill form—constrict blood vessels to shrink nasal swelling and open air passages, providing temporary relief of cold symptoms. Nasal sprays are more effective because they deliver a greater concentration of medicine to the nasal passages and give immediate relief.[16] But their overuse can cause a rebound effect, making congestion even worse. Nasal sprays should not be used for more than three consecutive days. Antihistamines are not effective for cold symptoms and may lead to drowsiness. Cough suppressants, which may offer relief from nagging coughing episodes, should be used with caution. On the positive side, the cough reflex is nature's way of clearing the lungs; on the negative side, persistent coughing may irritate the airway. A pharmacist or medical doctor should be consulted for help matching the appropriate cough medicine with the type of cough (dry or loose mucus).

The best advice for treating a cold is to take aspirin, ibuprofen, or acetaminophen (young children shouldn't take aspirin with cold symptoms because it may cause Reye's syndrome); drink plenty of fluids; eat a nutritious diet; and get plenty of rest.

Influenza

Influenza, or flu, is also caused by a virus. There are three primary strains of the influenza virus: A, B, and C. Most influenza develops from the A and B strains. These strains can change genetically, reappearing in an altered form every few years. Symptoms of all types of flu include chills, fever, weakness, headache, sore throat, dry cough, nausea, vomiting, and muscular aches and pains. All symptoms may not be present, and the severity varies greatly among people. Treatment for flu is the same as for the common cold. Aspirin should not be taken by children or teenagers because the potentially fatal Reye's syndrome can develop.

Vaccines can prevent particular types of influenza. Current recommendations are that priority in vaccination should be given to children and adults with chronic cardiovascular and lung disorders; residents of nursing homes; medical personnel who may transmit the virus to high-risk patients; everyone over 65; and anyone with conditions such as diabetes, kidney disease, hereditary anemias, and impaired natural immunity.

Headaches

One of the conditions that causes great discomfort is the headache. Some **headaches** may be the result of injury or brain disease, but most are caused by distress, tension, anxiety, and environmental factors. Tension

Washing your hands often is the best way to prevent the common cold.

headaches are the most common. Caused by involuntary contractions of the scalp, head, and neck muscles, tension headaches may be precipitated by anxiety, stress, and allergic reactions. Tension headaches can often be relieved by massaging the scalp and muscles in the neck. Aspirin or other pain relievers usually alleviate tension headaches.

Migraine headaches are characterized by throbbing pain that can last for hours or even days. Nausea and vomiting occasionally occur. Migraines, which seem to be initiated by stress, range from mild to severe. Migraines are considered a neurological disease with a hereditary link.[17] An abnormal drop in serotonin (a brain chemical that regulates blood vessel changes and controls pain) causes blood vessels near the surface of the brain to dilate, prompting nerve sensations perceived as pain. People who experience migraines may experience what is called an "aura"—flicker or jagged points of light that distorts vision. Other symptoms include a throbbing pain, usually on one side of the head and accompanied by nausea or vomiting.

Migraine sufferers have been able to get relief with the drug sumatriptan (Imitrex) since it was approved by the FDA in 1993. Recently, an easier-to-use nasal spray version of this drug became available. The nasal spray provides relief much more quickly than the pill, within fifteen minutes to two hours.[18] The drug is thought to work by mimicking the neurotransmitter serotonin.

Cluster headaches usually cause a knifelike pain behind the eye that quickly spreads to the forehead. The pain can spread to the neck, to the back of the head, and even into the teeth. The nose often runs, and the involved eye tears. The pain is often described as one of the worst pains a person can endure.

Cluster headaches get their name because they occur in clusters, at least one each day and sometimes several times a day. The attacks begin suddenly and may last from several minutes to several hours. In extreme cases they may last a few weeks or several months. Affected people may be symptom free for weeks or months. The cause of cluster headaches is unknown, but these headaches also appear to be related to arterial constriction and dilation.

A wide range of environmental factors may trigger headache pain. Exposure to smoke (including secondhand smoke), carbon monoxide (automobile exhaust, defective furnaces), alcohol, caffeine, and certain foods cause headaches in many people. Alcohol causes blood vessels to dilate, adding blood flow to irritated nerve endings. Caffeine in small amounts may help relieve headache pain by constricting blood vessels; in larger quantities (more than 2 cups), blood vessels dilate, which may lead to rebound headaches. Heavy coffee drinkers may experience withdrawal headaches if they

try to cut out caffeine cold turkey. A progressive reduction in caffeine over the course of a week or two should provide an appropriate acclimatization. Food triggers are most likely to be those containing amines. Amines cause blood vessels to constrict and dilate. Common dietary sources are aged cheeses, red wine, citrus fruits, and chocolates. Food additives, such as nitrates in hot dogs, smoked foods, and cold cuts, and flavor enhancers, such as monosodium glutamate (MSG), are often accused of provoking headaches.[20]

Many illnesses can cause a headache. Sinusitis, teeth and gum problems, high blood pressure, hypothyroidism, acute anemia, Cushing's disease, and Addison's disease are common offenders.[20] A complete physical exam can help identify specific medical causes. A headache should be evaluated by a physician if it is chronic, associated with a fever, accompanied by numbness or paralysis, associated with a stiff neck, interfering with thinking or memory, and/or continuing to get worse.

Treatment of headache pain includes a full gamut of interventions. Techniques such as deep breathing, progressive relaxation, biofeedback, meditation, and visualization seem to help relieve the pain in some sufferers. New drugs that block headache pain without negatively affecting other parts of the body are in the final stages of testing and could become available in the near future (see Real-World Wellness: Dealing with Headaches).

Real-World Wellness

Dealing with Headaches

I've heard about many remedies for headaches. What are the best ways to deal with the various types of headaches?

Here are some methods[19] for managing headaches:

• Migraines	Sumatriptan: an injectable, oral, or nasal application constricts the arteries of head. Can be used alone or in combination with the drugs ergotamine, tartrate, cafergot, or belladonna
• Tension	Over-the-counter analgesics; if chronic, antidepressants
• Cluster headaches	For acute attacks, sumatriptan or inhaled oxygen; preventive drugs such as methysergide, steroids, or lithium
• Sinus	Decongestants; antibiotics if needed

Inflammatory Bowel Disease

Inflammatory bowel disease (IBD) is a term that represents a variety of diseases that cause inflammation in the intestines. The two main types of IBD are Crohn's disease, which causes inflammation in the digestive tract, and ulcerative colitis, which creates severe ulcers in the inner lining of the colon and rectum. Both conditions can result in frequent and intense diarrhea, abdominal pain, gas, fever, and rectal bleeding.[21]

Crohn's disease affects men and women equally and seems to predominate in some families. About 20 percent of people with Crohn's disease have a blood relative with some form of IBD.[21] The cause of the disease is not fully understood, but in addition to a genetic predisposition, an autoimmune response may be responsible.[22] Researchers speculate that a viral or bacterial agent interacting with the body's immune system may be at fault. No evidence supports the theory that Crohn's disease is caused by tension, anxiety, or other psychological factors.[21] The success of treatment depends on the location, the severity, the complications, and the response to previous treatments. The goal of any treatment is to control inflammation, correct nutritional deficiencies, and relieve symptoms. Treatment may include drugs, nutritional supplements, surgery, or some combination of these options. Treatment can help control the condition, but no cure exists.

Ulcerative colitis is a chronic inflammation of the colon lining. It is different from Crohn's disease in that the inflammation affects only the colon.[23] The condition develops in fewer than one person in every 10,000 people. It typically appears in people between the ages of 15 and 35. The cause is unknown, but it is most common among Caucasians and seems to be familial. Controlling stress and avoiding any foods that cause discomfort may help relieve symptoms. To prevent flare-ups, anti-inflammatory drugs may be used. Researchers are testing nicotine patches after finding that they improve colitis symptoms.[23] Between 20 and 30 percent of people with ulcerative colitis need surgery. These are patients in whom complications have become severe and medication has not worked.

Summary

- Diabetes mellitus is a group of diseases with one of the following symptoms: The body does not make insulin, it doesn't make enough insulin, or it doesn't use insulin properly.
- The two major categories of diabetes are type 1 and type 2.
- Type 1 diabetes usually occurs early in life and requires insulin injections because the pancreas loses its ability to produce insulin.
- Type 2 diabetes occurs most often in people over 40 years of age who do not exercise and are obese.
- Arthritis is an inflammatory disease of the joints. The most common form of arthritis is osteoarthritis, characterized by deterioration of the cartilage covering the surfaces of the bones in certain joints.
- It is believed that rheumatoid arthritis is a disease of the immune system that results in joint swelling, pain, deformity, and decreased mobility.
- Asthma may be caused by extrinsic factors, such as pollen or dust, or intrinsic factors, such as stress.
- The common cold is caused by rhinoviruses, of which there are more than 200 varieties. Antibiotics do not cure colds.
- Influenza is caused by only three strains of virus, but these agents have the ability to change and reappear in different forms. Because influenza can range widely in severity, certain high-risk groups are encouraged to have an annual flu vaccine.
- Osteoporosis is a chronic disease characterized by a loss of mineral content of the bones, which makes them brittle and vulnerable to breakage.
- Mild to moderate exercises are effective in promoting bone strength in the elderly.
- Headaches are divided into three categories—tension, cluster, and migraine. People who experience migraines can use techniques such as deep breathing and meditation to alleviate pain or prevent the onset of a headache.
- Inflammatory bowel disease (IBD) is a group of diseases involving the gastrointestinal system.
- Crohn's disease is a type of IBD that results from erosion of the inner and middle layers of the intestinal tract wall.
- Ulcerative colitis is a type of IBD characterized by inflammation of the colon.
- Both conditions can trigger frequent and intense diarrhea, abdominal pain, gas, fever, and rectal bleeding.

Review Questions

1. Explain the difference between type 1 and type 2 diabetes.
2. Describe the main symptoms of diabetes.
3. What are the most serious potential complications of uncontrolled diabetes?
4. What steps can be taken to prevent the development of type 2 diabetes?
5. Explain the differences between the two most common forms of arthritis, their causes, and possible treatments.

6. Discuss the relationship between calcium, estrogen, exercise, and osteoporosis.

7. What are some measures and treatments that help reduce the severity and length of an asthma attack or prevent it altogether?

8. What behaviors may help prevent and treat the common cold?

9. Explain how the influenza viruses differ from the common cold viruses.

10. Explain the differences between tension headaches and migraine headaches. How do the causes, symptoms, and treatments differ?

11. What environmental factors can trigger headache pain?

12. What role does physical activity play in the various conditions discussed in this chapter?

References

1. Mayo Clinic. 1998. Diabetes—weight control and exercise may keep you off the road to high blood sugar. *Mayo Clinic Health Letter* 16(2).

2. Margolis, S., and C. D. Saudek. 1998. *The Johns Hopkins White Papers: Diabetes Mellitus—1998*. Baltimore, Md.: The Johns Hopkins Medical Institution.

3. Dinsmoor, R. S. 1994. Lifting the sugar embargo. *Harvard Health Letter* 19(12):7.

4. Editors. 1997. Dealing with diabetes: Diet and exercise hold key to control. *Environmental Nutrition—the Newsletter of Food, Nutrition and Health* 20(12).

5. Editors. 1994. Diabetic diet shifts emphasis from carbs toward "mono" fats. *Environmental Nutrition—The Newsletter of Food, Nutrition and Health* 17(10).

6. Helmrich, S. P., D. R. Ragland, and R. S. Paffenbarger. 1994. Prevention of noninsulin-dependent diabetes mellitus with physical activity. *Medicine and Science in Sports and Exercise* 26:824.

7. Margolis, S., and J. A. Flynn. 1998. *The Johns Hopkins White Papers: Arthritis*. Baltimore, Md.: The Johns Hopkins Medical Institution.

8. Harvard Medical School Publications Group. 1995. *Arthritis: A Harvard Letter Special Report*. Boston: Harvard Medical School.

9. Lamb, L. 1992. Exercise helps osteoarthritis. *Health Letter* 39(11):4.

10. Mayo Clinic. 1997. Rheumatoid arthritis. *Mayo Clinic Health Letter* 15(6):1.

11. Farrow, C. 1996. Estrogen, exercise aid bone density, study claims. *Commercial Appeal* 157(2):C4.

12. Alberts, N. 1995. Osteoporosis. *American Health* 14(9):70.

13. Willensky, D. 1995. Bone: How it works. *American Health* 14(9):87.

14. Liebman, B. 1994. Calcium: After the craze. *Nutrition Action Health Letter* 21(5):1.

15. Winker, M., and A. Flanagin. 1996. Infectious diseases—a global approach to a global problem. *Journal of American Medical Associates* 275(3):245.

16. Consumers Union. 1996. Finding the right cold medicine. *Consumer Reports* 61:62.

17. Editors. 1998. Managing migraines and other headaches: Diet's controversial role. *Environmental Nutrition—the Newsletter of Food, Nutrition, and Health* 21(6):1.

18. Editors. 1997. Healthnews—straight talk on the medical headlines: New options for migraines. *The New England Journal of Medicine Health News* 3(13):1.

19. Harvard University. 1998. Migraine—more than a headache. *Harvard Health Letter* 23(3):4.

20. Halpern, G. M. 1994. Headache can be a pain in the neck. *Healthline* 13(7):9.

21. National Digestive Diseases Information Clearinghouse. 1999. *Crohn's Disease.* Available online at **www.niddk.nih.gov/health/digest/pubs/crohns/crohns.htl**.

22. Doughty, D. B., and D. Jackson. 1993. *Gastrointestinal Disorders.* St. Louis: Mosby.

23. Mayo Clinic. 1995. Ulcerative colitis. *Mayo Clinic Health Letter* 13(12):1.

24. American Diabetes Association. 2001. *Type 2 diabetes.* Available online at **www.diabetes.org/ada/facts.asp**.

Suggested Readings

American Diabetes Association. 1997. *American Diabetes Association Complete Guide to Diabetes: The Ultimate Home Diabetes Reference.* ADA. Alexandria, VA.

This book is a comprehensive resource of information about diabetes self-care, covering nutrition, blood sugar, exercise, and potential complications.

Brody, J. 1995. *Jane Brody's Cold and Flu Fighter.* Scranton, Penn.: W. W. Norton.

This is an informative guide to preventing and treating colds and flu. The book dispels many age-old myths and contains a special section on treating children's colds and flu.

Kandel J., and D. B. Sudderth. 1998. *The Anti-arthritis Diet: Increase Mobility and Reduce Pain with This 30-Day Life-Changing Program.* Rocklin, Calif.: Prima Publishing.

This book provides over 100 recipes for the relief of the pain of arthritis.

Robbins, L. D., and S. S. Lang. 1995. *Headache Help: A Complete Guide to Understanding Headaches and the Medicines That Relieve Them.* St. Charles, Ill.: Houghton Mifflin.

The authors seek to narrow the doctor-patient communication gap by equipping headache sufferers with essential information to help stop pain. The book provides a guide to prescription and nonprescription headache drugs.

Name _____   Date _____   Section _____

Assessment Activity 14-1

Are You at Risk for Diabetes?

Directions: Check the appropriate column in response to the following questions to assess your probability of having diabetes. The more questions that you answer with a "yes," the higher the probability you have of becoming diabetic.

Taken alone, any "yes" answer does not necessarily indicate you are diabetic. However, if you have answered "yes" more than five times, consult your physician for a urine test.

	Yes	No
1. Is there a history of diabetes in your family?	_____	_____
2. Do you tire quickly or seem always to be fatigued?	_____	_____
3. Do you urinate frequently?	_____	_____
4. Are you constantly thirsty?	_____	_____
5. Is your vision blurry?	_____	_____
6. Have you suddenly lost weight?	_____	_____
7. Are you overweight?	_____	_____
8. Do you eat excessively?	_____	_____
9. Do wounds heal slowly?	_____	_____
10. Is your skin frequently itchy?	_____	_____

Name _____ Date _____ Section _____

Assessment Activity 14-2

Managing Your Asthma

Directions: If you have asthma, there are many things you can do to help manage your condition effectively. To assess your personal health management, place a check mark next to each statement that applies to you.

Reducing or Avoiding Asthma Triggers

_____ I have identified my asthma triggers.

_____ I do not smoke and I avoid environmental tobacco smoke.

_____ I use and properly maintain an air filter and an air conditioner to keep my home cleaner and more comfortable.

_____ I avoid vacuuming or I use a dust mask when vacuuming.

_____ I avoid mowing the lawn or I use a dust mask when mowing.

_____ I avoid woodstoves and fireplaces.

_____ I use dust-proof encasings on my pillows, mattress, and box spring.

_____ I use a dehumidifier as necessary in my home to reduce indoor mold.

_____ I use window shades or curtains made of plastic or other washable material for easy cleaning.

_____ My closets contain only needed clothing. Anything I do not currently wear is stored in plastic garment bags.

_____ I do not sleep or lie down on upholstered furniture.

_____ If I have a pet, it does not sleep in or go into my bedroom.

_____ I avoid perfume and cologne, cleaning chemicals, paint, and talcum powder as much as possible.

Preventing and Managing Asthma Attacks

_____ I have learned everything I can about asthma.

_____ I take my medications as prescribed by my physician.

_____ I carry my inhaler with me at all times.

_____ I have a crisis plan for managing a severe asthma attack.

_____ I keep emergency numbers by the phone and with me at all times.

_____ I know how quickly my asthma medications should work.

_____ I use a peak-flow meter to anticipate and respond quickly to asthma attacks.

Interpretation

17 or more items checked: You are doing a great job avoiding asthma triggers and preventing and managing asthma attacks.

14–16 items checked: In many ways you are doing a good job of managing your asthma. However, you may be unnecessarily exposing yourself to common asthma triggers, or your plan for preventing and managing attacks may need some work.

13 or fewer items checked: You need to manage your asthma much more effectively. Remember that an asthma attack can be fatal.

Discuss this assessment with other members of your family or your roommates. Ask them to help you with your asthma prevention and management program.

15

Becoming a Responsible Health Care Consumer

Online Learning Center

Log on to our Online Learning Center (OLC) for access to these additional resources:

- Chapter key term flashcards
- Learning objectives
- Additional goals for behavior change
- Concentration game
- Self-scoring chapter quizzes

- Additional lab activities

The OLC also offers weblinks for study and exploration of wellness topics. Access these links through **www.mhhe.com/ anspaugh5e**, click on "Student Center," click on "Chapter 15," and then click on "Web Activities."

Goals for Behavior Change

- Apply criteria for determining whether health information is valid, reliable, and based on scientifically controlled studies.
- Identify specific strategies for enhancing communication with your physician.
- Determine the diagnostic tests and immunizations appropriate for your age, gender, and health status.
- Find a specific online newsgroup or patient support group that might be helpful to you.

Key Terms

alternative medicine
contraindications
defensive medicine
diagnostic laboratory tests
double-blind study
epidemiologic studies
false negative
false positive
health insurance
health maintenance organization (HMO)
iatrogenic condition
immunizations
implied consent
informed consent
periodic examinations

placebo
point of service (POS)
polypharmacy
preferred provider organization (PPO)
primary-care physician
reliability
risk factor
scientifically controlled studies
selective health examinations
self-care
statistical relationship
statistical significance
validity

Objectives

After completing this chapter, you will be able to do the following:

- Explain how to evaluate the accuracy, validity, and reliability of health information.
- Discuss criteria for determining when, where, and how to choose health care.
- Describe the functions and purposes of the major components of a physical examination.

raditionally, Americans have had a rather passive attitude toward health care. Whether taking medicine, purchasing health care products, undergoing surgery, or having a diagnostic test administered, people have operated as if following orders. Fortunately, this attitude is changing. People are viewing themselves as active participants in their health care. They are asking questions, placing demands on *health care providers* (people and/or facilities that provide health care services), getting second opinions, and sometimes even refusing treatments. People realize that they must assume more responsibility for safeguarding their health. With this responsibility, however, comes the challenge of knowing what one can and should do for oneself. The purpose of this chapter is to lay the groundwork to enable you to become an informed, active participant in the health care marketplace.

Understanding Health Information

The first and perhaps most difficult challenge for consumers is to make sense of the health-information explosion. Many popular magazines regularly print health articles, newspapers often devote entire sections to medicine, the publications of health newsletters abound, television programs feature numerous health stories, and thousands of scientific health-related studies are published daily. Interest in health information appears to have reached an all-time high.

The availability of so much health information has drawbacks; the major drawback is that so much of the information is confusing, sometimes even contradictory. Even medical experts have trouble separating fact from fiction. It is not unusual for a new finding to be headlined one day and completely refuted the next. For some people the seemingly endless contradictions and medical flip-flops lead to an attitude that carried to the extreme completely disregards new developments and information, even those with life-saving potential.

Two examples illustrate the point. Several years ago beta-carotene was so highly regarded that it was presented as a panacea for preventing lung cancer; then, a large-scale study found that smokers who took beta-carotene supplements were more likely to contract lung cancer than those who were not taking the supplement. Another nutrition example is vitamin C. It is an antioxidant that has long been thought to minimize the effects of free radicals on the development of heart disease and cancer; recently, newspaper headlines reported that vitamin C changes DNA in a way that

may cause cancer. What are we to believe? Countless other examples could be cited that explain the skepticism, even distrust, of many people toward medical information.

The challenge for most people is to keep an open mind and realize that health information is constantly evolving. Cholesterol is a good example. At one time cholesterol was thought to be the major risk factor for heart disease. Nothing else seemed to matter. Then it was learned that some people with high cholesterol levels had little sign of atherosclerosis; conversely, some people with advanced stages of atherosclerosis had normal levels of cholesterol. How could this be explained? Were medical scientists wrong about cholesterol? Yes and no. Yes, it is a risk factor but, no, cholesterol by itself doesn't tell the whole story (see Chapter 2 for in-depth discussion of this risk factor). Now we know it is the cholesterol carriers in the form of low-density (LDLs) and high density lipoproteins (HDLs) that earn our attention. Today's emphasis on LDLs and HDLs doesn't mean the early messages about cholesterol were completely wrong. They were the first steps in understanding a complex issue. Without the early interest in cholesterol, it is unlikely that we would have learned what we know today about cholesterol carriers. Will today's knowledge about LDLs and HDLs be obsolete tomorrow? Possibly. But if that is the case it is likely that it will have served as an important building block for the medical truths of tomorrow. Much of what is known about health and medicine is like this. The editor of a highly respected health newsletter states the dilemma clearly: "Science proceeds by one good article or study at a time. There's never a direct, final answer because our information keeps increasing. So consumers and doctors often need to make tough decisions amid incomplete, changing, and contradictory information."[1]

Given the mixed messages about health, it is perhaps a good idea to adopt a somewhat skeptical attitude, especially toward extreme and sensational health claims. The First Amendment to the U.S. Constitution, which guarantees freedom of the press, also guarantees Americans the right to publish health-related hogwash. The more you read, generally the more contradictions you will uncover (see Just the Facts: The Making of a Medical Flip-Flop). This should not make you feel uncomfortable but, to the contrary, make you realize that medicine is still as much art as science.

Guidelines for Evaluating Health Information

Adhering to the guidelines that follow should help your search for correct health information.

∼ *Just the Facts* ∼

The Making of a Medical Flip-Flop[2]

Many of the health contradictions, or medical flip-flops, can be explained by the differences in motives between journalists and researchers. Journalists often highlight unusual findings to grab your attention. The goal is to sell newspapers, magazines, or in the case of television, time. Researchers, on the other hand, typically view each new study as a stepping stone to the truth, well aware that the latest finding may not stand the test of time. It is the body of evidence—confirmed and reconfirmed—not the latest headlines, that should influence decisions.

Often, what seems like a flip-flop is a shift in emphasis for scientists. To the casual reader it may appear as a contradiction. For example, it is common knowledge that dietary fat, especially saturated fat, is bad for health. But now it appears that an extremely low-fat diet may be worse for some people than a moderately fat diet especially if much of it consists of monounsaturated and omega-3 fatty acids. To the layperson the fat message appears to be flip-flopping; in reality, it isn't. It became more complex, requiring researchers to refine the message.

Avoid Jumping to Conclusions

Most health misinformation is based on facts, not lies. The problem is that facts get exaggerated and sometimes lead people to wrong conclusions.

A good example involves potato chips, which have long been considered a junk food. Actually, the quick cooking process of potato chips preserves nutrients better than mashing, boiling, or baking potatoes. Ounce per ounce, potato chips provide more nutrients than do other forms of potatoes. This information alone might convince people to begin consuming large quantities of potato chips. However, because potato chips are cooked in oil, they are high in fat and calories and are not recommended for people trying to lose weight. This extra bit of information gives a completely different angle to the perspective on potato chips. By being aware that the truth of most health issues is not simple, the tendency to oversimplify and overgeneralize health information can be thwarted.

Remember That Health Discoveries Take Time

Health discoveries often make their way into media headlines, but a cardinal rule of science is that findings must be replicable. Health information based on

a dramatic discovery is not usually considered valid unless it is confirmed in several follow-up studies or experiments.

Beware of Headline Reading

Newspaper, magazine, and television headlines are intended to arouse your curiosity primarily for one purpose: to make you buy or watch. A headline might cleverly capture the essence of a story or it might present a partial truth that leads to wrong conclusions. A common media strategy is to sensationalize a story by crafting a headline that contradicts conventional wisdom. Consider some recent examples: "New Study Weighs In: More Fat, Fewer Strokes." "'Dirty Drug' Nicotine Has Positives, Research Shows." "Low Sodium Diets Increase Blood Pressure." "A Drink a Day Can Help You Live Longer." These headlines are fraught with possible deceptions. They may represent the results of isolated studies that run against mainstream medical thought. They may serve as punchlines for stories based on studies with many shortcomings. Or they may actually represent new trends in thinking supported by a medical consensus. The only way to know for sure is to become a well-informed, discriminating consumer of information the way you are a consumer of products, goods, and services. The challenge is to avoid the tendency toward headline reading and to apply the criteria for determining if health information is both valid and reliable.

Apply the Criteria for Determining Validity and Reliability of Health Information

Health information that can be trusted is based on studies that are valid, reliable, and reported in a way that includes research and statistics in their proper context. When assessing validity and reliability, know the type of study that serves as the basis for new information. Knowing the meanings of the following terms will help to put new information in a proper context.

Validity

In health research, **validity** means *truthfulness*. If a study is designed and conducted properly, its findings are likely to be valid. For example, it was found that adding vitamin E to human cells in the laboratory stimulated cell division and growth. This was used to support the erroneous conclusion that vitamin E would delay the aging process. This was not a proper generalization because a simple laboratory experiment is not a valid procedure for demonstrating something as complex as aging.

Reliability

Reliability is another key criterion for evaluating health information. It refers to the extent that health claims can be consistently verified. If a claim is reliable, it can be demonstrated to occur consistently in study after study. The test of time is perhaps the ultimate criterion for evaluating the trustworthiness of new information.

Statistical significance

Researchers and reporters often use the phrase **statistical significance** to give meaning and credibility to findings. For example, in one study a group of college students who ate breakfast every morning before going to class did better in school than a comparison group who skipped breakfast. The differences were reported to be "statistically significant." Does this mean that the differences between the two groups were large, maybe equivalent to a full letter grade? Does this mean that breakfast is the key to academic success? Statistical significance does not necessarily imply largeness, but it does imply probability. *Statistical significance* means that the probability that a study's findings are due to chance alone is less than 5 percent. That is, 95 of 100 times similarly designed studies would yield similar results. If the differences between two groups are not statistically significant, they may be due to chance findings and might not show up again if a study were repeated. Because so many studies are performed, some studies that yield statistically significant results eventually prove to be wrong. Consequently, it takes hundreds of studies, many of them conflicting, to create a consensus on a particular health issue. Any health claim worth considering should be based on numerous studies or experiments conducted over many years.

Statistical relationship

Statistical relationship refers to the extent that two or more variables or events are associated with each other. Much health literature is based on research involving statistical relationships or associations. For example, it is well known that a statistical relationship exists between the consumption of salt and high blood pressure for some people. In other words, an increase in salt intake is accompanied by an increase in blood pressure. Conversely, a drop in salt intake is associated with a decrease in blood pressure. This is helpful information, but does it mean that high salt intake causes high blood pressure? No. If this were true, then all Americans who eat too much salt would have high blood pressure. The mistake many people make is to conclude that one event in a statistical relationship causes the other. Relationships are important and help-

ful clues to health and they provide a basis for better understanding health risks. However, they cannot and do not establish cause and effect.

Risk factor

The term **risk factor** refers to health habits and/or practices that increase the risk of getting certain diseases. The emphasis in Chapter 2, for example, is on those risk factors related to heart disease. In the popular press, risk factors are often presented out of context. For example, consider the following headline: "Bicycle Deaths Quadruple Auto Deaths on College Campus." The basis for the headline was a study that reported that the risk of death from bicycling to school increased 100 percent over the previous year, whereas deaths caused by driving to school increased by only 25 percent. The reporter incorrectly concluded that bicycling is four times more risky than driving. What is missing is information about baseline risk. If the baseline risk of deaths from bicycling is 1 in 1000, a 100 percent increase would raise it to 2 in 1000. If the baseline risk for driving to school is 400 in 1000, then a 25 percent increase would increase the risk of death by 100 to 500 in 1000. Driving to school would then turn out to be 250 times more risky than bicycling to school, a complete reversal of the meaning of the headline. Although this example is hypothetical, it serves as a reminder of the importance of inquiring about the chances of getting a disease in the first place before drawing conclusions regarding risk factors, diseases, and death.

Ask the Following Questions About Information

Answers to four questions about the nature and type of study will help you sort through the contradictory findings and claims reported in the popular press.

What type of study was used?

There are several types of studies and each has certain advantages and limitations.

Epidemiologic studies are population studies (rather than scientifically controlled experimental studies) that observe the health habits and lifestyles of thousands of people for a period of time. The Framingham Study in Framingham, Massachusetts is perhaps the longest running and most famous epidemiologic study in the United States. It has yielded information that has been invaluable to our understanding of the risk factors associated with many diseases, especially heart disease. Epidemiologic studies may be *prospective* or *retrospective*. In a *prospective* study researchers follow a group of people at a specific point in time and identify relationships between lifestyle and diseases. In a *retrospective study* researchers look back in time to identify possible disease relationships. Retrospective studies are generally considered less reliable than prospective studies.

An advantage of epidemiologic studies is that they tend to be more generalizable to the population at large. A disadvantage is that they do not prove cause and effect.

Scientifically controlled studies are experiments conducted in controlled settings. The classic study is a **double-blind study** that includes at least two groups, one that is an experimental group and receives some form of experimental treatment and another that is a control group and receives no treatment. The double-blind feature of a study ensures that neither the researcher nor the subjects knows who is receiving an experimental treatment, and, therefore, will not influence the outcome with that knowledge. If a researcher wanted to prove, for example, that a particular brand of soap prevents athlete's foot, one group of subjects would use the experimental soap, and the other would use a **placebo** or soap substitute. Researchers administering the soap treatment would not know which soap each subject was using, nor would the subjects in the experimental and control groups know. If the experimental group has significantly fewer cases of athlete's foot, the results could then be attributed to the treatment.

The experimental-control, double-blind requirement of scientific research is a difficult standard to meet. Such studies are costly and require considerable resources and manpower. Typically, they are referred to in the press as *clinical trials* or *population intervention studies*. The advantage of scientifically controlled studies is that they control the variables so that it is often possible to establish cause-and-effect relationships. The disadvantage is that results usually apply to a narrowly defined population group and lack generalizability to the general population.

What were the characteristics of the people included in the study?

Scientific studies require random sampling of subjects to represent the diverse racial, religious, gender, and cultural characteristics of the population at large. Medical breakthroughs should not be based on a small number of homogeneous, or similar, subjects. Broadly designed human clinical trials that are randomized (a systematic sorting of subjects according to the laws of chance), placebo controlled, and include a double blind offer the strongest proof of reliable information.[3] If a study is limited to one gender or racial or ethnic group, its findings will not apply to anyone of a different gender, race, or ethnicity. If the study involves animals, avoid drawing conclusions until subsequent human studies are conducted.

If you are at low risk for a particular condition being studied, the results probably do not apply to you. The consumption of alcohol illustrates the point. A number of studies report that one drink per day for a woman and up to two drinks a day for a man may reduce the risks associated with heart disease. These studies affect only people who have heart disease and consume alcoholic beverages. If you do not have heart disease and if you do not drink beverages that contain alcohol, the study findings are not relevant to you.

Remember, true breakthroughs in medical research are the exception rather than the rule.

How many people were in the study?

In general, the more people included in a study, the better. Studies that report results based on a small number of subjects are seriously limited in their reliability and/or generalizability, regardless of how tightly controlled they are. Unfortunately, small research projects with intriguing results can make headlines that are just as big as those given to larger, more comprehensive studies.[6]

Who funded the study?

Businesses stand to gain or lose substantial sums of money (and reputation) from headline stories featuring their products. Consider the huge upswing in profits experienced by businesses in the pharmaceutical industry when several studies reported the weight loss benefits of new diet drugs. Profits were staggering; so were the losses when the drugs were later pulled off the market. Before jumping to conclusions, inquire about the funding source. The advice of the editor of the *New England Journal of Medicine* is appropriate: "You have to look at the motivations of everyone involved in telling you that there is some breakthrough that is going to change your life."[4]

Consider the Sources of Information

Valid and reliable health information comes from respected journals, magazines, and newsletters. Such publications have experienced health or medical editors who subject their articles to peer review and criticism by other scientists. Because little or no space is devoted to advertising, they are less inclined to be influenced by the need to protect the reputation or promote the product of a sponsor or advertiser. Several of these newsletters are available free online (see Just the Facts: Health Help You Can Trust on the Internet).

Just the Facts

Health Help You Can Trust on the Internet

The internet has grown so rapidly that it would take volumes to list all of the available websites that offer health information. Even if that were feasible, there would be little assurance that the information could be trusted. Fortunately, several respected health organizations have reviewed selected websites and identified the ones that are useful and reliable. A few of these sites are listed here. Remember that many more excellent sites are available. (A $$ sign indicates that the website may charge a fee for use.)

Newsletters
- Harvard Medical School Publications at **www.harvardhealth.org**
- HealthNews at **www.webmd.com**
- Johns Hopkins InteliHealth Newsletter at **www.intelihealth.com**
- Mayo Health Oasis at **www.mayoclinic.org**
- Nutrition Action Health Letter at **www.cspinet.org**
- Tufts University Health and Nutrition Newsletter at **http://healthletter.tufts.edu**

Medical Database, Links, and/or Search Engines
- Achoo at **www.achoo.com**
- Hardin Meta Directory of Internet Health Sources at **www.lib.uiowa.edu/hardin/md/pharm.html**
- Health-Resource at **www.thehealthresource.com** ($$)
- HealthAtoZ at **www.Healthatoz.com**
- Healthtouch at **www.healthtouch.com**
- Medical Matrix at **www.medmarix.org**
- MedicineNet at **www.medicinenet.com.**

- MEDLINE (also National Library of Medicine) at **www.medlineplus.gov**
- Medscape at **www.medscape.com**
- MedSearch at **www.medsearch.com** ($$)

Other Health Sites
- American Cancer Society at **www.cancer.org**
- American Dental Association at **www.ada.org**
- American Heart Association at **www.americanheart.org**
- American Medical Association at **www.ama-assn.org**
- American Psychiatric Association at **www.apa.org**
- Institute for Safe Medication Practices at **www.ismp.org**
- Nutrition information at **www.navigator.tufts.edu**
- U.S. Food and Drug Administration at **www.fda.gov**
- U.S. Pharmacopeia (pharmaceutical information) at **www.usp.org**

Other Health Sites
- Alternative medicine at **www.wholehealthmd.com**
- Children's health at **www.kidshealth.org**
- Department of Health and Human Services at **www.healthfinder.gov**
- Noncommercial health sites at **www.healthweb.org**
- Ratings of physicians at **www.healthgrades.com**
- The Merck Manual at **www.merck.com**
- The Merck Manual Home Edition at **www.merckhomeedition.com**

Health information and the Internet

People who have access to a computer and an internet service provider can obtain health and medical information that once was available only to those in the medical profession who had user privileges at major medical libraries and research centers. Websites provide information regarding most diseases and health conditions. Some sites provide access to news groups, chat rooms, bulletin boards, support groups, and even to medical specialists (see Nurturing Your Spirituality: Support Is Just a Click Away). Perhaps more than any other development of recent times, the internet has been the best means of empowerment for people who want and need information so that they can be actively involved in their health care. Armed with the latest information, people can be better prepared to ask questions and become partners with their physicians when serious health issues occur.

According to a recent study in which medical consultants reviewed selected webpages, much of the information available online is "as good as any you'll find

Nurturing Your Spirituality

Support Is Just a Click Away

Online patient support groups can be useful, especially for people with chronic illness. With the click of a mouse it is possible to interact with others who share health problems. One of the most direct methods of communicating with others on the internet is through newsgroups. Newsgroups are locations where electronic messages (e-mail) related to a medical topic are posted. These are usually plain text messages rather than sophisticated, color-graphic presentations. Newsgroups are not a collection of news items. Essentially, they are virtual bulletin boards open to anyone who wants to participate. Newsgroups make it possible to locate other people experiencing the same health concerns you are and to hear about their experiences as well as tell about yours.

Participating in a health-related newsgroup allows you to exchange information with people who share your concerns.

There are more than 15,000 newsgroups available on the internet.[5] To locate the name of a specific newsgroup that might be helpful to you, visit one of the following websites:

· Deja News at **www.dejanews.com**
· Dictionary.com at **www.dictionary.com**
· Self-Help Sourcebook at **www.mentalhelp.net/selfhelp/**
· Healthfinder at **www.healthfinder.gov**

Following are some popular newsgroups devoted to specific health issues:

· AIDS at **http://sdmc.cpcra.org/links.usenet.html**
· Arthritis at **misc.health.arthritis**
· Asthma at **alt.support.asthma**
· Cancer at **sci.med.diseases.cancer**
· Depression at **alt.support.depression**
· Diabetes mellitus at **misc.health.diabetes**
· Eating disorders at **alt.support.eating-disord**
· Headaches at **alt.support.headaches.migraine**
· Infertility at **misc.health.infertility**
· Stop smoking at **alt.support.stop-smoking**

A newsgroup may receive dozens and even hundreds of new postings each day. You can read all of them or select those that seem to be most relevant. Messages on a related topic often are grouped together in a *thread*, making it easier to follow a conversation. Often, participants share practical tips for daily living. Sometimes, experts offer medical advice. Some groups are managed by administrators who screen submissions. However, most groups are uncontrolled, which means that they may contain inaccurate information.

in a good medical library—and in some cases more complete than the information your own physician could provide."[5] But the same study called the internet a "wild frontier" mixed with all sorts of information—good and bad, true and false, complete and dangerously incomplete. Some information may be outdated and some may be presented in websites that are not managed by knowledgeable sources or have not been subjected to peer review. Asking the following questions[6] should help determine if the information found at a particular website can be trusted:

· *Where does the information come from?* Information that comes from established medical institutions

like hospitals, universities, or government organizations can generally be trusted. Reputation counts on the internet just as it does elsewhere. But be cautious of soundalike names. One website hosted by an organization whose name sounds very much like *American College of Sports Medicine* posted information about a questionable treatment for atherosclerosis that has never been proved effective.[6]

· *Does the site reflect more than one opinion?* Quality sites often feature more than one perspective.

· *How often is the information updated?* Check to see if the information you are reading has been updated since its original posting. Ideally, a website will update its information on a monthly, if not weekly, basis.

- *Does the site promote products or procedures?* Exercise caution if a site uses anecdotal records and testimonials to promote specific products or procedures. Also be suspicious of sites that dwell on the shortcomings of mainstream medical science.

Managing Health Care

A major theme throughout this text is that you can control many factors that influence your health. An outgrowth of this attitude is the **self-care** movement, the trend toward becoming an active partner in the management of one's health rather than a passive recipient of medical treatment. Armed with correct information, you can manage many aspects of your health care that were once thought to be solely within the realm of a physician. An added bonus of becoming actively involved in self-care is a shift from feelings of helplessness and despair to feelings of control, responsibility, and involvement (see Assessment Activity 15-3).

Answers to the following questions guide the use of health care services, providers, and products and facilitate the self-care approach to wellness:

- When should you seek health care?
- What can you expect from a stay in the hospital?
- How can you select a health care professional?

When to Seek Health Care

Many people tend to fall into two extreme groups regarding health care: those who seek health care for every ache and pain and those who avoid health care unless experiencing extreme pain. Both groups unwisely use the health care establishment. Those in the first group fail to understand that too much health care can be ineffective or even harmful. They also fail to recognize the powerful recuperative powers of the body. The reality is that the majority of people who seek medical care are unaffected by the treatment. Most of the time the body is capable of healing itself. Of course, sometimes medical treatment is essential. But, for every person who gets better from treatment another person experiences an **iatrogenic condition.** An iatrogenic condition is a health problem or condition caused by medical treatment. Several examples include drug reactions, medical mistakes, and infection. Sometimes the iatrogenic condition may be worse than the presenting symptom. This does not mean that symptoms should be disregarded on the assumption the body will heal itself or if treatment is sought there is a 50:50 chance of an unnecessary complication. People who avoid health care at all costs fail to recognize the

value of early diagnosis and detection of disease. The challenge, therefore, is to know when to seek health care and when to allow for the natural course of events that occurs in the healing process.

Perhaps the best way to find a balance between too much and too little health care is to establish a physician-patient relationship with a general practitioner. The general practitioner may be a family practice physician or an internist who specializes in internal medicine.

Visit your doctor while you are in good health. This permits your doctor to serve as a facilitator of wellness and provides him or her with a benchmark for interpreting symptoms when they occur.

A second important way to balance health care is to trust your instincts. Nobody knows when something is wrong with your body better than you do. Health and illness are subject to a wide variation in interpretation. If you are attuned to your body, you are your own best expert for recognizing signs and symptoms of illness.

Several signs and symptoms warrant medical attention without question. Internal bleeding, as shown by blood in the urine, bowel movement, sputum, or vomit, or blood from any of the body's openings require immediate attention. Abdominal pain, especially when it is associated with nausea, may indicate a wide range of problems from appendicitis to pelvic inflammatory disease and requires the diagnostic expertise of a physician. A stiff neck when accompanied by a fever may suggest meningitis and justifies immediate medical intervention. Injuries, many first aid emergencies, and severe disabling symptoms require prompt medical care[7] (see Just the Facts: When a Cut or Scrape Requires a Doctor at **www.mhhe.com/anspaugh5e** Student Center, Chapter 15, Just the Facts).

There is debate about when medical care is needed in the case of fever. An elevated temperature may be a sign that the body's immune system is responding to an infection and working to destroy pathogens or disease-producing organisms. If left untreated for an extended time, a fever may cause harm to sensitive tissues in the body, such as connective tissue found in joints and tissues in the valves of the heart. Body temperature is generally about 98.6° F. Body temperature varies with exercise, at rest, by climate, and by gender. *Fever* means a reading over 99° F. It is not usually necessary for an adult to seek medical care for a fever. Home treatment in the form of aspirin, acetaminophen, and sponge baths usually lowers fever. You should consult your physician if fever remains above 101° F despite your actions or, in the case of a low-grade fever (99° F to 100° F), if there is no improvement in seventy-two hours.[8] You should consult a physician if fever lasts more than five days, regardless of improvement. Some ailments such as sore throat, ear pain, diarrhea, urinary problems, and skin rash may be the cause of a fever and should be treated. Fever in young children should be discussed with a physician.

Unintended weight loss may trigger a doctor's visit. Some people's weight loss fluctuates more than others. But if you haven't been trying to lose weight and you lose weight outside your normal fluctuations, consult your physician. It might signify any number of problems such as thyroid problems, diabetes, cancer, or depression.[9]

Persistent heartburn may suggest something more serious than the occasional bout of indigestion. If you take antacids frequently, ulcers, acid reflux, or stomach cancer may be implicated. Seek medical advice.

Headaches are difficult to diagnose and suggest a wide range of conditions ranging from muscle tension to a brain tumor. If you haven't been prone to headaches before—or if you're experiencing a new type of headache—consult with your physician. Seek medical attention without delay if headache pain follows a head injury, occurs only on one side of your head, is made worse by lying down, or occurs together with weakness or numbness. All of these may indicate a significant underlying problem from a brain tumor to a blot clot.[9]

Dizziness may suggest one or more of sixty-four different conditions ranging from drug reactions to inner ear infection.[9] If dizziness is particularly severe or if it interferes with your daily activities, it should be checked by a medical doctor.

Entering a Hospital

A hospital is driven by the goal of saving lives. It may range in size and service from small units that provide general care and low-risk treatments to large, specialized centers offering dramatic and experimental therapies. You may be limited in your choice of a hospital by factors beyond your control, including insurance coverage, your physician's hospital affiliation, and the type of care accessible in your location.

The large majority of Americans benefit from the care and services provided by hospitals. People usually check in, receive treatment, and leave better off than they were when they were admitted. Still, you should be aware of possible dangers. Well-known hospital hazards are unnecessary operations, unexpected drug reactions, harmful or even fatal blunders, and hospital-borne infections. Each year at least half a million hospital patients are harmed or killed by mistakes that doctors, nurses, and other staff members make. Roughly half of those events are preventable. More people die each year from hospital errors than from car crashes, breast cancer, and AIDS combined.[10] One of the greatest dangers that a hospital presents is infection, largely preventable by the most basic of infection-control health practices: hand washing.

What can laypeople do to ensure proper and safe care while in the hospital? The following guidelines should be considered:

- If you have a choice of hospitals, inquire about their accreditation status. Hospitals are subject to inspection to make sure they are in compliance with federal standards.
- Before checking into a hospital, you need to decide on your accommodations. Do you want to pay extra for a single room? Do you want a nonsmoker for a roommate? Do you need a special diet? Do you need a place to store refrigerated medicine? If someone will be staying with you, will he or she need a cot? You should try to avoid going in on a weekend when few procedures are done. When you get to your room, speak up immediately if it is unacceptable.
- You need to be familiar with your rights as a patient (see Just the Facts: Do You Know Your Medical Rights?). Hospitals should provide an information booklet that includes a Patient's Bill of Rights. The booklet will inform you that you have the right to considerate and respectful care; information about tests, drugs, and procedures; dignity; courtesy; respect; and the opportunity to make decisions, including about when to leave the hospital.
- You should make informed decisions. Before authorizing any procedure, you must be informed about your medical condition, treatment options, expected risks, prognosis, and the name of the person in charge of treatment. Your agreement to a procedure based on your having been informed of these matters, is called **informed consent.** The only instances in which hospitals are not required to obtain informed consent are life-threatening emergencies, cases involving unconscious patients when no relatives are present, and compliance with the law or a court order such as those regulating sexually transmitted diseases. If you are asked to sign a consent form, you should read it first. If you want more information, you should ask before signing. If you are skeptical, you have the right to postpone a procedure and discuss it with your doctor.
- Authorization of a medical procedure may be given nonverbally, such as through your appearance at a doctor's office for treatment, your cooperation during the administration of tests, or your failure to object when you could easily refuse consent. Your agreement to a procedure in such situations is called **implied consent.**

~ *Just the Facts* ~

Do You Know Your Medical Rights?

The following is a short list of some of your rights as a patient in the health care system:

- You have the right as a parent to stay with your children during tests and treatments, provided you don't interfere with medical treatment or are not suspected of child abuse.

- You have the right to request that a relative or friend accompany you during a test or treatment or hospitalization unless you're in a semiprivate room.

- You have the right to see your medical records if your state law permits it. Some states allow you to copy parts of your record under certain conditions[11] (see Just the Facts: Are Your Medical Records Yours? at **www.mhhe.com/anspaugh5e** Student Center, Chapter 15, Just the Facts).

- You have the right to emergency care whether you have insurance or not.

- You have the right to refuse to sign any form. The health care provider can also refuse to provide treatment in the absence of your signed authorization.

- You have the right to a second opinion, but your doctor can also stop treating you for challenging him or her.

- You have the right to leave the hospital at any time, even against medical advice or without paying the bill.

- You have the right to refuse or stop any treatment, whether or not it is experimental.

- You have the right to an itemized, detailed bill for all medical services.

- You have the right to know the results of all tests unless the doctor has reason to believe that the information will be harmful (for example, cause you to commit suicide).

~ *Just the Facts* ~

"Brown Bag Solution" to Polypharmacy Problems

Polypharmacy refers to the administration of many drugs at the same time. Prescribed indiscriminately the combined interaction of multiple drugs has the potential to cause problems that are worse than the disease being treated. Studies indicate that nearly 75 percent of doctors caring for older people taking four or more medications are unaware of all the drugs their patients are taking. One out of five hospitalizations is linked to drug side effects.[31] Many factors contribute to polypharmacy:

1. Patients' expectations that a doctor's visit ends with a prescription. Seventy-five percent of patients who see a doctor go home with a prescription.[12]
2. Direct marketing of prescription drugs.
3. Increase use of herbs and supplements that interact with medicines.
4. Many people go to several doctors and pharmacies at the same time. No one claims ownerships for the overall administration of medicines.
5. Many people save unused medicines and take them on their own when symptoms return.
6. Side effects from one drug may lead to the prescription of another drug and promote a vicious cycle of multiple drug use.

What can patients do to prevent complications from polypharmacy? Some experts suggest a "brown bag" approach, in which patients put all their pills, including vitamins, in a bag and bring them to the doctor for review. Even if you always see the same doctor, a periodic review of what you take can help prevent polypharmacy problems.[12]

You need to weigh the risks of drug therapy (see Just the Facts! "Brown Bag" Solution to Polypharmacy Problems), X-ray examinations, and laboratory tests against their expected beneficial results. When tests or treatments are ordered, you should ask about their purpose, possible risks, and possible actions if a test finds that something is wrong. Finally, you should inquire about prescribed drugs. Avoid taking drugs, including pain and sleeping medication, unless you feel confident of their benefits and are aware of their hazards. This is particularly true for antibiotics, which in general have been overprescribed to the point that some bacteria no

longer respond to their use. Your chances of harboring drug-resistant bacteria are greater if you have taken many antibiotics or have not taken them as prescribed. Even if you have never had an antibiotic, you can still acquire drug-resistant bacteria from others.[13]

When scheduled for surgery, prepare for anesthesia. In rare cases, general anesthesia can cause brain damage and death. One cause of such catastrophes is vomiting while unconscious. To reduce the risk, refuse any food or drink that may be offered by mistake during the eight hours before surgery.[10]

You need to know who is in charge of your care and record his or her office number and note when you can expect a visit. If your doctor is transferring your care to someone else, you need to know who it

Wellness On the Web
Behavior Change Activities

How Can You Choose Quality Health Care?

If you're like most people, you want the best health care available—but you may not know how to evaluate the quality of care you're receiving. The Agency for Health Care Policy and Research (AHCPR), a part of the U.S. Department of Health and Human Services, is the lead agency charged with supporting research designed to improve the quality of health care, reduce its cost, and broaden access to essential services. AHCPR's research programs bring practical, science-based information to medical practitioners as well as consumers and other health care purchasers. The agency has published "Your Guide to Choosing Quality Health Care," which shows how you can rate the quality of health care services you and your family receive. It describes quality measures, including consumer ratings, clinical performance measures, and accreditation—what they are, where to find them, and how to use them. The Guide has checklists, questions, charts, and other tools to help you make the health care decisions that are right for you. Take a moment to read about this information, which you'll find online at **www.mhhe.com/anspaugh5e**, "Student Center," "Chapter 15," "Wellness on the Web," and "Activity 1."

Choosing a Physician Who's Right for You

The most important factor in the quality of health care you receive is your personal physician, or primary-care provider. At certain times in your life, you may need to choose a physician. You may have moved recently or perhaps have a new health care plan that doesn't work with your provider. You may have become dissatisfied with your current physician and want to make a switch. Whatever the reason, selecting a new physician can be a daunting task if you're unsure where to begin. How do you know who's right for you or your family if all you have to go on is a list of names? You could just call a doctor's office at random and make an appointment, but chances are you'll make a better choice if you do a little homework up front. Go to the website listed previously and click on "Activity 2" to learn more about choosing a physician who's right for you.

What Insurance Coverage Meets Your Needs?

The search for quality medical care can be challenging—and so can the search for comprehensive yet affordable health insurance. The cost of health care in the United States is high and continues to escalate. Few Americans can afford the cost of medicines, physicians' fees, or hospitalization without some form of health insurance. Health insurance is a contract between an insurance company and an individual or group for the payment of medical care costs. Choosing health coverage can be a complex and confusing task, because health plans differ greatly in services performed, choice of providers, and out-of-pocket costs. The more you know, the easier it will be for you to decide what insurance plan best fits your personal needs and budget. Go to the website listed previously and click on "Activity 3" to learn more about choosing a plan that meets your needs.

---

is. If your doctor is not available and you do not know what is happening, you can ask for the nurse in charge of your case.

You should keep a daily log of procedures, medicines, and doctor visits. When you get your bill, compare each item with your written record. Insist on an itemized bill.

You should stay active within the limits of your medical problem. Many body functions begin to suffer from just a few days' inactivity. Moving about, walking, bending, and contracting muscles help to clear body fluids, reduce the risk of infections (especially in the lungs), and minimize the stress of hospital procedures, which can add to the depression and malaise of hospitalization.

Ask questions until you know all you need to know. Know the three Ps: Be polite, be pleasant, and most of all be persistent. According to some experts, the best way to avert hospital errors can be summarized in two words: "Speak up!"[14] The more you assert yourself and the more questions you ask, the fewer mistakes that will result.

Insist that hospital workers who enter your room wash their hands for at least 15 seconds with soap in your presence. Infectious disease control experts suggest that this is one of the most important things a patient can do to prevent the spread of infection. Concern for this basic hygiene measure takes on added importance when patients are subjected to invasive diagnostic procedures and/or surgery.

Selecting a Health Care Professional

Choosing a physician for your general health care is an important and necessary duty. Only physicians are discussed here, but this information applies to the selection of all health care practitioners. You must select one who will listen carefully to your problems and diagnose them accurately. At the same time, you need a physician who can move you through the modern medical maze of technology and specialists (see Just the Facts: Selected Health Care Specialists [Allopathic]).

Just the Facts

Selected Health Care Specialists (Allopathic)

The following lists show the fields of specialty of selected health care specialists:

Name of specialist	Field of specialty
Medical specialists	
Allergist	Allergic conditions
Anesthesiologist	Administration of anesthesia (such as during surgery)
Cardiologist	Coronary artery disease, heart disease
Dermatologist	Skin conditions
Endocrinologist	Diseases of the endocrine system
Epidemiologist	Study of the causes and sources of disease
Family practice physician	General care physician
Gastroenterologist	Stomach, intestines, digestive system
Geriatrician	Diseases and conditions of the aged
Gynecologist	Female reproductive system
Hematologist	Study of blood
Immunologist	Diseases of the immune system
Internist	Treatment of diseases in adults
Neonatologist	Newborns
Nephrologist	Kidney disease
Neurologist	Nervous system
Neurosurgeon	Surgery of the brain and nervous system
Obstetrician	Pregnancy, labor, childbirth
Oncologist	Cancer, tumors
Ophthalmologist	Eyes
Orthopedist	Skeletal system
Otolaryngologist	Head, neck, ears, nose, throat
Otologist	Ears
Pathologist	Study of tissues and the essential nature of disease
Pediatrician	Childhood diseases and conditions
Plastic surgeon	Use of material to alter or rebuild tissues
Primary-care physician	General health and medical care
Proctologist	Disorders of the rectum and anus
Psychiatrist	Mental illnesses
Radiologist	Use of X-rays
Rheumatologist	Diseases of connective tissues, joints, muscles, tendons
Rhinologist	Nose
Surgeon	Surgery
Urologist	Urinary tracts of men and women and reproductive organs of men
Dental Specialists	
Dentist	General care of teeth and oral cavity
Endodontist	Diseases of teeth below the gum line (root canal therapy)
Orthodontist	Teeth alignment, malocclusion
Pedodontist	Dental care of children
Periodontist	Diseases of supporting structures
Prosthodontist	Construction of artificial appliances for the mouth

For most people, good health care means having a **primary-care physician,** a professional who assists you as you assume responsibility for your overall health and directs you when specialized care is necessary. Your primary-care physician should be familiar with your complete medical history as well as your home, work, and other environments. You will be better understood in periods of sickness if your physician has also seen you during periods of wellness.

For adults, primary-care physicians are usually family practitioners, once called "general practitioners," and internists, specialists in internal medicine. Pediatricians often serve as primary-care physicians for children. Obstetricians and gynecologists, who specialize in pregnancy, childbirth, and diseases of the female reproductive system, often serve as primary-care physicians to women. General surgeons may offer primary care in addition to the surgery they perform. In some states, osteopathic physicians also practice family medicine.

There are several sources of information about physicians in your area:

- Local and state medical societies can identify doctors by specialty and tell you a doctor's basic credentials. You should check on the doctor's hospital affiliation and make sure the hospital is accredited. Another sign of standing is the type of societies in which the doctor has membership. The qualifications of a surgeon, for example, are enhanced by a fellowship in the American College of Surgeons (abbreviated as FACS after the surgeon's name). An internist fellowship in the American College of Physicians is abbreviated FACP. Membership in academies indicates physicians' special interests.
- All physicians board certified in the United States are listed in the *American Medical Directory* published by the American Medical Association and available in larger libraries.
- The American Board of Medical Specialists (ABMS) publishes the *Compendium of Certified Medical Specialties* (**www.ama-assn.org**), which lists physicians by name, specialty, and location.
- Pharmacists can be asked to recommend names.
- Hospitals can give you names of staff physicians who also practice in the community.
- Local medical schools can identify faculty members who also practice privately.
- The American College of Surgeons (**www.facs.org**) can identify doctors who are a fellow of the college. This suggests that the surgeon has passed a peer-reviewed evaluation and is staying current with the latest developments in his or her field.
- Many colleges and universities have health centers that keep lists of physicians for student referral.
- Friends may have recommendations, but you should allow for the possibility that your opinion of a doctor may differ from theirs.
- Detailed reports on doctors including credentials, degrees, and possible disciplinary actions and malpractice judgments are available on line (**www.consumerinfocentral.com**) for a fee. You can also check your state department of health website for information on licensure for all health professionals.

Once you have identified a leading candidate, you can make an appointment. You need to check with the office staff about office hours, availability of emergency care at night or on weekends, backup doctors, procedures when you call for advice, hospital affiliation, and payment and insurance procedures. You should schedule your first visit while in good health. Once you have seen your doctor, reflect on the following: Did the doctor seem to be listening to you? Were your questions answered? Was a medical history taken? Were you informed of possible side effects of drugs or tests? Was respect shown for your need of privacy? Was the doctor open to the suggestion of a second opinion?

Patient-physician communication

Most doctors are not disinterested in you, but they are busy—so busy that many patients complain that their doctors cannot or will not listen to them. There isn't much time to state your problem: Doctor visits last 18 minutes on average.[15] This is a problem because, according to the American Society of Internal Medicine, correct diagnoses depend largely on what you tell your doctor. Patients who do not speak up and who do not insist on being heard may get plenty of medical advice and prescription drugs, but they do not necessarily get the best results. Studies have shown that patients trained to ask questions, interrupt when necessary, and explain how their symptoms affect their lives have better health outcomes than those who are passive. Research also shows that better communication between patients and doctors can lead to a more accurate diagnosis, fewer tests, increased adherence to treatment, and greater satisfaction with care. Patients who report that their doctors communicate well are more likely to say their conditions improved than those who feel their doctors communicate poorly.[15] (See Assessment Activity 15-1.)

Patients can do much to facilitate the development of a physician-patient partnership. Understanding the meaning of commonly used medical words, abbreviations, suffixes, and prefixes can enhance this communication (see Just the Facts: Communicating with Health Care Professionals). The following are some tips to ensure good communication:

- When you see your physician about a problem, you should state the most important problem first. Doctors tend to believe that the first thing a patient says is most important.
- You should be specific. If you have a headache, where does it hurt? How long does it last? How often does it occur?
- You should know your family history. Because many illnesses run in families, you may be at higher risk for certain diseases. Before your first visit, you should contact your parents and close relatives to learn of their health problems, especially heart disease, cancer, stroke, arthritis, diabetes, alcoholism, and tuberculosis.

Just the Facts

Communicating with Health Care Professionals

Here are some words, abbreviations, suffixes, and prefixes often used in health and medical care.

Term	Meaning
A (prefix)	Without
Aberration	Different from normal action
Acute	A condition that occurs suddenly
Adult	Developed fully
Affinity	Attraction
-algia (suffix)	Pain in
Angio- (prefix)	Vessels (veins or arteries)
Arrest	Stopping, restraining
Arthr- (prefix)	Joint related
Asymptomatic	Without symptoms
Bowel	Intestine
BP	Blood pressure
Cardiac (cardio-)	Relating to the heart
Carpo (prefix)	Wrist
CAT	Computerized assisted X-ray
CCU	Coronary care unit
Chronic	A condition that occurs for a long time
Coma	Complete loss of consciousness
Congenital	Existing at or before birth
Contraindication	A reason for not prescribing a drug, procedure, or treatment
Coronary	Relating to the heart
CVA	Cerebrovascular accident (stroke)
Degenerative	Deterioration of a part of the body
Diagnosis	Determining of a disease
Dilation	Stretching, increase in size
Distention	Widening or enlargement
DO	Doctor of osteopathy
Dose	Amount of medication to be given at one time
Dys (prefix)	Bad, difficult
Dysfunction	Impairment of function
Edema	Swelling from accumulation of fluid
EEG	Electroencephalogram
EKG, ECG	Electrocardiogram
Embolus	Blood clot floating free in the bloodstream
Emia- (prefix)	In the blood
Endemic	Disease prevalent in a particular area
Entero- (prefix)	Intestine
Epidemic	Disease prevalence that is higher than normal
ER/ED	Emergency room/emergency department
Etiology	Reference to the cause of a disease
Extra- (prefix)	Outside of
Gastr- (prefix)	Stomach
GP	General practitioner

continued

Just the Facts

continued

Term	Meaning
Hem- (prefix)	Blood
Hemorrhage	Bleeding
Hyper- (prefix)	Excessive
Hypo- (prefix)	Insufficient
Indication	Condition that leads to a prescribed drug, procedure, or treatment
ICU	Intensive care unit
Innate	Hereditary, congenital
Innocuous	Harmless
Insidious	Refers to a disease that does not show early symptoms of its advent
-ism (suffix)	Condition, theory, method
-itis (suffix)	Inflammation
IV	Intravenous (within a vein)
Jaundiced	Yellow
Macro	Large
Mal (prefix)	Bad, deficient
Malady	Illness
Malaise	Uneasiness
MD	Medical doctor
MI	Myocardial infarction
Micro (prefix)	Small
MRI	Magnetic resonance imaging
Myo- (prefix)	Muscle
Nephro- (prefix)	Kidney
-opothy (suffix)	Cause unknown
Pandemic	Disease that is prevalent over a large region
Pernicious	Severe, fatal
Phag- (prefix)	To eat
Philia (suffix)	Attraction, affinity
Presby (prefix)	Old
Primary	Principal, most important
Prognosis	Medical outlook of a disease
Pulmo- (prefix)	Lung
Renal	Kidney
Sepsis	Infection
Sign	Something tangible that can be observed
Stenosis	Constricted, decreasing in size
Symptom	Intangible evidence of a disease
Symptomatic	Relating to symptoms
Syndrome	Set of symptoms that occur together for unknown causes
Systemic	Affecting all systems of the body
Thrombus	Solid blood clot
TIA	Transient ischemic attack
TPR	Temperature, pulse, respiration
Trauma	Injury from external force
Tumor	Growth
Uria (suffix)	Urine, urination

In an effort to assume responsibility for their own health care, people sometimes go too far. This is especially true for older people—those over 65 years of age—who are taking medications, both over-the-counter and prescription drugs. Common mistakes include the following: (1) taking larger doses of over-the-counter medicines than called for on the label; (2) mixing different types of medicines, both over-the-counter and prescription, without understanding the potential impact of taking two different drugs at the same time (such as analgesics and alcohol); and (3) taking someone else's medicine.

The risks and potential dangers for self-medication mistakes increase for the elderly. Drug companies typically set dosages for new drugs high enough to be effective for 90 percent of the intended population. Many times this dosage is too high even for people under age 65, and for those over 65, the risk of harmful side effects increases significantly.[18] Three characteristics are used to determine dosages by drug companies: (1) how much of the drug is absorbed into the bloodstream from the intestine; (2) how much of the drug is broken down in the body; and (3) how quickly the drug is eliminated from the body. The tests used to determine these characteristics are usually completed on

Wellness Across the Generations
Older Adults Can Go Too Far with Self-Care

healthy, young volunteers with healthy, young intestines, livers, and kidneys.

Unfortunately, as humans age, their organs tend to decline in function and the processes responsible for eliminating drugs decrease, thus allowing an "overloading" effect on the user. This problem is made worse when an elderly person is taking more than one type of drug, as many elderly people do. The more drugs ingested, the greater the possibility of drug interactions. Drug interactions can increase the potency of a drug, render it ineffective, or cause other side effects that might be life threatening. Older people in particular seem to be highly sensitive to drugs that affect the central nervous system, such as tranquilizers, antidepressants, and sleeping pills. Generally, older people are at increased risk for side effects if they are taking antidepressants, arthritis medications, blood thinners, dementia drugs, diabetes drugs, muscle relaxants, pain relievers, or sedatives or tranquilizers.[18]

To avoid potential overdoses, elderly patients should make both the physician and the pharmacist aware of all medications being taken so that more appropriate dosages can be prescribed and closer monitoring of effects can occur.

You need to list medications and treatments you are receiving, including over-the-counter drugs. The possibility of overdosing on either prescription or over-the-counter drugs is a growing problem, especially for older people—those over 65 years of age (see Wellness Across the Generations: Older Adults Can Go Too Far with Self-Care).[16] You will also need to identify any allergies and drug reactions. Remember the "brown bag" approach to polypharmacy.

You should tell about dietary supplements including herbs, vitamins, and minerals. Just because supplements are advertised as "natural" doesn't mean they're safe. Like drugs, supplements can have side effects and interact with each other and medicines.

You should ask questions. You can bring a written list of questions but try to make them brief and specific. You should ask about anything that is unclear and repeat the answers in your own words.

Before leaving the doctor's office, you need to make certain you know the diagnosis or how to follow the recommended treatment. If drugs are prescribed, you should inquire about the possible con-traindications (reasons for not using a drug), side effects, and generic substitutions.

When appropriate, ask your physician to write down instructions or recommend reading material for more information on a particular subject. Finally, inquire about the next steps in the treatment, if and when a return visit is required, and danger signs to look for and report to your physician.

Second opinions

Chronic pain, recurring illnesses, and conditions involving elective surgery often benefit from a second opinion. A second opinion is often appropriate and peace of mind is a sufficient reason for seeking it.

In some cases, such as elective surgery, your health insurer may require a second or third opinion before authorizing payment for certain treatments. (See Real-World Wellness: How to Get a Second Opinion for advice on getting a second opinion.)

If you decide to ask for a second opinion, common courtesy dictates that you discuss it with your physician.

Real-World Wellness

How to Get a Second Opinion

I am considering elective surgery and want a second opinion. What are some good sources for referral?

Here are some options for finding second opinions:

• Ask your primary-care physician for the names of two or three experts in the field.

• Call a medical center or hospital and ask to talk to the chief of surgery for a surgical opinion or to the chief of medicine for a nonsurgical question.

• Call the county medical society.

• Call the Second Surgical Opinion Hotline (800-638-6833) for medical organizations, which provides referrals on surgical questions.

• Call Health Benefits Research Corporation, which offers a Second Opinion Hotline (800-522-0036, 800-631-1220 in New York) and referral service. Consultation with a board-certified specialist is available for a fee.

• Call the American Board of Medical Specialists to determine if the opinion you're getting is from a board-certified physician. The number is 800-776-CERT.

Your physician may suggest bringing in a consultant to assess your situation and discuss it with you and your physician. You can also ask your physician for the name of someone to see separately.

A physician may feel that a second opinion is a waste of time or money. Regardless, your wish for more information should be respected. Reputable physicians do not feel threatened by another opinion; to the contrary, they may welcome another perspective on a difficult case. If your physician expresses displeasure for or resists your wish to have a second opinion, you may want to consider looking for another doctor.

Alternative Medicine

Alternative medicine, also called *complementary medicine* or *integrative medicine,* is the body of therapies not taught in U.S. medical schools and generally unavailable from doctors or hospitals.[17] More than 40 percent of the public—and half of people ages 35 to 49—have tried alternative medical therapy despite the skepticism of many providers of traditional medical care (also called *allopathic* medicine, which refers to the treatment of diseases using scientifically proven and established measures).[17] These therapies vary consid-

erably in their approach and include herbal medicine, biofeedback, magnetic therapy, light therapy, sound therapy, reflexology, and prayer therapy, among others (see Just the Facts: Alternative Medicine at **www.mhhe.com/anspaugh5e** Student Center, Chapter 15, Just the Facts).

Proponents of alternative medicine acknowledge that allopathic medicine is superb when it comes to surgery, emergency, and trauma. But they claim that alternative approaches work better for almost everything else, especially chronic degenerative diseases, because they focus on prevention and target causes rather than symptoms. Many alternative methods are thought to work by helping the body heal itself instead of by introducing strong drugs often to compensate for the side effects of other drugs.[18]

Skeptics of alternative medicine claim that its effectiveness has not been proven and worry about the indiscriminate use of some therapies. They offer numerous reasons for their concerns:[19]

• Patients often delay starting conventional medical treatment that has a proven track record to try an alternative approach touted as a miracle cure.

• There is the false perception that "natural" remedies are risk free. Many herbal medicines may negate the effects of important medicines. St. John's Wort, for example, affects the action of drugs like warfarin (Coumadin), the anti-clotting drug, and indinavir (Crixivan), an AIDS drug. Ginkgo biloba and ginseng interact with warfarin; kava interacts with sedatives. These interactions aren't monitored closely because the FDA has little authority over alternative medicines.[20]

• There is a lack of evidence from scientifically controlled studies that demonstrate a therapy's effectiveness to make good on its promise.

• Proponents tend to rely on anecdotal records (isolated incidents) and testimonials to promote therapies.

• Because herbs and vitamins are processed and excreted primarily by the liver and kidneys, as are most drugs, they can cause serious drug interactions with prescription and over-the-counter medications.

Many health problems, such as chronic pain, lower-back problems, and stress-related problems such as anxiety and insomnia, don't respond well to conventional medical approaches. If at first conventional treatments aren't effective, alternative therapies may offer some benefit. If you consider using a form of alternative medicine, experts recommend you do the following:[21]

• Keep a diary to track symptoms. Writing down when symptoms begin and when they abate is a good way to determine if there is an association between treatment and relief.

- Add one therapy at a time. It is hard to know which therapy may be helping and which may be causing side effects when multiple therapies are used. Use the diary to track one treatment at a time.
- Discuss alternative therapies with your conventional physician. Potential interactions between conventional and alternative therapies can cause serious health problems.
- Discuss conventional therapies with your alternative physician. If an alternative physician suggests discontinuing a drug, check with your conventional physician first.

Assessing Your Health

Many tests, procedures, gadgets, and machines assess various aspects of health and wellness. They range from the hands-on physical examination to the use of sophisticated diagnostic tests.

The Physical Examination

Until recently the annual physical examination was viewed as a normal and necessary part of health care. Now, considerable debate exists among medical experts as to who needs a physical examination, how often it is needed, and what it should include. The emphasis today is on the use of selective health examinations and periodic examinations. **Selective health examinations** are specific tests used for specific problems. The assumption of this approach is that tests are more useful if they are matched to specific complaints. **Periodic examinations** are assessments given according to age, health habits, predisposition for certain conditions, and/or risk factors.

The periodic exam includes only those tests warranted by the information coming from a thorough medical history and discussion of those lifestyle factors related to diseases. The assumption is that behavior and habits are the best criteria for predicting disease risk.

Criticisms of the comprehensive annual physical examination for a healthy adult are not meant to undermine the doctor-patient relationship. They simply cast doubt about the efficacy of the physical examination. However, this does not nullify the value of regular visits to the doctor. To the contrary, seeing a physician for a limited examination at regular intervals can be good preventive medicine.

How often?

The need for a complete physical exam depends on a person's age, health, and lifestyle. People over the age of 45 benefit from a checkup every year. People in good health and under the age of 45 should see their physicians for routine tests at least every two years.[22]

Regardless of their age, people with family histories of heart disease, stroke, high blood pressure, cancer, and diabetes can benefit from periodic checkups, even if they are in good health. The same is true for people whose health habits or occupations put them at higher than normal risk for chronic diseases and disabling conditions. Even in these cases, good judgment and discretion should rule the choice of tests to be included in the physical examination.

Components

The three basic tools for completing a physical examination are medical history, hands-on examination, and diagnostic/laboratory tests.

A medical history is the most important part of the physical examination, especially during the first visit with your physician.[23] This includes information about health habits, lifestyle, family history, and symptoms. Many physicians use health-risk appraisals, detailed questionnaires that provide information about health habits. This is one area of the physical examination for which a patient can prepare. By following the guidelines for communicating with your physician presented earlier in this chapter, you can help your physician obtain an accurate health profile.

The hands-on examination is the second part of the physical examination. It consists of touching, looking, and listening. Physicians can feel or palpate for enlarged glands, growths, and tumors with procedures such as the breast examination, pelvic examination, rectal examination, and hernia examination. Thumping the back and chest lets the physician know whether any fluid has built up in or around the lungs. Tapping a knee for reflexes may reveal nervous system damage. A stethoscope is used to listen to the heart, lungs, abdomen, and glands located near the surface of the skin. Possible problems that can be detected with the stethoscope range from a heart murmur to poor circulation, lung infection, intestinal blockage, and an overactive thyroid gland.

Physicians have access to a number of instruments to visually inspect for problems. An ophthalmoscope is used to view the brain through the eye. The first sign of some brain diseases is an unhealthy-looking optic nerve. Leakage in the blood vessels of the eye may be a sign of diabetes or hypertension. An otoscope is used to inspect the ear, particularly the tympanic membrane. The proctoscope and sigmoidoscope are used to examine the rectum and colon. The laryngoscope and bronchoscope provide a look at the larynx and bronchial tubes.

The last part of the physical examination includes **diagnostic laboratory tests,** which may vary from a simple urinalysis to invasive dye tests. The effectiveness of these tests is being debated. Tests conducted for specific symptoms may be invaluable in pinpointing disabling conditions. They may be just as valuable for what they do not reveal as they are for what they do reveal. This can be reassuring to the patient and physician. On the negative side, many physicians rely too heavily on laboratory tests. Patients often demand or acquiesce to more tests than are necessary and sometimes than are good for them.

Many times tests are recommended more for the purpose of protecting the doctor against medical malpractice suits than for their diagnostic value. This practice, called **defensive medicine,** paints a sobering picture of the difficulty in making medical decisions for doctors and patients. A doctor may know with 99 percent certainty a particular diagnosis but order a test or procedure anyway as protection against liability should he or she be sued later. Malpractice suits are a reality; over 1 million hospital patients will suffer an injury as the result of a medical mistake. More than 10 percent of these patients die, partly as the result of the mistake.[24] To avoid the threat of a malpractice lawsuit it is not unusual for physicians to order a battery of extra tests. Of course, patients always have the right to decline prescribed tests. The decision must be made by patient and doctor and should be based on the test's potential for contributing to an effective medical intervention.

Thus, when you go for a physical examination, you can determine which tests you are willing to be subjected to by asking the right questions:

- *What do you expect to find?* You should start by asking why you need the test. How will it help facilitate a diagnosis? You need to ask about alternatives and the disadvantage of waiting and not testing. Sometimes the best test is the test of time. Agreeing to a test because it is routine procedure is not a satisfactory explanation.
- *What risks are associated with the test?* No test is risk free; you should compare potential benefits and risks.

One problem with tests is that they are not 100 percent accurate. An inaccurate result can lead to a wrong diagnosis. A **false positive,** in which a test incorrectly reveals an abnormality, may occur. False positives provoke needless anxiety, causing some people to feel and even act sick. Conversely, normal results do not necessarily indicate good health. A **false negative** in which a test indicates normality even though a person is sick, may occur. These results may lead to a false sense of health and may delay much-needed treatment at critical stages of a disease.

Statistically, test results are accurate for about 95 percent of the population. Thus, 5 percent of patients can be expected to have false positives or false negatives on any laboratory tests. Other factors that may cause test errors are the taking of certain medications, exercise,

stress, diet, time of day, and mistakes in handling or processing specimens.

Another problem with tests is that they may involve physical risks. Some of the more common risks are infection; bleeding; damage to vital structures; and reactions to anesthetics, drugs, and dye-contrast materials. Again, it is important to ask questions.

- *What are the options after the test?* If a test is positive, then what? If none of the options is plausible to you, why have the test administered? If it is impossible to treat a disease that a test reveals, the test is not justified. The diagnosis of a treatable disease, on the other hand, usually justifies the test.
- *What is the value of the test?* This question need not be perceived as confrontational. If approached with sincerity and courtesy, discussions about the physical examination in general and laboratory tests in particular can serve as a basis for forming an active partnership with your physician in making decisions about your health care.

Common Diagnostic Laboratory Tests

Americans are having many diagnostic tests performed. Home medical tests, available from most pharmacies, allow you to monitor a growing list of medical conditions including high blood pressure, high body temperature, asthma, allergies, urinary tract infections, pregnancy, diabetes mellitus, colon cancer, cholesterol, and HIV infection. The tests should not be viewed as substitutes for your doctor. The accuracy rates and reliability of over-the-counter medical kits vary considerably, and their instructions do not always explain how to interpret the results. These tests procedures are also subject to human error, but they provide a useful way to get involved in your health care.

Some other inexpensive items should be included in your medicine cabinet (see Just the Facts: Essentials for Your Medicine Cabinet). These items should help you cope with most common minor aches and pains.

Depending on your health status, gender, age, symptoms, and risk for a disease, some of the more common tests may be recommended when you go to your physician for a checkup.

Multiple blood screening tests check for high blood sugar, which indicates diabetes; blood urea nitrogen, an indicator of kidney function; an overactive parathyroid gland; blood count, a screen for anemia; and much more (see Assessment Activity 15-2).

Blood cholesterol screening is recommended every five years for women 45 to 65 and men 35 to 65.[22] The test should measure total cholesterol, lipoprotein, and triglyceride levels. (See Chapter 2 for a thorough discussion of cholesterol and lipoprotein.)

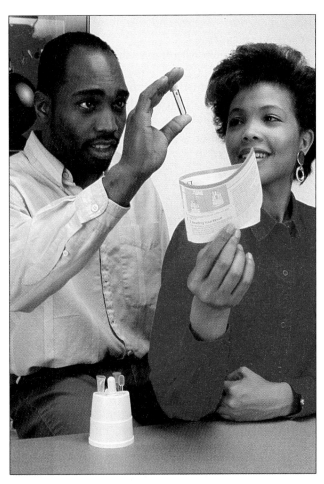

Self-care medical kits, such as home pregnancy tests, allow you to become more involved with your health care.

Fecal occult-blood tests, also called *hemoccult tests*, are used to detect hidden blood in bowel movements. If a test is positive, it may indicate signs of an early cancer of the colon. People over 50 should either test themselves (home screening kits are available in most pharmacies) or have their stools tested for blood every year.[28] (See Just the Facts: Fecal Occult-Blood Tests: Reducing False Positives at **www.mhhe.com/anspaugh5e** Student Center, Chapter 15, Just the Facts.)

Pulse rate may be an indicator of a health problem. The normal resting heart rate is between 60 and 80 beats a minute. Resting heart rates above 80 beats per minute put a person in a higher risk category for heart attacks and sudden death. The high heart rate does not increase the risk but is an indicator of basic problems, such as cigarette smoking, too much caffeine, stress, anxiety, hyperthyroidism, and most commonly a poor level of physical fitness.

Slow heart rates are normally found in physically fit people; in them slow heart rates are a sign of good health. Very slow rates below 50 beats per minute can

occur in people who are not fit and who have heart problems. These people should seek medical advice.

Blood pressure measurements should be monitored regularly, especially for people who have had previously high readings or have family histories of hypertension (high blood pressure). Inexpensive, accurate home blood pressure kits can be purchased at most drugstores. Because all kits are not equally reliable, you should ask your pharmacist for a recommendation. People who have measurements higher than 140 over 90 mmHg or lower than 100 over 60 mmHg should keep records of their blood pressure and present them to their physicians during periodic checkups.

Mammography, an X-ray examination of the breast, detects early signs of breast cancer. Women 50 and older should get mammograms yearly; for women between 40 to 49, a mammogram every one to two years is recommended.[22] High-risk women may be advised to have mammograms more often and at an earlier age.

Pelvic examinations and *Pap smears* detect abnormalities of the ovaries, uterus, and cervix. Pap smears should be performed annually for three years beginning at age 18 or the age of first intercourse. If they are normal, they may be performed every two to three years thereafter.[22] Pap smears should not be done during the menstrual period. The test is more accurate during the first half of the cycle if oral contraceptives are taken. Midcycle is preferred in most other menstruating women.

A complete *eye examination* includes a test for visual acuity; *tonometry,* a painless test for glaucoma; and a cataract check. The American Academy of Ophthalmology recommends a complete eye examination from puberty to age 40 only if eye discomfort or vision problems occur. After age 40 a glaucoma test and cataract (a clouding over the lens) check should be done every two to three years.

Electrocardiograms (ECGs) are used to detect irregularities of the heart. Although there is some debate about the use of ECGs as routine screening procedures for *asymptomatic* (without symptoms) low-risk people, periodic ECG readings starting at age 40 are recommended.[25] Chest pain, hypertension, and symptoms of cardiovascular disease justify earlier ECGs. *Stress tests* use ECGs to assess how the heart functions under the stress of exercise. They are routine when symptoms are present.

Chest X-ray examinations are valuable diagnostic tools for people with chest symptoms, respiratory diseases, and heart problems. For people without symptoms, their routine use is questionable. Several groups of experts, including those associated with the Food and Drug Administration, recommend discontinuation of routine chest X-ray examinations.[26] However, if you go to a hospital or often visit a doctor's office, you can anticipate a chest X-ray study more out of the need to comply with business policy than for diagnostic potential. Avoid a chest X-ray test if you may be pregnant.

Prostate cancer tests detect prostate cancer, a leading cause of cancer among men. Men 40 years and older should have an annual digital rectal examination. Combined with a blood test that looks for prostate-specific antigens (PSA), the digital examination significantly improves the chances of detecting early signs of cancer. The blood test for PSA should be performed annually on men starting at age 50 (45 for African Americans).[22,23] Because not all experts endorse this procedure, discuss the advantages and disadvantages of annual PSAs with your physician.

An *HIV test* is recommended for people who think they may have been infected with the HIV virus. This includes people who have had unprotected sex or a blood transfusion, have used IV drugs, or have participated in high-risk behaviors. After the blood test, these people should avoid high-risk behavior for six months to a year and then retest.

A *sigmoidoscopy* involves the insertion of a flexible viewing scope into the lower bowel to check for colorectal cancer. It should be performed every three to five years, starting at age 50.[22]

A visual *skin test* for skin cancer is recommended every three years for people 20 to 39 and annually for people over 40. An annual skin examination performed by a dermatologist is important for anyone with a history of many moles, pale skin, and a family history of melanoma.

A fasting *blood glucose test* is recommended to detect diabetes mellitus. The test requires a small blood sample following a twelve-hour fast. It is recommended for people with symptoms of diabetes, including excessive thirst and frequent urination, people who are overweight, and those who have strong family histories of the disease.

A *bone density* test detects bone thinning and/or loss and is recommended for women over age 65 or if beyond menopause at any age and at high risk for osteoporosis. The test involves the use of an X-ray type machine at two sites: spine and hip. Test results are reported in terms of a T-Score that describes how much bone density varies from what's considered normal. "Normal" is based on the typical bone mass of people in their 30s, when bone mass is at its peak.[27] (See Just the Facts: Interpreting Your T-Score.)

Ultrasound, also known as sonography, is a reliable, radiation-free imaging technique that can detect blood clots, assess heart valve and muscle function (*echocardiogram*), and determine the size and development of the developing fetus. Although ultrasound is useful in detecting fetal abnormalities, the American College of Obstetricians and Gynecologists has advised against its routine use in pregnancy.[27]

Immunizations for Adults

Many people believe that **immunizations** (administrations of preparations or vaccines, usually in the form of injections, for providing immunity or preventing a disease) are only for children. Consequently, many thousands of adults die every year of diseases they would not have acquired if they had received standard vaccines. For example, 60,000 people die prematurely each year because they fail to get pneumonia vaccines.[30] Adult immunization is recommended to prevent or ameliorate influenza, pneumonia, some forms of hepatitis, measles, rubella (German measles), tetanus, diphtheria, and chicken pox.

People born between 1957 and 1970 may need to be reimmunized for measles, mumps, and rubella (MMR) because the earlier vaccine may not have provided complete coverage.[30] A booster is not suggested for those born before 1957 because of the likelihood that they have natural immunity.

Booster shots should be given for tetanus and diphtheria every ten years (tetanus and diphtheria vaccines are usually combined). A booster shot is required annually for protection against common strains of influenza, whereas a pneumonia vaccine is usually good for life if administered after age 65.

Vaccines against hepatitis A, hepatitis B, and chicken pox are recommended for adults at risk because of their jobs, travel, or exposure to susceptible children or infected people. Hepatitis A vaccine lasts for several years. No booster shots are required for hepatitis B or chicken pox. If you are not sure whether you've had the disease, a blood test can check for antibodies.

Paying for Health Care

The cost of health care in the United States is expensive and is escalating. A majority of Americans cannot afford the cost of medicines, physicians' fees, or the cost of hospitalization without some form of health insurance. **Health insurance** is a contract between an insurance company and person or group for the payment of medical care costs. After the person or group pays a premium to an insurance company, the insurance company pays for part or all of the medical costs depending on the type of insurance and benefits provided. The type of insurance policy purchased greatly influences where a person goes for health care, who provides the health care, and what medical procedures can be performed.

Preferred Provider Organization (PPO)

A **preferred provider organization** (PPO) is a network of independent physicians, hospitals, and other health care providers who contract with an insurance company to provide medical care at discount rates. Subscribers are given incentives (reduced costs) if they use PPO-approved providers. This plan usually includes a *deductible,* an amount paid by the patient before being eligible for benefits from the insurance company. For example, if your expenses are $1000, you may have to pay $200 before the insurance company will pay the other $800. After the deductible is met, the insurance provider pays a percentage of the remaining balance. PPO subscribers can use out-of-network providers, but they then usually pay more because the care is not discounted. The advantages of this plan are that a patient usually has more options in choosing health care providers and is not required to obtain a referral from a primary care physician to seek the services of a specialist. Several disadvantages of this insurance option are that substantial costs may be incurred if unexpected illnesses or injuries occur and patients may not routinely receive comprehensive, preventive health care.

Point of Service (POS)

A **point of service** (POS) is an insurance plan in which subscribers use approved providers who have agreed to accept fixed copayments. The delivery of health care starts with and is coordinated by the primary-care physician. Before going to a specialist, a patient must first be referred by the primary-care physician. Out-of-plan providers can be seen but at a higher cost. Medical charges above the maximum allowed by the insurance company are the responsibility of the patient. Advantages of this insurance option are comprehensive health care coordinated by the primary-care physician, lower costs in the case of unexpected illnesses or accidents, and no deductibles. A disadvantage is the loss of accessibility to specialists without first obtaining referral approval.

Health Maintenance Organization (HMO)

A **health maintenance organization** (HMO) is a managed health care plan that provides a full range of medical services for a prepaid amount of money. For a fixed monthly fee, usually paid through pay-roll deductions by an employer, and often a small copayment, subscribers receive care from physicians, specialists, allied health professionals, and educators hired or contractually retained by the HMO.

HMOs provide an advantage in that they provide comprehensive care including preventive care at a lower cost than private insurance over a long period of coverage. One drawback is that patients are limited in their choice of providers to those who belong to the HMO.

Indemnity Plan

An indemnity plan is one in which a person pays a premium, which ensures health care on a fee-for-service basis. In addition to the premium, subscribers pay part of the cost for medical care. Typically, the insurance company pays 80 percent after the deductible has been met, and the subscriber pays 20 percent. Usually, there are fixed indemnity benefits, specified amounts paid for particular procedures. If your policy pays $500 for a tonsillectomy and the actual cost is $1000, you owe the health care provider $500. There are often exclusions, certain services not covered by the policy. Common examples of exclusions are elective surgery, dental care, vision care, and preexisting illnesses and injuries. An advantage of an indemnity plan is that there are no limits on the providers you can use or on how often you see them. A disadvantage is that this type of insurance usually costs more than PPOs, POSs, and HMOs.

Government Insurance

In a government insurance plan the government at the federal, state, or local level pays for health care costs of eligible participants. Two prominent examples of this plan are Medicare and Medicaid. Medicare is financed by Social Security taxes and is designed to provide health care for people 65 years of age and older, the blind, the severely disabled, and those requiring certain treatments such as kidney dialysis. Medicare Part A covers hospital, skilled nursing, and home health care costs. People who qualify for Social Security also qualify for Part A. Medicare Part B is optional for an extra premium and covers physician fees and costs of outpatient care and physical therapy. Medicaid is subsidized by federal and state taxes. It provides limited health care, generally for people eligible for benefits and assistance from two programs: Aid to Families with Dependent Children and Supplementary Security Income.

Summary

- Health information that can be trusted is based on scientifically controlled studies that yield consistent results over time.
- A study is considered reliable if its findings can be confirmed in repeated studies conducted over the course of many years.
- Scientifically controlled studies involve experimental and control groups, use randomly selected participants, and feature double-blind procedures.
- *Statistical significance* is a phrase health journalists and researchers use to indicate probability. If a finding is statistically significant, 95 of 100 times similar studies would yield similar findings.
- *Statistical relationship* is a phrase used to indicate the degree of association between two or more variables (e.g., dietary fat and heart disease). Statistical relationships do not demonstrate cause and effect.
- Epidemiologic studies are population studies that observe the health habits and lifestyles of many people over time. They may be prospective or retrospective.
- The discriminating use of the internet can yield helpful information for most health conditions.
- Signs and symptoms that warrant immediate medical attention are signs of internal bleeding, abdominal pain associated with nausea, a stiff neck accompanied by fever, and serious first aid emergencies and injuries.
- People can help to ensure proper and safe care while in a hospital by checking on the hospital's accreditation status, deciding on accommodations before admission, knowing their patient rights, discussing treatments and procedures with their physicians, asking questions, and staying active.
- Good health care means establishing a doctor-patient relationship while in good health.
- The doctor who manages the general care of patients and directs patients to specialized services is the primary-care physician.
- *Alternative medicine* is the use of therapies not taught in U.S. medical schools and generally unavailable from doctors or hospitals.
- When telling a physician about a problem, you can enhance good communication by presenting the most important problem first, being as specific as possible, being familiar with your family medical history, knowing the names of medicines you are taking, and asking questions.
- The three major components of a physical examination are the medical history, hands-on examination, and diagnostic laboratory tests.
- A medical history is the most important part of the physical examination, especially during the initial visit to a doctor.
- A selective health examination involves the use of specific tests for specific problems. A periodic exam involves the use of tests and procedures after a complete medical history and a discussion of personal lifestyle factors and risk factors.
- Defensive medicine is the practice of prescribing tests and procedures for the purpose of protecting doctors from medical-malpractice lawsuits.
- The eight diseases for which adults need to maintain immunization are influenza, pneumonia, hepatitis, measles, rubella, tetanus, diphtheria, and chicken pox.
- Health insurance options include the preferred provider organization (PPO), the point of service (POS), the health maintenance organization (HMO), the indemnity plan, and government insurance.

Review Questions

1. How does health fatalism negatively influence understanding of health information?
2. What are some examples of health information contradictions?
3. What criteria must a research study satisfy before its claims can be trusted?
4. What are some techniques and strategies that manufacturers and producers of health products use to mislead and deceive the public?
5. Explain the meaning and significance of *scientifically controlled, double-blind studies*. Cite an example.
6. What do the phrases *statistical significance* and *statistical relationship* mean in reference to health studies?
7. How do epidemiologic studies differ from scientifically controlled studies?
8. Why is it important to see a physician while in good health?
9. What can laypeople do while in a hospital to ensure that they receive safe and proper care?
10. Define the term polypharmacy. What can people do to prevent health complications caused by polypharmacy?
11. What is the major role and function of a primary-care physician?
12. Define *alternative medicine*. What reasons do conventional medical doctors give for being concerned about the indiscriminate use of alternative medicine?
13. List four sources of information for researching physicians and specialists in your geographical area.
14. Identify four techniques that facilitate communication between patient and physician.
15. Identify six rights patients have when in a hospital.
16. Differentiate between *selective health exam, periodic exam* and *comprehensive physical examination*.
17. Identify five items that should be included in the home medicine cabinet. What is the purpose of each?
18. In reference to medical tests, differentiate between the terms positive, negative, false positive, and false negative.
19. Define *defensive medicine*. Discuss its impact on both the quantity and quality of health care provided to patients.
20. Identify immunizations for adults.
21. Compare and contrast the basic plans of health insurance.

References

1. Sandroff, S. 2000. Frustrations of science. *Consumer Reports on Health* 12(8):2.
2. Forman, A. 2001. Why nutrition advice flip-flops all the time . . . or does it? *Environmental Nutrition* 24(3):1, 6.
3. Harvard University. 1999. Health information: turn of the news. *Harvard Health Letter* 24(11):1–2.
4. Consumers Union. 1997. Medical news: how to assess the latest breakthrough. *Consumer Reports* 62(6):62–63.
5. Consumers Union. 1997. Finding medical help online. *Consumer Reports* 62(2):27–31.
6. Mayo Foundation for Medical Education and Research. 1997. Health info on the internet. *Mayo Clinic Health Letter* 15(4):6.
7. Mayo Foundation for Medical Education and Research. 1999. Cuts and scrapes: when to see a doctor. *Mayo Clinic Health Letter* 17(7):7.
8. *New England Journal of Medicine.* 2001. Fever: friend or foe? *HealthNews* 7(2):5.
9. Tufts University. 2000. When nagging symptoms should trigger a doctor's visit. *Tufts University Health & Nutrition Letter* 18(5):4–5.
10. Consumers Union. 2000. Avoiding hospital blunders. *Consumer Reports on Health* 12(6):1, 3–5.
11. Sandroff, R. 1997. AHAdvocate. *American Health* 16(6):41–43.
12. Brody, J. August 9, 2000. A pill for this, for that; a body may revolt. *The Commercial Appeal* C1–2.
13. Poirot, C. June 9, 1999. Overuse is reducing effectiveness of antibiotics. *The Commercial Appeal* C1, C3.
14. Zuger, A. 1998. Having a safe hospital stay. *HealthNews* 4(2):4.
15. Consumers Union. 2001. Doctor, can we talk? *Consumer Report on Health* 13(7):7–8.
16. Consumers Union. 1998. Special report on health guide to medication. *Consumer Reports* 63(4):1–8.
17. Consumers Union. 2000. The mainstreaming of alternative medicine. *Consumer Reports* 65(5):17–25.
18. The Burton Goldberg Group. 1998. *Alternative Medicine, The Definitive Guide.* Puyallup, Wash.: Future Medicine Publishing, Inc.
19. Atkinson, H. 1997. Discussing alternative medicine. *HealthNews* 3(10):4–5.
20. Harvard University. 2000. Alternative medicine. *Harvard Health Letter* 25(11):1–3.
21. Harvard University. 1997. Alternative medicine, time for a second opinion. *Harvard Health Letter* 23(1):1–3.
22. Consumers Union. 1998. Checkups: are you getting what you need? *Consumer Reports* 63(8):17–19.
23. Harvard University. 1999. The physical exam: close encounter of a medical kind. *Harvard Health Letter* 24(10): 1–3.
24. Medical Malpractice Victims Organization. 2001. *Some startling facts about medical malpractice.* Available online at www.a-r-m.org.
25. Tufts University. 1997. Special report of mammograms, rectal exams, electrocardiograms. *Tufts University Health & Nutrition Letter* 15(6):4–5.
26. Lipman, M. 2001. Imaging tests: are more always better? *Consumer Reports on Health* 13(2):11.
27. Mayo Foundation for Medical Education and Research. 1999. Understanding your T-score. *Mayo Clinic Health Letter* 17(11):3.

28. Harvard University. 2001. The pros and cons of the screening tests. *Harvard Health Letter* 26(5):4–5.
29. *New England Journal of Medicine.* 1999. Home testing for colon cancer saves lives. *HealthNews* 5(5):5.

30. Mayo Foundation for Medical Education and Research. 1999. Immunizations. *Mayo Clinic Health Letter* 17(9):4–5.

31. Mayo Foundation for Medical Education and Research. 2001. Multiple medications: how to avoid interactions. *Mayo Clinic Health Letter* 19(1):7.

Suggested Readings

Chopra, D. 2001. *Perfect Health.* Three Rivers, Mich.: Three Rivers Press.

Perfect Health describes how to apply the ancient wisdom of Ayurveda to everyday life. Ayurveda maintains that freedom from sickness depends on contacting self-awareness, bringing it into balance, and then extending that balance to the body. *Perfect Health* provides a complete step-by-step program of mind body medicine tailored to individual needs. A quiz identifies the reader's mind body type: thin, restless Vata; enterprising, efficient Pitta; tranquil, steady Kapha; or any combination of these three. This body type becomes the basis for a specific Ayurvedic program of diet, stress reduction, neuromuscular integration, exercise, and daily routines.

Connolly, J. J. 2000. *America's Top Doctors.* New York: Castle Connolly Ltd.

This directory lists more than 4000 of America's top doctors in all specialties and with expertise in such areas as cancer, cardiac surgery, infectious diseases, arthritis, diabetes, cardiology, neurosurgery, orthopedics, and a host of rare diseases and conditions. Topics covered include what makes a doctor the best in a particular field, what criteria to go by when choosing a physician, and how to select a physician within the parameters of an HMO.

Griffith, H. W. 2001. *Complete Guide to Prescription and Non Prescription Drugs 2001.* New York: Berkely Publishing Co.

Comprehensive reference book provides information on all drugs including recently FDA-approved drugs. Includes easy-to-use chart format for quick access to data, advice on how to avoid dangerous interactions, and information on side effects of over 5,000 brand names and 700 generic names. Thorough guide that simplifies information for the layperson.

Name _____ Date _____ Section _____

Assessment Activity 15-1

Are You Communicating with Your Physician?

Directions: Using the following scale, circle the appropriate number for each question. Total your responses and find your score at the end of the activity.

When I go to my physician for a health problem,	Almost Always	Very Frequently	Frequently	Occasionally	Never
I plan ahead of time how I am going to describe my problem.	5	4	3	2	1
I describe my most important problem first.	5	4	3	2	1
I check with my immediate family to determine if my problem runs in the family.	5	4	3	2	1
I take a list of medications, over-the-counter drugs, and treatments I am receiving.	5	4	3	2	1
Before the visit, I prepare a written list of questions to ask.	5	4	3	2	1
I ask about anything that is unclear to me.	5	4	3	2	1
I repeat in my own words the physician's answers to my questions.	5	4	3	2	1
I understand the doctor's diagnosis of my problem.	5	4	3	2	1
I make sure I know the benefits and risks of prescribed treatments.	5	4	3	2	1
I know if and when to return for a follow-up visit.	5	4	3	2	1

Scoring
46–50 = Excellent communication
41–45 = Good
36–40 = Average
31–35 = Fair
Less than 30 = Poor

Name _____ **Date** _____ **Section** _____

Assessment Activity 15-2

Assessing the Results of Diagnostic Tests

Directions: Use this assessment to record the dates and results of commonly administered diagnostic med- ical tests. Refer to information in this chapter to review the purposes of these tests.

Test Name	Typical Reference Range	What's Being Tested	Your Results	Date
1. Alanine aminotransferase (ALT)	10–40 U/l	Heart, liver, muscle damage		
2. Albumin	3.5–5.2 g/dl	Kidneys		
3. Alkaline phosphate	35–128 mg/dl	Liver, parathyroid glands, bone disease		
4. Aspartate aminotransferase (AST)	10–59 U/l	Liver, heart, muscle damage		
5. Bilirubin	0.3–1.5 mg/dl	Liver, kidneys		
6. Blood urea nitrogen (BUN)	8–22 mg/dl	Kidneys		
7. Calcium	8.6–10.0 mg/dl	Parathyroid glands, cancer, bone disease		
8. Carbon dioxide	22–28 mEq/l	Lungs and heart		
9. Chloride	98–107 mEq/l	Dehydration		
10. Cholesterol (total)	<200 mg/dl	Heart and artery disease		
11. Creatinine	0.7–1.3 mg/dl	Kidneys		
12. Free T4 hormone	1.0–4.3 mg/dl	Thyroid gland		
13. Globulin	1.5–3.8 g/dl	Infections		
14. Glucose	<120 mg/dl	Diabetes mellitus		
15. Hematocrit	42–52%	Anemia		
16. High-density lipoprotein (HDL)	>40 mg/dl	Heart and artery disease		
17. Iron (total)	50–175 mg/dl	Anemia		
18. Lactic dehydrogenase	100–190 U/l	Liver		
19. Low-density lipoprotein (LDL)	<130 mg/dl	Heart and artery disease		
20. Lymphocyte	20–40%	Immune deficiency disorder		
21. Phosphorous	2.3–4.6 mg/dl	Kidneys		
22. Potassium	3.4–4.4 mEq/l	Kidneys		
23. Protein	6.4–8.3 g/dl	Kidneys, nutrition		
24. Red blood cells (RBC)	4.2–6.1 m/ml	Anemia		
25. Sedimentation rate	(<50) 15–20 mm/h	Infections		

Test Name	Typical Reference Range	What's Being Tested	Your Results	Date
26. Sodium	136–145 mEq/l	Kidneys, water retention		
27. Thyroid-stimulating hormone (TSH)	.4–4.2 mU/l	Pituitary gland, thyroid gland		
28. Total iron-binding capacity (TIBC)	250–425 mg/dl	Excessive iron		
29. Triglycerides	<250 mg/dl	Heart disease		
30. Uric acid	2.5–8.0 mg/dl	Gout		
31. White blood cell (WBC) count	4.8–10.8 thou/cumm	Infections		

Name _____ **Date** _____ **Section** _____

Assessment Activity 15-3

Self-Care Inventory

Directions: Using the following scale, circle the appropriate number for each statement. Total your responses and find your score at the end of the activity.

Statement	Never	Occasionally	Most of the Time	Almost All of the Time
1. I read health-related advertisements in a critical and careful manner.	1	2	3	4
2. I maintain a suspicious attitude about health claims.	1	2	3	4
3. I have a primary-care physician.	1	2	3	4
4. I know which hospitals my physician recommends.	1	2	3	4
5. I ask about fees before using health care services.	1	2	3	4
6. I ask about the risks and benefits of a medical test before its use.	1	2	3	4
7. I seek second opinions when I feel uncertain or uncomfortable with a recommended treatment.	1	2	3	4
8. I maintain adequate health insurance coverage.	1	2	3	4
9. I ask about the contraindications and side effects of prescription drugs before taking them.	1	2	3	4
10. I thoroughly read labels before taking nonprescription drugs.	1	2	3	4
11. I look for evidence of scientifically controlled studies when reading sensational health claims.	1	2	3	4
12. I am familiar with the medical history of close relatives.	1	2	3	4
13. I follow directions when taking medicines, including continuing their use for the prescribed duration.	1	2	3	4
14. I keep a supply of essential items in my medicine cabinet.	1	2	3	4
15. I keep records of the times, dates, and results of medical tests.	1	2	3	4
16. I keep a record of my immunizations.	1	2	3	4
17. I engage in appropriate medical self-care screening procedures.	1	2	3	4
18. I understand which health conditions are covered in my health insurance policy and which are not.	1	2	3	4
19. I know the deductible amount of my health insurance policy.	1	2	3	4
20. I go for selective health examinations according to the recommended schedule.	1	2	3	4

Scoring
70–80 = A highly skilled, discriminating, and assertive health consumer
60–69 = An adequately skilled health consumer
50–59 = A health consumer who tends to be passive
0–49 = A passive consumer

Appendix A

Food Composition Table

Nutritional Content of Common Foods

For this food composition table, foods are listed within the following groups:

1. breads, cereals, rice, and pasta
2. vegetables
3. fruit
4. milk, yogurt, and cheese
5. meat, poultry, fish, dry beans, eggs, and nuts
6. fats, oils, sweets, and alcoholic beverages.

Source: U.S. Department of Agriculture, Agricultural Research Service. 2001. <u>USDA Nutrient Database for Standard Reference, Release 14</u> (**www.nal.usda.gov/fnic/foodcomp**).

Breads, Cereals, Rice, and Pasta

Name	Amount	Weight (g)	Energy (calories)	Protein (g)	Carbohydrate (g)	Fiber (g)	Total Fat (g)	Saturated Fat (g)	Cholesterol (mg)	Sodium (mg)	Vitamin A (RE)	Vitamin C (mg)	Calcium (mg)	Iron (mg)
Bagel, plain	1 bagel, 4″ diameter	89	245	9.3	47.5	2.0	1.4	0.2	0	475	0	0	16	3.2
Barley, pearled, cooked	½ cup	79	97	1.8	22.2	3.0	0.3	0.1	0	2	1	0	9	1.0
Bulgar, cooked	½ cup	83	110	3.0	23.5	4.5	0.1	0	0	4	0	0	11	0.5
Biscuit	1 biscuit, 2½″ diameter	27	93	1.8	12.8	0.4	4.0	1.0	0	325	0	0	5	0.7
Bread, corn	1 piece	60	188	4.3	28.9	1.4	6.0	1.6	37	467	26	0	44	1.1
Bread, french	1 slice	64	175	5.6	33.2	1.9	1.9	0.4	0	390	0	0	48	1.6
Bread, oatmeal	1 slice	27	73	2.3	13.1	1.1	1.2	0.2	0	162	1	0	18	0.7
Bread, pita, white	1 pita, 6½′ diameter	60	165	5.5	33.4	1.3	0.7	0.1	0	322	0	0	52	1.6
Bread, pita, whole wheat	1 pita, 6½″ diameter	64	170	6.3	35.2	4.7	1.7	0.3	0	340	0	0	10	2.0
Bread, pumpernickel	1 slice	26	65	2.3	12.3	1.7	0.8	0.1	0	174	0	0	18	0.7
Bread, raisin	1 slice	32	88	2.5	16.7	1.4	1.4	0.3	0	125	0	0	21	0.9
Bread, rye	1 slice	32	83	2.7	15.5	1.9	1.1	0.2	0	211	0	0.1	23	0.9
Bread sticks	2 sticks, 7⅝″ × ⅝″	20	82	2.4	13.6	0.6	1.9	0.3	0	131	0	0	4	0.8
Bread stuffing	½ cup	100	178	3.2	21.7	2.9	8.6	1.7	0	543	81	0	32	1.1
Bread, white	1 slice	30	80	2.5	14.9	0.7	1.1	0.2	0	161	0	0	32	0.9
Bread, whole grain	1 slice	32	80	3.2	14.8	2.0	1.2	0.3	0	156	0	0.1	29	1.1
Bread, whole wheat	1 slice	28	69	2.7	12.9	1.9	1.2	0.3	0	148	0	0	20	0.9
Buckwheat groats, cooked	½ cup	84	77	2.8	16.8	2.3	0.5	0.1	0	3	0	0	6	0.7
Bun, hamburger/hotdog	1 roll	43	123	3.7	21.6	1.2	2.2	0.5	0	241	0	0	60	1.4
Cake, angelfood	1/12 of 10″ cake	50	129	3.1	29.4	0.1	0.2	0	0	255	0	0	42	0.1
Cake, chocolate w/frosting	⅛ of 18 oz cake	64	235	2.6	34.9	1.8	10.5	3.1	27	214	16	0.1	28	1.4
Cake, yellow w/icing	⅛ of 18 oz cake	64	243	2.4	35.5	1.2	11.1	3.0	35	216	21	0	23	1.3
Cereal, All-Bran	½ cup	30	53	3.7	22.7	15.3	0.9	0.2	0	127	260	17.3	116	5.2
Cereal, Bran Chex	⅔ cup	28	90	2.9	22.6	4.6	0.8	0.1	0	200	6	15.0	17	8.1
Cereal, Cheerios	1 cup	30	110	3.1	22.9	2.6	1.8	0.4	0	284	375	15.0	55	8.1
Cereal, cornflakes	1 cup	28	102	1.8	24.2	0.8	0.2	0.1	0	298	210	14.0	1	8.7
Cereal, Cream of Wheat	½ cup	126	67	1.9	13.8	0.9	0.3	0	0	168	0	0	25	5.1
Cereal, frosted flakes	¾ cup	31	119	1.2	28.3	0.6	0.2	0.1	0	200	225	15.0	1	4.5
Cereal, granola	½ cup	31	135	3.0	22.4	1.9	4.2	0.6	0	8	0	0.1	24	1.3
Cereal, raisin bran	1 cup	61	186	5.6	47.1	8.2	1.5	0	0	354	250	0	35	5.0
Cereal, Total	¾ cup	30	105	3.0	23.9	2.6	0.7	0.2	0	199	375	60.0	258	18.0
Cereal, Wheaties	1 cup	30	110	3.2	0.9	2.1	0.9	0.2	0	222	225	15.0	55	8.1
Coffee cake w/topping	1 piece	63	263	4.3	29.4	1.3	14.7	3.7	20	221	21	0.2	34	1.2
Cookie, chocolate chip	1 medium cookie	16	78	0.9	9.3	0.4	4.5	1.3	5	58	26	0	6	0.4
Cookie, fig bar	1 cookie	16	56	0.6	11.3	0.7	1.2	0.2	0	56	1	0	10	0.5
Cookie, fortune	1 cookie	8	30	0.3	6.7	0.1	0.2	0.1	0	22	0	0	1	0.1
Cookie, oatmeal	1 large cookie	18	81	1.1	12.4	0.5	3.3	0.8	0	69	0	0.1	7	0.5
Cookie, sandwich	1 cookie	10	47	0.5	7.0	0.3	0.3	0.4	0	60	0	0	3	0.4
Corn grits, cooked	½ cup	121	73	1.7	15.7	0.2	0.2	0	0	0	7	0	0	0.8
Corn meal, dry	¼ cup	35	126	2.9	26.8	2.6	0.6	0.1	0	1	14	0	2	1.4
Couscous, cooked	½ cup	79	88	3.0	18.2	1.1	0.1	0	0	4	0	0	6	0.3
Cracker, Crispbread, rye	3 crispbreads	30	110	2.4	24.7	5.0	0.4	0	0	79	0	0	9	0.7
Cracker, Goldfish	24 goldfish	12	70	1.0	8.0	1.0	4.0	0	0	100	0	0	8	0.4
Cracker, graham	3 squares	28	119	2.0	21.3	1.0	2.8	0.4	0	185	0	0	22	1.2
Cracker, matzo	1 matzo	28	112	2.8	23.7	0.9	0.4	0.1	0	1	0	0	4	0.9
Cracker, melba toast	6 pieces	30	117	3.6	23.0	1.9	1.0	0.1	0	249	0	0	28	1.1
Cracker, Ritz	5 crackers	16	79	1.2	10.3	0.3	3.7	0.6	0	124	0	0	24	0.6
Cracker, saltine	10 squares	30	130	2.8	21.5	0.9	3.5	0.9	0	390	0	0	36	1.6
Cracker, whole wheat	6 crackers	24	106	2.1	16.5	2.5	4.1	0.8	0	158	0	0	24	0.7
Croissant, butter	1 medium	57	231	4.7	26.1	1.5	12.0	6.6	38	424	106	0.1	21	1.2

Name	Amount	Weight (g)	Energy (calories)	Protein (g)	Carbohydrate (g)	Fiber (g)	Total Fat (g)	Saturated Fat (g)	Cholesterol (mg)	Sodium (mg)	Vitamin A (RE)	Vitamin C (mg)	Calcium (mg)	Iron (mg)
Danish pastry, cheese	1 pastry	71	266	5.7	26.4	0.7	15.5	4.8	11	320	32	0	25	1.1
Doughnut, glazed	1 medium	45	192	2.3	22.9	0.7	10.3	2.7	14	181	1	0	27	0.5
English muffin, plain	½ muffin	29	67	2.2	13.1	0.8	0.5	0.1	0	132	0	0	50	0.7
French toast	1 slice	65	149	5.0	16.3	0	7.0	1.8	75	311	86	0.2	65	1.1
Macaroni, cooked	½ cup	70	99	3.3	19.8	0.9	0.5	0.1	0	1	0	0	5	1.0
Muffin, blueberry	2″ by 2¾″	57	158	3.1	27.4	1.5	3.7	0.8	17	255	5	0.6	32	0.9
Muffin, oat bran	2¼″ by 2½″	57	154	4.0	27.5	2.6	4.2	0.6	0	224	0	0	36	2.4
Noodles, chow mein	½ cup	23	119	1.9	12.9	0.9	6.9	1.0	0	99	2	0	5	1.1
Noodles, egg, cooked	½ cup	80	106	3.8	19.9	0.9	1.2	0.2	53	6	5	0	10	1.3
Noodles, Japanese soba	½ cup	57	56	2.9	12.2	0	0.1	0	0	34	0	0	2	0.3
Oatmeal, instant	1 packet	155	153	4.1	31.4	2.6	1.8	0.4	0	234	302	0	105	3.9
Oats, uncooked	¼ cup	20	78	3.2	27.1	2.1	1.3	0.2	0	1	2	0	11	0.9
Pancake	4″ pancake	38	74	2.0	13.9	0.5	1.0	0.2	5	239	12	0.1	48	0.6
Pasta, cooked	½ cup	57	75	2.9	14.2	0	0.6	0.1	19	3	3	0	3	0.7
Popcorn, air-popped	2 cups	16	61	1.9	12.5	2.4	0.7	0.1	0	1	3	0	2	0.4
Popcorn, oil-popped	2 cups	22	110	1.9	12.6	2.2	6.2	1.0	0	194	3	0	2	0.6
Pretzels	10 twists	60	229	5.5	47.5	1.9	2.1	0.5	0	1029	0	0	22	2.6
Quinoa, uncooked	¼ cup	43	159	5.6	29.3	2.5	2.5	0.3	0	9	0	0	26	3.9
Rice, brown, cooked	½ cup	71	109	2.3	22.9	1.8	0.8	0.3	0	1	0	0	10	0.5
Rice cake	1 cake	9	35	0.7	7.3	0.4	0.3	0	0	29	0	0	1	0.1
Rice, white, cooked	½ cup	93	121	2.2	26.6	0.3	0.2	0.1	0	0	0	0	3	1.4
Rice, wild, cooked	½ cup	82	83	3.3	17.5	1.5	0.3	0	0	3	0	0	2	0.5
Roll, dinner	1 roll, 2″ square	28	84	2.4	14.1	0.8	2.0	0.5	0	146	0	0	33	0.9
Spaghetti, cooked	½ cup	70	99	3.3	19.8	1.2	0.5	0.1	0	70	0	0	5	1.0
Taco shell	1 medium	13	62	1.0	8.3	1.0	3.0	0.4	0	49	0	0	21	0.3
Tortilla chips	1 oz	28	142	2.0	17.8	1.8	7.4	1.4	0	150	6	0	44	0.4
Tortilla, corn	1 medium	26	58	1.5	12.1	1.4	0.7	0.1	0	42	0	0	46	0.4
Tortilla, flour	1 medium	49	159	4.3	27.2	1.6	3.5	0.9	0	234	0	0	61	1.6
Wheat germ, toasted	¼ cup	28	108	8.3	14.1	3.7	3.0	0.5	0	1	0	1.7	13	2.6

Vegetables

Name	Amount	Weight (g)	Energy (calories)	Protein (g)	Carbohydrate (g)	Fiber (g)	Total Fat (g)	Saturated Fat (g)	Cholesterol (mg)	Sodium (mg)	Vitamin A (RE)	Vitamin C (mg)	Calcium (mg)	Iron (mg)
Artichoke, cooked	1 medium	120	60	4.2	13.4	6.5	0.2	0	0	114	22	12.0	54	1.5
Arugula, raw	1 cup	20	5	0.5	0.7	0.3	0.1	0	0	3	24	3.0	16	0.1
Asparagus, cooked	6 spears	90	22	2.3	3.8	1.4	0.3	0	0	10	49	9.7	18	0.7
Bamboo shoots, canned	½ cup	66	13	1.1	2.1	0.9	0.3	0.1	0	5	1	0.7	5	0.2
Bean sprouts, raw	½ cup	35	43	4.6	3.3	0.4	2.3	0.3	0	5	0	5.4	23	0.7
*Beans, baked (plain)	½ cup	127	118	6.1	26.0	6.4	0.6	0.1	0	504	22	3.9	64	0.4
*Beans, black, cooked	½ cup	86	114	7.6	20.4	7.5	0.5	0.1	0	1	1	0	23	1.8
*Beans, fava, cooked	½ cup	85	94	6.5	16.7	4.6	0.3	0.1	0	4	2	0.3	31	1.3
Beans, green snap, cooked	½ cup	63	22	1.2	4.9	2.0	0.2	0	0	2	42	6.1	29	0.8
*Beans, kidney, cooked	½ cup	89	112	7.7	20.2	6.5	0.4	0.1	0	2	0	1.1	25	2.6
*Beans, lentils, cooked	½ cup	99	115	8.9	19.9	7.8	0.4	0.1	0	2	1	1.5	19	3.3
*Beans, lima, cooked	½ cup	94	108	7.3	19.6	6.6	0.4	0.1	0	2	0	0	16	2.2
*Beans, navy, cooked	½ cup	91	129	7.9	23.9	5.8	0.5	0.1	0	1	0	0.8	64	2.3
*Beans, pinto, cooked	½ cup	86	117	7.0	21.9	7.4	0.4	0.1	0	2	0	1.8	41	2.2
*Beans, refried	½ cup	126	118	6.9	19.6	6.7	1.6	0.6	10	377	0	7.6	44	2.1

*Dry beans and peas (legumes), which can be counted as servings of vegetables or as servings from the meat, poultry, fish, dry beans, eggs, and nuts group.

Name	Amount	Weight (g)	Energy (calories)	Protein (g)	Carbohydrate (g)	Fiber (g)	Total Fat (g)	Saturated Fat (g)	Cholesterol (mg)	Sodium (mg)	Vitamin A (RE)	Vitamin C (mg)	Calcium (mg)	Iron (mg)
Beans, yellow snap, cooked	½ cup	63	22	1.2	4.9	2.1	0.2	0	0	2	5	6.1	29	0.8
Beet greens, cooked	½ cup	144	39	3.7	7.9	4.2	0.3	0	0	347	734	35.9	164	2.7
Beets, cooked	½ cup	74	37	1.4	8.5	1.7	0.2	0	0	65	3	3.1	14	0.7
Broccoli spears, cooked	2 spears	78	22	2.3	3.9	2.3	0.3	0	0	20	108	58.2	36	0.7
Brussels sprouts, cooked	4 sprouts	84	33	2.1	7.3	2.2	0.4	0.1	0	18	60	52.1	30	1.0
Cabbage, cooked	½ cup	75	17	0.8	3.3	1.7	0.3	0	0	6	10	15.1	23	0.1
Cabbage, raw	½ cup	45	11	0.6	2.4	1.0	0.1	0	0	8	6	14.3	21	0.3
Carrot juice	¾ cup	177	71	1.7	16.4	1.4	0.3	0	0	51	1938	15.0	42	0.8
Carrots, cooked	½ cup	78	35	0.9	8.2	2.6	0.1	0	0	51	1915	1.8	24	0.5
Carrots, raw	1 medium	61	26	0.6	6.2	1.8	0.1	0	0	21	1716	5.6	16	0.3
Cauliflower, cooked	½ cup	62	14	1.1	2.5	1.7	0.3	0	0	9	1	27.4	10	0.2
Celery, raw	8 sticks	32	5	0.2	1.2	0.5	0	0	0	28	4	2.2	13	0.1
Chard, cooked	½ cup	88	18	1.6	3.6	1.8	0.1	0	0	156	275	15.8	51	2.0
Coleslaw, homemade	½ cup	60	41	0.8	7.4	0.9	1.6	0.2	5	14	49	19.6	27	0.4
Collards, cooked	½ cup	95	25	2.0	4.7	2.7	0.3	0	0	9	297	17.3	113	0.4
Corn, yellow, cooked	½ cup	82	89	2.7	20.6	2.3	1.1	0.2	0	14	18	5.1	2	0.5
Cucumber, raw	½ cup	52	7	0.4	1.4	0.4	0.1	0	0	1	11	2.8	7	0.1
Eggplant, cooked	½ cup	50	14	0.4	3.3	1.2	0.1	0	0	1	3	0.6	3	0.2
Endive, raw	½ cup	25	4	0.3	0.8	0.8	0.1	0	0	6	51	1.6	13	0.2
Hominy, canned	½ cup	83	94	1.2	11.8	2.1	0.7	0.1	0	173	0	0	8	0.5
Kale, cooked	½ cup	65	18	1.2	3.6	1.3	0.3	0	0	15	481	26.7	47	0.6
Lettuce, iceberg	1 cup	55	7	0.6	1.1	0.8	0.1	0	0	5	18	2.1	10	0.3
Lettuce, looseleaf	1 cup	56	10	0.7	2.0	1.1	0.2	0	0	5	106	10.1	38	0.8
Lettuce, romaine	1 cup	56	8	0.9	1.3	1.0	0.1	0	0	4	152	13.4	20	0.6
Mushrooms, cooked	½ cup	78	21	1.7	4.0	1.7	0.3	0	0	2	0	3.1	5	1.4
Mushrooms, raw	½ cup	35	9	1.0	1.4	0.4	0.1	0	0	1	0	0.8	2	0.4
Mustard greens, cooked	½ cup	70	11	1.6	1.5	1.4	0.2	0	0	11	212	17.7	52	0.5
Okra, cooked	½ cup	92	26	1.9	5.3	2.6	0.3	0.1	0	3	47	11.2	88	0.6
Onion, raw	½ cup	80	30	0.9	6.9	1.4	0.1	0	0	2	0	5.1	16	0.2
Parsnip, raw	½ cup	67	50	0.8	12.0	3.2	0.2	0	0	7	0	11.3	24	0.4
*Peas, blackeye, cooked	½ cup	86	100	6.6	17.9	5.6	0.5	0.1	0	3	1	0.3	21	2.2
*Peas, chickpeas (garbanzos)	½ cup	82	134	7.3	22.5	6.2	2.1	0.2	0	6	2	1.1	40	2.4
Peas, edible podded	10 peapods	34	14	1.0	2.6	0.9	0.1	0	0	1	5	20.4	15	0.7
Peas, green	½ cup	80	62	4.1	11.4	4.4	0.2	0	0	70	54	7.9	19	1.2
*Peas, split, cooked	½ cup	98	116	8.2	20.6	8.1	0.4	0.1	0	2	1	0.4	14	1.3
Pepper, green chili, canned	½ cup	70	15	0.5	3.2	1.2	0.2	0	0	276	9	23.8	25	0.9
Pepper, sweet green, raw	1 small	74	20	0.7	4.8	1.3	0.1	0	0	1	47	66.1	7	0.3
Pepper, sweet red, raw	1 small	74	20	0.7	4.8	1.5	0.1	0	0	1	422	140.6	7	0.3
Pickle, dill	1 medium	65	12	0.4	2.7	0.8	0.1	0	0	21	833	1.2	6	0.3
Potato, baked w/skin	1 medium	173	188	4.0	43.5	4.1	0.2	0	0	14	0	22.3	17	2.3
Potato, boiled	1 potato, 2½″ diameter	136	118	2.5	27.4	2.4	0.1	0	0	5	0	17.7	7	0.4
Potato, french fries	10 fries	50	109	1.7	17.0	1.6	4.1	1.9	0	141	0	4.8	5	0.7
Potato, mashed w/milk	½ cup	105	81	2.0	18.4	2.1	0.6	0.3	2	318	6	7.0	27	0.3
Potato salad	½ cup	125	179	3.4	14.0	1.6	10.3	1.8	85	661	41	12.5	24	0.8
Pumpkin, canned	½ cup	123	42	1.3	9.9	3.6	0.3	0.2	0	6	2702	5.1	32	1.7
Radish	13 medium	58	12	0.3	2.1	0.9	0.3	0	0	13.9	1	13.2	12	0.2
Rutabaga, mashed	½ cup	120	47	1.5	10.5	2.2	0.3	0	0	24	67	22.6	58	0.6
Sauerkraut, drained	½ cup	121	13	0.6	3.0	1.8	0.1	0	0	469	1	10.5	21	1.0
Soybeans, green, boiled	½ cup	90	127	11.1	9.9	3.8	5.8	0.7	0	13	14	15.3	131	2.3

Name	Amount	Weight (g)	Energy (calories)	Protein (g)	Carbohydrate (g)	Fiber (g)	Total Fat (g)	Saturated Fat (g)	Cholesterol (mg)	Sodium (mg)	Vitamin A (RE)	Vitamin C (mg)	Calcium (mg)	Iron (mg)
Spinach, cooked	½ cup	95	27	3.0	5.1	2.9	0.2	0	0	82	739	11.7	139	1.4
Spinach, raw	1 cup	30	7	0.9	1.1	0.8	0.1	0	0	24	202	8.4	30	0.8
Squash, summer, cooked	½ cup	90	18	0.8	3.9	1.3	0.3	0	0	1	26	5.0	24	0.3
Squash, summer, raw	½ small squash	59	12	0.7	2.6	1.1	0.1	0	0	1	12	8.7	12	0.3
Squash, winter	½ cup	100	39	0.9	8.8	2.8	0.6	0.1	0	1	356	9.6	14	0.3
Sweet potato, baked	½ cup	100	103	1.7	24.3	3.0	0.1	0	0	10	2182	24.6	28	0.5
Sweet potato, canned w/syrup	½ cup	100	108	1.3	25.4	3.0	0.3	0.1	0	39	716	10.8	17	1.0
Tomato juice	¾ cup	182	31	1.4	7.7	1.5	1.4	0	0	18	102	33.3	16	1.1
Tomato, raw	1 medium	123	26	1.0	5.7	1.4	0.4	0.1	0	11	76	23.5	6	0.6
Tomato sauce	½ cup	123	37	1.6	1.7	1.7	0.2	0	0	741	120	16.0	17	0.9
Turnip, cooked, mashed	½ cup	115	24	0.8	5.6	2.3	0.1	0	0	108	0	13.3	25	0.3
Vegetable juice	¾ cup	182	35	1.1	8.3	1.5	0.2	0	0	491	213	50.4	20	0.8
Vegetables, mixed	½ cup	91	54	2.6	11.9	4.0	0.1	0	0	32	389	2.9	23	0.7
Vegetable soup	1 cup	241	72	2.1	12.0	0.5	1.9	0.3	0	822	301	1.4	22	1.1
Water chestnuts	½ cup	70	35	0.6	8.7	1.8	0	0	0	6	0	0.9	3	0.6

Fruit

Name	Amount	Weight (g)	Energy (calories)	Protein (g)	Carbohydrate (g)	Fiber (g)	Total Fat (g)	Saturated Fat (g)	Cholesterol (mg)	Sodium (mg)	Vitamin A (RE)	Vitamin C (mg)	Calcium (mg)	Iron (mg)
Apple	1 medium	138	81	0.3	21.0	3.7	0.5	0.1	0	0	7	7.9	10	0.2
Apple juice	¾ cup	179	84	0.3	20.7	0.2	0.2	0	0	13	0	44.8	11	0.5
Applesauce, unsweetened	½ cup	122	52	0.2	13.8	1.5	0.1	0	0	2	4	25.9	4	0.1
Apricots	2 medium	70	34	1.0	7.8	1.7	0.3	0	0	1	183	7.0	10	0.4
Apricots, dried	9 halves	32	75	1.2	19.4	2.8	0.1	0	0	3	228	0.8	14	1.5
Avocado	1 medium	173	306	3.7	12.0	8.5	30.0	4.5	0	21	105	13.7	19	2.0
Banana	1 medium	118	109	1.2	27.6	2.8	0.6	0.2	0	1	9	10.7	7	0.4
Blackberries	½ cup	72	37	0.5	9.2	3.8	0.3	0	0	0	12	15.1	23	0.4
Blueberries	½ cup	73	41	0.5	10.2	2.0	0.3	0	0	4	7	9.4	4	0.1
Cantaloupe	¼ melon 5″ diameter	138	48	1.2	11.5	1.1	0.4	0.1	0	12	444	58.2	15	0.3
Carambola (starfruit)	1 small	70	23	0.4	5.5	1.9	0.2	0	0	1	34	14.8	3	0.2
Cherries, canned in syrup	½ cup	128	116	0.9	29.8	1.4	0.1	0	0	9	91	2.6	13	1.7
Cherries, sweet, raw	11 cherries	75	54	0.9	2.3	1.7	0.7	0.2	0	0	16	5.2	11	0.3
Cranberries, raw	½ cup	48	23	0.2	6.0	2.0	0.1	0	0	1	2	6.4	3	0.1
Cranberry juice cocktail	¾ cup	190	108	0	27.3	0.2	0.2	0	0	4	0	67.1	6	0.3
Cranberry sauce	¼ cup	139	105	0.1	26.9	0.7	0.1	0	0	20	1	1.4	3	0.2
Currants, dried	¼ cup	36	109	1.5	26.7	2.4	0.1	0	0	3	3	1.7	31	1.2
Dates, dried	¼ cup	45	122	0.9	32.7	3.3	0.2	0.1	0	1	2	0	14	0.5
Figs, raw	2 medium	100	74	0.8	19.2	3.3	0.3	0.1	0	1	14	2.0	35	0.4
Fruit cocktail, heavy syrup	½ cup	124	91	0.5	23.4	1.2	0.1	0	0	7	25	2.4	7	0.4
Fruit cocktail, light syrup	½ cup	121	69	0.5	18.1	1.2	0.1	0	0	7	25	2.3	7	0.4
Fruit cocktail, juice	½ cup	119	55	0.5	14.1	1.2	0	0	0	5	37	3.2	9	0.3
Grapefruit	½ medium	128	41	0.8	10.3	1.4	0.1	0	0	0	15	44.0	15	0.1
Grapefruit juice	¾ cup	185	70	1.0	16.6	0.2	0.2	0	0	2	2	54.1	13	0.4
Grapes	12 grapes	60	43	0.4	10.7	0.6	0.3	0	0	1	4	6.5	7	0.2
Guava	1 fruit	90	46	0.7	10.7	4.9	0.5	0.2	0	3	71	165.2	18	0.3
Honeydew	⅛ melon, 5¼″ diameter	125	44	0.6	11.5	0.8	0.1	0	0	13	5	31.0	8	0.1
Kiwifruit	1 large	91	56	0.9	13.5	3.1	0.4	0	0	5	16	68.3	24	0.4
Kumquats	5 fruits	100	63	0.9	16.4	6.6	0.1	0	0	6	30	37.4	44	0.4
Lemon, with peel	1 fruit	108	22	1.3	11.6	5.1	0.3	0	0	3	3	83.2	66	0.8

Name	Amount	Weight (g)	Energy (calories)	Protein (g)	Carbohydrate (g)	Fiber (g)	Total Fat (g)	Saturated Fat (g)	Cholesterol (mg)	Sodium (mg)	Vitamin A (RE)	Vitamin C (mg)	Calcium (mg)	Iron (mg)
Lemon juice	2 tablespoons	31	6	0.1	2.0	0.1	0.1	0	0	6	1	7.6	3	0
Mango	½ medium	103	65	0.5	17.0	1.8	0.3	0.1	0	2	389	27.7	10	0.1
Nectarine	1 fruit	136	67	1.3	16.0	2.2	0.6	0.1	0	0	101	7.3	7	0.2
Orange	1 medium	131	62	1.2	15.4	3.1	0.2	0	0	0	28	69.7	52	0.1
Orange juice	¾ cup	187	82	1.5	18.8	0.4	0.5	0.1	0	2	15	61.6	19	0.3
Papaya	½ medium	152	59	0.9	14.9	2.7	0.2	0.1	0	5	43	93.9	36	0.2
Passion fruit	½ cup	118	114	2.6	27.6	12.3	0.8	0.1	0	33	83	35.4	14	1.9
Peach, canned in juice	½ cup	124	55	0.8	14.3	1.6	0	0	0	5	47	4.4	7	0.3
Peach, raw	1 medium	98	42	0.7	10.9	2.0	0.1	0	0	0	53	6.5	5	0.1
Pear, canned	½ cup	124	62	0.4	16.0	2.0	0.1	0	0	5	1	2.0	11	0.4
Pear, raw	1 medium	166	98	0.6	25.1	4.0	0.7	0	0	0	3	6.6	18	0.4
Pineapple, canned in juice	½ cup	125	75	0.5	19.5	1.0	0.1	0	0	1	5	11.8	17	0.3
Pineapple, raw	1 slice 3½" × 3¼"	84	41	0.3	10.4	1.0	0.4	0	0	1	2	12.9	6	0.3
Plantain, raw	1 medium	179	218	2.3	57.1	4.1	0.7	0.3	0	7	6	2.3	5	1.1
Plums	1½ medium	99	55	0.8	13.0	1.5	0.6	0	0	0	32	9.5	4	0.1
Prune juice	¾ cup	192	136	1.2	33.5	1.9	0.1	0	0	8	0	7.9	23	2.3
Prunes, dried	5 prunes	42	80	1.1	26.3	3.0	0.2	0	0	2	84	1.4	21	1.0
Raisins	¼ cup	43	129	1.4	34.0	1.7	0.2	0.1	0	5	0	1.4	21	0.9
Raspberries	½ cup	62	30	0.6	7.1	4.2	0.3	0	0	0	8	15.4	14	0.4
Rhubarb, raw	1 stalk	51	11	0.5	2.3	0.9	0.1	0	0	2	5	4.1	44	0.1
Strawberries	5 large	90	27	0.6	6.3	2.1	0.3	0	0	1	3	51.0	13	0.3
Tangerine	1 medium	84	40	0.5	9.4	1.9	0.2	0	0	1	77	25.9	12	0.1
Watermelon	⅟₁₆ melon	286	92	1.8	20.5	1.4	1.2	0.1	0	6	106	27.5	23	0.5

Milk, Yogurt, and Cheese

Name	Amount	Weight (g)	Energy (calories)	Protein (g)	Carbohydrate (g)	Fiber (g)	Total Fat (g)	Saturated Fat (g)	Cholesterol (mg)	Sodium (mg)	Vitamin A (RE)	Vitamin C (mg)	Calcium (mg)	Iron (mg)
Buttermilk, lowfat	1 cup	245	98	8.1	11.7	0	2.2	1.3	10	257	20	2.5	284	0.1
Cheese, American	2 oz	57	186	11.1	4.1	0	13.9	8.8	36	905	124	0	325	0.5
Cheese, blue	1½ oz	43	150	9.1	1.0	0	12.2	7.9	32	593	97	0	225	0.1
Cheese, cheddar	1½ oz	43	171	10.6	0.5	0	14.1	9.0	45	264	118	0	307	0.3
Cheese, cottage, creamed	1 cup	210	216	26.2	5.6	0	9.5	6.0	32	850	101	0	126	0.3
Cheese, cottage, lowfat (1%)	1 cup	226	163	28.0	6.1	0	2.3	1.5	9	918	25	0	138	0.3
Cheese, cottage, fat free	1 cup	145	123	25.0	2.7	0	0.6	0.4	10	19	12	0	46	03
Cheese, cream	2 oz	57	198	4.3	1.5	0	19.8	12.5	62	168	216	0	45	0.7
Cheese, cream, fat free	2 oz	57	55	8.2	3.3	0	0.8	0.5	5	311	159	0	105	0.1
Cheese, feta	1½ oz	43	112	6.0	1.7	0	9.0	6.4	38	475	54	0	210	03
Cheese, mexican	1½ oz	43	151	9.6	1.2	0	12.0	7.6	45	279	27	0	281	0.2
Cheese, monterey	1½ oz	43	159	10.4	0.3	0	12.9	8.1	38	228	108	0	317	0.3
Cheese, mozzarella, part skim	1½ oz	43	108	10.3	1.2	0	6.8	4.3	25	198	75	0	275	0.1
Cheese, parmesan, grated	2 tablespoons	10	46	4.2	0.4	0	3.0	1.9	8	186	17	0	138	0.1
Cheese, process spread	2 oz	56	170	9.1	5.5	0	12.3	8.1	45	839	100	0.1	261	0.1
Cheese, provolone	1½ oz	43	149	10.9	0.9	0	11.3	7.3	29	373	112	0	321	0.2
Cheese, ricotta, part skim	½ cup	124	171	14.1	6.4	0	9.8	6.1	38	155	140	0	337	0.5
Cheese, swiss	1½ oz	43	160	12.1	1.4	0	11.7	7.6	39	111	19	0	409	0.1
Ice cream, chocolate	1 cup	132	285	5.0	37.2	1.6	14.2	9.0	45	100	151	0.9	144	1.2
Ice cream, vanilla, rich	1 cup	148	357	5.2	33.2	0	24.0	14.8	90	83	272	1.0	173	0.1
Ice cream, vanilla, light	1 cup	132	183	5.0	30.0	0	5.7	3.5	18	112	62	1.1	183	0.1
Ice cream, vanilla, soft serve	1 cup	172	370	7.1	38.2	0	22.4	12.9	157	105	265	1.4	225	0.4
Milk, chocolate	1 cup	250	208	7.9	25.9	2.0	8.5	5.3	30	150	73	2.3	280	0.6
Milk, fat free (nonfat)	1 cup	245	86	8.4	11.9	0	0.4	0.3	5	127	149	2.5	301	0.1

Name	Amount	Weight (g)	Energy (calories)	Protein (g)	Carbohydrate (g)	Fiber (g)	Total Fat (g)	Saturated Fat (g)	Cholesterol (mg)	Sodium (mg)	Vitamin A (RE)	Vitamin C (mg)	Calcium (mg)	Iron (mg)
Milk, lowfat (1%)	1 cup	244	102	8.0	11.7	0	2.6	1.6	10	124	144	2.4	300	0.1
Milk, reduced fat (2%)	1 cup	244	122	8.1	11.7	0	4.7	2.9	20	122	139	2.4	298	0.1
Milk, whole	1 cup	244	149	8.0	11.4	0	8.2	5.1	34	120	76	2.2	290	0.1
Pudding, made with milk	½ cup	142	158	4.5	25.6	1.4	4.8	3.0	17	146	37	1.0	158	0.5
Yogurt, frozen, vanilla	1 cup	144	229	5.8	34.8	0	8.1	4.9	3	125	82	1.2	206	0.4
Yogurt, lowfat, plain	8 oz container	227	143	11.9	16.0	0	3.5	2.3	14	159	36	1.8	415	0.2
Yogurt, lowfat, with fruit	8 oz container	227	238	11.0	42.2	0	3.2	2.1	14	148	136	1.6	384	0.2
Yogurt, nonfat, plain	8 oz container	227	127	13.0	17.4	0	0.4	0.3	5	175	5	2.0	452	0.2

Meat, Poultry, Fish, Dry Beans, Eggs, and Nuts

Name	Amount	Weight (g)	Energy (calories)	Protein (g)	Carbohydrate (g)	Fiber (g)	Total Fat (g)	Saturated Fat (g)	Cholesterol (mg)	Sodium (mg)	Vitamin A (RE)	Vitamin C (mg)	Calcium (mg)	Iron (mg)
Bacon	3 slices	19	109	5.7	0.1	0	9.4	3.3	19	303	0	0	2	0.3
Bacon, Canadian	2 slices	47	86	11.3	0.6	0	3.9	1.3	27	719	0	0	5	0.4
Beef, ½″ fat	3 oz	85	344	19.9	0	0	28.7	11.9	78	48	0	0	9	2.1
Beef, corned beef	3 oz	85	213	23.0	0	0	12.7	5.3	73	856	0	0	10	1.8
Beef, ground, extra lean, broiled	3 oz	85	218	21.6	0	0	13.9	5.5	71	60	0	0	6	2.0
Beef, ground, lean, broiled	3 oz	85	231	21.0	0	0	15.7	6.2	74	65	0	0	9	1.8
Beef, ground, regular, broiled	3 oz	85	246	20.5	0	0	17.6	6.9	77	71	0	0	9	2.1
Beef, lean, fat trimmed	3 oz	85	179	25.4	0	0	7.9	3.0	73	56	0	0	7	2.5
Beef liver, braised	3 oz	85	137	20.7	2.9	0	4.2	1.6	331	60	9011	19.6	6	5.8
Beef ribs, broiled	3 oz	85	306	18.7	0	0	25.1	10.2	70	53	0	0	10	1.8
Chicken breast, w/skin, roasted	½ breast	98	193	29.2	0	0	7.6	2.1	82	70	26	0	14	1.0
Chicken, dark meat, w/skin, roasted	3 oz	85	215	22.1	0	0	13.4	3.7	77	74	49	0	13	1.2
Chicken, dark meat, w/o skin, roasted	3 oz	85	168	22.2	0	0	7.9	2.2	76	76	18	0	12	1.1
Chicken, dark meat, w/skin, fried	3 oz	85	253	18.6	8.0	0	15.8	4.2	76	251	26	0	18	1.2
Chicken, drumstick, w/skin, roasted	1 drumstick	52	112	14.1	0	0	5.8	1.6	47	47	16	0	6	0.7
Chicken, light meat, w/skin, roasted	3 oz	85	189	24.7	0	0	9.2	2.6	71	64	27	0	13	1.0
Chicken, light meat, w/o skin, roasted	3 oz	85	147	26.3	0	0	3.8	1.1	72	65	8	0	13	0.9
Chicken, light meat, w/skin, fried	3 oz	85	235	20.0	8.1	0	13.1	3.5	71	243	20	0	17	1.1
Chicken liver, chopped	½ cup	70	110	17.1	0.8	0	3.8	1.3	442	36	3439	11.1	10	5.9
Chicken, thigh, w/skin, roasted	1 thigh	62	153	15.5	0	0	9.6	2.7	58	52	30	0	7	0.8
Chicken, wing, w/skin, roasted	1 wing	34	99	9.1	0	0	6.6	1.9	29	28	16	0	5	0.4
Egg white, large	1 egg white	33	17	3.5	0.3	0	0	0	0	55	0	0	2	0
Egg, whole, large	1 egg	50	75	6.2	0.6	0	5.1	1.6	213	63	97	0	25	0.7
Egg yolk, large	1 yolk	17	59	2.8	0.3	0	5.1	1.6	213	7	97	0	23	0.6

* Dry beans can be counted as servings from this group or the vegetables group; data on dry beans is listed under vegetables (see items marked with an asterisk).

Name	Amount	Weight (g)	Energy (calories)	Protein (g)	Carbohydrate (g)	Fiber (g)	Total Fat (g)	Saturated Fat (g)	Cholesterol (mg)	Sodium (mg)	Vitamin A (RE)	Vitamin C (mg)	Calcium (mg)	Iron (mg)
Fish, catfish, baked/broiled	3 oz	85	129	15.9	0	0	6.8	1.5	54	68	13	0.7	8	0.7
Fish, cod, baked/broiled	3 oz	85	89	19.5	0	0	0.7	0.1	40	77	9	2.6	7	0.3
Fish, halibut, baked/broiled	3 oz	85	119	22.7	0	0	2.5	0.4	35	59	46	0	51	0.9
Fish, salmon, baked/broiled	3 oz	85	175	18.8	0	0	10.5	2.1	54	52	13	3.1	13	0.3
Fish, salmon, canned	3 oz	85	130	17.4	0	0	6.2	1.4	37	457	45	0	203	0.9
Fish, salmon, smoked	3 oz	85	99	15.5	0	0	3.7	0.8	20	1700	22	0	9	0.7
Fish, sardine, canned in oil	1 can (3.75 oz)	92	191	22.7	0	0	10.5	1.4	131	465	62	0	351	2.7
Fish, snapper, baked/broiled	3 oz	85	109	22.3	0	0	1.5	0.3	40	48	30	1.4	34	0.2
Fish sticks	3 sticks	84	228	13.1	19.9	0	10.3	2.6	94	489	26	0	17	0.6
Fish, swordfish, baked/broiled	3 oz	85	132	21.6	0	0	4.4	1.2	43	98	35	0.9	5	0.9
Fish, trout, baked/broiled	3 oz	85	162	22.6	0	0	7.2	1.3	63	57	16	0.4	47	1.6
Fish, tuna, canned in oil	3 oz	85	158	22.6	0	0	6.9	1.4	26	337	20	0	3	0.6
Fish, tuna, canned in water	3 oz	85	109	20.1	0	0	2.5	0.7	36	320	5	0	12	0.8
Ham, extra lean	3 oz	85	116	18.0	0.4	0	4.1	1.4	26	965	0	0	5	0.8
Ham, regular	3 oz	85	192	17.5	0.4	0	12.9	4.3	53	800	0	11.9	7	1.2
Lamb, trimmed	3 oz	85	218	20.8	0	0	14.3	6.7	74	65	0	0	14	1.6
Lunch meat, beef pastrami	3 oz	85	297	14.7	2.6	0	24.8	8.9	79	1043	0	0	8	1.6
Lunch meat, beef, sliced	3 oz	85	151	23.9	4.9	0	3.3	1.4	35	1224	0	0	9	0.8
Lunch meat, bologna (beef)	3 slices	85	265	10.4	0.7	0	24.2	10.3	49	834	0	0	10	1.4
Lunch meat, bologna (turkey)	3 slices	85	169	11.7	0.8	0	12.9	4.3	84	747	0	0	71	1.3
Lunch meat, chicken breast	3 oz	85	108	14.3	1.9	0	4.7	1.2	50	1005	0	0	14	1.3
Lunch meat, franks (beef)	1 frank	57	180	6.8	1.0	0	16.2	6.9	35	585	0	0	11	0.8
Lunch meat, franks (chicken)	1 frank	45	116	5.8	3.1	0	8.8	2.5	45	617	17	0	43	0.9
Lunch meat, ham, lean, sliced	3 slices	85	111	16.5	0.8	0	4.2	1.4	40	1215	0	0	6	0.6
Lunch meat, liverwurst	3 oz	85	277	12.0	1.9	0	24.2	9.0	134	731	7059	0	22	5.4
Lunch meat, salami, dry	8 slices	80	334	18.3	2.1	0	27.5	9.8	63	1488	0	0	6	1.2
Lunch meat, turkey breast	3 oz	85	94	19.1	0	0	1.3	0.4	35	1216	0	0	6	0.3
Nuts, almonds	⅓ cup	47	274	10.1	9.3	5.6	24.0	1.8	0	0	0	0	117	2.0
Nuts, cashews, dry roasted	⅓ cup	46	262	7.0	14.9	1.4	21.2	4.2	0	7	0	0	21	2.7
Nuts, chestnuts, dry roasted	⅓ cup	48	117	1.5	25.2	2.4	1.0	0.2	0	1	1	12.4	14	0.4
Nuts, macadamia, dry roasted	⅓ cup	45	321	3.5	6.0	3.6	34.0	5.3	0	2	0	0.3	31	0.3
Nuts, pecans	⅓ cup	36	249	3.3	5.0	3.5	25.9	2.2	0	0	3	0.4	25	0.9
Nuts, pine	⅓ cup	45	257	10.9	6.4	2.0	23.0	3.5	0	2	1	0.8	12	4.2
Nuts, pistachios, dry roasted	⅓ cup	43	244	9.1	11.8	4.4	19.6	2.4	0	4	23	1.0	47	1.8
Nuts, walnuts	⅓ cup	40	262	6.1	5.5	2.7	26.1	2.5	0	1	2	0.5	39	1.2
Peanut butter, chunky	2 tablespoons	32	188	7.7	6.9	2.1	16.0	3.1	0	156	0	0	13	0.7
Peanut butter, smooth	2 tablespoons	32	190	8.1	6.2	1.9	16.3	3.3	0	149	0	0	12	0.6
Peanuts, dry roasted	⅓ cup	49	285	11.5	10.5	3.9	24.2	3.4	0	3	0	0	26	1.1
Pork chop, pan fried	3 oz	85	190	23.5	0	0	10.0	3.7	60	44	2	0.3	4	0.7
Pork ribs, braised	3 oz	85	337	24.7	0	0	25.8	9.5	103	79	3	0	40	1.6
Pork roast	3 oz	85	214	22.9	0	0	12.9	4.5	69	41	3	0	5	0.8
Pumpkin seeds, roasted	¼ cup	57	296	18.7	7.6	2.2	23.9	4.5	0	10	22	1.0	24	8.5
Sausage, beef	1 sausage	43	134	6.1	1.0	0	11.6	4.9	29	486	0	0	3	0.8
Sausage, pork	1 sausage	67	216	13.4	1.0	0	17.2	6.1	52	618	0	1.3	16	1.0
Sausage, smoked links	3 2″ links	48	161	6.4	0.7	0	14.6	5.1	34	454	0	0	5	0.7
Shellfish, clams, canned	3 oz	85	126	21.7	4.4	0	1.7	0.2	57	95	145	18.8	78	23.8
Shellfish, clams, steamed	10 clams	95	140	24.3	4.9	0	1.9	0.2	64	106	542	21.0	87	26.6
Shellfish, crab, steamed	3 oz	85	82	16.4	0	0	1.3	0.1	45	911	8	6.5	50	0.6
Shellfish, oysters, fried	6 medium	88	173	7.7	10.2	0	11.1	2.8	71	367	79	3.3	55	6.1
Shellfish, shrimp, canned	3 oz	85	102	19.6	0.9	0	1.7	0.3	147	144	15	2.0	50	2.3
Shellfish, shrimp, fried	4 large	30	73	6.4	3.4	0.1	3.7	0.6	53	103	17	0.5	20	0.4

Name	Amount	Weight (g)	Energy (calories)	Protein (g)	Carbohydrate (g)	Fiber (g)	Total Fat (g)	Saturated Fat (g)	Cholesterol (mg)	Sodium (mg)	Vitamin A (RE)	Vitamin C (mg)	Calcium (mg)	Iron (mg)
Sunflower seeds, dry roasted	¼ cup	32	186	6.2	7.7	3.6	15.9	1.7	0	1	0	0.4	22	1.2
Tempeh	½ cup	83	160	15.4	7.8	0	9.0	1.8	0	7	0	0	92	2.2
Tofu, firm	½ cup	126	183	19.9	5.4	2.9	11.0	1.6	0	18	21	0.3	861	13.2
Turkey, dark meat, w/o skin, roasted	3 oz	85	138	24.5	0	0	3.7	1.2	95	67	0	0	22	2.0
Turkey, dark meat, w/skin, roasted	3 oz	85	155	23.5	0	0	6.0	1.8	99	65	0	0	23	2.0
Turkey, light meat, w/o skin, roasted	3 oz	85	119	25.7	0	0	1.0	0.3	73	48	0	0	13	1.3
Turkey, light meat, w/skin, roasted	3 oz	85	139	24.5	0	0	3.9	1.1	81	48	0	0	15	1.4
Veal, sirloin, roasted	3 oz	85	172	21.4	0	0	8.9	3.8	87	71	0	0	11	0.8
Vegetarian bacon, cooked	1 oz	16	50	1.7	1.0	0.4	4.7	0.7	0	234	1	0	4	0.4
Vegetarian franks	1 frank	51	118	12.1	1.5	1.5	7.1	0.8	0	224	0	0	10	1.0
Vegetarian patties	1 patty	67	119	11.2	10.2	4.0	3.8	0.5	0	382	76	0	48	1.2
Vegetarian sausage	1 patty	38	97	7.0	3.7	1.1	6.9	1.1	0	337	24	0	24	1.4

Fats, Oils, Sweets, and Alcoholic Beverages

Name	Amount	Weight (g)	Energy (calories)	Protein (g)	Carbohydrate (g)	Fiber (g)	Total Fat (g)	Saturated Fat (g)	Cholesterol (mg)	Sodium (mg)	Vitamin A (RE)	Vitamin C (mg)	Calcium (mg)	Iron (mg)
Alcoholic beverage, beer	1 can or bottle	356	146	1.1	13.2	0.7	0	0	0	18	0	0	18	0.1
Alcoholic beverage, liquor	1.5 oz	42	97	0	0	0	0	0	0	0	0	0	0	0
Alcoholic beverage, wine	5 oz	148	103	0	2.1	0	0	0	0	12	0	0	12	0.5
Beverage, cola	1 can	370	152	0	38.5	0	0	0	0	15	0	0	11	0.1
Beverage, fruit punch	1 cup	247	114	0	28.9	0.2	0	0	0	10	2	108.4	10	0.2
Beverage, kiwi strawberry drink	1 cup	236	113	0.2	27.8	0	0	0	0	10	0	0	0	0
Beverage, lemon-lime soda	1 can	368	147	0	38.3	0	0	0	0	40	0	0	7	0.3
Beverage, tea, bottled, sweetened	1 bottle	480	178	0	40.8	0	0	0	0	0	0	0	0	0
Butter	1 tablespoon	14	102	0.1	0	0	11.5	7.1	31	117	107	0	3	0
Candy, caramels	1 piece	10	39	0.5	7.8	0.1	0.8	0.7	1	25	1	0.1	14	0
Candy, fudge	1 piece	17	65	0.3	13.5	0.1	1.4	0.9	2	11	8	0	7	0.1
Candy, jelly beans	10 large	28	104	0	26.4	0	0.1	0	0	7	0	0	1	0.3
Candy, milk chocolate	1 bar	44	226	3.0	26.0	1.5	13.5	8.1	10	36	24	0.2	84	0.6
Chocolate syrup	2 tablespoons	38	105	0.8	24.4	0.7	0.4	0.2	0	27	1	0.1	5	0.8
Cream, half and half	2 tablespoons	30	39	0.9	1.3	0	3.5	2.2	11	12	32	0.3	32	0
Cream, heavy, whipped	½ cup	60	206	1.2	1.7	0	22.1	13.8	82	23	252	0.4	39	0
Cream, sour	1 tablespoon	12	26	0.4	0.5	0	2.5	1.6	5	6	23	0.1	14	0
Frosting, chocolate	1/12 package	38	151	0.4	24.0	0.2	6.7	2.1	0	70	75	0	3	0.5
Honey	1 tablespoon	21	64	0.1	17.3	0	0	0	0	1	0	0.1	1	0.1
Jam/preserves	1 tablespoon	20	56	0.1	13.8	0.2	0	0	0	6	0	1.8	4	0.1
Lard	1 tablespoon	13	115	0	0	0	12.8	5.0	12	0	0	0	0	0
Marmalade	1 tablespoon	20	49	0.1	13.3	0	0	0	0	11	1	1.0	8	0
Margarine, hard	1 tablespoon	14	101	0.1	0.1	0	11.4	2.1	0	133	113	0	4	0
Margarine, liquid	1 tablespoon	14	102	0.3	0	0	11.4	1.9	0	111	113	0	9	0
Margarine, soft	1 tablespoon	14	101	0.1	0	0	11.3	2.0	0	152	113	0	4	0
Margarine-like spread	1 tablespoon	14	50	0.1	0.1	0	5.6	1.1	0	138	115	0	3	0
Mayonnaise, fat free	1 tablespoon	16	11	0	2.0	0.3	0.4	0.1	2	120	1	0	1	0
Mayonnaise, regular	1 tablespoon	15	57	0.1	3.5	0	4.9	0.7	4	105	12	0	2	0

Name	Amount	Weight (g)	Energy (calories)	Protein (g)	Carbohydrate (g)	Fiber (g)	Total Fat (g)	Saturated Fat (g)	Cholesterol (mg)	Sodium (mg)	Vitamin A (RE)	Vitamin C (mg)	Calcium (mg)	Iron (mg)
Oil, canola	1 tablespoon	14	124	0	0	0	14.0	1.0	0	0	0	0	0	0
Oil, corn	1 tablespoon	14	120	0	0	0	13.6	1.7	0	0	0	0	0	0
Oil, olive	1 tablespoon	14	119	0	0	0	13.5	1.8	0	0	0	0	0	0.1
Popsicle	1 single stick	88	63	0	16.6	0	0	0	0	11	0	9.4	0	0
Salad dressing, blue cheese	2 tablespoons	31	154	1.5	2.3	0	16.0	3.0	5	335	20	0.6	25	0.1
Salad dressing, French	2 tablespoons	31	134	0.2	5.5	0	12.8	3.0	0	427	40	0	3	0.1
Salad dressing, Italian	2 tablespoons	29	137	0.2	3.0	0	14.2	2.1	0	231	7	0	3	0
Salad dressing, Italian light	2 tablespoons	30	32	0	1.5	0	2.9	0.4	2	236	0	0	1	0.1
Sherbet	½ cup	74	102	0.8	22.5	0	1.5	0.9	0	34	10	2.3	40	0.1
Shortening, vegetable	1 tablespoon	13	113	0	0	0	12.8	3.2	0	0	0	0	0	0
Sugar, brown	1 tablespoon	14	52	0	13.4	0	0	0	0	5	0	0	12	0.3
Sugar, white	1 tablespoon	13	49	0	12.6	0	0	0	0	0	0	0	0	0
Syrup, corn	1 tablespoon	20	56	0	15.3	0	0	0	0	24	0	0	1	0
Syrup, maple	¼ cup	79	206	0	52.9	0	0.2	0	0	7	0	0	53	0.9

Appendix B

Nutritional Content of Popular Items from Fast-Food Restaurants

Arby's

	Serving Size	Calories	Protein	Total Fat	Saturated Fat	Total Carbohydrate	Sugars	Fibers	Cholesterol	Sodium	Vitamin A	Vitamin C	Calcium	Iron	% Calories from Fat
	g		g	g	g	g	g	g	mg	mg			% Daily Value		
Regular roast beef	154	388	23	19	7	33	N/A	3	43	1009	N/A	N/A	N/A	N/A	44
Super roast beef	247	523	25	27	9	50	N/A	5	43	1189	N/A	N/A	N/A	N/A	46
French dip	195	475	30	22	8	40	N/A	3	55	1411	N/A	N/A	N/A	N/A	41
Junior roast beef	126	324	17	14	5	35	N/A	2	30	779	N/A	N/A	N/A	N/A	39
Roast chicken Caesar sandwich	300	660	41	24	5	70	N/A	N/A	80	1900	N/A	N/A	N/A	N/A	33
Roast turkey & swiss	327	630	42	30	8	52	N/A	N/A	80	1670	N/A	N/A	N/A	N/A	43
Breaded chicken fillet	240	623	28	28	5	46	N/A	5	45	1016	N/A	N/A	N/A	N/A	40
Ham 'n cheese	169	359	24	14	5	34	N/A	2	53	1283	N/A	N/A	N/A	N/A	35
Jalapeño bites	110	330	7	21	9	29	N/A	2	40	670	N/A	N/A	N/A	N/A	57
Cheddar curly fries	120	333	5	18	4	40	N/A	0	3	1016	N/A	N/A	N/A	N/A	49
Potato cakes	85	204	2	12	2	20	N/A	0	0	397	N/A	N/A	N/A	N/A	53
Red ranch dressing	14	75	0	6	1	5	N/A	0	0	115	N/A	N/A	N/A	N/A	72
French-toastix	124	430	10	21	5	52	N/A	3	0	550	N/A	N/A	N/A	N/A	44
Jamocha shake	340	384	15	10	3	62	N/A	0	36	262	N/A	N/A	N/A	N/A	23

N/A: not available.

SOURCE: Triare Restaurant Group, 1998–2000, www.arbysrestaurant.com.

Burger King

	Serving Size	Calories	Protein	Total Fat	Saturated Fat	Total Carbohydrate	Sugars	Fibers	Cholesterol	Sodium	Vitamin A	Vitamin C	Calcium	Iron	% Calories from Fat
	g		g	g	g	g	g	g	mg	mg	% Daily Value				
Whopper®	278	680	29	39	12	53	9	4	80	940	10	15	10	30	52
Whopper Jr.®	172	420	20	24	8	32	6	2	55	520	4	8	8	20	51
Double Whopper® w/cheese	387	1020	53	65	25	55	9	4	170	1460	15	15	30	40	57
BK Big Fish™ sandwich	263	710	24	38	14	67	4	4	50	1200	2	0	8	20	48
BK Broiler® chicken sandwich	258	550	30	25	5	52	5	3	105	1110	6	10	6	20	41
Chicken Tenders® (8 pieces)	123	340	22	19	5	20	0	<1	50	840	0	0	0	4	50
Ranch dipping sauce	28	120	1	13	2	1	N/A	N/A	5	85	N/A	N/A	N/A	N/A	98
Barbecue dipping sauce	28	35	0	0	0	9	N/A	N/A	0	400	N/A	N/A	N/A	N/A	0
French fries, medium	116	370	4	17	5	49	0	4	0	760	0	2	0	6	41
Onion rings, medium	94	330	5	16	4	41	5	3	0	470	0	0	10	0	44
Chocolate shake, medium	397	440	12	10	6	75	67	4	30	330	8	0	30	15	21
Croissan'wich® w/sausage, egg & cheese	153	500	19	36	13	26	5	1	190	1020	8	0	15	15	65
French toast sticks	112	390	6	20	4.5	46	11	2	0	440	0	0	6	10	46
Dutch apple pie	113	340	2	14	3	15	23	1	0	470	2	0	0	8	37
Chicken club sandwich	242	620	30	32	8	54	6	4	75	1460	6	10	8	20	47

N/A: not available.

SOURCE: Burger King Corporation, 2001, www.burgerking.com. Burger King® trademarks, trade name, and Nutritional Guide are reproduced with permission from Burger King Brands, Inc.

Domino's Pizza

(1 serving = 2 of 8 slices or ¼ of 14-inch pizza; 2 of 8 slices or ¼ of 12-inch pizza; 1 6-inch pizza)

	Serving Size	Calories	Protein	Total Fat	Saturated Fat	Total Carbohydrate	Sugars	Fibers	Cholesterol	Sodium	Vitamin A	Vitamin C	Calcium	Iron	% Calories from Fat
	g		g	g	g	g	g	g	mg	mg	% Daily Value				
14-inch lg. hand-tossed cheese	219	516	21	15	7	75	6	4	32	1080	18	0	26	23	26
14-inch lg. thin crust cheese	148	382	17	17	7	43	6	2	32	1172	18	0	32	8	40
14-inch lg. deep dish cheese	257	677	26	30	11	80	9	5	41	1575	21	<1	33	31	40
12-inch med. hand-tossed cheese	159	375	15	11	5	55	5	3	23	776	13	0	19	17	26
12-inch med. thin crust cheese	106	273	12	12	5	31	4	2	23	835	13	0	23	5	40
12-inch med. deep dish cheese	181	482	19	22	8	56	6	3	30	1123	15	<1	24	22	41
6-inch deep dish cheese	216	598	23	28	10	68	7	4	36	1341	17	<1	30	30	42
Toppings: pepperoni	*	98	5	9	3	<1	<1	<1	20	364	†	†	†	†	83
ham	*	31	5	2	<1	<1	<1	<1	12	292	†	†	†	†	58
Italian sausage	*	110	5	9	3	3	<1	<1	22	342	†	†	†	†	74
bacon	*	153	8	13	4	<1	<1	<1	22	424	†	†	†	†	77
beef	*	111	6	10	4	<1	<1	<1	21	309	†	†	†	†	81
anchovies	*	45	9	2	<1	<1	<1	<1	18	791	†	†	5	6	40
extra cheese	*	68	7	6	3	<1	<1	<1	15	228	11	†	12	†	79
cheddar cheese	*	71	5	6	3	<1	<1	<1	18	110	4	†	13	†	76
Barbeque buffalo wings	25	50	5	2	<1	2	1	<1	26	175	†	†	†	†	36
Breadsticks (1 piece)	37	116	3	4	<1	16	<1	<1	0	152	†	†	†	†	31
Double cheesy bread	43	142	4	6	2	18	<1	<1	6	183	†	†	†	†	38

*Topping information is based on minimal portioning requirements for one serving of a 14-inch large pizza; add the values for toppings to the values for a cheese pizza. The following toppings supply fewer than 15 calories per serving: green and yellow peppers, onion, olives, mushrooms, pineapple.
†Contains less than 2% of the Daily Value of these nutrients.

SOURCE: Domino's Pizza, 2001 www.dominos.com. Reproduced with permission from Domino's Pizza LLC.

Jack in the Box

	Serving Size	Calories	Protein	Total Fat	Saturated Fat	Total Carbohydrate	Sugars	Fibers	Cholesterol	Sodium	Vitamin A	Vitamin C	Calcium	Iron	% Calories from Fat
	g		g	g	g	g	g	g	mg	mg	\% Daily Value				
Breakfast Jack®	126	280	17	12	5	28	3	1	190	750	8	6	15	20	39
Supreme croissant	164	530	21	34	10	37	6	0	225	1060	8	6	10	10	58
Hamburger	104	250	12	9	3.5	30	5	2	30	610	0	0	10	20	32
Jumbo Jack®	271	550	27	30	10	43	12	2	75	880	10	15	15	25	49
Sourdough Jack®	233	690	34	45	15	37	3	2	105	1180	15	15	20	25	59
Chicken fajita pita	230	320	24	10	4.5	34	6	3	55	850	20	25	20	15	28
Grilled chicken fillet	242	480	27	24	6	39	6	4	65	1110	8	15	20	25	45
Chicken supreme	305	830	33	49	7	66	5	3	65	2140	10	15	20	20	53
Jack Spicy Chicken®	252	570	24	29	2.5	52	9	2	50	1020	8	15	15	10	46
Garden chicken salad	253	200	23	9	4	8	4	3	65	420	70	20	20	4	41
Blue cheese dressing	57	210	1	15	2.5	11	4	0	25	750	0	0	2	0	64
Chicken teriyaki bowl	502	670	26	4	1	128	27	3	15	1730	130	40	10	25	5
Monster taco	138	270	12	17	6	19	2	4	30	630	10	4	20	8	57
Egg rolls (3 pieces)	170	440	15	24	6	40	5	4	30	1020	15	20	8	25	49
Chicken breast pieces (5)	150	360	27	17	3	24	0	1	80	970	4	2	2	10	43
Stuffed jalapeños (7 pieces)	168	530	16	31	12	46	5	4	60	1730	20	35	30	8	53
Barbeque dipping sauce	28	45	1	0	0	11	7	0	0	310	0	4	0	0	0
Seasoned curly fries	125	410	6	23	5	45	0	4	0	1010	6	0	4	10	51
Onion rings	120	450	7	25	5	50	3	3	0	780	4	30	4	15	50
Cappuccino classic ice cream shake	16 oz	630	11	29	17	80	58	0	90	320	15	0	35	0	41

SOURCE: Jack's Nutrition Facts, Rev. 2000. The following trademarks are owned by Jack in the Box, Inc.: Breakfast Jack,® Jumbo Jack,® Sourdough Jack,® Jack in the Box.® Reproduced with permission from Jack in the Box Inc.

KFC

	Serving Size	Calories	Protein	Total Fat	Saturated Fat	Total Carbohydrate	Sugars	Fibers	Cholesterol	Sodium	Vitamin A	Vitamin C	Calcium	Iron	% Calories from Fat
	g		g	g	g	g	g	g	mg	mg	\% Daily Value				
Original Recipe® breast	153	400	29	24	6	16	0	1	135	1116	*	*	4	6	54
Original Recipe® thigh	91	250	16	18	4.5	6	0	1	95	747	*	*	2	4	65
Extra crispy chicken breast	168	470	39	28	8	17	0	<1	160	874	*	*	2	6	54
Extra crispy chicken thigh	118	380	21	27	7	14	0	<1	118	625	*	*	2	6	64
Hot & spicy breast	180	505	38	29	8	23	9	1	162	1170	*	*	6	6	52
Hot & spicy thigh	107	355	19	26	7	13	0	1	126	630	*	*	2	4	66
Tender Roast sandwich w/sauce	211	350	32	15	3	26	1	1	75	880	4	*	4	10	39
Tender Roast sandwich w/o sauce	177	270	31	5	1.5	23	<1	1	65	690	*	*	4	10	17
Hot wings (6 pieces)	135	471	27	33	8	18	0	2	150	1230	*	*	4	8	63
Colonel's Crispy Strips™ (3)	115	300	26	16	4	18	1	1	56	1165	2	*	*	6	48
Chunky chicken pot pie	368	770	29	42	13	69	8	5	70	2160	80	2	10	10	49
Corn on the cob	162	150	5	1.5	0	35	8	2	0	20	2	6	*	*	9
Mashed potatoes w/gravy	136	120	1	6	1	17	0	2	<1	440	*	*	*	2	45
BBQ baked beans	156	190	6	3	1	33	13	6	5	760	8	*	8	10	14
Cole slaw	142	232	2	13.5	2	26	20	3	8	284	9	58	3	*	52
Biscuit (1)	56	180	4	10	2.5	20	2	<1	0	560	*	*	2	6	50
Potato salad	160	230	4	14	2	23	9	3	15	540	10	*	2	15	55

*Contains less than 2% of the Daily Value of these nutrients.

SOURCE: KFC Corporation, 2001, www.kfc.com. Reproduced with permission from Kentucky Fried Chicken Corporation.

Taco Bell

	Serving Size	Calories	Protein	Total Fat	Saturated Fat	Total Carbohydrate	Sugars	Fibers	Cholesterol	Sodium	Vitamin A	Vitamin C	Calcium	Iron	% Calories from Fat
	g		g	g	g	g	g	g	mg	mg		% Daily Value			
Taco	86	170	9	10	4	12	<1	3	30	330	8	0	8	4	53
Taco Supreme®	124	210	9	14	6	14	2	3	40	350	8	6	10	6	60
Double Decker Taco Supreme®	109	380	15	18	7	39	3	9	40	760	8	6	15	10	43
Beef soft taco	109	210	11	10	4	20	1	3	30	570	8	0	8	6	43
Chicken soft taco	109	190	13	7	2.5	19	1	2	35	480	4	2	8	4	33
Chicken Burrito Supreme	117	410	20	16	6	49	4	8	45	1120	45	8	15	10	35
Beef Double Burrito Supreme	319	510	23	23	9	52	4	11	60	1500	50	8	15	15	41
Chili cheese burrito	156	330	13	13	5	40	2	4	25	900	20	0	15	6	35
Bean burrito	218	370	13	12	3.5	54	3	12	10	1080	45	0	15	15	29
Nachos Supreme	218	440	14	24	7	44	3	9	35	800	0	6	15	15	49
Nachos BellGrande®	342	760	20	39	11	83	4	17	35	1300	10	8	20	20	46
Pintos 'n cheese	140	180	9	8	4	18	1	10	15	640	45	0	15	10	40
Mexican rice	148	190	5	9	3.5	23	<1	<1	15	750	100	2	15	8	43
Beef Fiesto Burrito	202	370	14	15	5	49	3	4	30	1110	30	0	10	10	36
Meximelt®	148	290	15	15	7	22	2	4	45	830	8	0	20	6	47
Chalupa Supreme,® beef	171	380	14	23	8	29	3	3	40	580	6	8	15	10	55
Chalupa nacho cheese, chicken	171	350	16	19	4.5	29	3	2	25	640	6	8	8	10	49
Gordita Supreme,® beef	171	300	17	14	5	27	4	3	35	550	2	6	15	10	42
Gordita Santa Fe,® chicken	171	370	17	20	4	30	3	3	40	610	4	6	15	10	49

SOURCE: Taco Bell Corporation, 2001, **www.tacobell.com**. Reproduced with permission from the Taco Bell Corporation.

Wendy's

	Serving Size	Calories	Protein	Total Fat	Saturated Fat	Total Carbohydrate	Sugars	Fibers	Cholesterol	Sodium	Vitamin A	Vitamin C	Calcium	Iron	% Calories from Fat
	g		g	g	g	g	g	g	mg	mg		% Daily Value			
Single w/everything	219	420	25	20	7	37	8	3	70	930	6	10	15	25	43
Big Bacon Classic	282	580	33	31	12	45	11	3	95	1500	15	20	25	30	48
Jr. hamburger	118	280	15	10	3.5	34	7	2	30	610	2	2	10	20	32
Jr. bacon cheeseburger	166	390	20	20	8	34	7	2	55	870	8	10	15	20	46
Grilled chicken sandwich	189	300	24	8	1.5	36	8	2	55	730	4	10	10	15	24
Caesar side salad (no dressing)	92	110	9	6	2.5	6	1	1	15	600	35	25	15	6	49
Grilled chicken salad (no dressing)	338	190	22	8	1.5	10	5	4	45	680	120	60	20	10	38
Taco salad (no dressing)	468	380	26	19	10	28	8	8	65	1040	45	45	35	25	45
Blue cheese dressing (2T)	28	180	1	19	3.5	0	0	0	15	170	0	0	2	0	95
Ranch dressing, reduced fat, calories (2T)	28	60	1	5	1	2	1	0	10	240	0	0	2	0	75
Soft breadstick	44	130	4	3	.5	23	N/A	1	5	250	0	0	4	9	21
Biggie fries	159	470	7	23	3.5	61	0	6	0	150	0	15	3	7	44
Baked potato w/broccoli & cheese	411	470	9	14	2.5	80	6	9	5	470	35	120	20	25	27
Baked potato w/chili & cheese	439	620	20	24	9	83	7	9	40	780	20	60	35	30	35
Chili, small, plain	227	210	15	7	2.5	21	5	5	30	800	8	6	8	6	30
Chili, large w/cheese & crackers	363	405	28	16.5	7	37	8	7	60	1380	14	10	22	26	37
Chicken nuggets (5)	75	230	11	16	3	11	0	0	30	470	0	2	2	2	63
Barbeque sauce	28	45	1	0	0	10	7	0	0	160	0	0	0	4	0
Frosty dairy dessert, medium	298	440	11	11	7	73	56	0	50	260	20	0	41	8	23
Chicken club sandwich	216	480	30	21	5	44	6	2	65	1000	4	10	10	15	39

N/A: not available.

SOURCE: Wendy's International, Inc., 2001, www.wendys.com. Reproduced with permission from Wendy's International, Inc.

Information on additional foods and restaurants is available online:

Arby's: www.arbysrestaurant.com
Burger King: www.burgerking.com
Domino's Pizza: www.dominos.com
Hardees: www.hardees.com
Jack in the Box: www.jackinthebox.com
KFC: www.kfc.com
McDonald's: www.mcdonalds.com
Subway: www.subway.com
Taco Bell: www.tacobell.com
Wendy's: www.wendys.com
White Castle: www.whitecastle.com

Appendix C

A Self-Care Guide for Common Medical Problems

This self-care guide will help you manage some of the most common symptoms and medical problems:

- Fever
- Sore throat
- Cough
- Nasal congestion
- Ear problems
- Nausea, vomiting, or diarrhea
- Heartburn and indigestion
- Headache
- Low-back pain
- Strains and sprains
- Cuts and scrapes

Each symptom is described here in terms of what is going on in your body. Most symptoms are part of the body's natural healing response and reflect your body's wisdom in attempting to correct disease. Self-care advice is also given, along with some guidelines about when to seek professional advice. In most cases, the symptoms are self-limiting; that is, they will resolve on their own with time and simple self-care strategies.

No medical advice is perfect. You will always have to make the decision about whether to self-treat or get professional help. This guide is intended to provide you with more information so you can make better, more informed decisions. If the advice here differs from that of your physician, discuss the differences with him or her. In most cases, your physician will be able to customize the advice to your individual medical situation.

The guidelines given here apply to *generally healthy adults*. If you are pregnant or nursing, or if you have a chronic disease, particularly one that requires medication, check with your physician for appropriate self-care advice. Additionally, if you have an allergy or suspected allergy to any recommended medication, check with your physician before using it.

If you have several symptoms, read about your primary symptom first, and then proceed to secondary symptoms. Use your common sense when determining self-care. If you are particularly concerned about a symptom or confused about how to manage it, call your physician to get more information.

Fever

Body temperature is generally about 98.6° F. Body temperature varies with exercise, at rest, by climate, and by gender. Fever means a reading over 99° F. It is most commonly a sign that your body is fighting an infection. Fever may also be due to an inflammation, an injury, or a drug reaction. Chemicals released into your bloodstream during an infection reset the thermostat in the hypothalamus of your brain. The message goes out to your body to turn up the heat. The blood vessels in your skin constrict, and you curl up and throw on extra blankets to reduce heat loss. Meanwhile, your muscles begin to shiver to generate additional body heat. The resulting rise in body temperature is a fever. Later, when your brain senses that the temperature is too high, the signal goes out to increase sweating. As the sweat evaporates, it carries heat away from the body surface.

A fever may not be all bad; it may even help you fight infections by making the body less hospitable to bacteria and viruses. A high body temperature appears to bolster the immune system and may inhibit the growth of infectious microorganisms.

Most generally healthy people can tolerate a fever as high as 103–104° F (39.5–40° C) without problems. Therefore, if you are essentially healthy, there is little need to reduce a fever unless you are very uncomfortable. Older adults and those with chronic health problems such as heart disease may not tolerate the increased metabolic demand of a high fever, and fever reduction may be advised.

Most problems with fevers are due to the excessive loss of fluids from evaporation and sweating, which may cause dehydration.

Self-Assessment

1. If you are sick, take your temperature several times throughout the day. Oral temperatures should not be measured for at least 10 minutes after smoking, eating, or drinking a hot or cold liquid. When using an oral glass thermometer, first clean it with rubbing alcohol or cool soapy water (hot water may break it). Then shake it down until it reads 95° F or lower. Place the thermometer under your tongue, and leave it in place for a *full 3 minutes.* (If you leave it in for only 2 minutes, the temperature reading will be off by at least half a degree.) To read the thermometer, notice where the colored column ends, and compare it with the degrees marked in lines on the thermometer. If you are using an electronic digital thermometer, follow the directions that came with it.

   "Normal" temperature varies from person to person, so it is important to know what is normal for you. Your normal temperature will also vary throughout the day, being lowest in the early evening. If you exercise or if it is a hot day, your temperature may normally rise. Women's body temperature typically varies by a degree or more through the menstrual cycle, peaking around the time of ovulation. Rectal temperatures normally run about 0.5–1.0° F higher than oral temperatures. If your recorded temperature is more than 1.0–1.5° F above your normal baseline temperature, you have a fever.

2. Watch for signs of dehydration: excessive thirst; very dry mouth; infrequent urination with dark, concentrated urine; and light-headedness.

Self-Care

1. Drink plenty of fluids to prevent dehydration—at least 8 ounces of water, juice, or broth every 2 hours.

2. Take a sponge bath using lukewarm water; this will increase evaporation and help reduce body temperature naturally.

3. Don't bundle up. This decreases the body's ability to lose excess heat.

4. Take aspirin substitute (acetaminophen, ibuprofen, or naproxen sodium). For adults, two standard-size tablets every 4–6 hours can be used to reduce the fever and the associated headache and achiness. Do not use aspirin in anyone younger than age 20 because some younger people with chicken pox, influenza, or other viral infections have developed a life-threatening complication, Reye's syndrome, after taking aspirin.

When to Call the Physician

1. Fever over 101° F despite self-care actions

2. Low-grade fever (99° F to 100° F) if there is no improvement in seventy-two hours

3. If fever last more than five days, regardless of improvement

4. Recurrent unexplained fevers

5. Fever accompanied by a rash, stiff neck, severe headache, difficulty breathing, cough with brown sputum, severe pain in the side or abdomen, painful urination, convulsions, or mental confusion

6. Fever with signs of dehydration

7. Fever after starting a new medication

Sore Throat

A sore throat is caused by inflammation of the throat lining resulting from an infection, allergy, or irritation (especially from cigarette smoke). If you have an infection, you may also notice some hoarseness from swelling of the vocal cords and "swollen glands," which are enlarged lymph nodes that produce white blood cells to help fight the infection. The lymph nodes, part of your body's defense system, may remain swollen for weeks after the infection subsides.

Most throat infections are caused by viruses, so antibiotics are not effective against them. However, about 20–30% of throat infections are due to streptococcal bacteria. This type of microbe can cause complications such as rheumatic fever and rheumatic heart disease and therefore should be diagnosed by a physician and treated with antibiotics. Strep throat is usually characterized by very sore throat, high fever, swollen lymph nodes, a whitish discharge at the back of the throat, and the absence of other cold symptoms such as a cough and runny nose (which suggest a viral infection). Allergy-related sore throats are usually accompanied by running nose, sneezing, and watery, itchy eyes.

Self-Assessment

1. Take your temperature.

2. Look at the back of your throat in a mirror. Is there a whitish, puslike discharge on the tonsils or in the back of the throat?

3. Feel the front and back of your neck. Do you feel enlarged, tender lymph nodes?

Self-Care

1. If you smoke, stop smoking to avoid further irritation of your throat.

2. Drink plenty of liquids to soothe your inflamed throat.

3. Gargle with warm salt water (1/4 tsp salt in 4 oz water) every 1–2 hours to help reduce swelling and discomfort.

4. Suck on throat lozenges, cough drops, or hard candies to keep your throat moist.

5. Use throat lozenges, sprays, or gargles that contain an anesthetic to temporarily numb your throat and make swallowing less painful.
6. Try aspirin substitute to ease throat pain.
7. For an allergy-related sore throat, try an antihistamine such as chlorpheniramine.

When to Call the Physician
1. Great difficulty swallowing saliva or breathing
2. Sore throat with fever over 101° F (38.3° C), especially if you do not have other cold symptoms such as nasal congestion or a cough
3. Sore throat with a skin rash
4. Sore throat with whitish pus on the tonsils
5. Sore throat and recent contact with a person who has had a positive throat culture for strep
6. Enlarged lymph nodes lasting longer than 3 weeks
7. Hoarseness lasting longer than 3 weeks

Cough

A cough is a protective mechanism of the body to help keep the airways clear. There are two types of cough: a dry cough (without mucus) and a productive cough (with mucus). Common causes of cough include infection (viral or bacterial), allergies, and irritation from smoking and pollutants. If you have a cold, the cough may be the last symptom to improve, because the airways may remain irritated for several weeks after the infection has resolved.

Your airways are lined with hairlike projections called cilia, which move back and forth to help clear the airways of mucus, germs, and dust. Infections and cigarette smoking paralyze and damage this vital defensive mechanism.

Self-Assessment
1. Take your temperature.
2. Observe your mucus. Thick brown or bloody mucus suggests a bacterial infection.

Self-Care
1. If you are a smoker, stop smoking. Smoking irritates the airways and undermines your body's immune defenses, leading to more serious infections and longer-lasting symptoms. Most people do not feel like smoking when they have a cold with a cough. If you want to quit, a cold may provide an excellent opportunity to do so.
2. Drink plenty of liquids (at least six 8-ounce glasses a day) to help thin mucus and loosen chest congestion.
3. Use moist heat from a hot shower or vaporizer to help loosen chest congestion.
4. Suck on cough drops, throat lozenges, or hard candy to keep your throat moist and help relieve a dry, tickling cough.

5. If you have a dry, nonproductive cough or the cough keeps you from sleeping, you can use a cough syrup or lozenge that contains the nonprescription cough suppressant dextromethorphan. Because a cough that produces mucus is protective, it is generally not advisable to suppress a productive cough.

When to Call the Physician
1. Cough with thick brown or bloody sputum
2. Cough with high fever—above 102° F (38.8° C)—and shaking chills
3. Severe chest pains, wheezing, or shortness of breath
4. Cough that lasts longer than 4 weeks

Nasal Congestion

Nasal congestion is most commonly caused by infection or allergies. With infection, the nasal passages become congested because of increased blood flow and mucus production. This congestion is actually part of the body's defense to fight infection. The increased blood flow raises the temperature of the nasal passages, making them less hospitable to germs. The nasal secretions are rich in white blood cells and antibodies to help fight and neutralize the invading organisms and flush them away. Nasal congestion associated with sore throat, cough, and fever usually indicates a viral infection. Green nasal discharge is common with viral infections; it does not mean you need an antibiotic.

Nasal congestion caused by allergies is often accompanied by a thin, watery discharge, sneezing, and itchy eyes; it is sometimes associated with a seasonal pattern. In an allergic reaction, the offending allergen (such as pollen, dust, mold, or dander) triggers the release of histamine and other chemicals from the cells lining the nose, throat, and eyes. These chemicals cause swelling, discharge, and itching. Antihistamine drugs block the release of these irritating chemicals.

Self-Assessment
1. Take your temperature.
2. Observe the color and consistency of your nasal secretions. A thick brown or bloody discharge suggests a bacterial sinus infection.
3. Tap with your fingers over the sinus cavities above and below the eyes. If the tapping causes increased pain, you may have a bacterial sinus infection.

Self-Care
1. If you smoke, stop smoking to prevent continuing irritation of the nasal passages.
2. Use moist heat from a hot shower or vaporizer to help liquefy congested mucus.
3. Use a decongestant nasal spray or drops to temporarily relieve congestion. However, if these

decongestants are used for more than 3 days, they can cause "rebound congestion" that actually creates more nasal congestion. As an alternative, use saltwater nose drops (1/4 tsp salt in 1/2 cup of boiled water, cooled before using).

4. Try an oral decongestant such as pseudo-ephedrine (60 mg every 6 hours) to help shrink swollen mucous membranes and open nasal passages. In some people, these medications can cause nervousness, sleeplessness, or heart palpitations. If you have uncontrolled high blood pressure, heart disease, or diabetes, check with your physician before using decongestants.

When to Call the Physician
1. Nasal congestion with severe pain and tenderness in the forehead, cheeks, or upper teeth and a high fever (above 102° F or 38.8° C)
2. Thick brown or bloody nasal discharge
3. Nasal congestion and discharge unresponsive to self-care treatment and lasting longer than 3 weeks

Ear Problems

Ear symptoms include earache, discharge, itching, stuffiness, and hearing loss. They may be caused by problems in the external ear canal, eardrum, middle ear, or eustachian tube (the passageway that connects the middle ear space to the back of the throat). The ear canal can become blocked by excess wax, producing hearing loss and a sense that the ear is plugged. An infection of the external ear canal due to excessive moisture and trauma is often referred to as "swimmer's ear." It can cause pain, a sense of fullness, discharge, and itching. Congestion and blockage of the eustachian tube by a cold or allergy can result in pain, a sense of fullness, and hearing loss. A middle ear infection often produces severe pain, hearing loss, and fever.

Self-Assessment
1. Take your temperature. A fever may be a sign of infection.
2. Have someone look into the ear canal with a flashlight or otoscope. Look for wax blockage or a red, swollen canal indicating an external ear infection.
3. Wiggle the outer part of the ear. If this increases the pain, an infection or inflammation of the external canal is the likely cause.

Self-Care
1. If blockage of the ear canal with wax is the problem, first try a hot shower to liquefy the wax, and use a wash cloth to wipe out the ear canal. You can also use a few drops of an over-the-counter wax softener and then flush the canal gently with warm water in a bulb syringe. Do not use sharp objects or cotton swabs; they can scratch the canal or push the wax in deeper.
2. To treat mild infections of the external ear canal, you must thoroughly dry the ear canal. A few drops of a drying agent (Burrow's solution) on a piece of cotton gently inserted into the canal can act as a wick to dry the canal.
3. To relieve congestion and blockage of the eustachian tube, try a decongestant like pseudoephedrine, a nasal spray (but for no longer than 3 days), or an antihistamine. Hot showers or a vaporizer may help loosen secretions, and yawning or swallowing may help open the eustachian tube. For a mild plugging sensation without fever or pain, pinch your nostrils and blow gently to force air up the eustachian tube and "pop" your ears.

When to Call the Physician
1. Severe earache with fever
2. Puslike or bloody discharge from the ear
3. Sudden hearing loss, especially if accompanied by ear pain or recent trauma to the ear
4. Ringing in the ears or dizziness
5. Any ear symptom lasting longer than 2 weeks

Nausea, Vomiting, or Diarrhea

Nausea, vomiting, and diarrhea usually are defensive reactions of your body to rapidly clear your digestive tract of irritants. These symptoms may be caused by a viral infection, foodborne illness, medications, or other types of infection. Vomiting dramatically ejects irritants from your stomach, and nausea discourages eating to allow the stomach to rest. With diarrhea, over-stimulated intestines flush out the offending irritants.

The major complications of vomiting and diarrhea are dehydration from fluid losses and decreased fluid intake and a risk of bleeding from irritation of the digestive tract.

Self-Assessment
1. Take your temperature. A fever is often a clue that an infection is causing the symptoms.
2. Note the color and frequency of vomiting and diarrhea. This will help you estimate the severity of fluid losses and check for bleeding (red, black, or "coffee grounds" material in the stool or vomit; iron tablets and Pepto-Bismol can also cause black stools).
3. Watch for signs of dehydration: very dry mouth; excessive thirst; infrequent urination with dark, concentrated urine; and light-headedness.
4. Look for signs of hepatitis, an infection of the liver: a yellow color in the skin and the white parts of the eyes.

Self-Care

1. To replace fluids, take frequent, small sips of clear liquids such as water, noncitrus juice, broths, flat ginger ale, or ice chips.
2. When the vomiting and diarrhea have subsided, try nonirritating, constipating foods like the BRAT diet: bananas, rice, applesauce, and toast.
3. For several days, avoid alcohol, milk products, fatty foods, aspirin, and other medications that might irritate the stomach. Do not stop taking regularly prescribed medications without discussing this change with your physician.
4. Medications are not usually advised for vomiting. For diarrhea, over-the-counter medications containing kaolin, pectin, or attapulgite may help thicken the stool. Loperamide, now available without a prescription, can be used to ease diarrhea.

When to Call the Physician

1. Inability to retain any fluids for 12 hours or signs of dehydration
2. Severe abdominal pains not relieved by the vomiting or diarrhea
3. Blood in the vomit (red or "coffee grounds" material) or in the stool (red or black tarlike material)
4. Vomiting or diarrhea with a high fever (above 102° F or 38.8° C)
5. Yellow color in skin or white parts of the eyes
6. Vomiting with severe headache and a history of a recent head injury
7. Vomiting or diarrhea that lasts 3 days without improvement
8. If you are pregnant or have diabetes
9. Recurrent vomiting and/or diarrhea

Heartburn and Indigestion

Indigestion and heartburn are usually a result of irritation of the stomach or the esophagus, the tube that connects the mouth to the stomach. The stomach lining is usually protected from stomach acids, but the esophagus is not. Therefore, if stomach acids "reflux," or back up into the esophagus, the result is usually a burning discomfort beneath the breastbone. The esophagus is normally protected by a muscular valve that allows food to enter the stomach but prevents stomach contents from flowing upward into the esophagus. Certain foods (such as chocolate), medications, and smoking can loosen and open this protective sphincter valve. Overeating, lying down, or bending over can also cause the stomach acids to gain access to the sensitive lining of the esophagus.

Self-Assessment

1. Look for a pattern in the symptoms. Do they occur after eating certain foods, taking certain medications, or when you bend over or lie down? Do certain foods or an antacid relieve the symptoms?
2. Observe your bowel movements. Black tarlike stools may indicate bleeding in the stomach (iron tablets and Pepto-Bismol can also cause black stools).

Self-Care

1. Avoid irritants such as smoking, aspirin, ibuprofen, naproxen sodium, alcohol, caffeine (coffee, tea, cola), chocolate, onions, carbonated beverages, spicy or fatty foods, acidic foods (vinegar, citrus fruits, tomatoes), or any other foods that seem to make your symptoms worse.
2. Take nonabsorbable antacids such as Maalox, Mylanta, or Gelusil every 1–2 hours and especially before bedtime, or try an acid reducer, now available without a prescription (Pepcid, Tagamet, or Zantac).
3. Avoid tight clothing.
4. Avoid overeating; eat smaller, more frequent meals.
5. Don't lie down for 1–2 hours after a meal. Elevate the head of your bed with 4- to 6-inch blocks of wood or bricks. Adding extra pillows usually makes things worse by creating a posture that increases pressure on the stomach. Using a waterbed also usually makes reflux worse. Try sleeping on your left side, which may reduce reflux compared to sleeping on your back or right side.
6. If you are overweight in the abdominal area, weight loss may help. Abdominal obesity can increase pressure on the stomach when you are lying down.

When to Call the Physician

1. Stools that are black and tarlike or vomit that is bloody or contains material that looks like coffee grounds
2. Severe abdominal or chest pain
3. Pain that goes through to the back
4. No relief from antacids
5. Symptoms lasting longer than 3 days

Recurrent or persistent abdominal pain may be a symptom of an ulcer, a raw area in the lining of the stomach or duodenum (the first part of the small intestine). About 1 in 5 men and 1 in 10 women develop an ulcer at some time in their lives. Most ulcers are linked to infection with the bacterium *Helicobacter pylori;* people who regularly take nonsteroidal anti-inflammatory drugs like aspirin or ibuprofen are also at risk for ulcers because these drugs irritate the lining of the stomach. *H. pylori* infection is relatively easy to diagnose and treat, and other medications are available to treat ulcers linked to other causes. Many of the self-care measures described above are also frequently recommended for people with ulcers.

Headache

Headache is one of the most common symptoms. There are four major types of headache: tension, migraine, cluster, and sinus. Tension headaches, migraines, and cluster headaches are described in Chapter 14. Sinus headaches are caused by blockage of the sinus cavities with resulting pressure and pain in the cheeks, forehead, and upper teeth. Headache caused by elevated blood pressure is very uncommon and occurs only with very high pressures.

Self-Assessment

1. Take your temperature. The presence of fever may indicate a sinus infection. Fever, severe headache, and a very stiff neck suggest meningitis, a rare but serious infection around the brain and spinal cord.
2. Tap with your fingers over the sinus cavities in your cheeks and forehead. If this causes increased pain, it may indicate a sinus infection.
3. For recurrent headaches, keep a headache journal. Record how often and when your headaches occur, associated symptoms, activities that precede the headache, and your food and beverage intake. Look for patterns that may provide clues to the cause(s) of your headaches.

Self-Care

1. Try applying ice packs or heat on your neck and head.
2. Gently massage the muscles of your neck and scalp.
3. Try deep relaxation or breathing exercises.
4. Take aspirin or aspirin substitute for pain relief. Over-the-counter products containing a combination of aspirin, acetaminophen, and caffeine are approved by the FDA for treating migraines.
5. If pain is associated with nasal congestion, try a decongestant medication like pseudoephedrine.
6. Try to avoid emotional and physical stressors (like poor posture and eyestrain).
7. Try avoiding foods that may trigger headaches, such as aged cheeses, chocolate, nuts, red wine, alcohol, avocados, figs, raisins, and any fermented or pickled foods.

When to Call the Physician

1. Unusually severe headache
2. Headache accompanied by fever and a very stiff neck
3. Headache with sinus pain, tenderness, and fever
4. Severe headache following a recent head injury
5. Headache associated with slurred speech, visual disturbance, or numbness or weakness in the face, arms, or legs
6. Headache persisting longer than 3 days
7. Recurrent unexplained headaches
8. Increasing severity or frequency of headaches
9. Severe migraine headaches. In recent years, many new prescription medications have been approved for the prevention and treatment of migraines.

Low-Back Pain

Pain in the lower back is a very common condition; it is most often due to a strain of the muscles and ligaments along the spine, often triggered by bending, lifting, or other activity. Low-back pain can also result from bone growths (spurs) irritating the nerves along the spine or pressure from ruptured or protruding discs, the "shock absorbers" between the vertebrae. Sometimes back pain is caused by an infection or stones in the kidney. Fortunately, however, simple muscular strain is the most common cause of low-back pain and can usually be effectively self-treated.

Self-Assessment

1. Take your temperature. Back pain with high fever may indicate a kidney or other infection.
2. Check for blood in your urine or frequent, painful urination, which may also indicate a kidney problem.
3. Observe for tingling or pain traveling down one or both legs *below* the knee with bending, coughing, or sneezing. These symptoms suggest a disc problem.

Self-Care

1. Lie on your back or in any comfortable position on the floor or a firm mattress, with knees slightly bent and supported by a pillow. Rest for 1–3 days if the pain persists.
2. Use ice packs on the painful area for the first 3 days, and then continue with cold or change to heat, whichever gives more relief.
3. Take aspirin or aspirin substitute for pain relief as needed.
4. After the acute pain has subsided, begin gentle back and stomach exercises. Practice good posture and lifting techniques to protect your back. Try to resume gentle, everyday activities like walking as soon as possible. Bed rest beyond 3 days is no longer advised. To learn more about proper back exercises and use of your back, consult a physical therapist or your physician.

When to Call the Physician

1. Back pain following a severe injury such as a car crash or fall
2. Back pain radiating down the leg *below* the knee on one or both sides
3. Persistent numbness, tingling, or weakness in the legs or feet
4. Loss of bladder or bowel control

5. Back pain associated with high fever (above 101° F or 38.3° C), frequent or painful urination, blood in the urine, or severe abdominal pain

6. Back pain that does not improve after 2 weeks of self-care

Strains and Sprains

Missteps, slips, falls, and athletic misadventures can result in a variety of strains, sprains, and fractures. A strain occurs when you overstretch a muscle or tendon (the connective tissue that attaches muscle to bone). Sprains are caused by overstretching or tearing ligaments (the tough fibrous bands that connect bone to bone). Depending on the severity and location, a sprain may actually be more serious than a fracture, because bones generally heal very strongly while ligaments may remain stretched and lax after healing. After a sprain, it may take 6 weeks for the ligament to heal.

After most injuries, you can expect pain and swelling. This is the body's way of immobilizing and protecting the injured part so that healing can take place. The goal of self-assessment is to determine whether you have a minor injury that you can safely self-treat or a more serious injury to an artery, nerve, or bone that should be treated by your physician.

Self-Assessment

1. Watch for coldness, blue color, or numbness in the limb beyond the injury. These may be signs of damage to an artery or a nerve.

2. Look for signs of a possible fracture, which would include a misshapen limb, reduced length of the limb on the injured side compared to the uninjured side, an inability to move or bear weight, a grating sound with movement of the injured area, extreme tenderness at one point along the injured bone as you press with your fingers, or a sensation of snapping at the time of the injury.

3. Gently move the injured area through its full range of motion. Immobility or instability suggests a more serious injury.

Self-Care

1. Immediately immobilize, protect, and rest the injured area until you can bear weight on it or move it without pain. Remember: If it hurts, don't do it.

2. To decrease pain and swelling, immediately apply ice (a cold pack or ice wrapped in a cloth) for 15 minutes every hour for the first 24–48 hours. Then apply ice or heat as needed for comfort.

3. Immediately elevate the injured limb above the level of your heart for the first 24 hours to decrease swelling.

4. Immobilize and support the injured area with an elastic wrap or splint. Be careful not to wrap so tightly as to cause blueness, coldness, or numbness.

5. Take aspirin or aspirin substitute for pain as needed.

When to Call the Physician

1. An injury that occurred with great force such as a high fall or motor vehicle crash
2. Hearing or feeling a snap at the time of the injury
3. A limb that is blue, cold, or numb
4. A limb that is bent, twisted, or crooked
5. Tenderness at specific points along a bone
6. Inability to move the injured area
7. A wobbly, unstable joint
8. Marked swelling of the injured area
9. Inability to bear weight after 24 hours
10. Pain that increases or lasts longer than 4 days

Cuts and Scrapes

Cuts and scrapes are common disruptions of the body's skin. Fortunately, the vast majority of these wounds are minor and don't require stitches, antibiotics, or a physician's care. An abrasion involves a scraping away of the superficial layers of skin. Abrasions, though less serious, are often more painful than cuts because they disrupt more skin nerves. There are two types of cuts: lacerations (narrow slices of the skin) and puncture wounds (stabs into deeper tissues).

Normal healing of a cut or abrasion is a remarkable process. After the bleeding stops, small amounts of serum, a clear yellowish fluid, may leak from the wound. This fluid is rich in antibodies to help prevent an infection. Redness and swelling may normally occur as more blood is shunted to the area, bringing white blood cells and nutrients to speed healing. There may also be some swelling of nearby lymph nodes, which are another part of your body's defense against infection. Finally, a scab forms. This is "nature's bandage," which protects the area while it heals.

The main concerns about cuts are the possibilities of damage to deeper tissues and the risk of infection. Damage to underlying blood vessels may lead to severe bleeding as well as blueness and coldness in areas beyond the wound. Injured nerves may produce numbness and a loss of the ability to move parts of the body beyond the injured area. Damaged muscles, tendons, and ligaments can also result in inability to move areas beyond the cut.

Wound infection usually does not take place until 24–48 hours after an injury. Signs of infection include increasing redness, swelling, pain, pus, and fever. One of the most serious, though fortunately uncommon, complications of puncture wounds is tetanus ("lockjaw"). This bacterial infection thrives in areas not exposed to oxygen, so it is more likely to develop in deep puncture wounds or dirty wounds. Tetanus is not likely to develop in minor cuts or wounds caused by clean objects like knives. You need a tetanus immunization shot following a cut under the following conditions:

- If you have never had the basic series of three tetanus immunization injections
- If you have a dirty or contaminated wound and it has been longer than 5 years since your last injection
- If you have a clean, minor wound and it has been longer than 10 years since your last injection

Self-Assessment

1. Look for warning signs of complications: persistent bleeding, numbness, an inability to move the injured area, or the later development of pus, increasing redness, and fever.
2. Measure the size of the cut. If your cut is shallow, less than 1/4 inch deep, less than an inch long, and not in a high-stress area (such as a joint, which bends) and you can easily hold the edges of the wound closed, it probably won't need stitches.

Self-Care

1. Apply direct pressure over the wound until the bleeding stops. The only exception is puncture wounds, which should be encouraged to bleed freely (unless spurting a large amount of blood) for a few minutes to flush out bacteria and debris.

2. Try to remove any dirt, gravel, glass, or foreign material from the wound with tweezers or by gentle scrubbing.
3. Wash the wound vigorously with soap and water, followed by an application of hydrogen peroxide solution as an antiseptic.
4. If it is an abrasion, cover the area with a sterile adhesive bandage until a scab forms. For minor lacerations, close the cut with a butterfly bandage or a sterile adhesive tape, drawing the edges close together but not overlapping. If there is an extra flap of clean skin, leave it in place for extra protection. Do not attempt to close a puncture wound. Instead, soak the wound in warm water for 15 minutes several times a day for several days. Soaking helps keep the wound open and thus prevents infection.

When to Call the Physician

1. Bleeding that can't be controlled with direct pressure
2. Numbness, weakness, or an inability to move the injured area
3. Any large, deep wound
4. A cut in an area that bends and with edges that cannot easily be held together
5. Cuts on the hands or face unless clean and shallow
6. A contaminated wound from which you cannot remove the foreign material
7. Any human or animal bite
8. If you need a tetanus immunization (see indications noted earlier)
9. Development of increasing redness, swelling, pain, pus, or fever 24 hours or more after the injury
10. If the wound is not healing well after 3 weeks

Appendix D

Resources for Self-Care

Books and Audiotapes

American College of Obstetricians and Gynecologists. 2000. *Encyclopedia of Women's Health and Wellness.* Washington, D.C.: American College of Obstetricians and Gynecologists. *A comprehensive look at women's health that includes checklists, questionnaires, and many other helpful tools.*

American Medical Women Association. 2001. *Complete Family Health Book.* New York: Golden Books. *A comprehensive guide to family health.*

Ammer, C. 2000. *The New A to Z of Women's Health: A Concise Encyclopedia,* 4th ed. New York: Facts on File. *An easy-to-use reference covering a wide variety of women's health topics.*

Brubaker, M., et al. 1999. *Surgery: A Patient's Guide from Diagnosis to Recovery.* San Francisco: UCSF Nursing Press. *A comprehensive look at surgery from diagnosis to the postsurgery recovery process at home.*

Griffith, H. W. 2000. *Complete Guide to Prescription and Nonprescription Drugs, 2001 Edition.* New York: Perigee. *A comprehensive guide to side effects, warnings, and precautions for the safe use of over 4000 brand-name and generic drugs.*

Griffith, H. W. 2000. *The Complete Guide to Symptoms, Illness, and Surgery,* 4th rev. ed. New York: Perigee. *An up-to-date reference covering signs and symptoms, illnesses and disorders, and surgeries.*

Hogan, R. W. 2000. *The PDR Pocket Guide to Prescription Drugs,* 4th ed. New York: Pocket Books. *An easy-to-use reference to over 1000 prescription drugs.*

Inlander, C. B., K. Morales, and the People's Medical Society. 2000. *Family Health for Dummies.* Foster City, Calif.: IDG Books. *Addresses a wide range of health topics.*

Kemper, D. W. 1999. *Healthwise Handbook: A Self-Care Manual for You.* Boise, Id.: Healthwise. *Practical guidelines for home care of common medical problems in adults and children.*

Komaroff, A. L., ed. 1999. *Harvard Medical School Family Health Guide.* New York: Simon & Schuster. *A comprehensive, easy-to-use guide to symptoms, disorders, treatments, medical emergencies, and the health care system.*

Lerner, P., and J. Lerner. 2000. *Lerner's Consumer Guide to Health Care.* Seattle, Wash.: Lerner Communications. *Presents advice on how to obtain quality medical care and to negotiate the bureaucracy of the health care system.*

Lorig, K., et al. 2000. *Living a Healthy Life with Chronic Conditions.* Palo Alto, Calif.: Bull. *A helpful guide to dealing with chronic illness.*

Medical Economics Staff, ed. 2001. *PDR Family Guide to Prescription Drugs,* 8th ed. New York: Three Rivers Press. *A comprehensive guide to prescription drugs.*

Medical Economics Staff, ed. 2001. *PDR for Nonprescription Drugs and Dietary Supplements,* 22nd ed. Montvale, N.J.: Medical Economics. *A clinical reference covering food and drug interactions, side effects, contraindications, costs, and other information on over-the-counter drugs and supplements.*

Men's Health Books, ed. 2000. *The Complete Book of Men's Health.* Emmaus, Pa.: Rodale Press. *An illustrated guide to men's health, with an emphasis on prevention.*

Muth, A. S. 2001. Surgery Sourcebook: *Basic Consumer Health Information About Major Surgery and Outpatient Surgeries.* Detroit: Omnigraphics. *A comprehensive, consumer-oriented look at surgery.*

Naparastek, B. *Health Journeys.* Akron, Ohio: Image Paths (800-800-8661; http://www.healthjourneys.com). *A selection of high-quality audiotapes for imagery for relaxation, mental health, illness management, and preparation for surgery.*

Pryor, J. L., and S. Glass. 2000. *It's in the Male: Everyone's Guide to Men's Health.* Minnetonka, Minn.: Appladay Press. *A concise guide to key men's health concerns.*

Rothenberg, M. A., and C. F. Chapman. 2000. *Dictionary of Medical Terms: For the Nonmedical Person,* 4th ed. Hauppauge, N.Y.: Barrons Educational Series. *Includes basic definitions of many medical terms.*

Rybacki, J. J., and J. W. Long. 2001. *The Essential Guide to Prescription Drugs.* New York: HarperResource. *A comprehensive drug reference that includes descriptions of how each drug works, possible side effects, and other precautions.*

Self-Care Advisor: The Essential Home Health Guide for You and Your Family. 2000. Alexandria, Va.: Time-Life. *Provides advice on more than 300 common health problems, including symptoms, suggestions for home care, advice on when to call the doctor, and tips for prevention.*

Shannon, J. B., ed. 1999. *Medical Tests Sourcebook.* Detroit: Omnigraphics. *Provides basic consumer information on a wide variety of medical tests.*

Silverman, H., ed. 2000. *The Pill Book,* 9th rev. ed. New York: Bantam. *Provides descriptions and illustrations of more than 1500 of the most commonly prescribed drugs.*

Sobel, D., and R. Ornstein. 1998. *Mind and Body Health Handbook.* Los Altos, Calif.: DRx. *Presents step-by-step instructions for how to use your mind to relieve stress, boost immunity, improve mood, and manage illness.*

See Chapter 1 for a list of general health-related newsletters and magazines.

Health Information Centers

Consumer Information Center (Pueblo, CO 81009, 888-8PUEBLO; http://www.pueblo.gsa.gov).

National Health Information Center (P.O. Box 1133, Washington, DC 20013, 800-336-4797); http://www.health.gov/nhic).

Office of Minority Health Resource Center (P.O. Box 37337, Washington, DC 20013, 800-444-6472; http://www.omhrc.gov).

Self-Help and Mutual Aid Groups

Self-help groups provide information and peer support for nearly every conceivable medical condition or problem. Look in the telephone book for a local chapter, or contact one of the following self-help clearinghouses for the names of self-help groups in your community.

American Self-Help Clearinghouse (St. Clare's Health Services, 25 Pocono Road, Denville, NJ 07834, 973-326-8853; http://www. mentalhelp.net/selfhelp).

National Self-Help Clearinghouse (365 5th Avenue, Suite 3300, New York, NY 10016, 212-817-1822; http://www. selfhelpweb.org).

Telephone Hotlines

For hotlines relating to the main topics of this text, see the For More Information sections at the end of each chapter. Additional hotlines are listed below. Extensive lists of health-related hotlines and clearinghouses are available from the National Health Information Center (800-336-4797; http://www.health. gov/nhic), the American Self-Help Clearinghouse (973-326-8853, http://www.mentalhelp. net/selfhelp/fonenums/helpline. htm), and Johns Hopkins Info-Net (http://infonet.welch.jhu.edu/advocacy.html).

Blindness: American Foundation for the Blind, 800-232-5463; National Library Service for the Blind and Physically Handicapped, 800-424-8567; Recording for the Blind and Dyslexic, 800-221-4792.

Chronic fatigue syndrome: CFIDS Association, 800-442-3437.

Consumer products: U.S. Consumer Product Safety Commission, 800-638-2772: FDA National Hotline, 888-463-6332.

Deafness/hearing problems: American Speech Language and Hearing Association, 800-638-8255; Dial-a-Hearing Screening Test, 800-222-EARS: National Institute on Deafness and Other Communication Disorders, 800-241-1044, 800-241-1055 (TTY).

Disabling conditions: Americans with Disabilities Act Hotline, 800-949-4232 (Voice/TTY); Job Accommodation Network, 800-232-9675 (Voice/TDD).

Down syndrome: National Down Syndrome Society, 800-221-4602.

Endometriosis: Endometriosis Association, 800-992-3636.

Epilepsy: Epilepsy Foundation of America, 800-EFA-1000; Epilepsy Information Service, 800-642-0500.

Gambling: National Council on Compulsive Gambling, 800-522-4700.

Headache: National Headache Foundation, 800-843-2256; American Council for Headache Education, 800-255-ACHE.

Hemophilia: National Hemophilia Foundation, 888-463-6643.

Irritable bowel syndrome: International Foundation for Functional Gastrointestinal Disorders, 888-964-2001.

Kidney disease: American Kidney Fund, 800-638-8299; National Kidney Foundation, 800-622-9010.

Lung disease/respiratory disorders: Lung Line, sponsored by the National Jewish Medical and Research Center, 800-222-LUNG, 800-552-LUNG (recorded information, 24 hours); American Lung Association, 800-LUNG-USA.

Lupus: Lupus Foundation of America, 800-558-0121.

Multiple sclerosis: Multiple Sclerosis Foundation, 800-441-7055.

Parkinson's disease: American Parkinson's Disease Association, 800-223-2732; National Parkinson Foundation, 800-327-4545.

Rare disorders: National Organization for Rare Disorders, 800-999-6673.

Self-abuse and self-mutilation: SAFE (Self-Abuse Finally Ends), 800-DONT-CUT.

Sickle-cell disease: Sickle Cell Disease Association of America, 800-421-8453.

Spina bifida: Spina Bifida Association of America, 800-621-3141.

Spinal cord injury: Christopher Reeve Paralysis Association, 800-225-0292.

Sports and sports injures: Women's Sports Foundation, 800-227-3988.

Sudden infant death: American SIDS Institute, 800-232-SIDS.

The Internet

The Internet is a global network of computers that links together commercial online communication services, such as America Online and CompuServe, with tens of thousands of university, government, and corporate networks. The Internet is composed of many parts, including World Wide Web documents, e-mail, newsgroups, mailing lists, and chat rooms. With access to the Internet, you can obtain in-depth information about hundreds of wellness topics and keep up with the latest research; you can also connect with people worldwide who share a medical problem or another challenge to wellness.

To reach the Internet, you need a computer, a modem, access to the network through a provider, and browser software, which allows you to navigate. Internet access is often available to students at little or no cost through college computer centers. If you have to obtain access through a commercial Internet service provider, choose one that suits your needs and your budget. Bare-bones access is available at low cost, but you may need to obtain additional software, including a browser such as Netscape Navigator or Microsoft Internet Explorer. Online services such as America Online, CompuServe, and Microsoft Network are often more expensive, but they provide all the necessary software and offer many features, including e-mail, newsgroups, and Web browsers.

The World Wide Web

The World Wide Web is made up of computer files called Web pages or Web sites that have been created by individuals, companies, and organizations. The Web is considered a user-friendly pan of the Internet because it offers easy access and navigation and has media capabilities, such as audio, video, and animation.

Each Web site is identified by an address or uniform resource locator (URL), such as http://www.healthfinder.gov. To access a site, you can type the URL into the appropriate screen of your browser or you can click on a *hyperlink*, a shortcut to another Web page or to a different part of the current page. When you view a Web page, hyperlinks may appear as images or as text that is a different color and/or is underlined. By clicking on links, you can jump quickly from one Web site to related sites, even if they are located on the other side of the world.

To search out information on a particular topic, you need to use a search engine or directory, such as one of the following:

AltaVista	http://www.altavista.com
Ask Jeeves	http://www.askjeeves.com
Excite	http://www.excite.com
Fast Search	http://www.alltheweb.com
Go/Infoseek	http://www.go.com
Google	http://www.google.com
Hotbot	http://www.hotbot.com
Lycos	http://www.lycos.com
Northern Light	http://www.northernlight.com
Yahoo!	http://www.yahoo.com

These search engines search a unique database of Web pages, so you will obtain different results from different search engines. A meta–search engine like the two listed below simultaneously submits your search to multiple search engines:

Dogpile	http://www.dogpile.com
MetaCrawler	http://www.go2net.com/search.html

To use a search engine, you may need to enter key words or navigate through a series of increasingly more specific directories; some search engines offer both key word and directory searches. Within seconds, the search engine will generate a list of sites (with hyperlinks) that match your search parameters, often with a brief description of each site.

When you are searching, it's best to make your searches as specific as possible. Searching for key words such as "AIDS" or "cancer" will yield thousands or even millions of matches. Use more specific phrases, such as "HIV vaccine" or "cervical cancer treatment." If the search engine has a help section, take a look at it. Different engines have different rules for how best to enter key words. For example, you may need to enclose phrases in quotation marks or put plus or minus signs between words to obtain an appropriate result. If you don't find the information you are looking for using one search engine, try another. In addition, there are search engines and directories that specialize in health and medicine:

Achoo	http://www.achoo.com
Health A to Z	http://www.healthatoz.com
Health on the Net	http://www.hon.ch
HealthWeb	http://healthweb.org
Karolinska Institutet	http://micf.mic.ki.se/Diseases
Medical Matrix	http://www.medmatrix.org
MedWeb	http://www.medweb.emory.edu/ MedWeb
MedWorld: Medbot	http://www-med.stanford.edu/ medworld/medbot

Listed next is a sampling of Web sites that contain information on a variety of wellness topics and/or links to many other appropriate sites. For Web sites dealing with a specific health topic, refer to the For More Information section in the appropriate chapter. Hyperlinks to all the sites in this text can be accessed from the *Core Concepts in Health* Online Learning Center (http://www.mhhe.com/insel9).

American Academy of Family Physicians
   http://aafp.org
   http://www.familydoctor.org
CDC Health Information A to Z
   http://www.cdc.gov/health/diseases.htm
Dr. Koop's Community
   http://www.drkoop.com
Duke University Healthy Devil On-Line
   http://gilligan.mc.duke.edu/h-devil
Go Ask Alice
   http://www.goaskalice.columbia.edu
Healthfinder
   http://www.healthfinder.gov
HealthTouch Online
   http://www.healthtouch.com
InteliHealth
   http://www.intelihealth.com
Mayo Health Oasis
   http://www.mayohealth.org
Medem
   http://www.medem.com
MedicineNet
   http://www.medicinenet.com
Merck
   http://www.merck.com
National Center for Health Statistics
   http://www.cdc.gov/nchs
National Women's Health Resource Center
   http://www.healthywomen.org
NetWellness
   http://www.netwellness.org
New York Online Access to Health
   http://www.noah-health.org
NIH Health Information Index
   http://www.nih.gov/health
NLM Medline Plus
   http://www.nlm.nih.gov/medlineplus
Thrive Online
   http://thriveonline.oxygen.com
U.S. Consumer Gateway: Health
   http://www.consumer.gov/health.htm
WebMD
   http://webmd.com
Wellnessweb
   http://wellweb.com

Usenet Newsgroups

Newsgroups consist of archived messages, articles, and postings about a particular topic; they are similar to bulletin boards. Commercial online services maintain members-only newsgroups, but many more are available on the Internet. To locate a newsgroup on a particular topic, use a search engine or visit a site devoted to newsgroups, such as Deja.com (http://www. deja.com).

You are free to browse any newsgroup's articles. Postings on related topics are often grouped together in a "thread," consisting of an original message that began a discussion and all the replies to that message. A busy newsgroup can receive thousands of postings a day, and older articles are deleted to make room for new ones. If you find an article of interest, print it or save it to your computer—it may be deleted from the newsgroup by your next visit.

In addition to browsing, reading, and saving newsgroup postings, you can also be an active participant. You can reply to a message, either to the person who posted it or to the entire newsgroup, or you can post a new message that starts a new thread of discussion. To ensure that your postings are appropriate, it's often a good idea to observe a newsgroup for a while or look at its "frequently asked questions" page prior to becoming an active member.

Listserv Mailing Lists

Listservs are similar to newsgroups, except that messages are delivered by e-mail to all subscribers to the mailing list rather than posted at a public site. Once you subscribe to a mailing list, you receive messages posted by other subscribers and you can post your own messages. As with newsgroups, it's a good idea to read messages for a while before joining the discussion. You can stop subscribing to a mailing list at any time.

To locate listservs for a particular topic, do a key word search using a search engine by entering the topic and the word *listserv*. Or try the extensive mailing list directory at Liszt (http:// www.liszt.com).

Real-Time Communication: Chat Rooms

With access to the Internet, you may also have the opportunity to participate in real-time communication with people from around the world. You can sign on to a particular chat group and communicate with others who are signed on to the same group at that time. You can have a "public" conversation, in which everyone in the chat room is included, or a "private" conversation between you and one other person. Many chat groups have a moderator who can kick people off and/or refuse them further access if they don't behave appropriately. For reasons of privacy and security, many people suggest that chat room participants avoid divulging too much personal information. See the sections on online relationships (p. 101) and cyberstalking (p. 664) for specific guidelines.

Evaluating Information from the Internet

Anyone can post information and advice on the Internet—true or false, good or bad. When evaluating information from the Internet, ask the following questions:

- *What is the source of the information? Who is the author or sponsor of the Web page?* Web sites maintained by government agencies, professional organizations, or established academic or medical institutions are likely to present trustworthy information. Many other groups and individuals post accurate information, but it is important to watch your sources carefully. Many sites will describe their sponsor on the home page; alternatively, they may have an "about us" or "who we are" link that provides this information. Take a look at the backgrounds, qualifications, and credentials of the people who are behind the information at the site. Beware of sites that don't indicate the sources of the information they post; if you don't know where it comes from, you can't assess it's validity.

  As you click on links and move from page to page, also pay attention to where you are. Even if you start out at a trustworthy site, the click of a button can catapult you into a completely different site. Learn how to read your current Web address so that you know when you've left one site and entered another. Look at the abbreviation in the server name in the URL, which will change according to the sponsor's purpose—for example, "org" for organizational, "gov" for governmental, "edu" for educational, and "com" for commercial.

- *How often is the site updated?* Most Web pages will indicate the date of their most recent modifications. Major organizations may update their Web sites on a daily or weekly basis. Look for sites that are updated frequently.

- *What is the purpose of the page? Does the site promote particular products or procedures? Are there obvious reasons for bias?* The same common sense you'd use to evaluate any factual claim applies to the Internet. Be wary of sites that sell specific products, use testimonials as evidence, appear to have a social or political agenda, or ask for money. Many sites sponsored by commercial companies and lay organizations do provide sound, useful information; however, it's a good idea to consider possible sources of bias in the information they present.

- *What do other sources say about a topic?* To get a broad perspective on a piece of information, check out other online sources or ask a professional. You are more likely to obtain and recognize quality information if you use several different sources. Be wary of claims that appear at only one site.

- *Does the site conform to any set of guidelines or criteria for quality and accuracy?* A number of organizations have developed codes of conduct or ethical standards for health-related sites; these codes include criteria such as use of information from respected sources and disclosure of the site's sponsors. These organizations include the following:

American Accreditation HealthCare Commission
 http://www.urac.org
American Medical Association
 http://www.ama-assn.org
Health Internet Ethics
 http://www.hiethics.com
Health on the Net Foundation
 http://www.hon.ch
Internet Healthcare Coalition
 http://www.ihealthcoalition.org

Look for sites that identify themselves as conforming to some code or set of principles.

- *Is the site easy to use? Does it have links to other sites?* In addition to strong content, good Web pages should be easy to use, be clearly organized, and have a good search capability. For more on finding and evaluating online wellness-related information, check out the following Web sites:

California Medical Association (select Health Care Links)
 http://www.cmanet.org
CDC: Internet Health Related Hoaxes and Rumors
 http://www.cdc.gov/hoax_rumors.htm
Oncolink Source Reliability Information
 http://www.oncolink.upenn.edu/resources/
 reliability
Science Panel on Interactive Communication and Health
 http://www.scipich.org
Search Engine Watch
 http://www.searchenginewatch.com
UC Berkeley Library Internet Tutorial
 http://www.lib.berkeley.edu/TeachingLib/Guides/
 Internet/FindInfo.html

Glossary

abstinence to refrain completely from engaging in a particular behavior.

acesulfame nonnutritive sweetener that is 200 times sweeter than sucrose and marketed as "sunette" in many food products.

acquaintance rape forced sexual intercourse between people who know one another well.

Acquired Immunodeficiency Syndrome (AIDS) viral destruction of the immune system, causing loss of ability to fight infections.

acute illness an illness that occurs suddenly, often has no identifiable cause, is usually treatable, and often disappears in a short time.

addiction a pathological need for a substance that has life-damaging potential.

addictive behavior behavior that is excessive, compulsive, and psychologically and physically destructive.

adipose cells fat cells.

adrenocorticotropic hormone (ACTH) hormone released by the hypothalamus during periods of stress that initiates various physiological responses.

aerobic literally "with oxygen"; when applied to exercise, refers to activities in which oxygen demand can be supplied continuously by individuals during performance.

aerobic capacity maximum oxygen consumption.

alcohol socially acceptable drug.

alcoholism disease in which an individual loses control over drinking; inability to refrain from drinking.

allergens substances that cause allergic reactions.

alternative medicine body of therapies that are not taught in the U.S. medical schools and are generally unavailable from doctors or hospitals.

amenorrheic cessation of menstruation.

amino acids chemical structures that form protein.

anabolic steroids drugs closely related to testosterone that increase muscle mass in humans.

anaerobic literally "without oxygen"; when applied to exercise, refers to high-intensity physical activities in which oxygen demand is greater than the amount that can be supplied during performance.

android deposition of fat that is characteristic of men; fat tends to accumulate in the abdomen and upper body.

aneurysm weak spot in an artery that forms a balloonlike pouch that can rupture.

angina chest pain that is the result of ischemia (see *ischemic*).

anorexia nervosa serious illness of deliberate self-starvation with profound psychiatric and physical components.

antioxidants compounds that block the oxidation of substances in food or the body (vitamins C and E and beta-carotene are examples).

arthritis inflammatory disease of the joints.

asthma chronic respiratory condition characterized by difficulties breathing.

asymptomatic without symptoms.

atherosclerosis slow, progressive disease of the arteries characterized by the deposition of plaque on the inner lining of arterial walls.

ATP adenosine triphosphate, the actual unit of energy used for muscular contraction.

atrophy a decrease in the size of organ, muscles, and body tissues from disease or disuse.

autogenics form of suggestion that precipitates relaxation.

autoimmune disease disease in which the immune system fails to recognize its own body parts and produces antibodies against them to the point of causing injury.

autonomic nervous system part of the nervous system that is concerned with control of involuntary bodily functions.

avoidance a behavioral strategy that emphasizes eliminating circumstances associated with undesirable behavior.

ballistic stretching repetitive contractions of agonist muscles to produce very quick, rapid stretches of antagonist muscles.

balloon angioplasty surgical procedure that involves the insertion of a catheter with a balloon at the tip used to compress fatty deposits and plaque against the walls of the artery.

basal cell carcinoma the most common type of skin cancer. It grows slowly and usually does not metastasize (spread).

basal metabolic rate (BMR) number of calories needed to sustain life.

behavior assessment process of counting, recording, observing, measuring, and describing behavior.

behavior substitution lifestyle change technique in which an incompatible behavior is substituted for a behavior being altered.

behavioral contract a written agreement in a lifestyle-change program.

benign noncancerous; refers to a growth that is unable to spread.

binge drinking consuming five or more drinks in a single session at least once during the previous two weeks, with the intent to become intoxicated.

binge-eating disorder practice of eating large amounts of food in a short period of time.

biofeedback educational tool used to provide information about an individual's physiological actions.

blood alcohol concentration (BAC) percentage of alcohol content in the blood.

body composition amount of lean versus fat tissue in the body.

body dysmorphic disorder (BDD) a psychiatric disorder characterized by a preoccupation with perceived imperfections in physical appearance that cause the person to withdraw from social activities.

body mass index (BMI) the ratio of body weight in kilograms to height in meters squared.

botanicals plants that are thought to have medicinal properties (also called *herbs* and *phytomedicinals*).

bulimia nervosa eating disorder characterized by episodes of secretive binge eating and purging.

Caesarean section delivery surgical removal of the fetus through the abdominal wall.

caffeine a stimulant that increases the heart rate.

caloric deficit occurs when the number of calories burned exceeds the number of calories consumed.

caloric expenditure calories expended by physical activity and metabolism.

caloric intake calories supplied by food.

calorie short for *kilocalorie*, which is the unit of measurement for food energy. A calorie is the amount of heat required to raise the temperature of 1 gram of water 1 degree Centigrade.

cancer group of diseases characterized by uncontrolled, disorderly cell growth.

carbon monoxide a colorless, tasteless, odorless gas that is the product of incomplete combustion of carbon-containing fuels.

carcinogens substances that cause cancer or enable the growth of cancer cells; cancer-causing agents.

carcinoma cancer of a body surface or body cavity, such as cancer of the breast, lung, skin, stomach, testis, or uterus.

cardia dysrhythmia irregular heart rate that is sometimes intractable.

cardiac output amount of blood ejected by the heart in 1 minute.

cardiorespiratory endurance ability to take in, deliver, and extract oxygen for physical work.

cariogenic refers to the promotion of dental caries, or cavities.

catheterization the process of examining the heart by introducing a thin tube (catheter) into a vein or an artery and passing it into the heart.

cause and effect in medical research, the type of a relationship in which one variable is scientifically proved to cause a certain effect.

cerebral hemorrhage bursting of a blood vessel in the brain.

chemoprevention nutritional intervention to prevent diseases, such as cancer, by bolstering the immune system.

chemotherapy use of drugs and hormones to treat various cancers.

child abuse physical, emotional, or sexual mistreatment of a child.

chlamydia one of the most common sexually transmitted diseases.

cholesterol steroid that is an essential structural component of neural tissue and cell walls and is required for the manufacture of hormones and bile.

chronic disease a disease that usually begins gradually and persists for an indefinite period of time, usually months or years.

chronic effects of exercise the physiological changes that result from cardiorespiratory training.

circuit resistance training a total of 8 to 15 exercises are usually used in a circuit. The exerciser goes through the circuit three times with minimum rest between exercise stations.

cocaine a stimulant used in powdered form.

cognitive dissonance an internal conflict that occurs when a person's behaviors are inconsistent with his or her beliefs, values, or knowledge.

communicable diseases diseases that can be transmitted from one person to another.

complete protein protein that contains all the essential amino acids.

complex carbohydrates polysaccharides, including starch and fiber.

concentric contraction shortening of the muscle as it develops the tension to overcome an external resistance.

condyloma warts on the genitalia.

contracting refers to a behavior change strategy that involves a written statement of health goals, target dates for completion of each goal, intervention strategies, rewards and incentives.

contraindication reason for not prescribing a drug or treatment.

control group in health research, the group receiving no treatment.

coping effort(s) made to manage or deal with stress.

coronary artery bypass surgery procedure involving the removal of a leg vein that is used as a shunt around the blocked area in the coronary artery.

countering the substitution of a new behavior for an undesirable one.

crack smokable form of cocaine that is extremely dangerous and very addictive.

Crohn's disease a type of inflammatory bowel disease whose cause is unknown. Crohn's disease is characterized by frequent and intense diarrhea, abdominal pain, gas, fever, and rectal bleeding.

cross-training the attainment of physical fitness by participating in a variety of activities regularly.

crude fiber residue of plant food following chemical treatment in the laboratory.

cunnilingus oral sex performed on the female genitalia.

daily values (DVs) provides nutritional guidelines for ingestion of carbohydrate, fat, saturated fat, cholesterol, sodium, potassium, and dietary fiber.

date rape forced sexual intercourse between people who are in a dating situation.

deceptive advertising advertising that misleads consumers by overstating or exaggerating the performance of a product.

deductible amount paid by a patient before being eligible for benefits from an insurance company.

defensive medicine practice of prescribing medical tests to protect doctors against malpractice lawsuits.

dehydration excessive loss of body water.

delta-9-tetrahydrocannabinol (THC) major psychoactive drug found in marijuana.

depressants known as sedatives and tranquilizers; these agents slow the central nervous system.

designer drugs illegally manufactured drugs that mimic controlled substances.

diabetes mellitus metabolic disorder involving the pancreas and the failure to produce insulin; a risk factor for cardiovascular disease.

diagnostic laboratory tests tests conducted for specific symptoms during a physical examination.

dietary fiber residue of plant food after digestion in the human body. One gram of crude fiber equals 2 to 3 grams of dietary fiber.

Dietary Reference Intakes (DRI) replaced the Recommended Dietary Allowance as the standards for presenting nutrient recommendations.

diet resistance the inability to lose weight by dieting.

disability insurance insurance that pays for income lost because of the inability to work due to an illness or injury.

disordered eating general term that entails sporadic eating, poor nutrition, unnecessary dieting, or occasional bingeing and purging but are not classified as full-blown problem areas by the American Psychiatric Association.

distress form of stress that results in negative responses.

diuretics substances that increase water output and the body's need for water.

diverticulitis infection of the diverticula of the intestines.

diverticulosis condition of having saclike swellings (diverticula) in the walls of the intestines.

double-blind study type of health research in which neither the researcher nor the subjects know who is receiving an experimental treatment.

drug chemical substance that has the potential to alter the structure and functioning of a living organism.

eating disorders refers to those eating disorders that meet specific criteria established by the American Psychiatric Association.

eccentric contraction the lengthening of a muscle as the weight or resistance is returned to the starting position.

echocardiography noninvasive technique that uses sound waves to determine the shape, texture, and movement of the valves of the heart.

ectomorph body shape characterized by thin body frame.

elderly abuse physical, emotional, sexual, or medical abuse of an elderly person. Most often the abuser is an adult child of the victim.

electrocardiograph (ECG) device for recording electrical variations in action of the heart muscle.

embolus mass of undissolved matter in the blood or lymphatic vessels that detaches from the vessel walls.

endomorph body shape characterized by rounded physical features and large body frame.

endorphins mood-elevating, pain-killing substances produced by the brain.

energy nutrients nutrients, such as carbohydrates, fat, and protein, that provide a source of energy for the body.

environmental dimension of wellness comprises aspects of wellness that improve quality of life in the community, including laws and agencies that safeguard the physical environment.

epidemiologic studies population studies that observe the health habits and diseases of large numbers of people.

epinephrine hormone produced by the adrenal medulla that speeds up body processes.

essential fat fat that is indispensable for individuals to function biologically and necessary to support life.

essential hypertension high blood pressure caused by unknown reasons.

essential nutrients nutrients that cannot be made by the body and must be supplied in the diet.

ethyl alcohol intoxicating agent in alcoholic drinks; colorless liquid with a sharp, burning taste.

eustress stress judged as "good" positive stress or stress that contributes to positive outcomes.

exclusion medical services that are not covered by an insurance policy.

experimental group in health research, the group receiving some form of experimental treatment.

false negative test results that incorrectly show a person is healthy when an abnormality actually exists.

false positive test results that incorrectly show an abnormality when a person is actually healthy.

family practitioner medical doctor who serves as a general practitioner for an individual or a family.

fasting complete starvation; avoidance of food consumption.

fat mixture of triglycerides.

fellatio oral sex performed on the male genitalia.

female athletic triad a condition characterized by disordered eating, lack of menstrual periods, and low age-adjusted bone density.

fiber substances in food that resist digestion; formerly called *roughage.*

fight-or-flight syndrome initial phase of the general adaptation syndrome (GAS); when a stressor is encountered, the body responds by preparing to stand and fight or run away depending on the situation; also called the *alarm phase* of the GAS.

fixed indemnity benefits specified amounts that are paid by an insurance company for particular medical procedures.

flexibility range of motion at a joint.

folate a vitamin B nutrient found primarily in leafy vegetables.

foodborne illness illness caused by ingestion of foods containing toxic substances produced by microorganisms.

fraternal twins twins who emanate from separate eggs and do not have identical genes.

freebasing smoking liquefied cocaine.

free radicals naturally produced chemicals that arise from cell activity.

fructose fruit sugar.

functional foods foods that provide a specific health benefit above and beyond their inherent nutritional value.

general adaptation syndrome (GAS) series of physiological changes that occur when a stressor is encountered; the GAS is conceived of as having three phases: alarm, resistance, and exhaustion.

genital warts warts on the genitalia.

glucose primary source of energy used by the body; blood sugar.

Glycemic Index (GI) an assessment of food in terms of its ability to increase blood sugar in the two to three hours after eating.

glyceride general term for fat compounds, including triglyceride, monoglyceride, and diglyceride.

Golgi tendon organ a proprioceptor that responds to muscle stretch and tension.

goniometer a protractor-like instrument used to measure the flexibility of various joints.

gonorrhea bacterial disease that is sexually transmitted and can lead to serious complications if left untreated, including sterility and scarring of the heart valves.

gynoid fat deposition characteristic of females, in whom fat tends to accumulate on the hips and thighs.

hardiness label used in describing a particular type of personality that tends to remain healthy even under extreme stress; the three components of hardiness are challenge, commitment, and control.

hate crimes crimes directed at individuals or groups solely because of their racial, ethnic, or religious background, sexual orientation, or other differences from the perpetrator.

headache a common discomfort that is often caused by distress, tension, and anxiety; may be the result of injury or brain disease.

health balancing of the physical, emotional, social, and spiritual components of personality in a manner that is conducive to optimal well-being and a higher quality of existence.

health behavior gap discrepancy between what people know and what they actually do regarding their health.

health care providers people and facilities such as physicians and hospitals that provide health care services.

health disparities the disproportionate prevalence of diseases and health problems among certain population groups.

health fatalism in health information the view that new information cannot be believed or trusted because it will inevitably be refuted.

health insurance a contract between an insurance company and an individual or a group for the payment of medical care costs.

health maintenance organization (HMO) prepaid group insurance program that provides a full range of medical services.

health-promoting behaviors things done to maintain and improve one's level of wellness.

health promotion art and science of helping people change their lifestyle to move toward a higher state of wellness.

health-related fitness components of fitness that include cardiorespiratory endurance, muscular strength, muscular endurance, flexibility, and body composition.

health risk appraisals questionnaires used to provide information about health habits, lifestyle, and medical history.

heat exhaustion serious heat-related condition characterized by dizziness, fainting, rapid pulse, and cool skin.

heat stroke heat-related medical emergency characterized by high temperature (106° F or higher) and dry skin and accompanied by some or all of the following: delirium, convulsions, and loss of consciousness.

hemoglobin substance in blood that carries oxygen.

hepatitis B one of five types of viral hepatitis. Hepatitis B is the most serious type and can be transmitted sexually.

herbs see *botanicals.*

herpes simplex virus (HSV) virus responsible for herpes genitalis, a sexually transmitted disease.

highly polyunsaturated fat fatty acid composed of triglycerides in which the carbon chain has room for many hydrogen atoms.

homeostasis state of balance or constancy; the body is continually attempting to maintain homeostasis.

homicide the intentional taking of another person's life; murder.

homocysteine amino acid that is thought to increase the risk of heart disease.

homogeneous group group of subjects with similar characteristics.

hypertrophy increase in the size of organs and muscle tissue.

human immunodeficiency virus (HIV) virus that is the source of AIDS.

human papilloma virus (HPV) causative agent of condyloma (genital warts).

hydrogenation process of adding hydrogen to unsaturated fatty acid to make it more saturated.

hyperglycemia high blood sugar.

hyperplasia increase in the number of cells.

hypertension high blood pressure.

hyperthermia excessive buildup of heat in the body.

hyperthyroidism disease caused by an overactive thyroid gland.

hypertrophy increase in the size of a cell.

hypokinesis physical inactivity.

hypothalamus part of the limbic system that contains the center for many bodily functions; in stressful situations the hypothalamus releases specific hormones to elicit appropriate bodily responses.

hypothermia cold weather-related condition that results in abnormally low body temperature.

hypothyroidism disease caused by an underactive thyroid gland.

iatrogenic condition condition caused as a result of receiving medical care.

identical twins twins who emanate from the same egg.

immunization a vaccine or other preparation administered to prevent disease.

immunotherapy in relation to cancer, technique for stimulating the body's immune system to destroy cancer cells.

implied consent nonverbal authorization of a medical procedure such as cooperation during the administration of tests.

incomplete protein protein that does not contain all the essential amino acids in the proportions needed by the body.

infarction death of heart muscle tissue.

inflammatory bowel disease (IBD) a variety of diseases that cause inflammation of the intestines. The two most common types are Crohn's disease and ulcerative colitis.

influenza commonly called *flu;* caused by a virus.

informed consent legal provision requiring patient's authorization of any medical procedure, therapy, or treatment.

inhalants substances that cause druglike effects when inhaled.

insoluble fiber fiber that does not dissolve in water; comes from wheat bran and vegetables.

insulin hormone secreted by the pancreas that increases the use of glucose by the tissues of the body.

intensity degree of vigorousness of a single bout of exercise.

internist medical doctor specializing in internal medicine and sometimes serving as a primary care physician.

ischemia diminished supply of blood to the heart muscle.

isoflavones phytoestrogens in soybeans that are thought to help prevent breast cancer by blocking natural estrogens.

isokinetic method for developing muscular strength that involves a constant rate of speed and changes in the amount of weight resistance.

isometric use of static contractions to develop strength.

isotonic method for developing muscular strength that involves a variable rate of speed and a constant weight resistance.

lactic acid metabolite formed in muscles as a result of incomplete breakdown of sugar.

lactose simple sugar; milk sugar.

lactovegetarian a person who eats plant foods and dairy products but excludes eggs, fish, poultry, and meat from their diet.

Leading Health Indicators (LHI) healthy lifestyle issues identified in the document *Healthy People 2010* as health priorities for Americans.

legumes foods that come from plants with seed pods that split on two sides when ripe.

leptin a protein made in fat cells that controls weight gain and loss.

leukemia cancer of the blood-forming tissues, including the bone marrow and spleen.

life insurance insurance that pays a death benefit.

lifestyle diseases diseases and/or health conditions largely caused by health habits and practices under the control of the individual.

limbic system large, C-shaped area that contains the centers for emotions, memory storage, learning relay, and hormone production (the pituitary gland, thalamus, and hypothalamus).

lipid class of nutrients more commonly referred to as *fat*.

lipoprotein fat-carrying protein.

locus of control perspective from which an individual views life. Individuals with an *internal* locus of control believe that their decisions make a difference and that they have control over their lives. People with *external* locus of control see themselves as "victims" and consider other people, situations, and conditions as being the controlling factors in their lives.

low-calorie diet diet that limits intake to 800 to 1000 calories a day; results in atrophy of heart muscle.

lymphoma cancer that develops in the lymphatic system, including the neck, armpits, groin, and chest.

macronutrients nutrients required by the body in large amounts. Usually refers to the energy nutrients: protein, fat, and carbohydrates.

mainstream smoke smoke that is inhaled and exhaled by smoker.

major minerals those minerals required in large amounts (more than 5 grams a day).

malignant cancerous; refers to a growth that has the ability to spread to other areas of the body.

mammography X-ray examination of the breast to detect cancer.

marijuana (cannabis) a plant that produces mild effects similar to both a stimulant and a depressant. Also labeled as a mild hallucinogen.

megadose large doses, usually in the form of supplements.

melanoma a dangerous form of skin cancer that has a strong tendency to spread to other areas of the body.

mesomorph body shape characterized by a muscular, athletic body build.

metabolism all chemical reactions that occur within the cells of the body.

metastasis process by which cancerous cells spread from their original location to another location in the body.

micronutrients nutrients required by the body in small amounts. Usually refers to vitamins and minerals.

migraine headaches headaches characterized by throbbing pain that can last for hours or days, sometimes accompanied by nausea and vomiting. Migraines are thought to be the result of dilation of blood vessels in the head.

minerals inorganic compounds in food necessary for good health.

mitochondria the cell's "powerhouse."

moderate-calorie diet diet that limits caloric intake to 1300 to 1600 calories a day.

monounsaturated fat fatty acid composed of triglycerides in which the carbon chain has room for two hydrogen atoms.

morbidity incidence of disease and/or sickness.

mortality incidence of death.

muscular endurance application of repeated muscular force developed by many repetitions against resistances considerably less than maximum.

muscular strength maximal force that a muscle or muscle group can exert in a single contraction.

myocardial infarction heart attack; death of heart muscle tissue.

narcotics powerful painkillers.

negative reinforcers avoidance of something unpleasant.

neoplasm abnormal mass of cells; also called a *tumor*; can be benign or malignant.

neutraceuticals natural ingredients intended to promote and maintain health.

newsgroup a location on the internet where electronic messages related to a medical topic are posted.

nicotine addictive substance and alkaloid poison found in tobacco.

novelty diets fad diets often based on gimmicks that typically promote certain nutrients or foods as having unique weight loss qualities.

nucleoside analogs a combination of drugs (AZT& ddl) that seems to prevent the development of opportunistic infections associated with AIDS.

nutrient substance found in food that is required by the body.

nutrient density ratio of nutrients to calories; also called the *index of nutritional quality*.

nutrition science that deals with the study of nutrients and the way the body ingests, digests, absorbs, transports, metabolizes, and excretes these nutrients.

obesity excessive amount of storage fat.

ob gene a gene found in fat cells that produces leptin. Also called the "fat gene."

occupational dimension of wellness comprises aspects of wellness that help achieve a balance between work and leisure in a way that promotes health and a sense of personal satisfaction.

Olestra a synthetic fat that has the flavor and taste of real fat but yields no calories.

omega-3 fatty acids type of fatty acid found in cold-water seafood and thought to lower the risks of heart disease.

oncogene cancer-causing gene.

osteoarthritis most common form of arthritis characterized by the deterioration of articular cartilage that covers the gliding surfaces of the bones in certain joints.

osteophyte another name for a bone spur.

osteoporosis progressive decrease in the mineral content of bone, making bones brittle.

overcompensatory eating an eating pattern characterized by over-consumption of low-fat foods, which causes an increase in total caloric intake.

overfat may or may not be within normal guidelines for weight but with an excessive ratio of fat compared with lean tissue.

overweight excessive weight for one's height without regard for body composition.

ovolactovegetarian a person who eats plant foods, eggs, and dairy products but excludes fish, poultry, and meat from the diet.

partner abuse physical or emotional abuse committed by an adult against his or her partner.

passive smoking inhalation of environmental cigarette smoke by a nonsmoker.

pathogen disease-producing organism.

pelvic inflammatory disease (PID) chronic condition of infection in the uterus, fallopian tubes, and upper reproductive areas; the leading cause of infertility in women.

performance-related fitness sports fitness; composed of speed, power, balance, coordination, agility, and reaction time.

periodic examination physical exam in which tests and assessments are prescribed according to risk factors.

pescovegetarian a person who eats plant foods, eggs, dairy products, and fish but excludes red meat from the diet.

phytochemicals plant chemicals that exist naturally in foods.

phytoestrogen plant hormone (estrogen) that exists naturally in foods.

phytomedicinals see *botanicals*.

placebo inactive substance, such as a fake drug.

point of service (POS) a type of health insurance plan in which subscribers use approved providers who have agreed to accept fixed co-payments.

pollovegetarian a persons who eats plant foods, eggs, dairy products, fish, and poultry but excludes red meat.

polypharmacy the administration of many drugs at the same time.

polyunsaturated fat fatty acid composed of triglycerides in which the carbon chain has room for four or more hydrogen atoms.

positive reinforcers rewards earned for achieving goals in a lifestyle-change program.

preferred provider organization (PPO) a group of private practitioners who sell their services at reduced rates to insurance companies.

preventive health behaviors health practices associated with the promotion of wellness and the prevention of sickness and death.

primary-care physician medical doctor who is responsible for an individual's overall health.

primary site (reference to cancer) original site of cancer cell formation.

proprioceptive neuromuscular facilitation (PNF) consists of several stretching techniques that involve some combination of contraction and static stretching and holding agonist and antagonist muscle groups.

prospective study an epidemiological study in which researchers predict possible disease relationships and patterns among groups of people.

protease inhibitor inhibits the enzyme protease, which allows HIV to develop.

protein complementing practice of combining plant protein with cereal/grain protein to provide complete protein.

psychoactives drugs that can alter feelings, moods, and/or perceptions.

psychosomatic disease diseases (physical symptoms) caused by psychological and emotional stressors.

psychoneuroimmunology (PNI) a medical discipline whose philosophy rests on the connections among brain function, the nervous system, and the body's response to infection and abnormal cell division.

radiotherapy use of radiation to either destroy cancer cells or destroy their reproductive mechanism so they cannot replicate.

rape trauma syndrome psychological reactions following a rape. Characterized by fear, nightmares, fatigue, crying spells, digestive upset and perhaps impaired sexual desire/functioning.

reactance motivation a behavioral response to force or coersion in which behavior is the opposite of that intended (e.g., a child refuses to eat a particular food because of parental force).

recidivism the tendency to revert to original behaviors/conditions after completing a behavioral change program.

recommended dietary allowances (RDAs) daily recommended intakes of nutrients for normal, healthy people in the United States.

reference daily intakes (RDI) represents minimum standards for essential nutrients and replaces the U.S. recommended daily allowance established in 1968.

relaxation techniques techniques used in coping with and managing stress.

reliability extent to which health studies yield consistent results.

reminders a behavioral strategy used to formulate action goals.

residual volume amount of air remaining in the lungs after expiration.

retrospective study an epidemiological study in which researchers review previously gathered data to identify possible disease relationships and patterns among groups of people.

reward deficiency syndrome a variety of disorders that have in common the traits of impulsiveness, addiction, and compulsiveness.

rheumatoid arthritis most crippling form of arthritis, characterized by inflammation of the joints, pain, swelling, and deformity.

risk factors conditions that threaten wellness and increase the chances of contracting a disease.

road rage overly aggressive driving that includes physical or verbal assault against another driver after a traffic dispute.

saccharides refers to sugars (general term).

safer sex a pattern of behavior in which steps are taken to protect oneself and one's partner from pregnancy and infection with HIV and sexually transmitted diseases. These steps can include using condoms or dental dams and having periodic medical tests and examinations.

sarcoma cancer of a connective tissue, such as bone and muscle.

saturated fat fatty acid composed of triglycerides in which all the fatty acids contain the maximum number of hydrogen atoms.

scientifically controlled study a study conducted in a controlled setting that involves a treatment (experimental) group and a placebo (control) group.

secondary site refers to the location of cancer cells after they have spread from the primary site.

sedentary physically inactive

selective health examination specific test used in response to specific symptoms or for diagnosing a specific problem.

self-care movement toward individuals taking increased responsibility to prevent or manage certain health conditions.

self-efficacy people's belief in their ability to accomplish a specific task or behavior; that belief then affects the outcome of the task or behavior; the theory that individuals who expect to succeed tend to succeed and those who expect to fail tend to fail.

self-help approach to lifestyle change that assumes individuals can plan and execute their own plans.

set point theory theory that the body has a preference for maintaining a certain amount of weight and defends that weight quite vigorously.

sexually transmitted diseases (STDs) diseases spread through sexual contact, such as AIDS, chlamydia, gonorrhea, and herpes.

shaping up a behavioral strategy in which a person acclimates to desired behaviors in small increments.

sidestream smoke smoke given off by burning tobacco products.

skinfold measures method for determining the amount of body fat by using skin calipers.

sleep apnea a condition characterized by loud snoring and brief periods during which breathing ceases.

soluble fiber fiber that dissolves in water; comes from fruit pectins and oat bran.

squamous cell carcinoma the second most common type of skin cancer. It rarely spreads to other areas, but it grows more quickly than basal cell carcinoma.

starch plant polysaccharides composed of glucose and digestible by humans.

static stretching passive stretching of antagonist muscles by slowly stretching and holding a position for 15 to 30 seconds.

statistical relationship an association between two or more variables or events.

statistical significance the probability that a study's findings are reliable and are not due to chance.

stimulants drugs that speed up the central nervous system.

stimulus control technique in lifestyle management involving the elimination and/or manipulation of stimuli related to a specific behavior.

stress nonspecific response of the body to any demands made on it.

stressor any physical, psychological, or environmental event or condition that initiates the stress response.

stretch reflex the myotatic reflex.

stroke volume amount of blood that the heart can eject in one beat.

subliminal advertising technique in which messages, words, and symbols are embedded or hidden in advertisements.

sucrose table sugar.

syndrome X combination of high blood pressure, high blood sugar, high blood lipids, and abdominal obesity.

syphilis a sexually transmitted disease.

tar black, sticky, dark fluid composed of thousands of chemicals and found in tobacco.

tension headaches most common kind of headache; caused by involuntary contractions of the scalp, head, and neck muscles and may be precipitated by anxiety, stress, and allergic reactions.

thermogenic effect of food (TEF) the amount of energy required by the body to digest, absorb, metabolize, and store nutrients.

thrombus stationary blood clot; can occlude an artery supplying the brain.

trace minerals those minerals required in small amounts.

transfatty acids saturated fat found in processed food that has been hydrogenated.

transmit time the time it takes food to move through the body.

transtheoretical model of behavior change a self-help approach to lifestyle change consisting of six well-defined stages. It is based on the principles of the behavior change model developed by James Prochaska.

triglyceride compound composed of carbon, hydrogen, and oxygen with three fatty acids.

tropical oils oils that come from the fruit of coconut and palm trees.

ulcerative colitis chronic inflammation of the colon lining. The symptoms are the same as those of Crohn's disease, but the only area affected is the colon lining.

unintentional injury any injury that occurs as a result of an accident or reckless behavior.

unsaturated fat fatty acid composed of triglycerides in which the carbon chain has room for more hydrogen atoms.

validity extent to which the research design of a health study permits the assertion of certain health claims.

variable resistance provides increasing resistance as a weight is lifted through the full range of motion.

vegan a person whose diet is limited to plant foods. Also called a *strict vegetarian.*

very low-calorie diets (VLCD) diets containing fewer than 800 calories a day.

viral hepatitis inflammation of the liver caused by one or more viruses.

visualization a form of meditation that makes use of the imagination.

vital capacity amount of air that can be expired after a maximum inspiration.

vitamin supplements natural and synthetic compounds taken orally to supplement the vitamins consumed in food.

vitamins organic compounds in food necessary for good health.

weight cycling potentially harmful pattern of repeated weight loss and weight gain.

wellness engaging in activities and behaviors that enhance quality of life and maximize personal potential.

Credits

Chapter 1: **Page 5:** © PhotoDisc/Vol. #58; p. 10: © PhotoDisc/Vol. #40;
p. 15: © PhotoDisc/Vol. #70; **Table 1-1:** Novartis Nutrition and McGraw-Hill. (2000). Obesity: A Modern Epidemic. *Innovations: Nutrition Updates and Applications,* McGraw-Hill. Murphy S.L. (2000). Deaths: Final data for 1998. *National Vital Statistics Reports,* 48(11):26.

Chapter 2: **Page 46:** © PhotoDisc/Vol. #40; **p. 54:** © PhotoDisc/Vol. #67; **Table 2-2:** Adapted from "Revised Cholesterol Guidelines." July, 2001. *Harvard Heart Letter,* 11(11):6–7.

Chapter 3: **Page 80:** © Michael Newman/PhotoEdit.

Chapter 4: **Table 4-1:** Adapted from Nieman, D.C. 1999. *Exercise Testing and Prescription.* Mountain View, CA. Mayfield Publishing Company.

Chapter 6: **Page 168:** © PhotoDisc/Vol. #67; **p. 171:** © PhotoDisc/Vol. #49; **p. 187:** © PhotoDisc/Vol. #48; **Table 6-2:** From American Dietetic Association. 1998. *Choosing Legumes: A Healthful and Versatile Food.* Available online at www.eatright.org/nfs45.html.
Fig 6-5: "How Hot is Hot Enough?" U.S. Department of Health and Human Services. (2000). *Nutrition and Health? Dietary Guidelines for Americans.* Washington, D.C. U.S. Government Printing Office.

Chapter 7: **Fig. 7-9(both):** Courtesy of Life Measurement Instruments. Concord, CA; **Table 7-1:** Adapted from Lohman, T.G., L.B. Houtkooper, and S.B. Going. 1997. Body composition assessment: Body fat standards and methods in the field of exercise and sports medicine. *ACSM Health Fitness Journal.* 1:30; **Table 7-2:** Adapted from Lohman, T.G., L.B. Houtkooper, and S.B. Going. 1997. Body composition assessment: Body fat standards and methods in the field of exercise and sports medicine. *ACSM Health Fitness Journal.* 1:30; **Table 7-4:** Adapted from NHLBI, 1998. "Obesity Education Initiative Expert Panel Clinical Guidelines on the Identification, Evaluation, and Treatment of Overweight and Obesity in Adults," National Heart Lung and Blood Institute. Washington D.C.

Chapter 8: **Page 244:** © PhotoDisc/Vol. #70; **p. 255:** © PhotoDisc/Vol. #70.

Chapter 9: **Page 281:** © PhotoDisc/Vol. #66; **p. 290:** © PhotoDisc/Vol. #103.
Wellness Across the Generations: The Time of Our Lives. Adapted from Johns Hopkins InteliHealth Online, www.intelihealth.com/ IH?ihtIH?d=dm.

Chapter 10: **Page 314:** © Bristol/Visuals Unlimited; **p. 320:** © PhotoDisc/Vol. #25; **Fig 10-1:** "Accident Types" From National Safety Council, *Accident Facts,* 1998.

Chapter 11: **Page 341:** © PhotoDisc/Vol. #48; **p. 343:** Missouri Chpt. of MADD and the parents of Jason Bitter; **p. 350:** Felicia Montirez/PhotoEdit.

Chapter 12: **Page 371:** © Phototake; **p. 373:** Phototake.

Chapter 13: **Fig 13-2:** "Cancer Incidence and Death by Site and Sex—1995 Estimates" American Cancer Society, Surveillance Research, 1998.
Just the Facts: Cancer-Related Checkup Guidelines, Adapted from American Cancer Society. Recommendations for the Early Detection of Cancer in Asymptomatic People. 1998. American Cancer Society, Inc.; **Fig 13-3a:** J.E. Wilson/Photo Researchers; **Fig. 13-3b:** Bio-Photo Assoc. SPL/Photo Researchers; **p. 393:** Will-Deni McIntyre/Photo Researchers.

Chapter 14: **Page 411:** David K. Crow/PhotoEdit; **p. 415:** Ron Chapple/FPG International.

Chapter 15: **Page 429:** Bill Lai/The Image Works; **p. 442:** © Aaron Haupt/Photo Researchers, Inc.

Index

A

Abdominal fat, negative health effects, 52, 219–220, 239
Abdominal muscles
  assessment of strength, 125
  and back pain, 141
Acquaintance and date rape, 321–322
  and college campuses, 321
  date rape drug, Rohypnol, 322
  prevention of, 321
Acute illnesses, nature of, 7–8
Addiction. *See also* Drugs, illegal
  causes of, 340
  definition of, 339, 340
Adenosine triphosphate (ATP), function of, 69
Adequate Intake (AI), meaning of, 156
Advertising, influence on behavior, 11–12
Aerobic capacity
  aerobic exercise, effects of, 68, 69
  definition of, 67
  detraining effects, 69
  genetic factors, 69
Aerobic exercise
  cardiorespiratory effects of, 67–70
  health benefits of, 72
  with resistance training, 98
  and weight loss, 254, 255
Aerobic, meaning of, 67
African-Americans, and hypertension, 40
Aggression, overaggressive drivers, 317–318
Aging
  body composition changes, 222, 240–241
  and flexibility exercises, 139
  and heart attacks, 40
  inevitable illness issue, 410
  and metabolism, 254
  and nutrient gap, 180
  and protein intake, 161
  and quality of life, 284
  and resistance training, 100
  and self-care, 438
  and weight control, 254
Agonist muscle contraction, 135–136
AIDS (acquired immunodeficiency virus).
    See HIV/AIDS
Air-displacement plethysmography, 226–227
Air pollution
  and jogging, 82
  types of pollutants, 315

Alcohol use, 189–190, 341–346
  absorption, affecting factors, 343–344
  and automobile accidents, 316, 345
  binge drinking, 345–346
  health benefits, 190
  moderation, meaning of, 189–190
  negative health effects, 45, 47, 190, 342
  reasons for use, 341
  responsible drinking guidelines, 343, 346
  and violence, 345
Alcoholic drink, definition of, 45, 189–190
Alcoholism
  alcoholic hepatitis, 390
  definition of, 344
  self-assessment, 359
  theories of, 344
  treatment of, 344
Alternative medicine, 439–440
  cancer treatment, 399
  decision-making about use, 439–440
  proponent/opponent views, 439
Amenorrhea, and female athletes, 260
Amino acids, and protein, 160
Anabolic-androgenic steroids, 115–116
  negative effects of, 116
Anaerobic exercise, strength training as, 99
Analog drugs, types of, 340
Android pattern, fat distribution, 219–220
Anemia, and iron deficiency, 171
Aneurysm, and stroke, 38
Angel dust, 354
Angina pectoris (chest pain), 36
Anorexia nervosa, 257–258
  diagnosis of, 258
  treatment of, 258
Antagonist muscle contraction, 135–136
Antioxidants, 166–167
  functions of, 157, 166
  vitamins as, 166–167
Anxiety, about body weight, 237
Art therapy, focus of, 5
Arthritis, 411–412
  and obesity, 238
  osteoarthritis, 411–412
  rheumatoid arthritis, 412
  strength training for, 98
Aspirin therapy, heart disease prevention, 56

Asthma, 413–414
  exercise-induced, 414
  intrinsic and extrinsic, 414
  management assessment, 421
  management of, 414
  triggers of, 414
Atherosclerosis
  C-reactive protein for diagnosis, 55
  development of, 36, 43–45
  lipid oxidation theory of, 43–44
Athrophy, of muscle, 98
Autogenics, relaxation method, 287–288
Automated teller machine (ATM), crime/violence at, 319–320
Automobile accidents
  aggressive drivers, 317–318
  and alcohol use, 316, 345
  drowsiness, prevention of, 316
  motorcycle safety, 318–319
  pedestrian safety, 319
  prevention of, 315–319
  safety and type of vehicle, 317
  types of accidents, 315

B

B vitamins, 166, 168–169
  for vegetarians, 182–183
Back pain
  flexibility exercises for, 140–141
  lower, causes of, 141
Ballistic stretching, 140
Balloon angioplasty, 56, 57
Basal cell carcinoma, 391
Basal metabolic rate (BMR). *See also*
    Metabolism
  estimation of, 271
  meaning of, 254
  stimulation by exercise, 254
Behavior assessment
  and behavior change, 16
  tools for, 16
Behavior change
  contracting strategy, 17
  countering strategies for, 17
  self-help approach, 11–18
  shaping up strategy, 18
  stages of, 13–18
  theoretical model of, 12–13
Behavior, influences on, 11–12

Benign tumors, 383
Bicycling, safety measures, 313
Bilberry, pros/cons of use, 175
Binge drinking, 345–346
    college students, 345–346
    definition of, 339, 345
Binge-eating disorder, 259
    diagnosis of, 259
Bioelectrical impedance analysis (BIA), 224
Biofeedback
    focus of, 5
    relaxation method, 288–289
Bioterrorism, precautions to take, 325
Biotin, 166
Blood, components of, 35
Blood pressure, 442
    high. *See* Hypertension
    measurement of, 46, 442
    nature of, 46
    readings for normal/high pressure, 47
    systolic and diastolic, 47
Blood screening tests, 441
Blood volume, and aerobic exercise, 68
Boating, safety measures, 314
BodPod, 228–229
Body composition
    definition of, 216
    essential fat, 216
    and growth process, 222
    regional fat distribution, 218–220
Body composition measures
    air-displacement plethysmography, 226–227
    bioelectrical impedance analysis (BIA), 224
    skinfold measurements, 224–228
    underwater weighing, 223
Body dysmorphic disorder (BDD), 236, 237
Body image
    assessment of, 267
    body dysmorphic disorder (BDD), 236, 237
    influencing factors, 236
Body mass index (BMI), 220–221, 231, 238
Body shape
    genetic factors, 242
    types of, 242
Body weight
    American obsession with, 236–237
    caloric intake recommendations, 157,
        159, 237–238
    increases, reasons for, 237–238
Body weight measures, 220–222, 226
    body mass index (BMI), 220–221
    desirable body weight from percent body
        fat, calculation of, 226, 233
    height/weight tables, 220, 222
    practical measure, 218
Bone density test, 443
Botanicals. *See* Herbs
Brain, stress effects, 282
Breast cancer, 393, 395
    drug treatments, 393
    exercise, benefits of, 388
    risk factors, 393
    self-examination for, 396–397
Breathing technique, relaxation method, 287
Bulimia nervosa, 258–259
    diagnosis of, 259
    treatment of, 259

C

Caffeine
    caffeinism, 341
    as drug, 341
    negative health effects, 341
    and osteoporosis, 413
Calcium
    for bone health, 413
    food sources of, 170, 171
    health benefits, 170
    increasing intake, tips for, 171
    in pregnancy, 191
    recommended intake, 171
Calories
    caloric deficit and weight loss, 245
    definition of, 157
    expended in daily activities, 253, 272
    expended in exercise, 75, 253–254, 269
    on food labels, 193–194
    increased need and stress, 283
    recommended caloric intake, 157, 159,
        237–238
Campylobacker jejuni, and foodborne
    illness, 186
Canadian Trunk Strength Test, 125
Cancer
    breast cancer, 393, 395
    childhood cancers, 382
    colorectal cancer, 389
    deaths by site/sex, 387
    leukemia, 390
    liver cancer, 390
    lung cancer, 388–389
    lymphoma, 390
    oral cancer, 392
    ovarian cancer, 395
    pancreatic cancer, 390
    prostate cancer, 397–398
    skin cancer, 391
    stomach cancer, 390
    testicular cancer, 395
    uterine cancer, 395
Cancer development
    cell growth, 383, 386
    and cigarette smoking, 48, 346–347, 389
    common sites for, 384, 387–388
    early detection guidelines, 394
    environmental causes, 386
    genetic factors, 385
    as immune system dysfunction, 385
    and obesity, 238
    and stress, 386
    and sun exposure, 387
    and viral disease, 387
    warning signs, 394
Cancer prevention
    early detection assessments, 403–405
    and exercise, 388
    guidelines for, 383, 394
    and nutrition, 383
Cancer treatment
    alternative treatments, 399
    chemotherapy, 398
    immunotherapy, 398
    radiotherapy, 398
    surgical, 398
    survival and social support, 386, 399

Candidiasis, signs/treatment of, 375
Car jacking, 320–321
Carbohydrate intake
    assessment of, 201
    pre-physical activity, 191–192
    recommended intake, 160
Carbohydrates, 159–160
    complex carbohydrates, 159
    and glucose production, 159, 244
    simple carbohydrates, 159
Carbon monoxide
    in cigarette smoke, 346
    home detection devices, 311–312
Carcinogens
    meaning of, 346, 384
    types of, 384
Carcinoma, 384
Cardiac catheterization, cardiovascular
    disease diagnosis, 56
Cardiac output, and aerobic exercise, 67–68
Cardiorespiratory endurance, 67–70
    and aerobic exercise, 67–70
    definition of, 67
    health benefits of, 70–71
    training effects, 67–69
Cardiovascular disease
    atherosclerosis, 36, 43–45
    and cholesterol, 41–46
    and cigarette smoking, 48, 347
    coronary heart disease, 36–38
    and diabetes mellitus, 52, 411
    diagnosis of, 55–56
    and hypertension, 46–48
    as modern disease, 36
    and obesity, 52, 220, 238, 239
    and physical inactivity, 50–51
    prevention of, 48, 53–54, 56
    risk assessment, 61–63
    risk factors, 38, 54–55
    and stress, 52–53, 281
    stroke, 38
    surgical treatment, 56–57
Caries, and sugar intake, 188
Carotenoids, 167–168
Catheterization, coronary stent implant, 56
Cellular phones, and driving safety, 317
Cerebral hemorrhage, and stroke, 38
Chancroid, signs/treatment of, 375
Chemoprevention, meaning of, 173
Chemotherapy, 398
    new drugs for, 398
Child abuse, 323
Children
    body fat, changes over time, 222
    childhood cancers, 382
    and flexibility exercises, 139
    and type 2 diabetes, 409
Chlamydia
    signs of, 373
    treatment of, 373
Cholesterol, 41–46
    and cardiovascular disease, 42, 162
    dietary sources of, 42, 162
    high-density lipoprotein cholesterol
        (HDL) cholesterol, 44–46
    low-density lipoprotein (LDL) cholesterol,
        43–44

lowering, guidelines for, 41, 43
manufacture by body, 41
risk profile, 43
triglycerides, 46, 161
very-low density lipoprotein (VLDL) cholesterol, 43
Cholesterol screening, 441
Chromium picolinate, and resistance training, 114
Chronic disease
nature of, 7
and quality of life, 413
Cigar smoking, dangers of, 50, 348, 392
Cigarette smoking
and back pain, 142
clove cigarettes, 348
harmful substances of, 48–49, 346
negative health effects, 48, 49, 50, 346–348, 392
passive smoking, 49–50, 347
and premature death, 9–10, 48
Cigarette smoking cessation, 49, 262, 348–350
benefits of, 348–349
nicotine-containing aids, 350
plan for, 349
Circuit resistance training, 111–112
Circulatory system, and heart, 34–35
Clinical trials, health research, 427
Clostridium botulinum, and foodborne illness, 186
Clove cigarettes, 348
Club drugs, 351
Cluster headaches, 416
Cocaine, 352
Cocktail, AIDS therapy, 371
Cognitive dissonance, meaning of, 15
Cold weather and exercise, 81–82
frostbite, 81
hypothermia, 81–82
Colds
management of, 415
spread of, 415
College campuses
acquaintance/date rape, 321
binge drinking, 345–346
Colorectal cancer, 389
exercise, benefits of, 388
prevention of, 389
Communication
about sexually transmitted disease, 366
patient-physician communication, 435, 439, 449
and relationships, 324
Complementary medicine. *See* Alternative medicine
Complete protein, 160
Complex carbohydrates, benefits of, 159
Concentric muscle contraction, 100, 108
Conditioning
benefits of, 348
components of, 71–76
Condoms, guidelines for use, 366
Conduction, heat loss or gain, 79
Conflict, cognitive dissonance, 15
Congenital heart defects, incidence of, 36

Conjugated linoleic acid (CLA), and weight-loss, 252
Contracting, for behavior change, 17
Controlled Substance Act of 1970, 339
Convection, heat loss or gain, 79
Cooldown
flexibility exercises, 134–135
purposes of, 77
Coping
elements of, 286
styles, positive and negative, 301–302
Coronary artery bypass surgery, 56
Coronary heart disease, 36–38
childhood origins of, 37
ischemia, 37
and myocardial infarction (heart attack), 36
risk factors, 36
Countering, for behavior change, 17
Crack, 352
Creatine, and resistance training, 114
Crohn's disease, 417
Cross-training, benefits of, 76

D
Daily References Intakes (DRI), 156–157
Daily Values (DVs)
food labels, 193–194
meaning of, 156, 193
Dance therapy, focus of, 5
Death
and cigarette smoking, 9–10, 48
leading causes of, 9–10
nonphysical causes of, 8
and obesity, 238
physical causes of, 7–8
Deductibles, health insurance, 444–445
Defensive medicine, 441
Dehydration
and heat stress, 80
prevention of, 81
Dependence, definition of, 339
Depressant drugs, 340
Depression
and cardiovascular disease, 53
and chronic stress, 281
Designer drugs, 340, 351
Diabetes mellitus
and abdominal fat deposition, 219–220
and cardiovascular disease, 52, 411
complications of, 52, 411
diagnosis/testing, 410
exercise, positive effects, 52, 409–410
genetic factors, 409
and Glycemic Index (GI), 188–189
metabolic abnormality in, 408
and obesity, 52, 238, 409
risk assessment, 419
signs of, 408
treatment of, 409–410
Type 1 diabetes, 52, 408
Type 2 diabetes, 52, 408–409
Diagnostic laboratory tests, 440–443
assessment of results, 451–452
common tests, 441–443
false positives and false negatives, 441
Diet drugs, 252, 261
Diet resistance, and obesity, 243

Dietary fat, 161–165
fish oils, 162
food label information, 194, 195
food sources, listing of, 163, 164
hydrogenation, 161–162
monounsaturated fat, 161
and physically active person, 193
polyunsaturated fat, 161–162
saturated fat, 161, 162, 163
sources of cholesterol/saturated fat, 42, 211–212
stress, effects on synthesis, 283
synthetic fats, 162
transfatty acids, 162, 163, 165
unsaturated fat, 161, 162
Dietary fat intake
assessment of, 203
excess intake, negative health effects, 162, 164
food label information about, 194, 195
high/medium/low fat foods, 211–212
of monosaturated fat, 165
of polyunsaturated fat, 165
recommended intake, 162, 164–165
reducing, guidelines for, 187–188
of saturated fat, 164–165
Dietary Guidelines for Americans (2000), guidelines of, 178, 197
Dieting. *See* Weight-loss
Distress, definition of, 276
Diuretics, herbal, 252
Domestic violence
child abuse, 323
elderly abuse, 323
partner abuse, 323
Drug abuse, definition of, 339
Drug misuse, definition of, 339
Drug use
addiction, causes of, 340
drug terminology, 339
prevention programs, 355
reasons for use of, 338–339
self-assessment, 361
Drugs
alcohol, 341–346
caffeine, 341
depressants, 340
over-the-counter drugs, 354
polypharmacy, 432
schedules I through V drugs, 339
tobacco products, 346–350
Drugs, illegal
analog drugs, 340
club drugs, 351
cocaine, 352
designer drugs, 340, 351
Ecstacy (MDMA), 351
GHB (gammahydroxbutrate), 351
heroin, 353–354
inhalants, 340
ketamine, 340
LSD (lysergic acid diethylamide), 354
marijuana, 340, 352–353
methamphetamine (crank), 354
narcotics, 340
phencyclidine (PCP), 340
psychoactive drugs, 340

Drugs, illegal—*Cont.*
    rohypnol, 351
    stimulant drugs, 340
Duration of exercise, 74–75
    FIT principle, 74–75
    and resistance training, 113
Dynamic exercise, forms of, 108
Dynamic muscle contraction, 100

E

E. coli, and foodborne illness, 186
Eating disorders, 257–260
    anorexia nervosa, 257–258
    binge-eating disorder, 259
    bulimia nervosa, 258–259
    female athlete triad, 260
    underweight, 260
Eccentric muscle contraction, 100, 108
Echinacea, pros/cons of use, 175
Echocardiography, cardiovascular disease
        diagnosis, 56
Ecstasy (MDMA), 340, 351
Ectomorph, 242
Elderly abuse, 323
Electrocardiograms (ECGs), 443
ELISA testing, for HIV/AIDS, 370
Emotional arousal, and behavior change, 15
Emotional wellness
    and immune system, 280–281
    and physical health, 5–6
    psychosomatic disease, 7
Endomorph, 242
Endorphins, and stress response, 280
Environmental toxins, and cancer risk, 386
Environmental wellness, and physical
        health, 6–7
Ephedra, 252
Epidemiologic studies, health research, 426–427
Epinephrine, and stress response, 280
Ergogenic aids, 114–115
    anabolic-androgenic steroids, 115–116
    nutritional supplements, 114–115
Essential hypertension, 47
Essential nutrients, types of, 157
Estrogen replacement therapy (ERT)
    heart disease prevention, 40
    for osteoporosis, 413
Ethnic foods
    Americanization of, 184
    types of, 185
Eustress, 276
Evaporation, heat loss, 80
Exercise
    cardiorespiratory endurance, 67–70
    and cold weather, 81–82
    cooldown, 77
    cross-training, 76
    duration of exercise, 74–75
    excessive (hypergymnasia), 259
    fluid consumption, 81
    frequency of, 74
    home fitness equipment, selection of, 79
    and hot weather, 78–81
    injuries from, 71
    intensity of, 71–74
    motivational tips, 76, 256

outdoors, safety measures, 320
    overload, 75
    overtraining, effects of, 74
    safe workout guidelines, 71
    specificity, 75–76
    sports/exercise, rating of, 78
    stimulation of metabolism by, 254
    stopping, effects of, 69
    in urban environment, 82
    warm-up, 67, 76–77
Exercise and health/illness
    arthritis, 98, 412
    asthma, 414
    cancer prevention, 388
    diabetes mellitus, 52, 409–410
    hypertension, 48
    osteoarthritis, 98
    osteoporosis, 98–99, 413
    stress management, 290–291
    stress reduction, 53
    weight-loss, 254–256, 260–261

F

Fad diets, 250
False negatives, 441
False positives, 441
Fast foods
    negative nutritional aspects, 195
    nutritional content tables, 465–469
    pre-physical activity, 192
Fasting, and weight-loss, 226, 253
Fast-twitch muscle fibers, 111
Fat, body fat
    body weight measures, 220–222, 226
    distribution of, 218–220
    essential fat, 216
    obesity, 216–217
    overweight, 218
Fat distribution, 218–220
    android pattern, 219–220
    gender differences, 219–220, 240
    gynoid pattern, 219
    negative health effects, 219–220
    and syndrome X, 52, 220
    waist-to-hip ratio (WHR) measure, 219
Fat genes, 242
Fat substitutes, 162, 248
Fat-free foods, food labeling for, 194, 195
Fats in foods. *See* Dietary fat; Dietary fat
        intake
Fat-soluble vitamins, 165–166
Fecal occult-blood tests, 442
Female athlete triad, 260
Fen-phen, 252
Feverfew, pros/cons of use, 175
Fiber, 176–178
    food sources of, 176, 177
    health benefits, 176, 177
    insoluble fiber, 176–177
    recommended intake, 177–178
    soluble fiber, 176
    and weight control, 261
Fibrinogin levels, and heart disease, 55
Fight-or-flight syndrome, stress response,
        52–53, 277–278
Fire detection devices, 310–311

Fish oils
    fatty acids, sources of, 162
    health benefits, 162
    omega-3 fatty acids, 41, 162
FIT principle, 74–75
Flexibility assessment
    goniometer for, 140
    shoulder flexion test, 149
    sit-and-reach test, 147
    sling test, 151
    trunk extension, 153
Flexibility exercises
    ancient methods, 135
    for back and neck pain, 140–142
    ballistic stretching, 140
    benefits of, 134
    frequency of, 67
    illustrations of, 136–141
    proprioceptive neuromuscular facilitation
        (PNF), 138–140
    safety guidelines, 137–138
    static stretching, 136–140
    for stress management, 291
    for warm-up and cool-down, 67, 77,
        134–135
Flexibility, importance of, 134
Fluid consumption
    deyhdration, prevention of, 82
    and exercise, guidelines for, 81
    water intake, 172–173
Folate, 166, 168–169
Food Guide Pyramid (FGP), 179–181
Food labels, 193–195
    Daily Values (DV), 193–194
    example of, 194
    and low-fat/fat-free foods, 194, 195
Foodbourne illness, 184–186
    pathogens/symptoms of illness, 186
    prevention of, 185–186
Fortified foods, 173
Framingham Heart Disease Study, 35, 36
Free radicals, production of, 166
Free-weight training, 110
Frequency of exercise, 74
    overtraining effects, 74
    and resistance training, 113
Fruits, adding to daily intake, 184
Functional foods, 173

G

Gallbladder disease, and obesity, 238
Garlic, pros/cons of use, 175
Gender differences
    arthritis, 411
    body fat distribution, 219–220, 240
    cancer types, 387
    heart disease, 40, 46
    high-density lipoprotein cholesterol
        (HDL) cholesterol levels, 46
    obesity measure, 216–217
    stress response, 284
General adaptation syndrome, stress
        response, 52–53, 277–278
Genetic factors
    aerobic capacity, 69
    alcoholism, 344

body shape, 242
body weight, 217
cancer, 385
diabetes mellitus, 409
drug addiction, 340
heart disease, 40
obesity, 242–243
Genital warts, 372–373
treatment of, 373
GHB (gammahydroxbutrate), 351
Ginger, pros/cons of use, 175
Ginkgo, pros/cons of use, 175
Ginseng, and resistance training, 114
Glucosamine, pros/cons of use, 175
Glucose production, and carbohydrates, 159, 244
Glycemic Index (GI), 188–189
Goal-setting
assessment of goals/priorities, 305–306
realistic goals, 285
short and long term goals, 289
Golgi tendon organ, 136–137
Goniometer, flexibility assessment, 140
Gonorrhea, 373–374
signs of, 373
treatment of, 374
Graded exercise tests, cardiovascular disease diagnosis, 55
Grains. *See* Whole-grains
Granuloma inguinale, signs/treatment of, 375
Guns in home, safety measures, 311
Gynoid pattern, fat distribution, 219

H
Hallucinogenic drugs, 340
Hardy personality
assessment of, 303
paths to hardiness, 303
traits of, 284–285
Hate crimes, 323–324
Headaches, 415–416
cluster headaches, 416
migraine headaches, 416
and stress, 281
treatment of, 416
Health assessment
diagnostic laboratory tests, 440–443
immunizations, 444
physical examination, 440–441
Health behaviors, health-promoting/health-inhibiting behaviors, 31
Health care
alternative medicine, 439–440
hospital care, 431–433
patient rights, 432
quality care, choosing quality care, 433
situations for use of, 430–431
terms used in, 436–437
Health care professionals, 433–439
defensive medicine, 441
information sources on, 435
patient-physician communication, 435, 439, 449
primary-care physicians, 434
second opinions, 438–439
specialties of, 434

Health care providers, meaning of, 424
Health, continuum for, 3
Health disparities, of racial and ethnic minorities, 7, 8
Health information
changing information, 424
from health research, 425–427
on Internet, 428–430
Health insurance, 444–445
health maintenance organization (HMO), 444
indemnity plans, 445
Medicare and Medicaid, 445
point of service (POS), 444
preferred provider organization (PPO), 444
Health Locus of Control Scales, 29
Health maintenance organization (HMO), 444
Health research
clinical trials, 427
epidemiologic studies, 426–427
reliability of, 426
risk factors, 426
scientifically controlled studies, 427
statistical relationship, 426
statistical significance, 426
validity of, 425
Health-promoting behaviors, examples of, 14
Health-related fitness, 66–67
Healthy People 2010, 9
Healthy Weight Pyramid, 246–247
Heart, 34–35
and circulation, 34–35
disease. *See* Cardiovascular disease
electrical conduction system, 35
Heart attack. *See* Myocardial infarction
Heart rate
and aerobic exercise, 67
calculation of, 72–74, 93
cardiac output, 67–68
Heart transplantation, survival rate, 56
Heart volume, and aerobic exercise, 68–69
Heat loss, physiological mechanisms of, 79–80
Heat stress. *See* Hot weather and exercise
Height/weight tables, 220, 222
Hemoccult tests, 442
Hemochromatosis, iron overload, 171
Hemoglobin, and iron, 171
Hepatitis
hepatitis A, and foodborne illness, 186
hepatitis B, 372, 390
and liver cancer, 390
signs of, 372
types of, 372
Herbs, 174–176
guidelines for use, 176
herbal diet remedies, 252–253
listing of nutritional supplements, 175
Herceptin, 393
Heroin, 353–354
Herpes, 371–372
herpes simplex types 1 and 2, 371
transmission of, 372
treatment of, 372
triggers of, 372
and women, 372

High sensitivity C-reactive protein (hs-CRP), and heart disease, 55
High-density lipoprotein (HDL) cholesterol, 44–46
gender differences, 46
increasing, guidelines for, 45–46
levels, meaning of, 46
protective effect of, 44
HIV/AIDS, 367–371
diagnosis of, 368, 370, 443
HIV types 1 and 2, 368
information sources on, 371
and IV drug use, 353–354
prevention of, 370
signs of, 367
transmission of, 369, 370
treatment of, 371
and women, 369
Hodgkin's disease, 390
Home safety, 310–312
assessment of, 329–330
carbon monoxide detection devices, 311–312
fire detection devices, 310–311
general safety guidelines, 310
gun safety, 311
Homeostasis, meaning of, 277
Homocysteine
dietary control of, 55
and heart disease, 54–55
Hospital care, 431–433
choosing hospital, 431–433
Hot weather and exercise, 78–81
heat exhaustion, 79
heat stroke, 79
safety guidelines, 80–81
Human papilloma virus, genital warts, 372–373
Humor, and stress-reduction, 289
Hydrogenation
dietary fat, 161–162
and transfatty acids, 162
Hyperglycemia, and diabetes, 408
Hypergymnasia, 259
Hyperplasia, 239–240
Hypertension, 46–48
control of, 47
essential hypertension, 47
exercise, positive effects, 48
and obesity, 238
and stroke, 47
Hypertrophy, 239–240
Hypnosis, focus of, 5
Hypothermia, 81–82
prevention of, 82

I
Illegal drugs. *See* Drugs, illegal
Imagery, focus of, 5
Immune system
psychoneuroimmunology (PNI), 281, 399
stress, effects on, 280–282
and Vitamin C, 283
Immunizations. *See also* Vaccinations
purpose of, 444
Immunotherapy, cancer treatment, 398

Incomplete protein, 160
Indemnity plans, 445
Infections
        colds, 415
        influenza, 415
        and obesity, 242
Infectious disease, as past cause of death, 7
Infertility, and stress, 281
Inflammatory bowel disease
        Crohn's disease, 417
        ulcerative colitis, 417
Influenza, vaccine for, 415
Inhalants, 340
In-line skating, safety measures, 313
Intellectual wellness, and physical health, 6
Intensity of exercise, 71–74
        heart rate, calculation of, 72–74
        levels of, 72, 73
        and resistance training, 113
        and weight loss, 255
Internet
        health information on, 428–430
        support groups on, 429
Inverted U-theory, stress, 276–277
Iron
        deficiencies, 171
        food sources of, 170, 172
        health benefits, 170, 171
        overload, negative health effects, 54, 171
Ischemia, and heart attack, 37
Isoflavones, 161
Isokinetic training, 108, 110
Isometrics. *See* Static training (isometrics)
Isotonic training, 108–109

J

Jet skis, safety measures, 314
Joint flexibility, importance of, 134

K

Karvonen formula, heart rate calculation,
        73, 93
Ketamine, 340
Kidney disease
        and diabetes mellitus, 411
        and high-protein diets, 161

L

Laboratory tests. *See* Diagnostic laboratory
        tests
Lactic acid, exercise and production of, 77
Lactovegetarians, 183
Laughter, and stress-reduction, 289
Leading Health Indicators, listing of, 9
Learned helplessness, 283
Legumes, as protein source, 160–161
Leptin, and body weight, 242
Leukemia, 384, 390
Life expectancy, age of Americans, 7
Lifestyle
        change, self-help approach, 11–18
        diseases of, 7
        lifestyle assessment inventory, 23–28
Limbic system, functions of, 279–280
Lipoproteins
        and heart disease, 55
        high-density lipoprotein (HDL), 44–46

increasing, guidelines for, 55
        low-density lipoprotein (LDL), 43–44
        very-low density lipoprotein (VLDL), 43
Listeria monocytogenes, and foodborne
        illness, 186
Liver cancer, lifestyle causes, 390
Logs, resistance training log, 116, 117, 131
Low-carbohydrate diets, 250–251
Low-density lipoprotein (LDL) cholesterol,
        43–44
        lowering, guidelines for, 44
Low-fat diet, 187–188
        and cholesterol control, 41
        fat-free food problem, 247–248
        guidelines for, 187–188
        heart disease risk from, 164
        maximum fat intake, 162
Low-fat foods
        food labeling for, 194, 195
        and overcompensatory eating, 248
LSD (lysergic acid diethylamide), 354
Lung cancer, 388–389
        prevention of, 389
Lymphatic system, functions of, 383
Lymphoma, 384, 390
        categories of, 390

M

Ma huang, 252
Macronutrients, 157
Malignant melanoma, 391
Malpractice, avoiding, 441
Mammograms, 395, 442
Marijuana, 340, 352–353
Massage therapy, relaxation method, 289
Medicare and Medicaid, 445
Medication, polypharmacy, 432
Medicine cabinet, essential items, 442
Meditation
        focus of, 5
        process of, 288
Mediterranean diet, health benefits of, 165
Menopause
        estrogen replacement therapy (ERT), 40
        and osteoporosis, 99, 412
Meridia, 252
Mesomorph, 242
Metabolic syndrome, and heart disease, 41
Metabolism
        and aging, 254
        basal metabolic rate (BMR), 254
        stimulation by exercise, 69, 254
Metal healing, focus of, 5
Methamphetamine (crank), 354
Micronutrients, 157
Migraine headaches, 416
Minerals, 170–172
        calcium, 171
        functions of, 170
        iron, 171
        major minerals, 170
        and physically active person, 193
        selenium, 172
        sodium, 170
        trace minerals, 170
        zinc, 171–172
Monogamy, serial monogamy, 364

Monosaccharides, 159
Monounsaturated fat
        chemical composition of, 161
        food sources of, 163
        recommended intake, 165
Moonrock, 354
Morbidity, meaning of, 7
Mortality, meaning of, 7
Motorcycles, safety measures, 318–319
Muscle contraction
        agonist and antagonist contractions,
                135–136
        concentric and eccentric contractions,
                100, 108
        and resistance training, 100, 110–112
        static and dynamic contractions, 100
        and stress, 281
Muscle endurance
        assessment of, 123, 125, 127–129
        definition of, 112
        and resistance training, 112
Muscle soreness
        causes of, 109
        prevention of, 108–109
Muscle spindle, 136–137
Muscle strength, 99–100
        assessment of, 121–122, 127–129
        definition of, 99
        disuse atrophy, 98
        and resistance training, 99–100
Muscles
        fiber types, 111
        names/location, illustration of, 110
        stretch reflex, 136–137
Music, for relaxation, 289
Music therapy, focus of, 5
Myocardial infarction (heart attack)
        nature of, 36
        silent type, 36–37
        sudden cardiac death and fitness, 70
        warning signs, 38

N

Narcotics, 340
Nautilus equipment, 109
Neck pain, flexibility exercises for, 140–142
Niacin, 166
Nicotine, 48–49, 346–347
        addictive effect of, 346–347
        negative health effects, 48–49, 346
Nicotine gum, 350
Nicotine-containing aids, cigarette smoking
        cessation, 350
Nicotrol inhaler, 350
Nongonococcal urethritis, signs/treatment
        of, 375
Non-Hodgkin's lymphoma, 390
Norepinephrine, and stress response, 280
Novelty diets, 251
Nucleoside analogs, AIDS therapy, 371
Nutrients
        botanicals/phytomedicinals, 174–176
        carbohydrates, 159–160
        common foods, nutritional content tables,
                456–464
        dietary fat, 161–165
        essential nutrients, 157

fiber, 176–178
intake assessment, 205–207
macronutrients and micronutrients, 157
minerals, 170–172
phytochemicals, 174
protein, 160–161
values/upper limits, chart of nutrients, 158
vitamins, 165–170
water, 172–173
Nutrition
alcohol use, 189–190
assessment of diet, 201–213
calorie intake, 157, 159
for cancer prevention, 383
ethnic foods, 185
fast foods, 195, 465–469
Food Guide Pyramid (FGP), 179–181
food labels, 193–195
foodbourne illness, 184–186
fruits/vegetables/grains, adding daily, 184
low-fat diet, 187–188
moderation/serving size, 181–182
nutrient density of foods, 182
-physical activity relationship, 191–193
and pregnancy, 190–191
prepackaged convenience dinners, 196
salt, limiting use of, 189
snacking, 195
sugar, limiting consumption, 188–189
variety of foods, 179–181
vegetarianism, 182–183
wellness nutrition strategy, 196–197
Nutritional guidelines
Adequate Intake (AI), 156
Daily References Intakes (DRI), 156–157
daily values (DVs), 156
Recommended Dietary Allowances
(RDA), 156
tolerable upper intake levels (UL), 156
Nutritional status
and health, 156
nutrient gap and older age, 180
and resistance training, 114
and stress, 281–282, 283

O

Obesity, 216–217
abdominal fat and disease, 52,
219–220, 239
biological theories of, 241–242
and cardiovascular disease, 52, 220,
238, 239
chronic diseases related to, 238–239
classification of, 240
development of, 239–241
and diabetes mellitus, 52, 409
and diet resistance, 243
dietary fat versus calories, 244
gender differences, 216–217
genetic factors, 242–243
leptin theory, 242–243
overeating as cause, 243–244
and physical inactivity, 244–245
set point theory, 243
syndrome X, 52, 220, 239
and thermogenic effect of food (TEF), 244
Occupational wellness, benefits of, 6

Older persons. *See* Aging
Olestra, 162, 248
Omega-3 fatty acids
food sources of, 162, 165
for healthy heart, 41, 162, 165
Omega-6 fatty acids
food sources of, 165
for healthy heart, 165
Oncogenes, 385
1.5 Run/Walk Test, 70, 89
Optimism
benefits of, 282–283
development of, 283
Oral cancer, 392
Ornish program, 54, 164
Osteoarthritis, 411–412
risk factors, 412
treatment of, 412
Osteoporosis, 98–99, 412–413
causes of, 412–413
exercise, benefits of, 99, 413
risk factors, 413
treatment of, 413
Outdoor safety. *See* Recreational/outdoor
safety
Ovarian cancer, 395
Overcompensatory eating, and low-fat
foods, 248
Overeating, and obesity, 243–244
Overload
and aerobic exercise, 76
and resistance training, 113–114
Over-the-counter drugs, safety guidelines, 354
Overtraining, effects of, 74
Overweight. *See also* Obesity
definition of, 218
and overfat, 218
overweight fit persons, 239
Ovolactovegetarians, 183
Ozone, air pollution, 315

P

Pancreatic cancer, 390
Pantothenic acid, 166
Pap smears, 442–443
Parasites, in food, 185
Partner abuse, 323
Passive smoking, 49–50, 347
Pedestrians, accidents involving, 319
Pediculosis, signs/treatment of, 375
Peer pressure, and drug use, 338–339
Pelvic inflammatory disease, signs/treatment
of, 375
Perfectionism, meaning of, 289
Performance-related fitness, 66
Personality
and drug addiction, 340
stress-related personality types, 284–285
Pescovegetarians, 183
Phencyclidine (PCP), 340
Physical activity. *See also* Exercise
amount per day, 178–179
definition of, 51
forms of, 51
health benefits of, 12, 51
-nutrition relationship, 191–193
nutritional guidelines, 191–193

staying active, tips for, 11
and weight-loss, 253
Physical Activity and Health, 10–11
Physical fitness
definition of, 66
health-related fitness, 66–67
performance-related fitness, 66
Physical inactivity
and cardiovascular disease, 50–51, 70
negative health effects, 10–11, 50, 98, 140
and obesity, 244–245
Physical injuries, recreational injuries, 312
Phytochemicals, 157
as antioxidants, 166–167
food sources of, 174
health benefits of, 174
Phytoestrogens, in soy foods, 161
Phytomedicinals, 157. *See also* Herbs
Plaque, in atherosclerosis, 36, 43–45
Point of service (POS) plan, 444
Pollovegetarians, 183
Polypharmacy, 432
Polysaccharides, 159
Polyunsaturated fat, 161–162
chemical composition of, 161
food sources of, 162, 163, 165
recommended intake, 165
Portion size
regulation of, 249, 261
supersize portions, 248–249
Positive reinforcement, for weight control, 257
Potentiating effect, of drug, 339
Prayer, focus of, 5
Preferred provider organization (PPO), 444
Pregnancy
folate in, 168–169
herpes and childbirth, 372
HIV transmission to newborn, 369
nutritional guidelines, 190–191
vitamin supplementation, 191
weight gain, 190
Prepackaged convenience dinners, evaluation
of, 196
Procrastination, as time waster, 289
Progression of exercise
principle of, 75
and resistance training, 114
Progressive muscle relaxation, 287
Proprioceptive neuromuscular facilitation
(PNF), 138–140
methods of, 139–140
Prostaglandins, 283
Prostate cancer, 397–398
diagnosis of, 397, 443
exercise, benefits of, 388
Prostate-specific antigen (PSA) test, 397
Protease inhibitor, AIDS therapy, 371
Protein, 160–161
amino acids, 160
complete and incomplete proteins, 160
increased need and stress, 283
legumes as source of, 160–161
Protein intake
assessment of, 201
high intake, dangers of, 161
and physical activity, 192
recommended intake, 161

Protein supplementation, and resistance training, 114
Proto-oncogenes, 385
Psychoactive drugs, 340
Psychoneuroimmunology (PNI)
    cancer research, 399
    focus of, 281
Psychosomatic disease, nature of, 7
Psychotherapy, focus of, 5
Psyllium, 252
Pulse rate
    as health diagnosis, 442
    taking pulse, guidelines for, 74
Pyridoxine, 166

R

Racial and ethnic minorities
    health disparities of, 7, 8
    and heart disease, 40
Radiation, heat loss, 79–80
Radiotherapy, cancer treatment, 398
Raloxifene, 393
Rape
    acquaintance and date rape, 321–322
    actions to take, 323
    psychological effects of, 322
Recidivism, meaning of, 15
Recommended Dietary Allowances (RDA),
    meaning of, 156
Recreational/outdoor safety, 312–315
    air pollution/air quality, 315
    assessment of, 331–332
    bicycling, 313
    boating, 314
    exercise safety, 320
    general safety guidelines, 312
    in-line skating, 313
    physical injuries, 312
    skateboarding, 313
    snowmobiling, 314–315
Redux, 252
Relationships
    and communication, 324
    monogamous, 364
Relaxation techniques, 286–291
    autogenics, 287
    biofeedback, 288–289
    deep breathing, 287
    humor, 289
    hypertension control, 47
    massage therapy, 289
    music as, 289
    progressive muscle relaxation, 287
    spiritual practices, 5
    visualization, 288
Reliability, of health research, 426
Repetitions (reps), resistance training, 100
Resistance training
    as anaerobic exercise, 99
    benefits of, 98–99
    circuit resistance training, 111–112
    ergogenic aids, 114–115
    exercises, illustrations of, 101–109
    free-weight training, 110
    guidelines for, 115
    isokinetic training, 108, 110

isotonic training, 108–109
and muscle endurance, 112
muscle soreness, 108–109
and muscular strength, 99–100
principles of, 113–114
repetitions (reps), 100
static training (isometrics), 100, 110
training log, 116, 117, 131
variable resistance training, 109–110
Respiration
    and aerobic exercise, 69
    and obesity, 238
Restaurant dining, supersized portions, 249
Reward deficiency syndrome, and
    addiction, 340
Rheumatoid arthritis, 412
Riboflavin, 166
Risk factors, in health research, 426
Ritalin, 338, 340
Road rage, 317–318
    prevention of, 318, 333
Rockport Fitness Walking Test, 70, 85–87
Rohypnol, date rape drug, 322, 351

S

Safety
    automobile safety, 315–319
    home safety, 310–312
    recreational/outdoor safety, 312–315
    violent events, 319–325
St. John's wort, pros/cons of use, 175
Salmonella, and foodborne illness, 186
Salt intake
    and hypertension, 47, 189
    limiting use of, 189
    negative health effects, 189
    sodium and nutrition, 170
Sarcoma, 384
Saturated fats
    chemical composition of, 161
    food sources of, 162, 163
    maximum recommended intake, 164–165
Saw palmetto, pros/cons of use, 175
Scientifically controlled studies, health
    research, 427
Seat belts, 316
Sedentary lifestyle. *See* Physical inactivity
Selenium
    food sources of, 172
    health benefits of, 172
Self-blame, of rape victim, 322
Self-care
    assessment inventory, 453
    and older people, 438
Self-esteem
    and drug use, 339
    and stress, 282
Self-examination
    of breasts, 396–397
    of testicles, 397
Self-monitoring, for weight control,
    256–257
Self-suggestion, relaxation method, 287–288
Serial monogamy, 364
Serving size, calculation of, 181
Set point theory, of obesity, 243

Sexuality
    engaging in, decision-making about, 365,
        379–380
    safe sex, 364–366
Sexually transmitted diseases (STDs)
    chlamydia, 373
    communicating with partner, 366
    genital warts, 372–373
    gonorrhea, 373–374
    hepatitis B, 372
    herpes, 371–372
    HIV/AIDS, 367–371
    incidence of, 367
    prevention of, 364–366
    risk assessment, 377
    syphilis, 374
Shaping up, and behavior change, 18
Shoulder flexion test, 149
Sidestream smoke, 347
Sigmoidoscopy, 443
Single-use diagnostic system (SUDS), 370
Sit-and-reach test, 147
Skateboarding, safety measures, 313
Skin cancer
    ABCDs of, 391
    basal cell carcinoma, 391
    malignant melanoma, 391
    prevention of, 392, 443
    risk factors, 391
    squamous cell carcinoma, 391
    and sun exposure, 387, 392
Skinfold measurements, 224–226, 227–228
Sleep apnea, and obesity, 238
Sling test, 151
Slow-twitch muscle fibers, 111
Smokeless tobacco, 50, 348
Snacking, healthy snacks, 195, 196
Snowmobiling, safety measures, 314–315
Social contacts. *See also* Support groups
    and wellness, 4
Sodium. *See also* Salt intake
    health benefits of, 170
Soy foods, types of, 161
Specificity of exercise
    and cross-training, 76
    principle of, 75–76
    and resistance training, 114
Spinal column, structure of, 142–144
Spirituality
    meaning of, 3
    ritual drug use, 338
    spiritual practices, 5
    and wellness, 3–5
Staphylococcus, and foodborne illness, 186
Static muscle contraction, 100
Static stretching, 136–140
Static training (isometrics), 100, 110
    limitations of, 100, 110
Statistical relationship, of health research, 426
Statistical significance, of health
    research, 426
Steady state, and aerobic exercise, 67
Stimulant drugs, 340
Stomach cancer, 390
    prevention of, 390
Strength training. *See* Resistance training

Stress
  assessment of, 297–299
  and attitude, 282–283
  and cancer risk, 386
  and cardiovascular disease, 53, 281
  definition of, 276
  distress, 276, 278–279
  eustress, good stress, 276
  excessive distress, signs of, 278–279
  exercise, positive effects, 52
  fight-or-flight syndrome, 52–53, 277–278
  gender differences in reaction to, 284
  and hardy personality, 284–285
  and immune system, 280–282
  inverted U-theory, 276–277
  and nutritional status, 281–282, 283
  physiological responses to, 52–53, 277, 279–280
  positive effects of, 277
  and self-esteem, 282
  sources of, 276, 278, 279
  stressors, acute and chronic, 53
  and Type A personality, 284
Stress management
  basic guidelines, 285
  coping, elements of, 286
  exercise, 290–291
  relaxation techniques, 286–291
  time management, 289–290
Stressors
  assessment of life stressors, 295–296
  types of, 276
Stretch reflex, 136–137
Stroke
  causes of, 38, 238
  and hypertension, 47
  prevention of, 38
  warning signs, 38
Stroke volume, and aerobic exercise, 67
Sudden cardiac death, 70
Sugar, 188–189
  forms of, 159
  terms on food labels, 188
Sugar intake
  Glycemic Index (GI), 188–189
  negative health effects, 188
Sun exposure, and skin cancer, 387, 392
Support groups
  and behavior change, 18
  and cancer survival, 386, 399
  focus of, 5
  on Internet, 429
Syndrome X, 52, 220, 239
Synergistic effect
  definition of, 339
  of drugs, 339
  of foods and vitamins, 399
Syphilis
  stages of, 374
  treatment of, 374

T

Tai chi, benefits of, 135
Talk Test, 74
Tamoxifen, 393
Tanning devices, negative effects of, 392

Taxol, 393
Terrorism, bioterrorism, precautions to take, 325
Testicular cancer, 395
  self-examination for, 397
Thermogenic effect of food (TEF), 244
Thiamine, 166
3-Minute Bench Step Test, 70, 91
Thyroid disease, and body weight, 241–242
Time management, 289–290
  strategies for, 289–290
  time wasters, 289
  use of time, assessment of, 307–308
Tobacco products, 346–350
  cigarettes, 49–50
  cigars, 50, 348
  designer drugs, 351
  nicotine in, 48–49, 346–347
  pipes, 348
  smokeless tobacco, 50, 348
To-do list, 290
Tolerable upper intake levels (UL), meaning of, 156
Tonometry, 443
Trace minerals, 170
Transdermal patches, nicotine withdrawal, 350
Transfatty acids
  on food labels, 163, 187
  negative health effects, 162, 165
Treadmill test, cardiovascular disease diagnosis, 55–56
Trichomoniasis, signs/treatment of, 375
Triglycerides
  and cardiovascular disease, 46
  fatty acids of, 161
  lowering, guidelines for, 46
Type A personality, traits of, 284
Type B personality, traits of, 284
Type 1 diabetes, 52, 408
Type 2 diabetes, 52, 408–409

U

Ulcerative colitis, 417
Ultrasound, 443
Underwater weighing, 223
Underweight, 260
Universal Gym, 109
Unsaturated fats
  chemical composition of, 161
  examples of, 162
Urban environment, exercise safety, 82
Uterine cancer, 395

V

Vaccinations
  for adults, 444
  for influenza, 415
  and past diseases, 7
Valerian, pros/cons of use, 175
Validity, of health research, 425
Variable resistance training, 109–110
  equipment for, 109
Vegetables, adding to daily intake, 184
Vegetarianism, 182–183
  forms of, 183
  health benefits, 184

and nutritional deficiencies, 171, 182–183
  in pregnancy, 191
  vegans, 182–183
Ventricular assist devices, 56
Very-low-calorie diets (VLCDs), 247, 261–262
Very-low density lipoprotein (VLDL) cholesterol, 43
Violent events, 319–325
  acquaintance and date rape, 321–322
  and alcohol use, 345
  assessment of personal safety, 335–336
  at automated teller machine (ATM), 319–320
  car jacking, 320–321
  domestic violence, 323
  hate crimes, 323–324
  homicide, 322–323
  statistics on crime, 319
Viral disease, and cancer, 387, 390
Vision loss, and diabetes, 411
Visualization, relaxation method, 288
Vitamin A, 166, 283
  megadoses and birth defects, 191
Vitamin C, 166, 167, 283
Vitamin D, 166
Vitamin E, 166, 168, 283
Vitamin K, 166
Vitamins, 165–170
  antioxidants, 166–167
  B vitamins, 166, 168–169
  buying guidelines, 170
  carotenoids, 167–168
  versus dietary nutrients, 399
  fat-soluble vitamins, 165–166
  folate, 168–169
  food sources/benefits chart, 166
  functions of, 165
  and immune system, 283
  megadoses, 191, 193
  and physically active person, 192–193
  during pregnancy, 191
  supplements, indications for use, 169
  water-soluble vitamins, 165, 166

W

Waist-to-hip ratio (WHR) measure, of fat distribution, 219
Warm-up, 76–77
  flexibility exercise, 67, 77, 134–135
  goals of, 76–77
Water, 172–173
  bottled water, types of, 172
  daily requirements, 172, 173
  deficiency, signs of, 173
  physiological functions of, 172
Water-soluble vitamins, 165, 166
Weight-gain
  guidelines for, 260
  and pregnancy, 190
  and quitting smoking, 49, 262
Weight-loss
  caloric deficits and loss, 245, 253–254
  and conjugated linoleic acid (CLA), 252
  diet drugs, 252, 261
  diet-only strategies, 245–246
  and exercise, 254–256, 260–261

Weight-loss—*Cont.*
 fad diets, 250
 and fasting, 253, 262
 healthier weight, meaning of, 238
 healthy food substitutions, 251
 Healthy Weight Pyramid, 246–247
 herbal diet remedies, 252–253
 low-carbohydrate diets, 250–251
 low-fat diets, 247
 low-fat foods, 248
 maintenance of, 255–257, 260–262
 meal skipping, avoiding, 262
 novelty diets, 251
 and physical activity, 253
 plateau phase, 261
 and portion size, 248–249, 261
 realistic loss, guidelines for, 217
 use of term, 239

 very-low-calorie diets (VLCDs), 247,
  261–262
 weekly loss recommendations, 245
 weight cycling, 246
Wellness
 benefits of, 2
 components of, 2–7
Western blot test, for HIV/AIDS, 370
Whole-grains
 adding to daily intake, 184
 daily servings, 182
 fiber from, 176–177
Women. *See also* Gender differences
 alcohol and tobacco use, 344, 345
 and herpes complications, 372
 and HIV/AIDS, 369
 work-household roles and stress, 282
Workaholism, 289

Workplace activities, and musculoskeletal
  problems, 140–141
World Trade Center terrorist attack, 325

X
X-rays, chest, 443

Y
Yesism, meaning of, 289
Yoga
 benefits of, 135
 focus of, 5
Yo-yo dieting, 246

Z
Zinc, 171–172
 functions of, 172
 in pregnancy, 191